Obstetric Emergencies

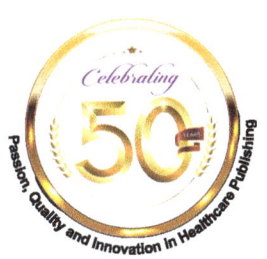

Obstetric Emergencies

THIRD EDITION

Editor

Kamini A Rao
DGO DORCP DCh FRCOG (UK) MCh (UK) FRCOG PGDMLE (Law) FNAMS
Medical Director
Milann—The Fertility Center
Bengaluru, Karnataka, India

Co-Editor

Vyshnavi A Rao
MBBS MS (Obs & Gyn) Fellowship in Reproductive Medicine
Consultant IVF Specialist
Department of Reproductive Medicine
Milann—The Fertility Center
Bengaluru, Karnataka, India

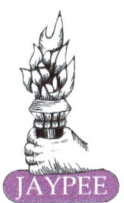

JAYPEE BROTHERS MEDICAL PUBLISHERS
The Health Sciences Publisher
New Delhi | London

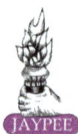 **Jaypee Brothers Medical Publishers (P) Ltd**

Headquarters
Jaypee Brothers Medical Publishers (P) Ltd
4838/24, Ansari Road, Daryaganj
New Delhi 110 002, India
Phone: +91-11-43574357
Fax: +91-11-43574314
E-mail: jaypee@jaypeebrothers.com

Overseas Office
JP Medical Ltd
83 Victoria Street, London
SW1H 0HW (UK)
Phone: +44 20 3170 8910
Fax: +44 (0)20 3008 6180
E-mail: info@jpmedpub.com

Website: www.jaypeebrothers.com
Website: www.jaypeedigital.com

© 2020, Jaypee Brothers Medical Publishers

The views and opinions expressed in this book are solely those of the original contributor(s)/author(s) and do not necessarily represent those of editor(s) of the book.

All rights reserved. No part of this publication may be reproduced, stored or transmitted in any form or by any means, electronic, mechanical, photocopying, recording or otherwise, without the prior permission in writing of the publishers.

All brand names and product names used in this book are trade names, service marks, trademarks or registered trademarks of their respective owners. The publisher is not associated with any product or vendor mentioned in this book.

Medical knowledge and practice change constantly. This book is designed to provide accurate, authoritative information about the subject matter in question. However, readers are advised to check the most current information available on procedures included and check information from the manufacturer of each product to be administered, to verify the recommended dose, formula, method and duration of administration, adverse effects and contraindications. It is the responsibility of the practitioner to take all appropriate safety precautions. Neither the publisher nor the author(s)/editor(s) assume any liability for any injury and/or damage to persons or property arising from or related to use of material in this book.

This book is sold on the understanding that the publisher is not engaged in providing professional medical services. If such advice or services are required, the services of a competent medical professional should be sought.

Every effort has been made where necessary to contact holders of copyright to obtain permission to reproduce copyright material. If any have been inadvertently overlooked, the publisher will be pleased to make the necessary arrangements at the first opportunity. The **CD/DVD-ROM** (if any) provided in the sealed envelope with this book is complimentary and free of cost. **Not meant for sale.**

Inquiries for bulk sales may be solicited at: jaypee@jaypeebrothers.com

Obstetric Emergencies

First Edition: 2003

Second Edition: 2011

Third Edition: **2020**

ISBN 978-93-89587-19-7

CONTRIBUTORS

A Shilpa Reddy MS (Obs & Gyn)
Fellow in Obstetrics and Gynecology Ultrasound
Mediscan, Chennai, Tamil Nadu, India
Consultant, Lakshmi Kishore Hospital
Proddatur, Andhra Pradesh, India

Aishwarya Yerram
MBBS (Osm) DNB (Obs & Gyn) FRM
Senior Consultant, Iswarya Fertility Center
Hyderabad, Telangana, India

Akhila Vasudeva MD DNB MRCOG
Professor and Unit Chief
Chief Consultant, Division of Fetal Medicine
Department of Obstetrics and Gynecology
Kasturba Medical College, Manipal
Manipal Academy of Higher Education
Udupi, Karnataka, India

Anju Dogra MBBS MD
Senior Resident
Government Medical College
Jammu, Jammu and Kashmir, India

Aparna Jha
MBBS MS (Obs & Gyn) DNB (Obs & Gyn) MRCOG (UK)
Gynecologist and Obstetrician
Department of Obstetrics and Gynecology
Apollo Cradle
Bengaluru, Karnataka, India

Arathi Sreedhara MBBS DMCH DGO FMIS
Consultant, Obstetrician and Laparoscopic Gynecologist
BSOG, FOGSI
Karnataka Medical Council, Indian Medical Association
Neiya Speciality Clinic, Vasvi Hospital
Visiting Consultant, Cloudnine Hospital
Aster RV, Apollo Cradle
Milann—The Fertility Centre
Bengaluru, Karnataka, India

Arya Rajendran
MD (Obs & Gyn) DNB (Obs & Gyn) FNB (Reproductive Medicine)
Consultant
Department of Reproductive Medicine
NIMS Fertility Center
Palakkad, Kerala, India

BS Susheela Rani MD PGDMLE FICOG
Medical Director, Manjushree Speciality Hospital
Bengaluru, Karnataka, India
Past President
Bangalore Society of Obstetrics and Gynecology
Chairperson, Postgraduate Forum of Bangalore Society of Obstetrics and Gynecology

Chandana C MBBS MS DNB
Associate Professor
Department of Obstetrics and Gynecology
Vydehi Institute of Medical Sciences and Research Centre
Bengaluru, Karnataka, India

CS Sushma Madhuprakash
MBBS DGO Fellowship in Maternal Fetal Medicine
Consultant
Division of Maternal and Fetal Medicine
Dr Jyothi's Health Care Pvt Ltd
Mysuru, Karnataka, India

Deepa Nambiar
MBBS MS (Obs & Gyn) DNB (Obs & Gyn) PGDMLS PGDHHM CCGDM
Consultant
Department of Obstetrics and Gynecology
Shanthi Women's Healthcare Center
Bengaluru, Karnataka, India

Deepa Patil MBBS MS FRM
Consultant
Vijayapur-assisted Conception Center
Bijapur, Karnataka, India

Haritha Mannem
MS (Obs & Gyn) FRM
Consultant Infertility Specialist
Milann—The Fertility Center
Bengaluru, Karnataka, India

Harleen Kour MBBS MD
Senior Resident
Government Medical College
Jammu, Jammu and Kashmir, India

Jyothirmayi Kunam
MBBS MS (Obs & Gyn) FRM (BACC)
Milann—The Fertility Center
Bengaluru, Karanataka, India

Karthigayeni Rathinam
MBBS MS (Obs & Gyn) DNB (Obs & Gyn) MRCOG FRM
Consultant
Department of Reproductive Medicine
Milann—The Fertility Center
Bengaluru, Karnataka, India

Komal Unadkat
MBBS DNB (Obs & Gyn) Fellowship in Reproductive Medicine
Consultant
Poojan IVF Centre
Ahmedabad, Gujarat, India

Mahesh Koregol MBBS MS (Obs & Gyn) FICOG Fellowship in Reproductive Medicine
Consultant Reproductive Medicine Specialist
Andrologist and Laparoscopic Surgeon
NOVA IVI Fertility
Bengaluru, Karnataka, India

Meghana V Nyapathi MS (Obs & Gyn) FRM
Consultant
Department of Reproductive Medicine
Milann—The Fertility Center
Bengaluru, Karnataka, India

Neha Tyagi
MBBS DNB (Obs & Gyn) FRM
Infertility Specialist
Milann—The Fertility Center
Bengaluru, Karnataka, India

Nilofer MBBS MS FMAS
Assistant Professor
Dr Pinnamaneni Siddhartha Medical College and Research Center
DR NTR University of Health Sciences
Vijayawada, Andhra Pradesh, India

Nisha Singh
MBBS MS (Obs & Gyn) DNB (Obs & Gyn) FNB (Reproductive Medicine) PGDMLE
Consultant
Reproductive Medicine and Assisted Conception
Amaira Urology and Fertility Center
Surat, Gujarat, India

Priyadharsini S MBBS MS OG FRM
Consultant, Obstetric, Gynecology and Infertility Specialist
The Hosur Women's Hospital and Infertility Center
Hosur, Tamil Nadu, India

Priyanka Yadav MBBS DGO DNB
Attending Consultant, Fortis Escorts
Department of Reproductive Medicine
Jaipur, Rajasthan, India

Rahul Wani DNB DGO LLM LLB PGDMLS
Consultant
Department of Obstetrics and Gynecology
Archana Maternity Nursing Home
Navi Mumbai, Maharashtra, India

Rajitha Yarlagadda MBBS MS (Obs & Gyn) FRM
Reproductive Medicine Specialist
Marvel Hospital
Bengaluru, Karnataka, India

Ravi Kumar IR MBBS MD
Consultant Anesthesiologist
Milann—The Fertility Center
Bengaluru, Karnataka, India

Ravishankar P
MBBS MS (Obs & Gyn) FRM DMAS (Germany)
Consultant
Reproductive Medicine
The Nest Woman Wellness and Fertility Clinic
Thiruvananthapuram, Kerala, India

Contributors

Rekha Viswanath MBBS MS (Obs & Gyn) DNB (Obs & Gyn) Fellowship in Reproductive Medicine (RGUHS)
Former Fellow in Reproductive Medicine
Milann—The Fertility Center
Bengaluru, Karnataka, India

Revathi S Rajan MBBS DGO DNB (Obs & Gyn)
Fellowship in Fetomaternal Medicine (RGUHS)
Chief Consultant
Division of Maternal Fetal Medicine
Managing Director, Mirror Health
Bengaluru, Karnataka, India

Rinke S Tiwari
FRM (Reproductive Medicine) MS (Obs & Gyn)
Consultant
Department of Reproductive Medicine
Oasis Fertility Center
Hyderabad, Telangana, India

Roopa PS MBBS MS
Associate Professor
Manipal Academy of Higher Education (MAHE)
Kasturba Medical College and Hospital
Manipal, Karnataka, India

Shalini MA
MBBS MS (Obs & Gyn) FMAS FRM
Consultant
Department of Reproductive Medicine
Garbhagudi IVF Center
Bengaluru, Karnataka, India

Shashikala KT
MBBS DGO Fellowship in Reproductive Medicine
(Fellowship in Minimal Access Surgery)
Infertility Specialist, Obstetrician and Gynecologist
Department of Reproductive Medicine
Milann—The Fertility Center
Bengaluru, Karnataka, India

Shravya Tallapureddy
MBBS MS (Obs & Gyn) FNB (Reproductive Medicine)
Fellow in Reproductive Medicine
Milann—The Fertility Center
Bengaluru, Karnataka, India

Smitha Avula MBBS DNB FFM
Consultant, Division of Maternal Fetal Medicine
Milann—The Fertility Center
Bengaluru, Karnataka, India

Sneha MBBS MD DNB FRM
Consultant
Department of Reproductive Medicine
NU Hospitals
Bengaluru, Karnataka, India

Sonal Agarwal
MBBS MS DNB (Obs & Gyn) FMAS MNAMS FNB (REP MED)
Consultant Infertility Specialist
SMH Infertility IVF Center
New Delhi, India

Soumya Mahesh Koregol
MBBS MS (Obs & Gyn) FIAOG
Consultant, Fertility Specialist and Gynecologist
Hospitec Multispecialty Hospital
Bengaluru, Karnataka, India

Sowmya Davuluri
MBBS MS (Obs & Gyn) FRM DMAS
Consultant
Department of Reproductive Medicine
Milann—The Fertility Center
MS Ramaiah Memorial Hospital
Bengaluru, Karnataka, India

Sowparnika SN
DGO DNB FRM (Reproductive Medicine)
Fellow in Reproductive Medicine
Milann—The Fertility Center
Bengaluru, Karnataka, India

Srividhya GK MS Fellowship in Fetal Medicine
Consultant, Department of Fetal Medicine
Milann—The Fertility Center
Bengaluru, Karnataka, India

Sudeepti Mummadi MBBS MS FRM
Consultant
Department of Reproductive Medicine
Neelima Mom Fertility Center
Sainath Hospital
Hyderabad, Telangana, India

Sumi Maria
MBBS MS (Obs & Gyn) DNB (Obs & Gyn) FNB (Obs & Gyn)
Consultant
Department of Reproductive Medicine
Milann—The Fertility Center
Bengaluru, Karnataka, India

Sunil Gupta
MD FRCP (Edinburgh) (Glasgow) FACP (USA) FICP FIAMS FIACM
Managing Director
Sunil's Diabetes Care n' Research Centre Pvt Ltd
Nagpur, Maharashtra, India

Sunitha B
MBBS DGO DNB FFMM PGDU PGDHHM PGDMLE
Senior Consultant
Department of Maternal Fetal Medicine
Milann—The Fertility Center
Bengaluru, Karnataka, India
Executive Committee Member of Bangalore Society of Obstetrics and Gynecology and Society of Maternal Fetal Medicine

Surbhi Gupta
MBBS MS (Obs & Gyn) DNB FNB (Reproductive Medicine)
Consultant
Reproductive Medicine
Milann—The Fertility Center
Gurugram, Haryana, India

SV Joga Rao ML Mphil PhD Maxplanck Fellowship
Advocate, Solicitor and Healthcare
Consultant, Legalexcel
Visiting Professor
National Law School of India University (NLSIU)
Bengaluru, Karnataka, India

Swetha MBBS DA (DNB)
Anesthesiologist
Mallya Hospital
Bengaluru, Karnataka, India

Taswin Kaur Reddy MBBS DGO FRM FMAS
Consultant
Department of Obstetrics and Gynecology, Reproductive Medicine
Chandra Superspecialty Hospital
Anantapur, Andhra Pradesh, India

Thejaswini J MBBS MS PGDRSM
Consultant Gynecologist
Columbia Asia Hospital
Bengaluru, Karnataka, India

Vignata N MBBS MS (Obs & Gyn) FRM Dip in USG
Fertility Consultant
Janardani Hospital
Guntur, Andhra Pradesh, India

Vinay Kumar
MBBS MD Fellowship in Reproductive Medicine
Diploma in Minimal Access Surgery
Consultant
Government Medical College
Jammu, Jammu and Kashmir, India

Vyshnavi A Rao
MBBS MS (Obs & Gyne) Fellowship in Reproductive Medicine
Infertility Specialist, Gynecologist and Obstetrician
Department of Reproductive Medicine
Milann—The Fertility Center
Bengaluru, Karnataka, India

PREFACE TO THE THIRD EDITION

The word "emergency" means a serious, unexpected and dangerous event, which requires immediate medical attention. Although pregnancy and labor are physiological processes, obstetric emergencies are often unexpected and can develop rapidly. *Obstetric Emergencies* provides the obstetrician with insights regarding optimum care for the mother and the unborn child and how to deal with emergency situations in obstetric practice.

With the advent of technology, practicing obstetricians need to keep updating themselves with current advances in their clinical practice. The book will serve as an indispensable reference guide to all the clinicians and postgraduate students, since it provides a practical and accessible guide to all emergency situations from the immediately life-threatening to the smaller but urgent problems that could arise, thus ensuring a better prognosis.

Special topics that include medicolegal issues in obstetrics, pregnancy as a result of rape, diabetic ketoacidosis in pregnancy and labor and role of imaging modalities in obstetric emergencies are some of the topics which have been covered.

Evidence-based knowledge and current scientific evidence form the cornerstone for any successful treatment. The contributors have taken time out from their busy schedule in order to do thorough research into their topic thus, putting each topic into proper perspective and providing readers with unambiguous practice guidelines to help them achieve their goals.

The first and second editions of this book was well received. With the third edition we have updated the contents, keeping in mind the algorithm of the topic to help in easy understanding of the subject.

It is our hope that the book will be a reference guide for all busy practitioners, providing a scientific and evidence-based approach, leading to best clinical practices.

Kamini A Rao
Vyshnavi A Rao

PREFACE TO THE FIRST EDITION

The dictum "A healthy mother and a healthy baby" has been spearheading advances in the field of Obstetrics and Gynecology, into areas thought implausible in yesteryears. At this stage, it would do well to review the basics of treatment, many of which have stood the test of time and continue to be the gold standards in obstetric care.

This handbook, without much ado addresses the obstetric problems faced in daily practice. It encompasses the basic principles of diagnosis and management in practical detail.

This book has been conceived as an aid to doctors working at the primary health centers and at institutions where no sophisticated facilities exist. Theoretical details have intentionally been omitted, so as to serve as a quick reference when encountered with a problem.

I hope that this handbook serves as a guide to all those involved in the care of the pregnant woman, so as to make unsafe obstetric practices a thing of the past.

Kamini A Rao

ACKNOWLEDGMENTS

This book is a culmination of the sincere efforts of all the authors who very enthusiastically came forward to write the chapters. We would like to express our sincerest thanks to all of them for their time, effort and commitment to sharing their knowledge and expertise. As always, the publication team of M/s Jaypee Brothers Medical Publishers (P) Ltd, New Delhi, India has gone out on a limb to bring out the book and ensure its timely release. We thank Shri Jitendar P Vij (Group Chairman), Mr Ankit Vij (Managing Director), Ms Chetna Malhotra Vohra (Associate Director-Content Strategy) for their constant support in making this happen. Special thanks to Mrs Kala Diwakar for coordinating the entire effort, interacting with both the contributors and the publishers at every stage, and generally following up with all stakeholders until the book becomes finally a reality. Lastly of course to our families—thank you for standing by us and supporting our every effort.

CONTENTS

1. **Antenatal Care** 1
   Aparna Jha

2. **Miscarriages** 4
   Vyshnavi A Rao

3. **Hyperemesis Gravidarum** 14
   Vyshnavi A Rao

4. **Ectopic Pregnancies: Diagnosis and Management** 19
   Deepa Nambiar

5. **Retroverted Gravid Uterus** 51
   CS Sushma Madhuprakash

6. **Hydatidiform Mole** 55
   Nisha Singh

7. **Trauma in Pregnancy** 71
   Haritha Mannem

8. **Shoulder Dystocia** 86
   BS Susheela Rani

9. **Hypertensive Emergencies in Pregnancy and Labor** 95
   Sunitha B

10. **Cardiac Failure in Pregnancy** 108
    Shalini MA

11. **Acute Fatty Liver and Jaundice in Pregnancy** 114
    Chandana C

12. **Infections in Pregnancy** 119
    Deepa Patil, Shravya Tallapureddy

13. **Deep Vein Thrombosis in Pregnancy** 129
    Rinke S Tiwari

14. **Preterm Labor** 141
    Shravya Tallapureddy

15. **Antepartum Hemorrhage** 155
    Chandana C, Srividhya GK

16. **Retained Placenta** 168
    Sowparnika SN

17. **Intrauterine Growth Restriction**.. 173
    Rekha Viswanath

18. **Management of Amniotic Fluid Emergencies** 181
    Arya Rajendran

19. **Intrauterine Fetal Death** 189
    Mahesh Koregol, Soumya Mahesh Koregol

20. **Amniotic Fluid Embolism** 193
    Thejaswini J

21. **Breech Presentation and its Complications** 198
    Ravishankar P

22. **Abnormal Fetal Heart Trace on Cardiotocography**................................... 208
    Revathi S Rajan

23. **Anesthetic Complications in Pregnancy and Labor**................................. 216
    Swetha, Ravi Kumar IR

24. **Cesarean Delivery** 229
    Aishwarya Yerram

25. **Perimortem Cesarean Delivery** 239
    Aishwarya Yerram

26. **Postpartum Hemorrhage**... 243
    Meghana V Nyapathi

27. **Perineal Tears** 253
    Nilofer

28. **Vaginal Birth after Cesarean Section** 258
    Sonal Agarwal

29. **Drug Therapy in Pregnancy**... 269
    Vignata N

30. **Peripartum Cardiomyopathy** 278
    Shalini MA

31. **Uterine Inversion** 288
    Priyadharsini S

32. **Peripartum Collapse** 293
    Smitha Avula

33. **Acute Abdomen in Pregnancy** 297
    Smitha Avula

34. **Umbilical Cord Prolapse**.. 303
    Taswin Kaur Reddy

35. **Epilepsy in Pregnancy**.. 311
    Surbhi Gupta

36. **Diabetic Ketoacidosis in Pregnancy**.. 322
    Sunil Gupta

37. **Laparoscopy in Pregnancy** 327
    Arathi Sreedhara

38. **Pregnancy as a Result of Rape** 331
    Rahul Wani

39. **Obstetric Emergencies: Medicolegal Issues and Implications** 339
    SV Joga Rao

40. **Puerperal Sepsis** 358
    Sudeepti Mummadi

41. **Obstructed Labor**.. 365
    Rajitha Yarlagadda

42. **Retained Mop in Abdomen/Gossypiboma in Abdomen** 372
    Shashikala KT

43. **Malpresentations**.. 379
    Sneha

44. **Acute Asthma in Pregnancy**.. 385
    A Shilpa Reddy

45. **Scar Dehiscence** 393
    Sumi Maria

46. **Disseminated Intravascular Coagulation in Obstetrics** 398
    Vinay Kumar, Harleen Kour, Anju Dogra

47. **In Utero Transfer** 407
    Vinay Kumar, Anju Dogra, Harleen Kour

48. **Delivery in Emergency Department** 417
    Sowmya Davuluri

49. **Induction of Labor**.. 423
    Karthigayeni Rathinam

50. **Abnormal Progress of Labor**.. 436
    Komal Unadkat

51. **Transfusion Reactions**.. 441
    Rekha Viswanath

52. **Anaphylaxis** 444
    Neha Tyagi

53. **Sickle Cell Crisis** 454
    Priyanka Yadav

54. **Severe Anemia in Pregnancy and Labor** 459
    Jyothirmayi Kunam

55. **Role of Imaging Modalities in Obstetric Emergencies** 472
    Roopa PS, Akhila Vasudeva

56. **Uterine Rupture** 486
    Sudeepti Mummadi

Index *491*

CHAPTER 1

Antenatal Care

Aparna Jha

■ DEFINITION

Systematic supervision of women during pregnancy to monitor the progress of fetal growth and to ascertain the well-being of the mother and the fetus, also to detect pregnancy-related complications at the earliest.

■ OBJECTIVES OF ANTENATAL CARE

- To promote, protect, and maintain the health of mother during pregnancy
- To detect high-risk cases and give them proper attention
- To foresee complications and prevent them
- To ensure that antenatal care (ANC) is used as opportunity to detect and treat the existing health issues in pregnant females
- To make sure that services are available to manage obstetric emergencies
- To protect pregnant women and their families for the eventuality of any emergency
- To remove anxiety associated with pregnancy and delivery
- To teach the mother about the elements of child care, nutrition, personal hygiene, and environmental sanitation
- To reduce maternal and infant mortality and morbidity
- To sensitize the mother about the need of spacing the birth and family planning
- To attend the under-fives accompanying the mother.

■ COMPONENTS OF ANTENATAL CARE

- Antenatal visits
- Prenatal advises
- Specific health protection
- Mental preparation
- Family planning.

■ PROTOCOLS OF ANTENATAL VISITS

Every country's ANC protocols are different. Based on the base-line health of the pregnant females, following are the antenatal protocols by Indian Health Governing Bodies. They are divided into:

- Essential components of ANC checkup
- Desirable component of ANC checkup.
  Antenatal care starts from the first visit of the pregnant female by the healthcare provider.

Schedule of essential antenatal visits are:
- Below 12 weeks of pregnancy
- Between 14 weeks and 26 weeks of pregnancy
- Between 28 weeks and 34 weeks of pregnancy
- About 36 weeks till term.

Schedule of desired antenatal visits is:
- *From conception till 28 weeks*: Monthly visits
- *About 28–36 weeks*: Fortnightly visits
- *About 36 weeks till delivery*: Weekly visits.

2 Obstetric Emergencies

▍ PRENATAL ADVICE

History taking: Detailed history of pregnant female to be taken under following headings:
- *Pregnancy scoring*:
  - *Gravida*: Number of times patient has become pregnant
  - *Parity*: Living number of existing children
  - *Abortion*: Number of times abortions occurred
  - Any kind of complication in previous pregnancies.
- History of medical, surgical, or obstetric complication that may affect the present pregnancy
- Any familial disease that may affect the current pregnancy
- Menstrual history to calculate the expected date of delivery (EDD) by Naegele's formula (EDD = 1st date of last menstrual period + 9 months 7 days)
- History of drug allergies or any drug intake.

▍ PHYSICAL EXAMINATION

Weight: Prepregnancy weight has to be recorded.
- Total weight gain during pregnancy for a normal pregnancy should be 10–12 kg.
  - *First trimester*: 1–2 kg
  - *Second trimester*: 2–3 kg
  - *Third trimester*: 5–7 kg.
- *In obese patients*:
  - Body mass index > 30, weight gains should be 6–8 kg
  - Body mass index > 35, weight gain should be 3–4 kg.
- Excessive weight gain that is more than 3 kg per month or more than 500 g per week, preeclampsia, gestational diabetes mellitus (GDM), and twin pregnancies should be ruled out.

Pallor

To rule out anemia, pallor should be checked at lower palpebral conjunctiva, nails, tongue, oral mucosa, and palms. If pregnant female is pale of anemic, its causes should be determined by laboratory investigations and treatment should be started.

Edema

Physiological edema of pregnancy is seen in normotensive pregnant females. It is of pitting type, nontender, extends generally till ankle which appears in evening and disappears by morning is not related to albuminuria.

Pathological Edema

Pathological edema is edema above the ankle/hand/face/abdominal wall/vulva. It could be pitting or nonpitting and tender. It does not disappear completely after taking rest. If there is a presence of pathological edema, then hypertension, anemia, hypothyroidism, and filariasis should be ruled out.

Blood Pressure Monitoring

Regular blood pressure (BP) monitoring should be done in seated position with feet supported. BP should be taken in both the arms in 1st antenatal visit. The right arm should be used thereafter if there is no significant difference between the readings between left and right. Any BP of more than or equal to 140/90 over several readings is considered hypertension during pregnancy.

Breast Examination

Thorough breast examination should be carried out to rule out any existing breast lump. Also, nipple examination should be done to rule out flat, retracted nipple, or skin infection of areola. In case of retracted or flat nipples, corrective measures should be taught to the pregnant female to facilitate breastfeeding upon birth.

SPECIFIC HEALTH PROTECTION

Tetanus Toxoid

According to Ministry of Health and Family Welfare of India, administration of two dosage of tetanus toxoid (0.5 mL IM) is mandatory. The first dose should be given as soon as the pregnancy is registered. The second dose should be given 4-6 weeks apart preferably at least 1 month before the EDD. If a woman receives the first dose after 38 weeks of pregnancy, then the second dose may be given in postnatal period after a gap of 4 weeks. If a woman has been previously immunized with two doses of TT during her previous pregnancy within past 3 years, then she should be given only 1 dose of TT in present pregnancy.

Flu Vaccination

Flu vaccination should be given to all the pregnant women who are at risk of the disease.

Tetanus, Diphtheria, and Pertussis

According to the latest international recommendations, pregnant women should be given 1 dose of tetanus, diphtheria, and pertussis vaccination intramuscular (IM) in between 27 weeks and 36 weeks of pregnancy.

Folic Acid Supplementation

All women in the reproductive age group should be advised to have folic acid (*recommended dose:* 400 µg) for 2-3 months preconception and continue during pregnancy in the first 12 weeks to reduce the incidence of neural tube defect in the fetus.

Iron-folic Acid Supplementation

- *Prophylactic dosage*: All pregnant females should be given one tablet of iron-folic acid (IFA) (100 mg elemental iron and 0.5 mg folic acid) every day for at least 100 days starting after the first trimester.
- *Therapeutic dosage*: If hemoglobin is less than 11 g/dL, then the patient needs to take two IFA tablets per day for 3 months and also investigation should be carried out and specific treatment should be given.

MENTAL PREPARATION

Pregnant woman should be talked to about the normal changes during pregnancy, mode of delivery, process of delivery, breastfeeding, and newborn care. Healthcare provider should also educate the family members of the pregnant woman to give supportive care as and when required.

FAMILY PLANNING

During antenatal checkups, pregnant women should be counseled about the spacing between births and various methods of family planning—temporary and permanent. She should be given the cafeteria choice of family planning methods and she should be helped to choose one in order to keep her health and her children's health in good condition.

CHAPTER 2

Miscarriages

Vyshnavi A Rao

▌ DEFINITION

Abortion is defined as the spontaneous or induced termination of pregnancy before the period of fetal viability or expulsion of an embryo or fetus weighing 500 g or less[1] before the period of viability before 20 weeks (28 weeks in India).

The terms Abortion or Miscarriage are often used synonymously.

On the other hand, induced abortion implies surgical or medical termination.

Serum human chorionic gonadotropin (hCG) measurements can identify very early pregnancies. With the advent of transvaginal sonography:

- The earlier detection of pregnancy in which no products are seen in ultrasonography (USG)
- Pregnancy that displays a gestational sac but no embryo
- Those in which a dead fetus can be detected.

▌ ETIOLOGY

Cause of spontaneous abortion is multifactorial:

- Chromosomal anomalies[2]
- Metabolic and endocrine abnormalities
- Anatomical factors—cervical incompetence, congenital anomalies of the uterus, uterine adhesions and uterine fibroids
- *Others*: Infections (5–10%), immunological causes (5–10%), ABO blood group incompatibility, advanced maternal age, stress-related factors, extremes of age can lead to abortions.[3-5]

There are a few terminologies which need to be defined:

- *Biochemical pregnancy*: It denotes a positive serum beta-hCG with pregnancy not being located on scan.
- *Fetal loss*: Previous crown-rump length (CRL) measurement with loss of fetal cardiac activity.
- *Early pregnancy loss*: Confirmation of an empty sac or fetus on USG but no fetal cardiac activity <12 weeks of gestation.
- *Delayed miscarriage/late pregnancy loss*: Loss of fetal cardiac activity >12 weeks of gestation.
- *Pregnancy of unknown location (PUL)*: Serum beta-hCG being positive with no identifiable pregnancy on scan.

▌ TYPES OF MISCARRIAGES

Types of miscarriages have been shown in Table 1.

▌ IMPLANTATION BLEEDING

Cyclical bleeding that may happen up to 12 weeks of pregnancy until the decidual space is obliterated by the fusion of decidua capsularis with decidua vera.

Miscarriages

TABLE 1: Types of miscarriages.

Type	Definition	Clinical presentation
Spontaneous miscarriage	Miscarriage occurring without medical (or) mechanical intervention to empty the uterus	• Bleeding per vagina • Cramping pain abdomen
Threatened miscarriage	Miscarriage which causes minimal spotting/bleeding but has not progressed to a stage where recovery is impossible	• Light bleeding • Cervical os closed • Uterus corresponds to dates • Scan: fetal cardiac activity present
Inevitable miscarriage	Miscarriage where the changes have progressed to a state from where continuation of pregnancy is impossible	• Cramping lower abdominal pain, uterus being tender on examination • Heavy bleeding, uterus corresponds to dates, dilated cervix
Incomplete miscarriage	Miscarriage where products of conception are partially expelled	Heavy bleeding, dilated cervix, uterus smaller than dates
Complete miscarriage	Miscarriage where the products of conception are completely expelled	Light bleeding, closed cervical os, uterus smaller than dates, softer than normal
Missed miscarriage	When the fetus is dead in utero and retained inside for a variable length of time	Cervical os closed, no bleeding, fetal cardiac activity which was previously present but presently no cardiac activity seen on USG
Septic miscarriage	Miscarriage associated with clinically detectable infection of uterus and its contents	• Tachycardia and fever • General malaise, sweating, headache, features suggestive of endotoxic shock, reduced urine output, dryness of tongue

Bleeding is minimal lasts for lesser duration than her usual and usually corresponds to the date of the expected period.

PREREQUISITES ON APPROACHING A CASE OF MISCARRIAGE

- Detailed history with respect to last menstrual period to ascertain the period of gestation, whether the pregnancy occurred due to a contraceptive failure (use of emergency contraception) or whether it was a planned one
- Previous obstetric and gynecological procedures
- Contraceptive history and to educate the woman regarding repeated abortions/dilatation and evacuation (D&E) can result in infertility in the later years to be emphasized upon
- Drugs taken either over the counter or anticoagulant medication
- Complete medical/surgical history
- Any concomitant comorbidities for which the patient is already on medications has to be enquired into.

CLINICAL EXAMINATION

- General physical examination—to look for pallor, icterus, cyanosis, clubbing, lymphadenopathy and edema
- Examination of breast, thyroid, and spine along with vitals like pulse rate, blood pressure, respiratory rate, and temperature is must to be performed
- Pelvic examination—to determine the size of the pregnant uterus, uterus anteverted/retroverted, presence of any other pelvic pathology (leiomyoma/ectopic pregnancy or adnexal mass) has to be ruled out

6 Obstetric Emergencies

- With the advent of ultrasound, the diagnosis and management of abortions have become much more precise.

■ LABORATORY INVESTIGATIONS

- Blood grouping and Rh typing
- Complete blood picture determining the hemoglobin, total leukocyte count, differential count, erythrocyte sedimentation rate (ESR), packed cell volume and RBC indices, thyroid-stimulating hormone (TSH)
- To look for infection and the general health of the patient has to be considered
- Urine routine and microanalysis along with urine albumin and sugar
- Serology—human immunodeficiency viruses (HIV), hepatitis B surface antigen (HBsAg), hepatitis C virus (HCV), venereal disease research laboratory (VDRL)
- Vaginal swabs if there is suspicion of reproductive tract infection
- Pelvic ultrasound is a must, in order to confirm the pregnancy is intrauterine in origin, and pelvic USG is mandatory before performing a Medical Termination of Pregnancy (MTP).

■ COMPLETE ABORTION

Clinical Presentation

- Pregnancy test is positive
- Cervical os is closed as the products of conception are expelled completely
- Pain may be present or absent
- Vaginal bleeding is present/absent
- Signs and symptoms of pregnancy coincide with the weeks of gestation.

Management

- A pelvic USG is required in order to check if the uterine cavity is empty
- If patient complains of pain, analgesics may be prescribed
- Contraception advice.

■ THREATENED ABORTION

Clinical Presentation

- Ultrasound shows a live fetus
- Pregnancy test is positive
- Cervical os is closed
- Pain is absent or slight
- Vaginal bleeding is minimal, bright red color, bleeding followed by pain
- Signs and symptoms coincide with the weeks of gestation.

Management

- Bed rest is advocated until bleeding subsides
- Intercourse should be avoided
- Progestogens, e.g. hydroxyprogesterone caproate 250 mg intramuscular (IM) one dose if excessive bleeding is detected
- The meta-analysis of all women suggests that there is probably a reduction in the number of miscarriages for women given progestogen supplementation compared to placebo/controls [average risk ratio (RR) 0.69, 95% confidence interval (CI) 0.51–0.92, 11 trials, 2,359 women, moderate-quality evidence][6,7]
- Micronized progesterone 400 mg vaginal BID up to 16 weeks if conception as occurred as a result of assisted reproductive techniques (ARTs)
- Role of hemostatics: First trimester decidual hemorrhage leads to adverse outcomes including pregnancy loss, pre-eclampsia, abruption, intrauterine growth restriction (IUGR) and preterm births (PTBs). Decidual hemorrhage generates excess thrombin that binds to decidual cell-expressed protease-activated receptors (PARs) to induce chemokines

promoting shallow placentation; such bleeding later in pregnancy generates thrombin to downregulate decidual cell progesterone receptors and upregulate cytokines and matrix metalloproteinases (MMPs) linked to PTB. Endometria of progestin-only, long-acting, reversible contraception (pLARC) users display ischemia-induced excess vasculogenesis and progestin inhibition of spiral artery vascular smooth muscle cell proliferation and migration leading to dilated fragile vessels prone to bleeding
- Perivascular decidualized human endometrial stromal cells (HESCs) promote endometrial hemostasis during placentation yet facilitate menstruation through progestational regulation of hemostatic, proteolytic, and vasoactive proteins. Pathological endometrial hemorrhage elicits excess local thrombin generation, which contributes to pLARC-associated abnormal uterine bleeding (AUB), endometriosis and adverse pregnancy outcomes through several biochemical mechanisms.[8]

INEVITABLE ABORTION

Clinical Presentation

- Symptoms and signs of pregnancy coincide its duration
- Vaginal bleeding is excessive, and may be associated with clots
- Colicky pain is present in the suprapubic region which radiates to the back
- Dilated internal os with products of conception may be felt through the os
- Rupture of membranes between 12 weeks and 28 weeks which represents a sign of inevitability
- USG may or may not show a live fetus.

Management

- Any attempt to continue pregnancy may be not useful
- On per speculum examination—products at os are present—remove using sponge holding forceps/ovum forceps, check curettage may be required
- USG pelvis to confirm if there are retained products of conception (PROC)
- Prophylactic antibiotics are to be administered
- Postmiscarriage counseling—grief counseling and correction of anemia if present
- Contraception advice.

INCOMPLETE ABORTION

When there is presence of PROC in the uterine cavity, it is called incomplete abortion.

Clinical Presentation

- Patient gives history of passage of a part of products of conception
- Bleeding per vaginam (PV) is continuous
- USG shows products of conception retained inside uterine cavity
- On examination, uterus is less than the period of amenorrhea.

Treatment

- On speculum examination, if products of conception are seen, it is removed using sponge holding/ovum forceps
- Misoprostol 400 µg vaginal/sublingual dose or 600 µg orally/rectally
- Products of conception need to be expelled completely
- Analgesics, antipyretics should be given if needed
- Postmiscarriage counseling
- Repeat scan in order to confirm that the uterine cavity is empty
- Contraceptive advice.

MISSED ABORTION

Clinical Presentation

- Regression of pregnancy associated symptoms like nausea, vomiting and breast tenderness
- Fetal movements are not perceived or ceases if present before
- Uterus does not correspond to the period of gestation
- Cervical os is closed
- Dark brownish vaginal discharge is present.

Management

- USG will reveal a collapsed gestational sac, absent fetal heart/movement
- Diagnosis—based on two transvaginal/transabdominal (TV/TA) USG at least 7 days apart shows an embryo >7 weeks of gestation (CRL >6 mm diameter and gestational sac >20 mm in diameter) with absent fetal cardiac activity
- Complete blood picture to rule out sepsis and disseminated intravascular coagulation (DIC).

Evacuation of uterus becomes essential when:
- There is presence of excessive bleeding PV
- Spontaneous expulsion does not occur within 5 weeks
- Infection or DIC sets in:
  - Dilatation and evacuation is the treatment of choice in first trimester missed abortions
  - Medical management:
    - Misoprostol 600 µg vaginal/sublingually 3 hourly maximum of two doses
    - 800 µg vaginally 3 hourly maximum of two doses
    - Prophylactic antibiotics to be administered for 5 days
    - Analgesics, antipyretics may be needed
    - Postmiscarriage counseling
    - Contraceptive advice.

SEPTIC ABORTION

Septic abortion is characterized by infection of uterus and its contents, which usually follows unsafe abortion or incomplete abortion. The infection may spread to and involve myometrium, parametrium, tubes, ovaries and peritoneum.

Retained products of conception form a good culture media for organisms like *Escherichia coli*, streptococci and anaerobes responsible for causing septic abortion.

It may occur due to criminal interference.

Types of Septic Abortion

Grade 1: The infection is confined to decidua—80%.

Grade 2: The infection extended to myometrium—15%.

Grade 3: The infection extends to pelvis, generalized peritonitis, endotoxic shock present.

- Detailed history of the patient needs to be obtained—where, how, by whom was the case previously handled, use of abortifacients
- Pyrexia, tachycardia, general malaise, sweating, headache, joint aches
- Bleeding—duration, amount and presence of clots
- Cramping—duration severity, any history of fainting episodes (suggestive of ectopic pregnancy)
- Previous obstetric/gynecological history.

On Clinical Examination

- Suprapubic pain and tenderness
- Absent bowel sound as in paralytic ileus
- Abdominal rigidity and distention indicate peritonitis due to bowel perforation.

Local Examination

- Vaginal bleeding
- Offensive vaginal discharge
- Uterus is tender
- Fullness and tenderness of pouch of Douglas (POD) point out toward pelvic abscess associated with diarrhea.

Investigations and Management of a Case of Septic Abortion

Investigations:
- Complete blood count, blood grouping and Rh typing
- Cervical swabs for culture and sensitivity
- Coagulation profile, serum electrolytes blood culture if pyrexia >38.5°C

↓

Treatment:
- Isolate patient, bed rest in semi prone position
- Establish an IV line, In case of shock, CVP line to help in administering
- Fluid/ blood products if needed

↓

Monitoring vital signs:
- Pulse rate, blood pressure, temperature
- Intake output chart

↓

Antibiotics:
- Effective against gram negative, gram positive, anaerobic organism and *Chlamydia*

Uterine evacuation:
- Vaccum aspiration is avoided if there is prior interference
- Oxytocin (20 Units in 500 mL of IV fluid) and methyl ergometrine (0.2 mg IM) for uterine atony
- Products of conception are sent for histopathology

- Close monitoring of pulse rate, blood pressure, temperature, bleeding PV is mandatory
- Intravenous therapy is continued until patient is afebrile for 48 hours and has to be followed by oral medication, Tablet doxycycline 100 mg twice a day for 2 weeks
- Tetanus immunoprophylaxis is recommended
- Follow-up and contraception advice
- Anti-D immunoglobulin is given to Rh-negative women, 300 µg[9]
- Ampicillin 1 g IV every 6 hours
- Gentamicin 80 mg IV every 12 hours
- Metronidazole 500 mg IV every 8 hours.
- Retained products of conception were evacuated under antibiotic cover and sent for histopathology
- A booster dose of tetanus toxoid 0.5 mL to be given.

Septic abortion is complicated mostly with septic shock, generalized peritonitis and suspected renal failure.

Management of Shock[10,11]

- Universal measures:
  - Airway—should be open
  - Keep the patient nil per oral
  - Keep the patient warm
  - Maintain circulation by leg elevation so that the vital organs remain perfused.
- Oxygen—by mask at 6–8 L/minute
- Fluid therapy—to be maintained for hydration. Normal saline or Ringer's lactate started at the rate of 1 L in 20–30 minutes, gradually titrated as per requirement
- Blood transfusion—to maintain hemoglobin between 7–9 g%[10]
- Vasopressors—used to maintain mean arterial pressure of at least 65 mm Hg

- Dopamine is started at the rate of 5–10 µg/kg/minute IV and the infusion is adjusted according to blood pressure
- Epinephrine is used when blood pressure is poorly responsive to norepinephrine or dopamine.
- Inotropes—recommended when cardiac output remains low despite fluid resuscitation and vasopressors[10]
- Steroids—used when blood pressure is poorly responsive to fluid and vasopressor therapy hydrocortisone 200 mg/day in four divided doses for 7 days or more[12]
- Monitoring—pulse rate, blood pressure, respiratory rate and intake/output charting. Central venous pressure (CVP) is monitored and maintained at 8–10 cm of water
  - Injection ceftriaxone 2 g IV every 12 hours and injection metronidazole 500 mg IV every 8 hours were started
  - A booster dose of tetanus toxoid was given
  - In view of suspected gut/uterine perfusion, patient was taken up for urgent laparotomy.

Prognosis

- Prognosis depends upon the degree of infection present, intervention and presence of complications
- In India, 13–25% of the cases admitted to hospital succumb to complications due to septic shock, DIC and hepatorenal failure[3,4]
- Late complications include tubal block and infertility, pelvic inflammatory disease and chronic pelvic pain.

INDUCED ABORTION

Indications

- Pregnancy as a result of rape
- When continuation of pregnancy endangers the life of a pregnant woman in conditions like:
  - Persistent heart disease after cardiac decompensation
  - Invasive carcinoma of cervix.
- When continuation of pregnancy may cause severe physical deformities or mental retardation of the child.

Medical Methods

Antiprogesterone (RU486).

Contraindications

- Intrauterine device (IUCD) in situ
- Hypertension, glaucoma, asthmatic, anemia
- Lactating women
- Previous uterine scar.

Complications

- Nausea, vomiting and gastrointestinal cramping
- Failure to abort—1%
- Möbius syndrome—in fetus (congenital facial palsy, limb defects, hydrocephalus)
- Termination of pregnancy is mandatory if medical methods fail
- In case the woman bleeds profusely, emergency evacuation is mandatory
- Subsequent menstruation may be delayed.

Prostaglandins

- The prostaglandins (PGs) are a group of physiologically active lipid compounds having diverse hormone-like effects
- Prostaglandins have been found in almost every tissue in humans and other animals
- They are derived enzymatically from fatty acids.

MEDICAL TERMINATION OF PREGNANCY PROTOCOL

- Obtaining an informed consent is mandatory
- Performing a USG prior to administration of MTP drugs is vital in order to confirm

Miscarriages

the presence of intrauterine pregnancy, its duration and to rule out ectopic pregnancy.

For Pregnancies up to 9 Weeks of Gestation (63 Days)

- Medical termination with mifepristone 200 mg orally followed by vaginal misoprostol 24–48 hours later
- For vaginal route, the recommended dose is 800 µg. It can also be administered through the sublingual/buccal routes
- Up to 7 weeks of gestation, misoprostol can be administered by vaginal, buccal, sublingual routes. After week 7, oral misoprostol should not be used
- Up to 9 weeks of gestation, misoprostol is given by vaginal, buccal/sublingual routes.

For Pregnancies between 9 Weeks and 12 Weeks (63–84 Days)

- 200 mg mifepristone orally followed by 36–48 hours later by 800 µg of misoprostol vaginally
- Misoprostol should be given 400 µg vaginally or sublingually every 3 hours up to four doses until products of conception are expelled.

For Pregnancies above 12 Weeks of Gestation

- 200 mg mifepristone orally followed by 36–48 hours later administration of misoprostol
- Gestations between 12 weeks and 24 weeks, the initial misoprostol dose followed by oral mifepristone should be either 800 µg vaginally or 400 µg orally
- Subsequent doses of misoprostol 400 µg given by the vaginal/sublingual routes every 3 hours up to four doses
- For pregnancies beyond 24 weeks, because of greater sensitivity of the uterus to PGs, misoprostol usage must be decreased.

Recommended Methods for Medical Abortion in Situations Where Mifepristone is not Available

- For pregnancies of gestational age up to 12 weeks (84 days):
  - *For medical abortions*: The recommended dose of misoprostol is 800 µg given either vaginally or sublingually, up to three doses of 800 µg can be administered at a given gap of 3–4 hours but not longer than 12 hours.
- For pregnancies of gestational age over 12 weeks:
  - 400 µg of misoprostol given vaginally or sublingually repeated every 3 hourly up to five doses is acceptable
  - For pregnancies beyond 24 weeks, misoprostol dose should be decreased considerably due to the higher sensitivity of the uterus to PGs, but lack of clinical studies precludes specific dosing recommendations.
- Between 12 weeks and 24 weeks:
  - Dilatation and evacuation and medical methods (mifepristone and misoprostol; misoprostol alone) are both recommended for miscarriages for gestation over 12–14 weeks.

THE MEDICAL TERMINATION OF PREGNANCY ACT, 1971

- An Act to provide for the termination of certain pregnancies by registered medical practitioners and for matters connected therewith or incidental thereto. Be it enacted by Parliament in the Twenty-second Year of the Republic of India
- Aims to improve the maternal health scenario by preventing large number of unsafe abortions and consequent high incidence of maternal mortality and morbidity
- Legalizes abortion services

- Promotes access to safe abortion services to women.

Medical Grounds

When the continuation of pregnancy is likely to:

Endanger the life of the pregnant women or cause grievous injury to her physical and/or mental health, as in cases of severe hypertension, cardiac disease, diabetes, psychiatric illnesses, genital and breast cancer.

Eugenic Grounds

When there is an increased risk of the child being born with serious physical or mental abnormalities.

Humanitarian Grounds

When the pregnancy is caused by rape or incest.

Social Grounds

When in the actual or reasonably foreseeable future, her environment (social/economic) might lead to risk of injury to her health or pregnancy has resulted due to a failure of a contraceptive device/method.

Authorized Place for Conducting an MTP

- A hospital established or maintained by Government.
- A place for the time being approved for the purpose of this Act by Government.

DEPARTMENT OF HEALTH AND FAMILY WELFARE DRAFT: MTP (AMENDMENT) BILL, 2014

The Government took cognizance of the challenges faced by women in accessing safe abortion services and in 2006 constituted an expert group to review the existing provisions of the MTP Act to propose draft amendments. A series of expert group meetings were held from 2006 to 2010 to identify strategies for strengthening access to safe abortion services. In 2013, a national consultation was held which was attended by a range of stakeholders further emphasized the need for amendments to the MTP Act. The proposed amendments to the MTP Act were primarily based on increasing the availability of safe and legal abortion services for women in the country.

- Expanding the provider base
- Increasing the upper gestation limit for legal MTPs
- Increasing access to legal abortion services for women
- Increasing clarity of the MTP law.

CONTRACEPTION ADVICE: POSTABORTION

- The informed choice of the available methods of contraception needs to be offered to the patient after detailed counseling regarding the side effects and failure rates of each method. This is called Cafeteria approach
- With the advent of an active sexual life, particularly in adolescent age group, advice regarding contraception is the need of the hour
- Pregnancy, abortion and gynecological pathology including sexually transmitted infections (STIs) and acquired immuno-deficiency syndrome (AIDS) must be discussed in detail as each can have a significant impact on long-term physical, mental and social well-being of women.

CONCLUSION

- Abortion is a process where the fetus is expelled either spontaneously or induced as discussed above causing tremendous physical, mental and emotional turmoil in

women. As clinicians we need to address all aspects involved in a very sympathetic yet scientific and rational manner
- Safe abortion saves lives.

REFERENCES

1. Abortion. In: Cunningham FG, Leveno KJ, Bloom SL, Hauth JC, Gilstrap LC, Wenstrom KD (Eds). Williams Obstetrics, 22nd edition. India: McGraw Hill; 2005. pp. 232-51.
2. Kajii T, Ferrier A, Niikawa N, et al. Anatomic and chromosomal anomalies in 639 spontaneous abortuses. Hum Genet. 1980;55:87-98.
3. Arck PC, Rucke M, Rose M, et al. Early risk factors for miscarriage: a prospective cohort study in pregnant women. Reprod Biomed Online. 2008;17:101-13.
4. Maconochie N, Doyle P, Prior S, et al. Risk factors for first trimester miscarriage results from a UK population-based case-control study. BJOG. 2007;114:170-86.
5. Gracia CR, Sammel MD, Chittams J, et al. Risk factors for spontaneous abortion in early symptomatic first trimester pregnancies. Obstet Gynecol. 2005;106:993-9.
6. Haas DM, Hathaway TJ, Ramsey PS. Progestogen for preventing miscarriage in women with recurrent miscarriage of unclear etiology. Cochrane Database Syst Rev. 2018;10: CD003511.
7. Ku CW, Allen JC Jr, Lek SM, et al. Serum progesterone distribution in normal pregnancies compared to pregnancies complicated by threatened miscarriage from 5 to 13 weeks gestation: a prospective cohort study. BMC Pregnancy Childbirth. 2018;18(1):360.
8. Schatz F, Guzeloglu-Kayisli O, Arlier S, et al. The role of decidual cells in uterine hemostasis, menstruation, inflammation, adverse pregnancy outcomes and abnormal uterine bleeding. Hum Reprod Update. 2016;22(4): 497-515.
9. FOGSI. Clinical guidelines—ICOG Guideline Committee. Guidelines for the use of anti-D immunoglobulin for Rh prophylaxis. [online] Available from: https://www.scribd.com/document/22713246/Anti-D-Ig-Prophylaxis-Guidelines-FOGSI [Last accessed September, 2019].
10. Dellinger RP, Levy MM, Carlet JM, et al. Surviving sepsis campaign: international guidelines for management of severe sepsis and septic shock: 2008. Crit Care Med. 2008;36: 296-327.
11. Clinical management of abortion complications: a practical guide. Geneva, World Health Organization; 1994.
12. Marik PE, Pastores SM, Annane D, et al. Recommendations for the diagnosis and management of corticosteroid insufficiency in critically ill adult patients: consensus statements from an international task force by the American College of Critical Care Medicine. Crit Care Med. 2008;36:1937-49.

CHAPTER 3

Hyperemesis Gravidarum

Vyshnavi A Rao

INTRODUCTION

Nausea and vomiting [nausea and vomiting of pregnancy (NVP)] are the most common symptoms seen in early pregnancy in most pregnant women usually requiring no treatment. It affects about 75–85% of all pregnant women,[1] 50% of whom experience both nausea and vomiting, 25% have nausea only, and 25% remain unaffected.[2]

DEFINITION

Hyperemesis gravidarum is defined as the occurrence of more than three episodes of vomiting per day with ketonuria and more than 3 kg or 5% weight loss. The diagnosis is established clinically following exclusion of other causes.[3,4]

Hyperemesis gravidarum is seen in about 0.5–2% of pregnancies,[5] with an average of 2–4 days of hospital stay.

Peak incidence is seen between 8 and 12 weeks of gestation and symptoms resolve by 20 weeks of gestation resulting in weight loss, nutritional deficiencies abnormalities in fluids, electrolytes levels, and acid base balance.

Grades of severity[6] include:
- *Grade 1*: Nausea and vomiting without metabolic imbalance
- *Grade 2*: Pronounced feeling of sickness with metabolic imbalance.

DIFFERENCE BETWEEN MORNING SICKNESS AND HYPEREMESIS GRAVIDARUM

The differences between morning sickness and hyperemesis gravidarum have been provided in Table 1.

PATHOGENESIS OF HYPEREMESIS GRAVIDARUM

Hyperemesis gravidarum may be related to:
- Elevated levels of human chorionic gonadotropin (hCG) during pregnancy
- Studies also suggest that *Helicobacter pylori* infection may play a role in hyperemesis[3]
- *A genetic basis*: Sisters and daughters of women with hyperemesis have an increased incidence
- Biological, physiological, psychological, and sociocultural factors may also contribute.

TABLE 1: Differences between morning sickness and hyperemesis gravidarum.

Morning sickness	Hyperemesis gravidarum
Nausea sometimes with vomiting	Nausea with severe vomiting
Nausea subsides after 12 weeks or even before that	Nausea which does not subside at all
Dehydration does not occur	Dehydration occurs
Vomiting but small frequent meals can be taken	Intractable vomiting unable to take orally

RISK FACTORS[7]

- Nulliparity
- Obesity
- Hyperemesis in past pregnancy
- Female gestation
- Twin pregnancy
- Triploidy and trisomy 21
- Prepregnancy weight—underweight[8]
- Previous or present molar pregnancy
- Hydrops fetalis
- Women with history of migraine headaches, psychiatric illness, pregestational diabetes, hyperthyroidism, pyridoxine deficiency, gastrointestinal disorders, and prior history of motion sickness.

Transient Hyperthyroidism of Hyperemesis Gravidarum

It is a spontaneously resolving type of hyperemesis gravidarum, which persists up to 18 weeks of pregnancy and needs no treatment.[9]

Protective factors appear to be cigarette smoking and maternal age above 30 years.

HISTORY AND CLINICAL EXAMINATION

- Period of amenorrhea
- Number of episodes of vomiting, amount, and contents
- Altered sense of taste and sensitivity to odors
- Urine output
- Complaints of fatigue and exhaustion
- Complaints of headache, epigastric pain, pyrexia, diarrhea, and flank pain—to rule out other causes.

General Examination Reveals

- Signs of dehydration—decreased skin turgor, positional change in pulse, blood pressure, and sunken eyeballs
- Acetone like odor in breath
- Loss of weight
- Temperature and respiratory rate
- Pallor and jaundice
- Goiter
- Cardiovascular and respiratory system.

Abdominal Examination

- Whether uterus is palpable or not
- Tenderness—other causes to be ruled out.

INVESTIGATIONS

- Complete blood picture
- *Liver function tests*: Mildly elevated (enzymes < 00 U/L, serum bilirubin <4 mg/dL)
- Blood urea nitrogen (BUN) and creatinine and serum electrolytes
- *Urinalysis*: May show increased specific gravity and also to rule out, e.g. pyelonephritis, urine-albumin, sugar, and ketones
- *Imaging modalities*: Ultrasonography to rule out molar pregnancy or multifetal gestation.

MANAGEMENT

Management of the hyperemesis is based on the severity of the symptoms and needs to be addressed by a multidisciplinary team, if severe.

Diet and Lifestyle Modifications

- Pregnant women must be advised to have small frequent meals—nuts, dry biscuits, and increase intake of fluids in order to prevent dehydration.
- High protein intake and decrease oil consumption.
- Emotional support and psychosomatic medications may be advised if need be.

Medications[10]

Single Therapy

Prescribing only vitamin B6 10-25 mg/day which can be increased to 200 mg/day given either TID/QID.[11]

Dual Therapy

- Along with pyridoxine adding Tab. doxylamine (antihistamine H1 receptor blocker) 12.5 mg, three or four times daily dose to be modified based on severity of symptoms[12]
- Low dose antiemetics—ondansetron (5 hydroxy tryptamine 3 receptor agonist)—starting dose of 4 mg either IV or PO depending on severity of symptoms, may be repeatedly administered every 15-minutes until improvement of symptoms are seen
- Drugs such as antihistaminics and anticholinergics like diphenhydramine and meclizine have be proven to be more effective to placebo and can be used safely to treat hyperemesis gravidarum.[13]
- Minor side effects of the above mentioned drugs include: dizziness, drowsiness, dry mouth, and constipation
- Major adverse effects may include— decreased alertness, hallucinations, convulsions, headache, muscular pains, fever, or tremors may occur.

Severe Hyperemesis Gravidarum

- In severe cases, hospitalization may be required (Flowchart 1).
- Steroids are to be considered as a last option in patients, who require enteral or parenteral nutrition due to weight loss
- Patients who do not respond to therapy within 3 days and not likely to respond.
- If response is seen, then course of the treatment needs to be tapered over 2 weeks

Flowchart 1: Algorithm to be followed on hospitalization.[2]

When patient has intractable vomiting, cannot tolerate orally and has failed out patient regimen, or has developed severe dehydration or, hospitalization becomes mandatory for evaluation and further management

↓

To maintain hydration, establish an intravenous (IV) line for easy access to fluid therapy in the form of (IV) fluid replacement. Continue the same until vomiting stops or limits to less than 2–3 times a day

↓

IV fluids–normal saline or ringer lactate solution along with IV multivitamin
Continue treatment until patient is able to tolerate orally
or till no/minimal ketones present in urine
Correction of electrolyte imbalance

↓

Drugs: Dimenhydrinate 50 mg (in 50 mL saline, over 20 minutes) every 4–6 hours
(OR)
Metoclopramide 5–10 mg every 8 hours, IV
(OR)
Promethazine 12.5–25 mg every 4 hours, IV
Ondansetron 8 mg, over 15 minutes, every 12 hours, IV

- Corticosteroids have to be used with caution and avoided before 10 weeks gestation due to the risk of developing oral clefts.[2]

Total Parenteral Nutrition

- Useful in highly refractory cases in order to ensure sufficient calorie intake
- Complications include—infections, thrombosis, or endocarditis.

DIFFERENTIAL DIAGNOSES OF VOMITING IN PREGNANCY[7]

Pregnancy-associated Causes

- Multiple pregnancy
- Gestational trophoblastic disease
- Preeclampsia.

Gynecological Cause

Twisted ovarian cyst.

Gastrointestinal Cause

- Cholecystitis, pancreatitis, fatty liver of pregnancy, peptic ulceration, and appendicitis
- *When associated with diarrhea*: Gastroenteritis and medicines(iron tablets)

Urinary Cause

- Urinary tract infection
- *When accompanied with flank pain*: pyelonephritis and nephrolithiasis.

Neurological Cause

Increased intracranial pressure.

Metabolic Cause

- Thyrotoxic crisis
- Addison's disease
- Diabetic ketoacidosis.

CONCLUSION

- Early treatment of NVP is mandatory in order to prevent progression to hyperemesis gravidarum
- Administering a multivitamin at the time of conception may decrease the severity of nausea and vomiting in pregnancy
- Hyperemesis gravidarum is a self-limiting condition usually resolving by 20 weeks gestation but can like be associated with more serious complications such as Mallory–Weiss syndrome, esophageal rupture, peripheral neuropathy, Wernicke's encephalopathy, preeclampsia, and fetal growth retardation.[11]

REFERENCES

1. Bottomley C, Bourne T. Management strategies for hyperemesis. Best Pract Res Clin Obstet Gynaecol. 2009;23:549-64.
2. American College of Obstetrics and Gynecology. ACOG Practice Bulletin : nausea and vomiting of pregnancy. Obstet Gynecol. 2004;103: 803-14.
3. Golberg D, Szilagyi A, Graves L. Hyperemesis gravidarum and Helicobacter pylori infection: a systematic review. Obstet Gynecol. 2007;110: 695-703.
4. Gadsby R, Barnie-Adshead AM, Jagger C. Pregnancy nausea related to women's obstetric and personal histories. Gynecol Obstet Invest. 1997;110:695-703.
5. Goodwin TM. Hyperemesis Gravidarum. Obstet Gynecol Clin N Am. 2008;35:401-17.
6. Mylonas I, Gingelmaier A, Kainer F. Nausea and vomiting in pregnancy. Dtsch Arztebl. 2007;104:A1821-26.
7. Jueckstock JK, Kaestner R, Mylonas I. Managing Hyperemesis gravidarum: a multimodal challenge. BMC Med. 2010;8:46.
8. Cedergren M, Brynhildsen J, Josefsson A, et al. Hyperemesis gravidarum that requires hospitalisation and the use of antiemetic drugs in relation to maternal body composition. Am J Obstet Gynecol. 2008;198:412.e1-5.

9. Glinoer D. The regulation of thyroid function in pregnancy: pathways of endocrine adaptation from physiology to pathology. Endocr Rev. 1997;18:404-33.
10. Levichek Z, Atanackovic G, Oepkes D, et al. Nausea and vomiting of pregnancy. Evidence based treatment algorithm. Can Fam Physician. 2002;48:267-8, 277.
11. Sheehan P. Hyperemesis gravidarum—assessment and management. Aust Fam Physician. 2007;36:698-701.
12. Neutel CI, Johansen HL. Measuring drug effective by default: the case of Bendectin. Can J Public Health. 1995;86:66-70.
13. Leathem AM. Safety and efficacy of antiemetics used to treat nausea and vomiting in pregnancy. Clin Pharm. 1986;5:660-8.

CHAPTER 4

Ectopic Pregnancies: Diagnosis and Management

Deepa Nambiar

DEFINITION

An ectopic pregnancy is one in which the blastocyst implants itself anywhere else, other than the endometrium of the uterine cavity. It is derived from the Greek word *ektopos* which implies being "out of place".[1]

The ectopic pregnancy has an insidious and potentially cataclysmic nature which has made it one of the most dangerous conditions to occur in the reproductive age group of women, this has been proven historically. Heterotopic pregnancy is a rare phenomenon and it is a unique dual presentation of pregnancy, one is a normal intrauterine gestation (Fig. 1) and other is an ectopic pregnancy (incidence: 1:17,000–30,000).

EPIDEMIOLOGY[1,2]

- *Incidence*: 2% in 1st trimester pregnancies
- *Fatality rate*: 10% in pregnancy-related mortality.

CLASSIFICATION[3]

The most common site of implantation in ectopic pregnancies accounting for 95% is in the fallopian tube, which are mostly ampullary implantations.[1] Bilateral ectopic pregnancies are extremely rare, and their estimated prevalence is 1 of every 200,000 pregnancies.[3]

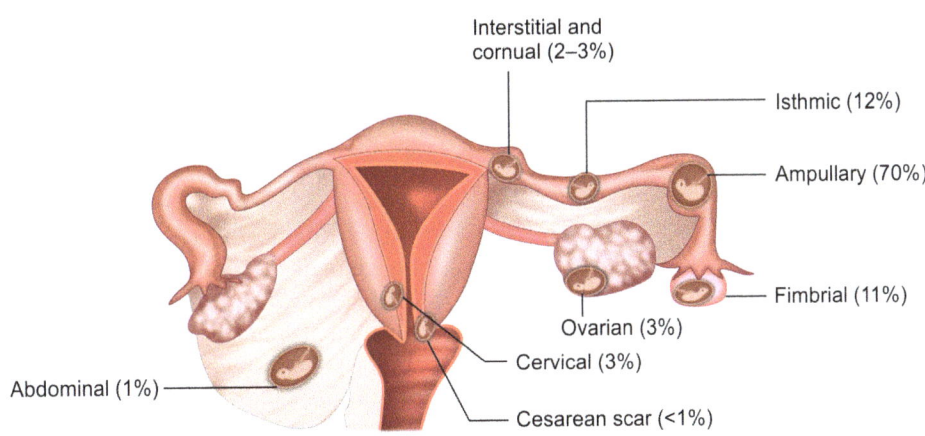

Fig. 1: Various frequencies and sites of ectopic pregnancy.

ETIOLOGY[4,5]

Factors that are responsible for the fertilized ovum to remain in the fallopian tube

- *Pelvic inflammatory disease*: Causes impairment of the muscular peristalsis, loss of cilia lining, and narrowing of the tubal lumen, peritubal adhesions resulting in kinking and angulation of the tube, and formation of pockets of adhesion between mucosal folds.
- *Iatrogenic*: Contraception devices (Cu-T), tubal sterilization, tubal recannulation, and pelvic surgery
- Previous ectopic pregnancy, previous abortion, and previous cesarean section
- Assisted reproductive technology (ART)
- Transperitoneal migration of the ovum.
- Developmental defects of the tube.

Factors that facilitate nidation of the fertilized ovum into the tubal mucosa

- Increased decidual reaction
- Tubal endometriosis
- Premature degeneration of zona pellucida causing early resumption of trophoblastic activity.

RISK FACTORS FOR ECTOPIC PREGNANCY[1]

Factor	Relative risk (%)
Prior ectopic pregnancy	3–13
Prior tubal surgery	4
Tubal sterilization	9
Tubal pathology	3.8–21
Prior medical or surgical abortion	0.6–3
Assisted reproductive technology	2–8
Prior cesarean delivery	1–2.1
Infertility >1 year	2.5–3
Lifelong sexual partners >5	1.6–3.5
Prior IUD use	1–4.2
Smoking >20 cigarettes per day	1.7–4
Pelvic inflammatory disease (PID) confirmed by laparoscopy or positive test for *Chlamydia trachomatis*	2–4

PATHOPHYSIOLOGY[3]

In an ectopic pregnancy, changes occur in the tube as well as in the uterus. The corpus luteum produces progesterone and estrogen which changes the secretory endometrium into decidua (the endometrium may produce a mixed proliferative and secretory pattern called as Arias-Stellar reaction. Uterus enlarges to 8 weeks size).

- Tubal pregnancy does not usually prolong beyond 8–10 weeks due to:
  - The inadequacy of tubal lumen to accommodate the pregnancy
  - Lack of decidual reaction in the fallopian tube
  - Bleeding in the site of implantation as the trophoblast invades into the tubal musculature.
  - The thin wall of the fallopian tube.
- Acute inflammation has been indicated in the tubal damage that predisposes to ectopic pregnancies. Salpingitis isthmica nodosa and chronic salpingitis also contribute to such tubal damage.
- Embryo progress is arrested due to inflammation within the fallopian tube and this provides a premature preimplantation signal. Primarily, oviduct interstitial cells of Cajal are specialized pacemaker cells responsible for egg transport and oviduct motility.

- Cannabinoid receptor (CB1) is yet another factor involved with oviductal transport of embryos; it is mediated by endocannabinoid signaling. Endocannabinoid levels are elevated in smokers, where there is a chronic exposure to nicotine which causes fallopian tube dysfunction.
- In artificial reproductive techniques, the mechanism for ectopic pregnancy in women has been a dilemma as the fallopian tube is bypassed. Only in women who underwent in vitro fertilization (IVF), E-cadherin, an adhesion molecule, was evidently localized to the tubal embryo implantation site. This implies a biological factor that accounts for the ectopic pregnancies in IVF.
- The absence of a submucosal layer beneath its epithelium in a fallopian tube plays an important role in the tubal pregnancy genesis after the disruption of the normal tubal transport, so the embryo effortlessly burrows through the epithelium and implantation occurs within tube's muscularis layer (Figs. 2A and B), which leads to hemorrhaging into the trophoblastic space/adjacent tissues.
- The extent of damage can be predicted by the site of ectopic pregnancy. Implantations that take place in the isthmic or ampullary portion of the fallopian tubes rupture earlier than the interstitial portion. Rupture is unpredictable and spontaneous, but it can also be caused by a coitus or bimanual pelvic examination.
- Ectopic pregnancy development that happens after implantation explains the typically divergent clinical manifestations between acute and chronic ectopic pregnancies.

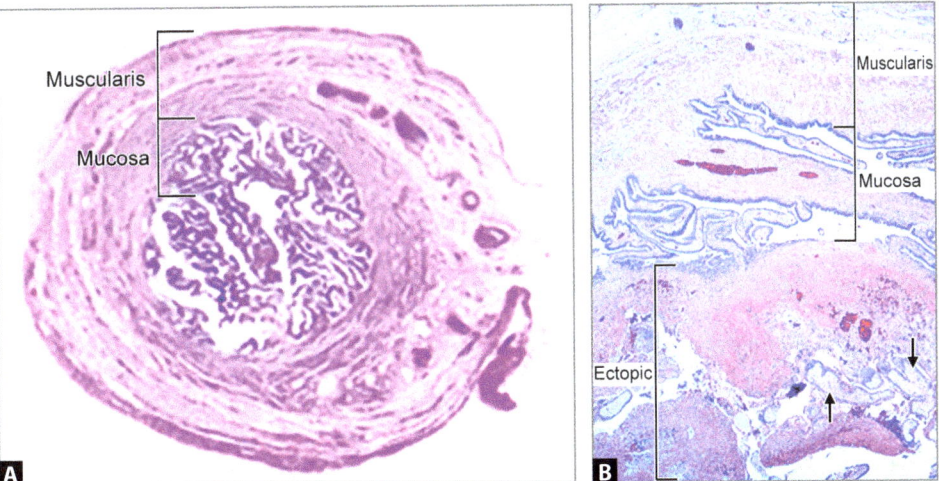

Figs. 2A and B: (A) Fallopian tube with normal ampullary lumen; (B) Ectopic tubal pregnancy—chorionic villi (arrows) within the lumen.
Source: Hoffman BL, O Schorge J, Bradshaw KD et al. Ectopic pregnancy. Williams gynecology, 3rd edition. New York: McGraw-Hill Education; 2016.
https://obgynkey.com/wp-content/uploads/2016/06/m_p9780071849081-ch007_f002.png

Obstetric Emergencies

Acute ectopic pregnancies[2]
- High serum beta-human chorionic gonadotropin (β-hCG) level at presentation corresponds with the depth of trophoblastic invasion into the tubal wall.
- Greater invasion promotes associated severe ischemic changes and eventually tubal wall rupture.
- Rapid pregnancy growth leads to painful tubal distention or rupture and aids immediate diagnosis.

Chronic ectopic pregnancy
- An inflammatory response caused due to minor repeated ruptures or tubal abortion leads to formation of a pelvic mass.
- Negative or lower, serum β-hCG levels are found as the abnormal trophoblasts die early.
- Chronic ectopic commonly forms a complex pelvic mass and typically ruptures late.

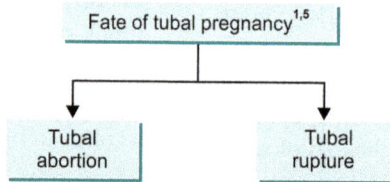

Fate of tubal pregnancy[1,5]: Tubal abortion | Tubal rupture

- Common in ampullary pregnancies
- Chorio decidual hemorrhage causes placental separation and results in:
  - *Complete tubal abortion*: Through the fimbrial end into the peritoneal cavity
  - *Incomplete tubal abortion*: Hematosalpinx is formed in cases of blocked tubes
  - *Complete tubal absorption*
  - *Missed tubal abortion*: Products of conception are retained in the tubal lumen and repeated chorio decidual hemorrhages converts it into a carneous/tubal mole, that partly gets absorbed resulting in a small symptomless hydrosalpinx.

In rare cases, calcification of the fetus occurs, which is called lithopedion.

- Common in isthmic pregnancies
- Signs of hypovolemia are common
- Rupture that occurs in the antimesenteric border of the fallopian tube results in profused intraperitoneal hemorrhage.
- Rupture that occurs in the mesenteric boundary of the tube causes a broad ligament hematoma that progresses slowly and ultimately ruptures into the peritoneal cavity.
- Rupture is impetuous and impulsive, but may occur following trauma caused by coitus/bimanual examination.

CLINICAL MANIFESTATIONS

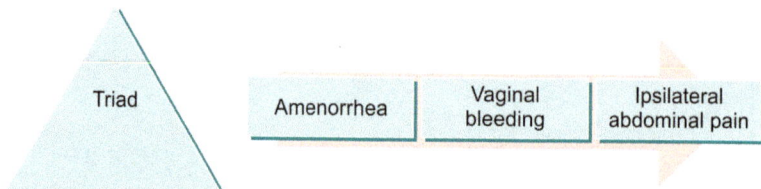

Triad: Amenorrhea | Vaginal bleeding | Ipsilateral abdominal pain

The classic symptom triad of ectopic pregnancy is amenorrhea followed by vaginal bleeding and ipsilateral abdominal pain. Unfortunately, only about 50% of patients present with all three symptoms. However, as women nowadays seek care earlier, the ability to diagnose ectopic pregnancy before rupture—even before the onset of symptoms is not unusual.

Early pregnancy discomforts such as breast tenderness, nausea, and urinary frequency may accompany more ominous findings.

Symptoms and signs of ectopic pregnancy are often subtle or even absent.

ACUTE ECTOPIC PREGNANCY: AN OBSTETRIC EMERGENCY[1]

Rupture of a tubal ectopic pregnancy, which results in a massive intraperitoneal hemorrhage leads to an acute presentation.

Pain	Abnormal bleeding	Abdominal and pelvic tenderness	Uterine changes	Vital signs
• 95% report with pelvic and abdominal pain. • Shoulder pain worsened by inspiration, which is caused by phrenic nerve irritation from sub-diaphragmatic blood • Acute retention of urine caused due to upward displacement of the uterus by the mass causing obstruction can cause severe suprapubic pain.	• Amenorrhea with some degree of vaginal bleeding/spotting is seen in 60–80% patients	• With unruptured ectopic tenderness is uncommon. • Three-fourth women with ruptured ectopic pregnancies have exquisite tenderness on abdominal and pelvic examination, especially with cervical motion. • Patients have symptoms of painful defecation.	• In later stages, the uterus can be pushed to one side by the ectopic mass. • Uterus is enlarged to 8 weeks due to hormonal stimulation.	• It is generally normal before rupture. • Responses in moderate hemorrhage include no change in vital signs; a slight rise in systolic BP or a vasovagal response with hypotension and bradycardia, which manifests as a syncope/shock. • In eminent rupture: Blood pressure will fall and the pulse rate will only rise.

Signs[4,5]

General examination: Signs of shock.

Extreme pallor, restlessness, air hunger, thready pulse with marked tachycardia, hypotension, subnormal temperature, and cold extremities.

Shock index (heart rate/systolic BP) is greater than 0.85.

Breast signs of pregnancy usually are not present.

Per abdominal (PA) examination: Mild abdominal distension (distension is not always due to intraperitoneal blood, but due to localized ileus of the gut caused by blood).

Periumbilical bluish discoloration (Cullen's sign is a late sign) due to absorption of intra-peritoneal blood into the lymphatics.

On palpation: Extreme tenderness in the lower abdomen and slight rigidity.

Local examination: Vagina is pale and tender.

Per speculum (P/S) examination: Cervix has a bluish discoloration (rarely seen in early pregnancy), bleeding may/may not be seen through os.

Per vaginal (P/V) examination: Cervix is soft and tender.

Due to the severe abdominal pain, a bimanual examination may not be accurate, but if possible uterus is bulky and soft. A tender bulge or fullness in the pouch of Douglas (POD) is suggestive of a pelvic hematocele.

Very gentle forniceal examination may reveal soft tender mass, but it is discouraged to prevent the possibility of rupture.

Differential Diagnosis in Cases of Acute Abdomen[2]

A woman who belongs to the reproductive age group and presenting with complaints of abdominal pain, should be investigated as a whole keeping the mind alert for other conditions also, such as:

Conditions within the reproductive system	Conditions involving other organs
• Incomplete abortion in retroverted uterus • Pyosalpinx • Ovarian torsion • Rupture of an ovarian cyst (endometrial/corpus luteal cyst) • Salpingitis • Septic abortion • Pelvic abscess • Uterine fibroid.	• Acute appendicitis • Urinary tract infections • Diverticulitis • Intestinal intussusception.

■ CHRONIC ECTOPIC PREGNANCY[4]

It is the most common variety, which occurs due to small recurrent intraperitoneal bleeding that results from a tubal abortion.

Symptoms: Amenorrhea + vaginal bleeding + pain.

Pain may manifest as the following:
Constant dull pain: Due to distension and tearing of the fallopian tube.

Cramping pain: Due to peristalsis and dilatation of the fimbrial end of the fallopian tube.

Sharp pain: Due to cervical movement on the uterine body.

Gross abdominal pain: Due to peritoneal irritation by the blood.

Signs: Findings may be normal.

A chronic leaking ectopic may rupture and produce acute symptoms.

Diagnosis and Management

Ectopic pregnancy is a potentially life-threatening condition. Patients with abnormal bleeding, pelvic pain, or both, who are found to have ectopic pregnancy or those who are strongly suspected of having ectopic pregnancy require establishment of a diagnostic and management plan and close follow-up to avoid the potentially catastrophic complication of tubal rupture with massive hemorrhage and shock that with delay increases the chances of morbidity and mortality.

Multimodality Diagnosis[1]

Clinical findings + serum analyte testing + transvaginal ultrasonography (TVS) + laparoscopic diagnosis.

- *Laboratory tests*:
    - Beta-Human Chorionic Gonadotropin:[1,6]

Accurate and rapid determination of pregnancy is essential, current blood serum analytical tests that use ELISA for β-hCG is sensitive to levels as low as 10–20 mIU/mL.

Kadar Principle: Doubling time.
In an intrauterine pregnancy, the β-hCG doubles with every 48 hours during the 1st

42 days' period of gestation; but in an ectopic pregnancy, there is less than 66% increase in β-hCG levels within 48 hours.

This alone cannot be taken in diagnosing an ectopic pregnancy as it is not specific only to ectopic pregnancies since similar fall in β-hCG levels are seen in failing intrauterine pregnancies also.
- *Serum progesterone*: Value >25 ng/mL excludes an ectopic pregnancy with a 92.5% sensitivity. Values <5 ng/mL are suggestive of a failing intrauterine pregnancy/ectopic pregnancy.
- *Culdocentesis*: Presence of microclots in the blood aspirated from the POD justifies laparotomy.
- *Hemogram*: After hemorrhage, the depleted blood volume is restored by hemodilution over a period of 24 hours/longer; thus even after a substantive hemorrhage, the hematocrit value may be within normal, hence after an acute hemorrhage, a drastic decrease in the values of hemoglobin and hematocrit over several hours is a more valuable index of blood loss than compared to the initial level. Leukocytosis varying up to 30,000/μL may be documented.
- *Novel serum markers (ongoing trials)*: Vascular endothelial growth factor (VEGF), cancer antigen 125 (CA 125), insulin-like growth factor (IGF), pregnancy-associated plasma protein A (PAPP-A), creatine kinase, fetal fibronectin, and mass spectrometry-based proteomics.
- Sonography:[2,3]
    - *Transabdominal sonography*:
        - *Discriminatory zone*: 6,000 mIU/mL. Discriminatory zone1 is the value of serum β-hCG level above which failure to visualize an intrauterine pregnancy indicates with high reliability that the pregnancy either is ectopic or is not viable.
        - *Ectopic pregnancy is certain*: Where a sonographic absence of a uterine pregnancy, positive assay for β-hCG, free fluid in the POD, and an abnormal pelvic mass (Fig. 3). Transabdominal scan helps to image other neighboring organs and the extent of the hemoperitoneum. Blood (seen as fluid with altered hyperechogenicity) is seen in the Morison's pouch.
    - *Transvaginal sonography*:
        - *Discriminatory zone*: 2,000 mIU/mL
        - *Ultimate diagnostic tool*:
            - *Endometrial cavity*: Trilaminar pattern is unique for diagnosis.
            - *Anechoic fluid collections*: Pseudogestational sac is formed due to decidual reaction and sloughing, and lies in the midline and is contiguous with the endometrial stripe, unlike a normal gestational sac that is eccentrically located. Decidual cyst is formed due to decidual breakdown and predates formation of a decidual cast. It lies in the endometrial cavity at endo-myometrial border (Fig. 4).
            - *Adnexa*: An ectopic pregnancy is established when the fallopian tubes and the ovaries are visualized along with the products of conception as an extrauterine yolk sac or embryo, but such findings are seen in only 15–30% of such cases.
            - *Bagel sign*: Characteristic ring pattern.
            - *Tubal ring*: Halo—surrounded by a thin hypoechoic area which is accounted for due to subserosal edema. *Differentiation of an ectopic pregnancy from a*

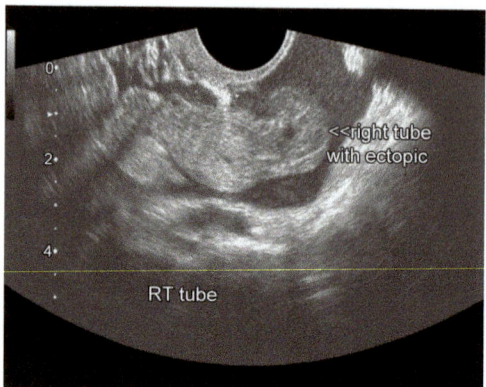

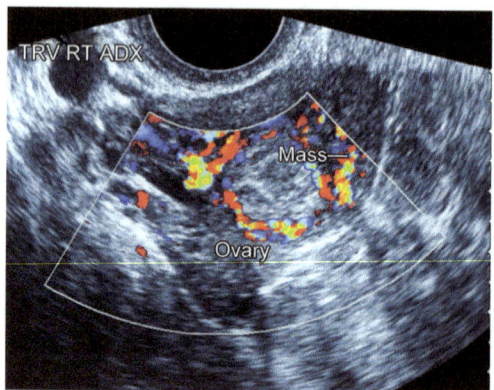

Fig. 3: Ultrasound picture of the right tube showing a ruptured ectopic pregnancy with free fluid in POD.
Source: https://3.imimg.com/data3/PO/KI/MY-12206051/sonography-of-ruptured-ectopic-500x500.jpg

Fig. 5: Ring of fire—ectopic pregnancy.
Source: Hoffman BL, O Schorge J, Bradshaw KD et al. Ectopic pregnancy. Williams gynecology, 3rd edition. New York: McGraw-Hill Education; 2016.
https://obgynkey.com/wp-content/uploads/ 2016/06/m_ p9780071849081-ch007_f005.png

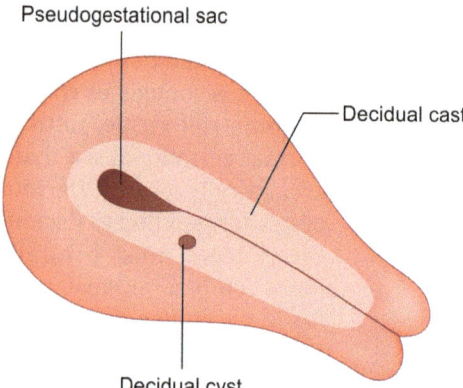

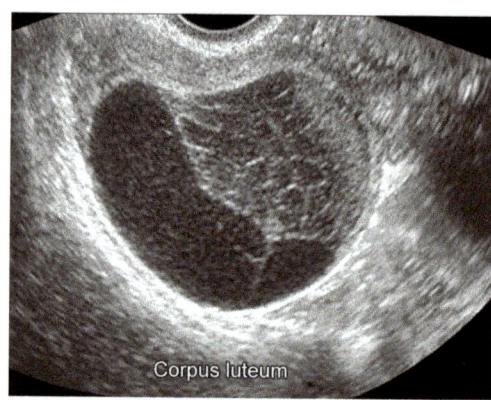

Fig. 4: Trilaminar pattern of endometrium with a centrally located pseudocyst.

Fig. 6: Cobweb appearance (due to fibrin strands)—corpus luteum.
Source: https://i.pinimg.com/originals/30/bf/bf/30bfbf304c579e90597f17e30f400c55.jpg

corpus luteum is challenging. With TVS Doppler imaging, placental blood flow within the periphery of the complex adnexal mass (ring of fire) can be seen (Figs. 5 to 7).

Classical appearance of a CL cyst: Spongiform and lace-like/reticular pattern.

- *Diagnostic laparoscopy:* In cases where an ectopic pregnancy is suspected and ultrasound is inconclusive, a diagnostic laparoscopy is required. This is believed to be the "gold standard" investigation in ectopic pregnancy. Indeed delay or reluctance in performing a diagnostic laparoscopy has been highlighted as a factor in fatal cases. An alternative to diagnostic laparoscopy may involve serial repeat ultrasound examinations,

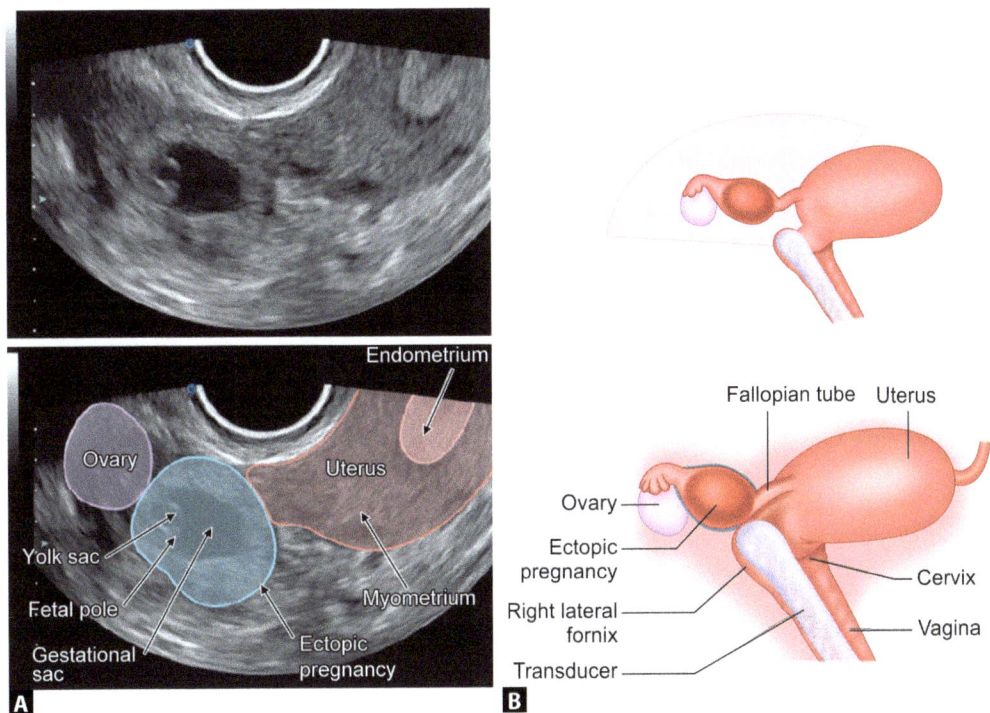

Figs. 7A and B: Picture of uterus without a fetal pole and a complex adnexal mass consistent with ectopic pregnancy.
Source: Simel DL, Rennie D. The Rational Clinical Examination: Evidence-based Clinical Diagnosis. Mayo Clin Proc. 2009;84(11):1045

particularly when β-hCG concentrations are close to 1,500 IU/L.
- *Endometrial biopsy*: In selected cases of pregnancy of unknown location (PUL), an endometrial biopsy may be taken and analyzed for the presence or absence of chorionic villi.

The absence of chorionic villi in the presence of a positive serum β-hCG is suggestive of an ectopic pregnancy. Dilatation and curettage is useful when performed in association with a "negative" diagnostic laparoscopy for a suspected ectopic pregnancy.

Heterotopic Pregnancy[1,3]

Heterotopic pregnancy, a rare phenomenon in the past, is now becoming more common

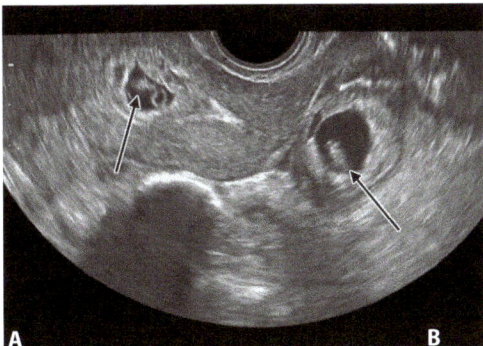

Figs. 8A and B: (A) Intrauterine gestation seen along with a (B) right tubal ectopic gestation.
Source: http://www.ultrasound-images.com/s/cc_images/cache_4215718788.jpg?t=1450776546

because of assisted reproductive technique (Fig. 8).

The most important aid in the diagnosis of heterotopic pregnancy is the utilization of high-resolution TVS. The management of heterotopic pregnancy still remains controversial. Operative management is still a mainstay, but it involves surgical and anesthetic risk to both the mother and fetus.

Laparoscopy is preferred in the diagnosis and treatment. Methotrexate with its potential adverse effects on the intrauterine gestation and RU486, a prostaglandin, with their potential effect on uterine contractility, are not options in the treatment of ongoing heterotopic pregnancy. The injection of potassium chloride to selectively reduce multiple intrauterine gestations has been widely used.

Adequate counseling and judicious follow-up of the patient are the essential components of expectant management. The use of more stringent selection criteria results in increase in the efficacy of expectant management to approximately 70%.

Evaluation Algorithm[1]

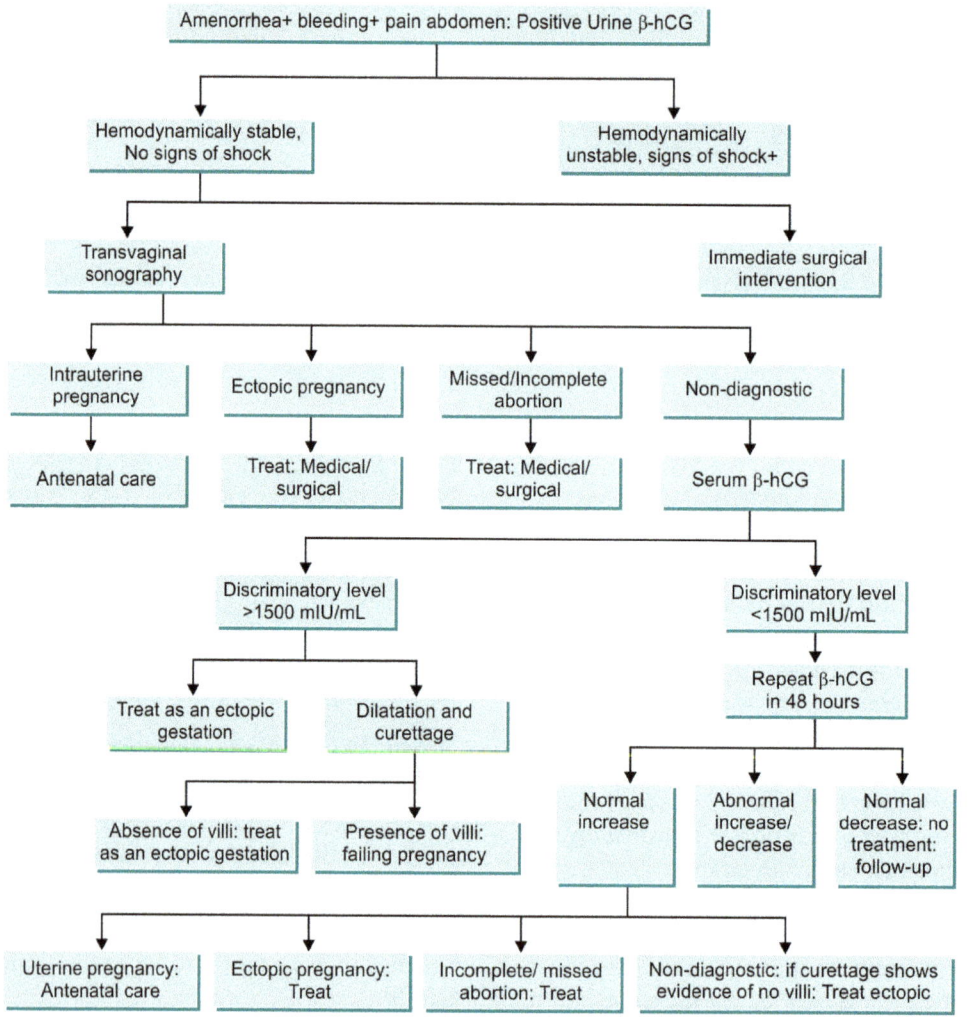

MANAGEMENT

After a conclusive diagnosis has been made, treatment options comprise:
- Medical management
- Expectant management
- Surgical management

- Acute ruptured ectopic pregnancy is an obstetric emergency requiring immediate surgical management.
- *Postoperatively*: In an Rh-negative woman—not yet sensitized to the Rh antigen. Anti-D gamma-globulin of 50 µg should be given intramuscularly (IM) (deltoid), if gestation <12weeks and a 300 µg dose should be given if the gestation >12 weeks.

Indications for active surgical intervention in ectopic pregnancy are as follows:
- The patient is hemodynamically unstable.
- The patient is diagnosed with a heterotopic pregnancy—containing a viable intrauterine gestation.
- Failed medical therapy
- The patient does not meet the criteria for medical therapy.

Preparation[7-9]

Preoperative orders to be followed:
- Relevant investigations
- Secure a large-bore venous cannula and establish fluid resuscitation
- Ascertain the availability of cross-matched blood
- There should be no delay in the operation, if the patient has an active bleeding site/is in evident shock
- Under aseptic precautions, catheterize the patient before starting the procedure
- In case of unavailability of blood, make arrangements required for autotransfusion. Take informed consent from the patient after counseling (chances of conversion of a laparoscopy into a laparotomy, unilateral/bilateral salpingectomy if required, chances of bowel and bladder injuries in the presence of adhesions).

Technique

As early diagnosis is aimed for and often achieved in these cases in today's era with the help of faster and accurate laboratory results and technology, it is followed up with a prompt treatment plan.

A multidisciplinary mode of management involving conservative microsurgery has replaced the once-standard laparotomy hence minimalizing tubal damage and maintaining its function.

Laparotomy is only indicated for patients with complicated ectopic pregnancies and patients who present with features of hemorrhagic shock.

Advantages of laparoscopic approach over laparotomy
- Laparoscopic surgery is associated with significantly less blood loss
- It results in fewer postoperative adhesions
- Laparoscopy is more economical for the patient as the period of hospitalization is reduced
- Reduced need for analgesia and fast recovery

Risk factors for converting laparoscopy to laparotomy
- Dense pelvic adhesions
- Surgical experience and skill of the team
- Convenient obtainability of the equipment
- Deteriorating condition of the patient
- History of multiple abdominal surgeries

Conservative laparoscopic surgery, usually salpingotomy is opted procedure for in the absence of the below indications. Since salpingectomy is a radical procedure, adequate counseling and informed consent must be obtained prior to the surgery.

Conditions in which salpingectomy is indicated in:
- Patient has completed her family and sterilization is requested and given consent for
- Ruptured ectopic pregnancy
- Ectopic pregnancy after a failure of sterilization or also after a prior partial salpingectomy
- Ectopic pregnancy in a previously reconstructed fallopian tube
- Hemostasis is not achieved after a salpingotomy
- In case of findings conclusive of a chronic tubal pregnancy.

In case the ectopic pregnancy is at the fimbrial end, then gentle evacuation from the fimbria is opted for. Partial salpingectomy is suggested if the pregnancy has implanted in mid portion of the fallopian tube and she is cooperative and is a willing candidate for later tubal reanastomosis (if required).

Aim: Active resuscitation and surgical intervention, as time is of the essence in these cases.

Emergency laparotomy: Abdomen is opened in layers.

Findings: Peritoneum appears bluish in color—blood and clots are suctioned out [it may be collected in acid citrate dextrose (ACD) bottles in 1:5 ratios for autotransfusion if required].

Primary aim is to stop the bleeding, inspect the uterus, and adnexa for the site of rupture. Apply two clamps on ectopic side with the tips meeting the center of the mesosalpinx, examine the area well and rule out (R/O) a broad ligament hematoma. Always inspect the opposite tube and ovary. Carefully cut and remove the section of the tube containing the ectopic pregnancy and ligate the ends. Attain good hemostasis.

Milking out of the sac from the *tube should never be done* as it lacerates the endosalpinx and causes further damage. Intra-abdominal drain should be kept and monitored closely postoperatively. The effected tube and products of conception should be sent for histopathological examination to rule out tuberculous salpingitis for medicolegal reasons.

Procedures:[2,3,10,11]

- *Linear salpingotomy/salpingostomy*: It is the surgery opted for in unruptured (ampullary) ectopic pregnancies (Fig. 9).

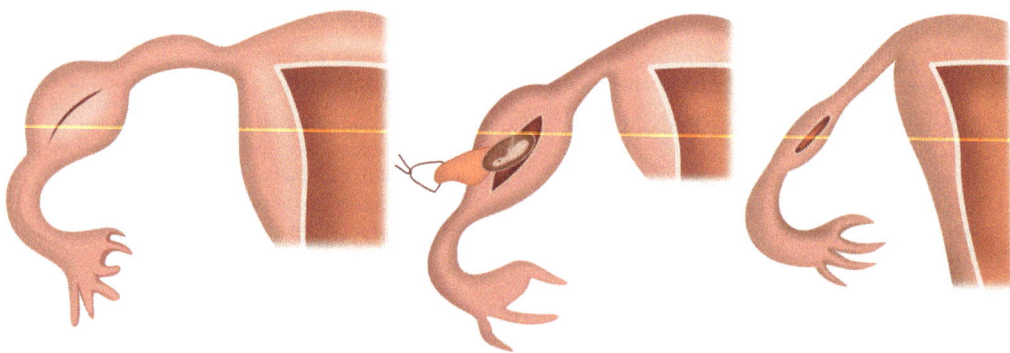

Fig. 9: Technique of salpingostomy.

Ectopic pregnancies in the ampulla are usually located between the lumen and the serosa, hence are ideal candidates for linear salpingostomy. Studies have not found primary closure of the tubal incision (salpingotomy) to have any significant advantages over healing by secondary intention (salpingostomy).

- *Open technique*:
  - Identify the tube containing the ectopic pregnancy and free it from surrounding structures.
  - The tube is held with a non-traumatic Babcock's forceps. In order to minimize the bleeding, a dilute solution consisting 20 U of vasopressin in 20 mL of isotonic (Nalco) sodium chloride solution may be injected into the mesosalpinx just below the site of ectopic gestation. Aspirate before injecting to ascertain that the needle is not in a blood vessel, as intravascular injection of vasopressin causes bradycardia and acute arterial hypertension.
  - An absolute contraindication of vasopressin is in patients with H/O ischemic heart disease.
  - Using a microelectrode or scalpel, 1–2 cm linear incision is made over the antimesenteric side—choosing the thinnest segment of the tube containing the gestation.
  - Aqua dissection is a method used in which pressurized irrigation helps dislodge the ectopic pregnancy and clots with minimal damage to the surrounding tissues, hence better hemostasis.
  - Even if minimal trophoblastic tissue persists, the vasopressin eventually leads to anoxia and death of the trophoblast.
  - Bleeding at the site is managed initially by applying pressure with gauze held in some blunt tissue forceps for about 3–5 minutes. Continuous ooze suggests an arterial bleed that requires bipolar cauterization, whereas diffused venous bleeding is well controlled by using monopolar current, only is absolutely indicated.
  - Application of hemostatic ligatures to the mesosalpingeal vessels must be attempted if the hemostasis is not adequate.
  - The incision over the fallopian tube is left open to heal and is not sutured/repaired.
- *Laparoscopic technique (Figs. 10 and 11)*:
  - *Three-port laparoscopy*: 1 optic port (10 mm), 2 accessory lateral ports (5 mm), after creating pneumoperitoneum. All the blood and clots in the peritoneal cavity is suctioned and the affected tube is identified.
  - Mesosalpinx is infiltrated with diluted vasopressin and with a needle electrode, a 1–2 cm incision

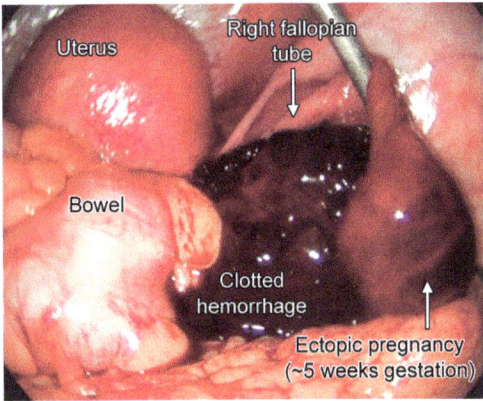

Fig. 10: Laparoscopic view of the 5 week tubal ectopic pregnancy surrounded by clots.
Source: http://www.sharinginhealth.ca/multimedia/images/ectopic_laproscopy_pre.jpg

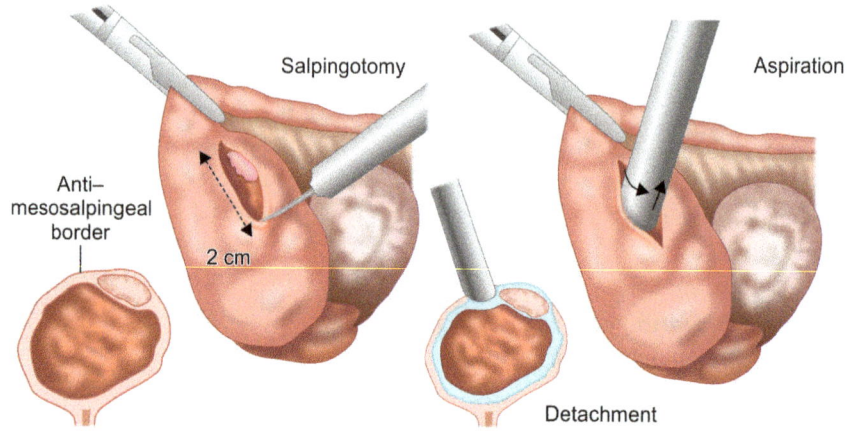

Fig. 11: Laparoscopic salpingostomy procedure.
Source: http://www.pregnancyproblem.co.uk/wp-content/uploads/2012/04/Screen-Shot-2012-04-29-at-20.57.452.png.

is made on the antimesenteric side of the tube.
- The aqua dissector is inserted deep into the incision to aid maximum removal of the pregnancy.
- The products are retrieved through the 10 mm optic port to prevent spillage and prevent the chance for persistent trophoblastic disease.
- Bleeding can be controlled by applying pressure with gauze in an atraumatic forceps for 2–5 minutes.
- Intractable bleeding would require the application of an endoscopic loop to provide adequate compression through the ligature for around 5–10 minutes after which it is released. Failure of which would lead to an attempt to secure the mesosalpingeal vessels to achieve adequate hemostasis.

Total Salpingectomy (Fig. 12B)

Patients with isthmic pregnancies usually have a damaged endosalpinx, hence do poorly with salpingostomy and they have higher chances of recurrence, hence either a total/partial salpingectomy is preferred.

- *Open technique*: Clamp should be applied on either sides of the fallopian tube, one clamp applied 2 cm lateral from the uterus and the other from the fimbrial end until it meets the tip of the 1st clamp. Clamp, cut, and ligate the tubo-ovarian artery while care should be taken to preserve the utero-ovarian artery. This process is done to free the fallopian tube from its mesenteric attachments. Cut the pedicle free and excise the tube. Ligate the stump and check for hemostasis.
- *Laparoscopic technique*: Using bipolar cautery, the portion of the fallopian tube between the uterus and the ectopic pregnancy is cauterized carefully. The tubo-ovarian artery is also cauterized preserving the utero-ovarian artery. Followed by dissecting along the desiccated path, closer to the specimen, making sure to leave a pedicle for hemostasis. This is repeated cautiously until the fallopian tube is free from its attachments and can be excised completely.

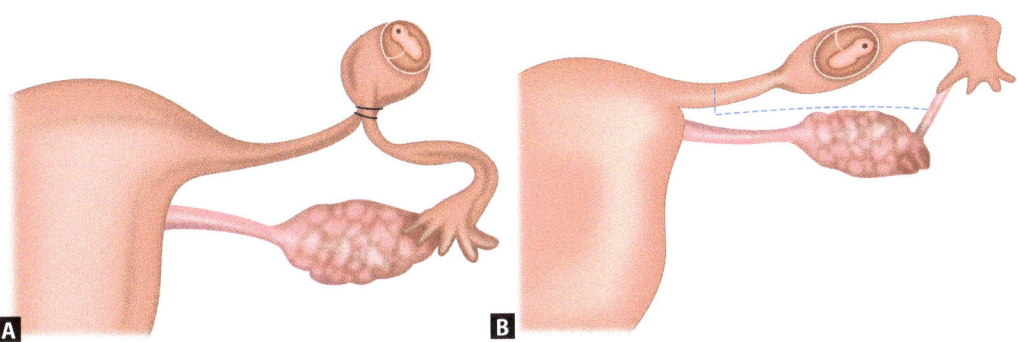

Figs. 12A and B: (A) Partial salpingectomy; (B) Total salpingectomy.

Partial Salpingectomy (Fig.12A)

Involves resection of a segment of the fallopian tube containing the ectopic gestation.
- *Open technique*: Hold the fallopian tube at the distal and proximal ends with a Babcock's forceps. Identify an avascular area in the mesosalpinx and create a space in order to place two ties on either side of the affected segment and ligate each side. Cut and isolate the segment carefully. Attain hemostasis.
- *Laparoscopic technique*: Bipolar cauterization is performed across the segment of the tube containing the ectopic pregnancy. The tube is then separated at the sites of cauterization. The mesosalpinx lying under the ectopic pregnancy should be checked for bleeders and judicious cauterization to attain hemostasis should be implemented.

Postoperative Plan

Postoperative care:
- Adequate analgesia and postoperative hemodynamic stability are very essential requirements.
- Patients who are treated by laparoscopy could be discharged within 24 hours after the surgery, if there were no complications and she had good postoperative recovery.
- Follow-up on the histopathology is important.
- In conservative surgeries: A β-hCG follow-up is done to R/O persistent trophoblastic disease.
- Counselling on contraception for 3 months is essential.

Psychological counselling should also be provided as the patient is usually anxious and depressed.

Expected outcomes: The general prognosis for women with an early diagnosis of an ectopic pregnancy is good. The earlier the diagnosis is made along with prompt resuscitation and treatment, the higher the likelihood of subsequent fertility. Maternal mortality due to ectopic pregnancies have reduced to 0.05%.

The chance of recurrence of an ectopic pregnancy is 1 in 10, and a chance of viable live birth in such patients is that of 1 in 3.[12]

An important factor that has been the cause of improved fertility rate is related to the increase in salpingectomies due to advances in imaging and due to laparoscopic conservative surgeries.

Postoperative β-hCG monitoring:
- *Postsurgical excision (laparoscopic/laparotomy) of the ectopic gestation*: Weekly monitoring of quantitative β-hCG levels is essential until the level reaches zero to ensure complete successful treatment (The average clearance time for

β-hCG from the system is 2–3 weeks, but in some cases, it may take up to 6 weeks).
- Salpingostomy carries a 5–15% rate of persistent trophoblastic tissue than a total salpingectomy.
- A fall in β-hCG levels of <20% every 72 hours represents incomplete treatment after a conservative surgical removal of an ectopic pregnancy.
- The occurrence of persistent trophoblastic tissue is much greater with higher initial β-hCG levels (>3,000 IU/L).
- The possibility of persistent trophoblastic tissue is very significant in cases with the following findings:
  - *Hematosalpinx*: Exceeding 6 cm in diameter
  - *Serum β-hCG value*: More than 20,000 IU/L
  - *Hemoperitoneum*: >2 L.

Medical management:[1,2,5]
- Medical treatment is the choice of intervention when the ectopic pregnancy has been diagnosed with non-doubling β-hCG levels and ultrasonography, without need for a diagnostic laparoscopy.
- Medical management is cost-effective and potent, it avoids the risk of morbidity associated with surgery and anesthesia.
- Methotrexate is a folic acid antagonist that prevents DNA synthesis and thus inhibits cell replication.
- Methotrexate is the preferred choice of drug used for medical treatment of ectopic pregnancy since 1982 from when it was first used.

The mechanism of action:
- *Methotrexate is a potent drug that selectively kills the target*: Cytotrophoblasts, which are the rapidly dividing trophoblastic cells at the fallopian tube implantation site, after which the body spontaneously resorbs it.

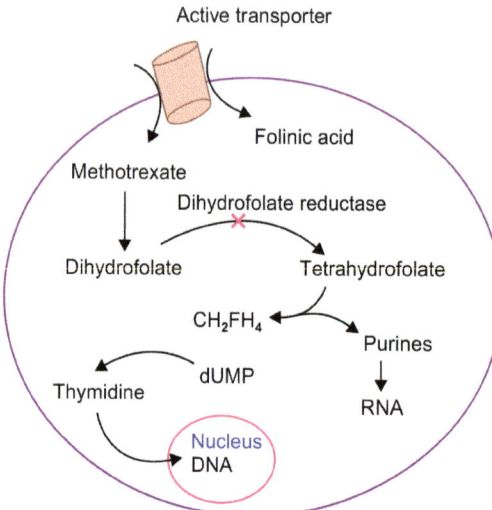

The mechanism by which methotrexate inhibits cellular proliferation. (Ch_2FH_4: methylenetetrahydrofolate; dUMP: deoxyuridine monophosphate; RNA: ribonucleve acid; DNA: deoxyribonucleic acid)

Patient selection:[1,2]
Patient selection is critically important when medical treatment is used for ectopic pregnancy.

The criteria for medical treatment:
- A gestational sac measuring less than 3.5 cm with an absent cardiac activity
- Unruptured ectopic pregnancy
- *Stable vital parameters*:
  - *Pulse*: 60–100 beats per minute
  - *Blood pressure*: 90/60 mm Hg to 120/80 mm Hg
  - *Breathing*: 12–18 breaths per minute
  - *Temperature*: 97.8–99.1°F
- Less than 100 mL of fluid (blood) in the POD.
- Patient who is willing and available for follow-up
- There should be no contraindication for methotrexate therapy.
- Serum β-hCG should not exceed 6,500–10,000 mIU/mL.

Studies have revealed success rates of methotrexate therapy for ectopic pregnancy based on initial β-hCG level,[13] which indicates that a serum β-hCG value of <1,000 mIU/mL has a potentially good success rate of 88%, and a β-hCG value of >4,000 mIU/mL is relatively is less—42%, than compared to the latter.

Contraindications to methotrexate therapy for ectopic pregnancy:[2]
- History of sensitivity to methotrexate
- Acute pulmonary disease
- Breastfeeding
- Hematologic dysfunction (bone marrow hypoplasia, leukopenia, thrombocytopenia, or severe anemia)
- Peptic ulcer disease
- Laboratory evidence of immunodeficiency syndromes
- Gestational sac >3.5 cm and presence of cardiac activity
- *Abnormal renal function tests*: Serum creatinine level >1.3 mg%
- Chronic liver disease and H/O alcoholism
- *Liver function tests*: SGOT and SGPT >50 IU/L
- Low hemoglobin levels and low platelet counts.

Patients who are fit to undergo medical treatment with methotrexate must be screened for the following: Complete blood count, blood group and type, liver and kidney function tests, in addition to serial measurements of serum β-hCG levels.

Regimens:[1]
After much research, many treatment protocols have been advocated for medical therapy in ectopic pregnancy. With the evolution of these protocols, trials have proved (3 general schemes) single-dose, two-dose, and multidisk regimens, to be the most successful regimens.

Regimen	Surveillance
Single dose: On Day 1: Administration of a single dose of injection methotrexate 50 mg/m² or 1 mg/kg IM	*Measure β-hCG level on days 4 and 7*: If β-hCG level decreases <15%—repeat the regimen from Day 1. If β-hCG level decreases >15%—repeat B β-hCG weekly until untraceable. If cardiac activity develops and persists even on day 7—repeat the regimen from day 1. If β-hCG levels do not decrease/fetal cardiac activity still persists, then active surgical intervention should be carried out.
Two dose: On Day 0 and Day 4 Administration of 2 doses of injection methotrexate (50 mg/m² or 1 mg/kg) IM	Follow-up is similar as that of the single-dose regimen
Variable dose regimen (up to 4 doses): Administration of intramuscular injection methotrexate 1 mg/kg on days 1, 3, 5, and 7 along with injection leucovorin 0.1 mg/kg IM on days 2, 4, 6, and 8.	Serum β-hCG levels are measured on days 1, 3, 5, and 7. Continue the alternate day injections until β-hCG levels decrease >15% in 48 hours of after the 4 doses of methotrexate is given. Weekly follow-up with serum β-hCG is continued until it is undetectable.

The single-dose regimen is usually opted for because it is cost-effective, has a much lesser rate of adverse effects, does not require folinic acid rescue, and necessitates less frequent β-hCG monitoring.

Adverse effects:
- Methotrexate acts faster on rapidly dividing cells hence gastrointestinal adverse effects, such as nausea, vomiting, gastric pain, and stomatitis are the most common side effects.
- Other rare adverse effects include reversible alopecia, severe neutropenia, and acute pneumonitis.

Persistent Ectopic Pregnancy[8]

The failure rate is similar for medical and surgical management. Rupture of persistent ectopic pregnancy occurs in 5-10% women who are treated medically; it is the worst form of primary therapy failure.

Persistence in level of serum β-hCG is diagnostic and usually a single dose of injection methotrexate resolves most of persistent ectopic pregnancies.

Recurrent ectopic pregnancy is seen in 10% cases; no matter whatever method was used for the previous treatment for ectopic pregnancy. In such cases, it is vital to counsel the patient about the poor prognosis and is prudent to perform bilateral (B/L) salpingectomy and offer IVF, if the cost permits.

Expectant Management[9,13]

Expectant management should be undertaken only in select cases after careful evaluation and counseling of the patient. It is quite reasonable to observe very early tubal pregnancies that are associated with stable or falling β-hCG levels, as many as one-third of such women will present with declining β-hCG levels.

The criteria required for expectant management are:
- Decreasing β-hCG levels
- Tubal ectopic pregnancies only
- Diameter of the ectopic mass <3.5 cm
- No evidence of intra-abdominal bleeding due to tubal rupture by TVS.

In cases where the initial serum β-hCG values <1,000 IU/mL gradual resolution usually takes place, without any treatment. However, the patient should be counseled to follow up until the serum β-hCG value drops to zero.

ABDOMINAL PREGNANCY[1,11]

An abdominal pregnancy is an uncommon form of ectopic pregnancy with very high maternal and fetal morbidity. Diagnosis in such conditions are often challenging, it requires a high index of suspicion while encountering such cases for a prompt early diagnosis, which is extremely vital (Figs. 13 and 14).

An abdominal pregnancy is usually caused by a secondary implantation, meaning that it originated from a tubal (rarely ovarian) pregnancy and in due course of time, it has re-implanted itself into a neighboring organ with good blood supply to help it thrive. There have been reports of abdominal pregnancies reaching term.

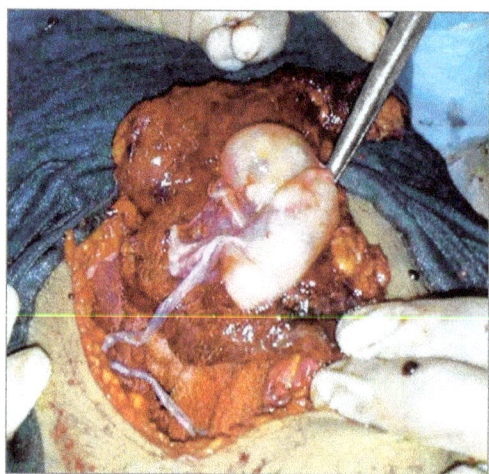

Fig. 13: Abdominal pregnancy
Source: https://upload.wikimedia.org/wikipedia/commons/0/09/Intra-abdominal_fetus_being_delivered.png

Epidemiology: Abdominal pregnancies constitute 1.4% of all ectopic pregnancies.

Symptoms: History of amenorrhea/mild vaginal irregular bleeding, abdominal pain, and gastrointestinal symptoms are not uncommon.

Abdominal pregnancy has a high maternal mortality rate by itself, but other factors that cause death in women with an abdominal pregnancy include moderate-to-severe anemia, infection, coagulopathies, and pulmonary embolism.

Risk factors are similar to that of a tubal pregnancy with sexually transmitted diseases playing a major role.

- Implantation sites in an abdominal pregnancy can be present in any component within the abdomen, but mostly occurs in:
  - Peritoneum outside of the uterus, the peritoneum of the pelvic wall and the abdominal wall
  - Pouch of Douglas
  - Momentum small/large bowel and its mesentery
  - The growing placenta may encroach gradually onto the neighboring organs and its structures too
  - Uncommon sites have been reported: Liver, spleen, and diaphragm.

Differences in primary versus secondary implantation[1,2,5]

Primary abdominal pregnancy	Secondary abdominal pregnancy
It is a pregnancy that is first implanted directly in the peritoneum; such kind of pregnancies are very rare to encounter.	It is a pregnancy that develops after a fimbrial abortion, a uterine rupture or rupture of a uterine rudimentary horn causing a deviation in the normal path of the embryo and promoting the chance of implantation elsewhere. *Intraligamentary pregnancy* is an extraperitoneal pregnancy that develops between the anterior and posterior leaves of the broad ligament that occurs after rupture of a tubal pregnancy in the mesosalpingeal border/lateral rupture of intramural pregnancy.

Diagnosis: Patients usually present with a period of amenorrhea, complaints of dull aching pain that can be persistent and gradually increases followed by an attack of sharp abdominal pain which is relieved temporarily with the help of analgesics and symptoms of irregular bouts of minimal vaginal bleeding that subsides spontaneously. Some patients may however have no complaints at all, other than that of normal pregnancy related symptoms.

On examination (O/E):

In a patient who is hemodynamically stable	In a patient who is hemodynamically unstable
In this scenario, the pregnancy grows normally till a capacity and gets its blood supply from the organ attached.	In cases of intra-abdominal bleeding/premature placental separation: Patient goes into hemorrhagic hypovolemic shock.
PA: Lie is usually transverse or oblique	O/E: Signs of shock evident
Fetal parts are felt very superficially	PA: Distension + rigidity + tenderness + dullness on percussion
Lower Extremity (LE): No bleed PV	
P/S: Cervical position can be displaced	Lower Extremity (LE): Minimal bleed PV may/may not be present
PV: Cervix (Cx) soft, and uterus may be 8 weeks palpable separately from that of the fetus	No time should be wasted and a multidisciplinary approach of treatment should be initiated.

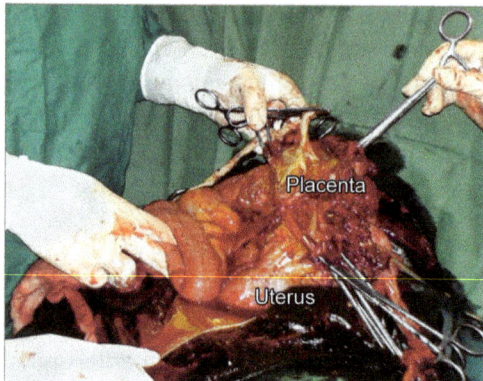

Fig. 14: Normal sized uterus and Placenta seen feeding off the Momentum and segment of the bowel. *Source:* Baffoe P, Fofie C, Gandau BN. Term Abdominal Pregnancy with Healthy Newborn: A Case Report. Ghana Medical Journal. 2011;45(2):81-3.

Investigations:
- X-rays can be used to aid diagnosis: It confirms abnormal lie, abnormally high position of the fetus, in lateral view, the fetus overshadows the maternal spine.
- *Sonography* can accurately demonstrate that the pregnancy is outside an empty uterus, there is reduced or no amniotic fluid between the placenta and the fetus, absence of a uterine wall surrounding the fetus, fetal parts are very close to the abdominal wall, the fetus has an abnormal lie, the placenta looks abnormal, and there is evident free fluid in the abdomen.
- *Magnetic resonance imaging (MRI)* is the most accurate and has been used to diagnose abdominal pregnancy and plan for surgery. Preoperative detection of placental anatomical relations is very important.
- Elevated *alpha-fetoprotein* levels have also aided in the diagnosis of an abdominal pregnancy.

Studdiford's criteria[1-3] *need to be fulfilled*:
- The tubes and ovaries should be normal
- There should be no abnormal connection (fistula) between the uterus and the abdominal cavity
- The pregnancy should solely be related to the peritoneal surface, without signs that there was a tubal pregnancy first.

Studdiford's criteria were refined in 1968 by Friedrich and Rankin to include microscopic findings.

Differential diagnosis: Ruptured uterus

Treatment: Ideally the management of abdominal pregnancy should be done by a multidisciplinary team that consist of an anesthesiologist, obstetrician, and gynecologist, gastrointestinal surgeon/urosurgeon, neonatologist in complicated or term abdominal pregnancies.

In early detected uncomplicated abdominal pregnancies, surgical intervention is the choice of treatment which involves removal of the pregnancy (through laparoscopy or laparotomy), using methotrexate, embolization or both adjunctively.

Conservative treatment is also possible, only if the following criteria are met:
1. The fetus is healthy and alive
2. There are no major congenital malformations
3. Continuous hospitalization in a well-equipped and well-staffed maternity unit at a tertiary center, which has immediate blood transfusion facilities available.
4. If the placental implantation is in the lower abdomen away from the liver, spleen, and diaphragm.
5. Patient should be counseled regarding the probable course of the treatment plan and prognosis, and is willing to go ahead and is willing for surveillance.

The treatment is indicated as soon as the diagnosis is made, however the choice is largely controlled by the clinical scenario.

Advanced Abdominal Pregnancy[11]

Advanced abdominal pregnancy implies to abdominal pregnancies that continue to grow

beyond 20 weeks of gestation. Women with a viable/nonviable abdominal pregnancy never go into labor. Laparotomy is the only mode of delivery in a case of an advanced abdominal pregnancy. There is a high rate of morbidity and the perinatal mortality rates range between 40% and 95%.
- Babies of abdominal pregnancies are liable to multiple birth defects which are cause due to the following reasons:
  - Due to compression in the absence of the uterine wall
  - Reduced amount of amniotic fluid
  - Inadequate development and failure to reach its growth potential due to the inadequacy of placental blood supply. The rate of malformations and deformations is about 21%, which are usually facial and cranial asymmetries, limb defects, joint abnormalities, and malformation in the central nervous system.
- Delivering the baby is not complicated, but placental management becomes an issue as in an abdominal pregnancy, the placenta is located over highly vascularized and friable tissues that cannot contract and attempts of its removal may lead to life-threatening blood loss. Unless the placenta can be easily ligated away from the vital structures and retrieved without any collateral damage, it is wise to leave it in place and allow autolysis and natural regression to take over. This may take several months, and hence patient should be counseled for follow-up through clinical examination, serial serum β-hCG levels and Doppler ultrasonography, until there is no evidence of any remnant.
- Blood transfusion is vital for the resuscitation and management of patients with an abdominal pregnancy. In order to reduce blood loss agents such as tranexamic acid and recombinant factor VIIa are also used.
- The role of methotrexate/mifepristone in treatment of placental regression in such cases is highly contentious as the large amount of necrotic tissue is a definite site for infection.
- Angiographic embolization is another method option to cut off blood supply to the placenta.
- There are complications that develop even when the placenta is left behind such as intestinal obstruction, secondary/residual bleeding, infection at the placental site and surrounding tissues, inhibition of lactation due to placental hormones and preeclampsia (which necessitates further surgical intervention).

OVARIAN PREGNANCY[2,3]

- Ovarian pregnancy is another uncommon form of ectopic pregnancy which often ends with rupture during the first trimester way before it reaches 12 weeks itself.
- *Incidence*: 0.5–3% of all the ectopic gestations.

Symptoms include the TRIAD: Abdominal pain, vaginal bleeding, and amenorrhea, but the distinguishing symptom is that of persistent pelvic pain.

On pelvic examination, an adnexal mass may be appreciated and forniceal fullness is felt in 60% of cases.

Ovarian pregnancies are very unlikely to be diagnosed preoperatively, due to the proximity to the tube and on ultrasound they may resemble any other ovarian cyst. Diagnosis is usually incidental and is confirmed at surgery, since the patient undergoes a diagnostic laparoscopy for a tubal ectopic or ruptured corpus luteal cyst which rarely turns out to reveal an ovarian pregnancy. Confirmation of the diagnosis is following the pathological diagnosis only.

Ultrasound findings:
- A wide, echogenic ring with an internal echo lucent area as compared to a tubal pregnancy which has a thin tubal ring.
- A yolk sac or fetal pole with cardiac activity could be identified on occasion. It is rare to correctly identify the embryo or trophoblastic tissue even intraoperatively.
- Ovarian pregnancies look like complex adnexal masses or solid cystic masses, with or without fluid in cull de sac, fluid surrounding the ovary, and ovarian enlargement.

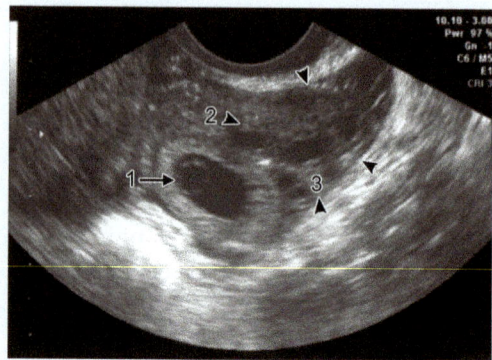

Sonography findings of ovarian pregnancy
Source: https://image.slidesharecdn.com/pregnancy of unkown location-150203121610-conversion-gate01/95/pregnancy-of-unknown-location-25-638.jpg?cb=1438360399

Treatment:
- The most common surgical treatment consists of ovarian wedge resection or oophorectomy either laparoscopic or via minilaparotomy.
- The outcome of subsequent pregnancy is successful, with a low rate of subsequent ectopic pregnancy
- Ovarian pregnancy can be treated by injecting methotrexate into the sac at laparoscopy, and have had successful outcomes, however surveillance is needed.
- Specimen should be sent for histopathology for confirmation of diagnosis.

Intraoperative findings should fulfill Spielberg's criteria[1]

- An intact ipsilateral tube which is clearly separate from the ovary
- A gestation that occupies the normal position of the ovary
- A gestational sac that is connected to the uterus by the utero-ovarian ligament;
- Ovarian tissue present in the wall of the gestational sac (Fig. 15).

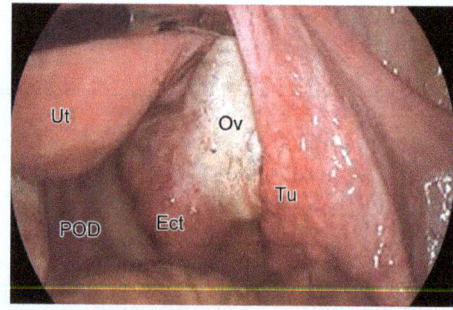

The Laparoscopic view of an unruptured right ovarian ectopic pregnancy. (Ut: uterus, POD: pouch of Douglas, Ect: ectopic pregnancy, Ov: right ovary, Tu: Fallopian tube).
Soure: Gebeh AK, Amoako AA, Olakanmi Joseph O, et al. Laparoscopic Surgery for Ovarian Pregnancy using Diathermy Hook with Conservation of Ovary: A Case Report and Literature Review. J. Clin. Med. 2013;2(4):214-9. http://www.mdpi.com/jcm/jcm-02-00214/article_deploy/html/images/jcm-02-00214-g002-1024.png

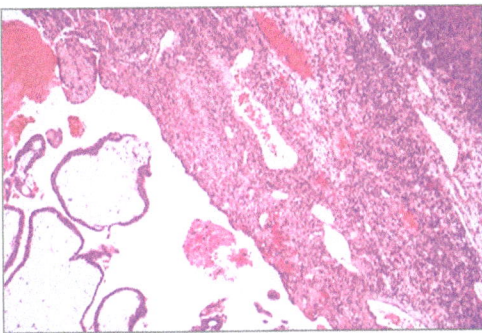

Fig. 15: Histopathology depicting ovarian tissue with immature chorionic villi consistent with ectopic pregnancy. On the left lower field there are immature chorionic villi. On the right side is ovarian stroma with a primordial follicle.
Source: https://www.hindawi.com/journals/criog/ 2012/934571.Figure.003.jpg

■ CERVICAL PREGNANCY[1,2,14]

- An ectopic pregnancy that has implanted in the endocervix of the uterus is referred to as a cervical pregnancy. This kind of pregnancy does not grow beyond the first trimester and the rate of abortion is high, however, if it is implanted closer to the uterine cavity it is called a cervico-isthmic pregnancy and it may progress for a longer duration. Pregnancies involving the isthmus are more common than true cervical pregnancies. Risk Factor: Development of cervical pregnancy.
  To uterine instrumentation, specifically repeated dilatation and curettage procedures.
- Cervical pregnancies are to be differentiated from pregnancies that start from an implantation in a scar
- Of a previous cesarean section, so-called *scar pregnancies*
- In cervical pregnancy, the typical most common symptom is that of sudden painless vaginal bleeding.
- Diagnosis is made in these situations after taking a detailed history and on gentle speculum examination the cervix appears to have a bluish discoloration, rarely a mass is seen.
- Transvaginal sonography is the best imaging modality to diagnose this condition, findings show the location of the gestational sac in the cervix and an "empty" uterine cavity.
- MRI is also a useful modality to confirm and know the extent of the cervical pregnancy and its attachment and extent to the surrounding tissues.
- True cervical pregnancies eventually abort in the 1st trimester itself, but if the pregnancy is located higher in the cervical canal and the placenta attaches itself into the uterine cavity, then it can grow beyond 12 weeks. Due to the abnormal site of placental implantation catastrophic bleeding is expected at the time of delivery and placental separation.[14]
- Palman and McElin (1959)[14] proposed five additional clinical criterias for the diagnosis of this condition which are as follows:
  1. Period of amenorrhea followed by uterine bleeding without cramping pain
  2. Soft and enlarged cervix equal to or larger than the fundus ("hour glass" uterus) (Fig. 16A).
  3. Products of conception entirely confined within and firmly attached to the endocervix.
  4. A closed internal os (Fig. 16B)
  5. A partially opened external os.

Methods used in the management of cervical pregnancies are discussed below:

- *Surgical excision of trophoblast:* Curettage and hysterectomy are the classical methods for surgical excision of trophoblast tissue. Curettage is the trusted fertility-preserving procedure; but due to the high risk of

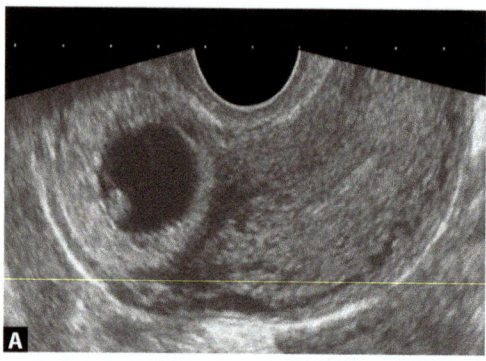 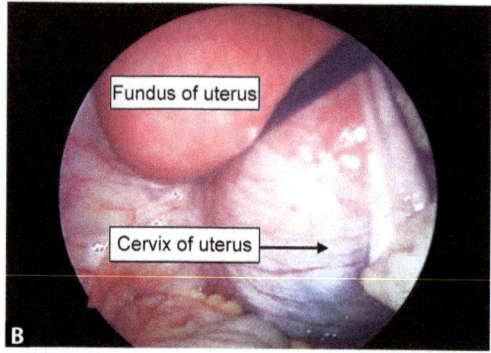

Figs. 16A and B: (A) The ultrasound appearance of ballooning cervical pregnancy with a gestational sac containing a yolk sac and fetal pole, along with an empty uterus with a closed internal os. (Hour-glass appearance); (B) Laparoscopic view of the cervical pregnancy.
Source: Bolaji I, Singh M, Goddard R. Sonographic signs in ectopic pregnancy: Update. Ultrasound. 2012;20:192-210. https://www.researchgate.net/profile/Ibrahim_Bolaji/publication/258198598/Figureure/Figure19/AS:297385482833932@1447913632916/a-Cervical-pregnancy-b-laparoscopic-view-of-cervical-ectopic-pregnancy-and-c-live.png

uncontrollable hemorrhage, it is done only in selected cases and adequate measures to limit hemorrhage like tamponade and cervical artery ligation/embolization are used prior to the procedure.

In patients diagnosed with a cervical pregnancy who present with or develop torrential bleeding, the patient and husband is counseled regarding the best approaches to tackle the situation and explained that primary hysterectomy is the best modality in uncontrollable hemorrhage. Cervical pregnancies that manage to grow into the 2nd/3rd trimester ultimately requires an emergency hysterectomy.

- *Tamponade*: A Foley catheter (size 16) is gently placed beyond the internal os and the bulb is inflated with 30 mL of NS. This technique is used during a curettage in order to help control the bleeding.
- *Reduction of blood supply*: It is obtained by the following methods—cervical cerclage, vaginal ligation of cervical arteries, uterine artery ligation, internal iliac artery ligation and/or angiographic embolization of the cervical, uterine or internal iliac arteries. These methods are carried out mostly preoperatively in order to reduce the risk of hemorrhage and aim at preserving future fertility by conservative treatment of such pregnancies.
- *Intra-amniotic feticide*: The following procedure requires good skill and expertise. Intra-amniotic instillation of potassium chloride and/or methotrexate via ultrasound guidance has been used as a conservative approach.
- *Systemic chemotherapy*: The most commonly used agent in management of ectopic pregnancy is methotrexate, it may be used in a single dose or multiple doses, with or without folinic acid. However, methotrexate may be associated side effects (as discussed earlier). In clinically stable patients, if ultrasound findings show absent cardiac activity and the gestational age is <9 weeks, systemic methotrexate may be tried. Whereas with a gestational period >9 weeks with the presence of cardiac activity on ultrasound in a clinically stable patient may require the addition of

Ectopic Pregnancies: Diagnosis and Management

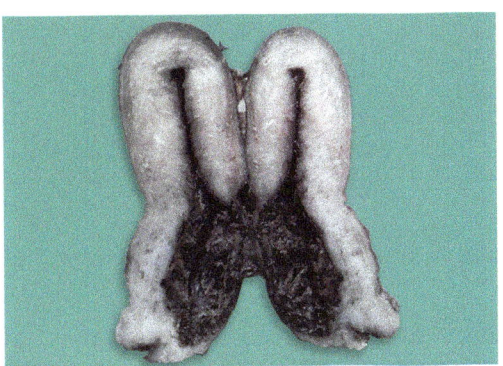

Fig. 17: Gross appearance of a specimen of the uterus with a cervical pregnancy extending up to the ectocervix.
Source: Khatib Y, Khashikar A, Wani R, et al. Cervical ectopic pregnancy: A case report of missed diagnosis. Med J DY Patil Univ 2016;9:741-3.
http://www.mjdrdypu.org/articles/2016/9/6/images/MedJDYPatilUniv_2016_9_6_741_194201_f3.jpg

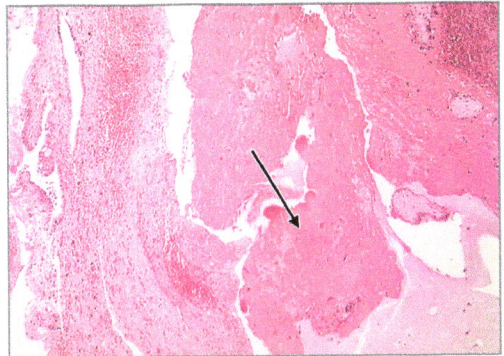

Fig. 18: Chorionic villi and trophoblastic tissue are seen in juxtaposition to the endocervical glands.
Source: Khatib Y, Khashikar A, Wani R, et al. Cervical ectopic pregnancy: A case report of missed diagnosis. Med J DY Patil Univ 2016;9:741-3.
http://www.mjdrdypu.org/articles/2016/9/6/images/MedJDYPatilUniv_2016_9_6_741_194201_f4.jpg

intra-amniotic potassium chloride in addition to systemic methotrexate for a better outcome.
- Recently, a combination of laparoscopy-assisted uterine artery ligation followed by hysteroscopic endocervical resection is making progress in the treatment of such pregnancies.

Final diagnosis is made by the histopathology report of the specimen (Fig. 17).

Histologically the diagnosis is made by Rubin's criteria:
1. Presence of cervical glands opposite to that of the trophoblastic tissue
2. Presence of trophoblastic attachment, below the anterior peritoneal reflection.
3. Absence of fetal elements in the uterine corpus (Fig. 18).

CESAREAN SCAR PREGNANCY[12]

- Cesarean scar pregnancy (CSP) is an ectopic pregnancy implanted in the myometrium of the uterus at the site of a previous cesarean section scar. It is the rarest kind of ectopic pregnancy and may lead to severe complications like uterine rupture and severe hemorrhage, therefore early and accurate diagnosis is obtained in order to avoid complications and preserve fertility.
- The increasing rate of cesarean sections in the last two decades has increased the rates of complications as well, mainly CSP.
- *Definition*: CSP is an ectopic gestation completely surrounded by myometrium and fibrous tissues of the cesarean section scar and is well away from the endometrium cavity and endocervical canal.
- It results in a pregnancy that loses its vascular connections while growing, thus causing a spontaneous abortion, or it may continue to grow gaining new stronger vascular connections ending into a low-lying adherent placenta with or without invasion of surrounding organs.
- The most common symptom is painless massive vaginal bleeding (with associated hemoperitoneum).

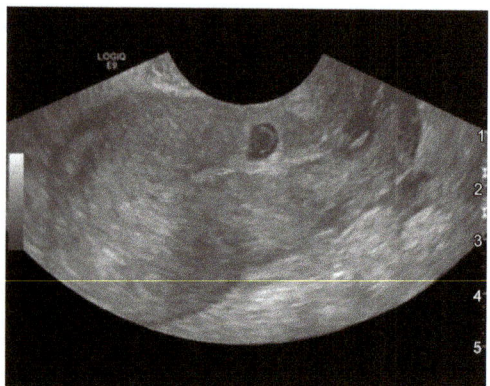

Fig. 19: Ultrasound findings in a cesarean scar pregnancy.
Source: Kim DJ Welch M, Kendall JL. A case of cesarean scar ectopic: a rare but important form of ectopic pregnancy. Crit Ultrasound J. 2011;3: 55.
https://media.springernature.com/original/springer-static/image/art%3A10.1007%2 Fs13089-011-0064-5/MediaObjects/ 13089_2011_64_Figure1_HTML.jpg

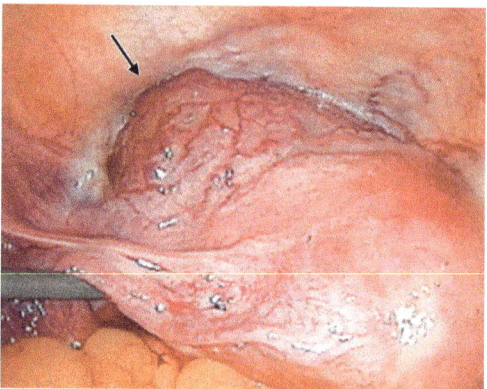

Fig. 20: Laparoscopic view of a caesarian scar pregnancy.
Source: https://2.bp.blogspot.com/Jx4t2nsVdws/UbddRB7F03I/AAAAAAAABaU/DqiMUOLQDBw/s320/cesarean+scar+pregnancy+Kung+2006.jpg

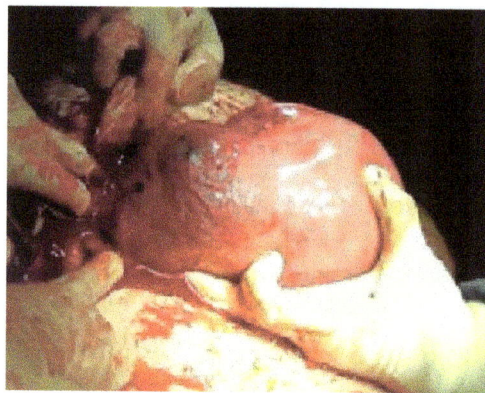

Fig. 21: Ruptured cesarean scar ectopic pregnancy during laparotomy.
Source: Hong SC, Lau MS, Yam PK. Ectopic pregnancy in previous Caesarean section scar. Singapore medical journal. 2011;52. e115-7.
https://www.researchgate.net/profile/Matthew_Lau3/publication/51470010/Figureure/Figure1/AS:305969335685121 @1449960182441/Photograph-shows-ruptured-Caesarean-scar-pregnancy-during-laparotomy.png

- Since there is no specific clinical sign of the CSP, TVS and color flow Doppler are essential for diagnosis.
- The sonographic criteria[12] for diagnosis are:
    - An empty uterus and empty cervical canal
    - The development of the sac occurs in the anterior wall of the isthmic portion
    - Presence of a discontinuity on the anterior wall of the uterus
    - Diminished or absent healthy myometrium between the bladder and the sac
    - Peritrophoblastic vascular flow showing high velocity with low impedance surrounding the sac (Figs. 19 to 21).

Treatment:
- *Medical treatment:* It consists of methotrexate administration locally or systemically, or a combination of methotrexate injected into the sac and potassium chloride injected locally into the fetal heart. It requires a prolonged follow-up (up to 4 months) and implies a high cost, hence adequate counseling of the couple is essential.
- Uterine artery embolization (UAE) has been successful in the treatment of select hemodynamically stable patients.
- *Surgical treatment includes:*

Radical procedures	Conservative procedures
• Total hysterectomy: When the uterus is ruptured or if bleeding is uncontrollable.	• Evacuation of the pregnancy by genlte dilatation and curettage (D and C) and repair of the uterine defect by laparotomy or laparoscopy • Bilateral hypogastric artery ligation associated with dilatation and curettage (D and C) under

The immediate complications are severe hemorrhage, uterine rupture, need for total hysterectomy, maternal morbidity, and maternal mortality if active intervention is not executed. Long-term outcomes to be considered after medical, UAE, or conservative surgical treatments, are decreased successful outcomes of future fertility and recurrence of CSP.

CORNUAL/INTERSTITIAL PREGNANCY[15]

It is an uncommon version of an ectopic pregnancy, its incidence is that of 2–3% of all ectopic pregnancies, which often poses a diagnostic and therapeutic challenge to the clinician and is associated with a significant risk of rupture and bleeding.

- *Predisposing factors*: Previous salpingectomy, rudimentary horn, and proximal intratubal adhesions.
- Despite accurate TVS findings and β-hCG assays, early identification of a cornual ectopic pregnancy remains a difficult task. Diagnosis of a cornual pregnancy can be made TVS when the classic endometrial stripe is visualized, with the pregnancy located laterally in the uterine fundus.
- Rupture typically occurs later than 9 weeks, usually seen between 14 weeks and 16 weeks, but with newer accurate modalities, diagnosis is made way before rupture.
- Rupture causes life-threatening internal hemorrhage, hence early diagnoses and prompt plan of management should be commenced.
- Surgical intervention if the only mode of successful treatment, but there have been recent reports of the efficacy of methotrexate in managing such cases, and hysteroscopic removal of the sac in cases diagnosed early.
- Traditionally cornual resection via laparotomy is the mode of intervention but in the recent year's laparoscopic surgery is the choice of surgical approach, even in emergent rupture cases. Laparoscopic cornuotomy or cornual resection is the mode of treatment, where a good laparoscopic team and anesthetic team can manage this condition. However, the patient should always be counseled regarding the chance for a conversion into a laparotomy.
- Harmonic scalpel and bipolar cautery are used while separating the cornual pregnancy; after the resection is done, the uterine musculature is sutured with 8-0 polyglactin (vicryl), the round ligament is used to cover the cornual defect to prevent scarring to the site, hence giving excellent coverage of the closure site of the cornu.
- With any surgery on the uterus, the scar of a previous laparoscopic cornual resection may become the site of a uterine rupture in future pregnancy and hence is an indication for a cesarean section.
- The occurrence of an angular pregnancy, which is different from a cornual/interstitial pregnancy anatomically by its position in relation to the round ligament, should also be taken into the diagnostic consideration. An angular pregnancy is

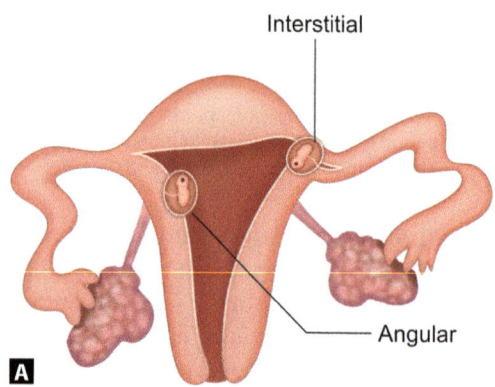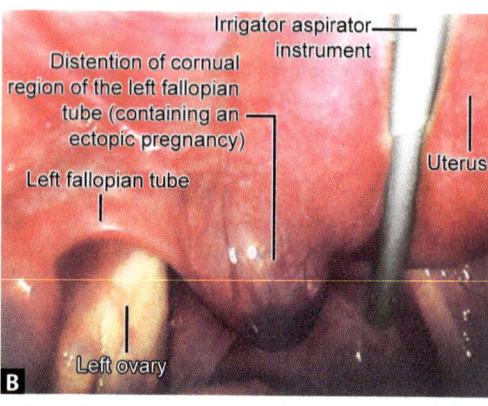

Figs. 22A and B: (A) Diagram representing the site of implantation in an angular pregnancy and an interstitial ectopic pregnancy; (B) Laparoscopic view of a interstitial pregnancy.
Source: http://www.thenewjerseyectopicpregnancycenter.com/images/p_cornual_01.jpg

defined as a pregnancy which implants in one of the lateral angles of the uterine cavity. It has been classified as ectopic, nearly ectopic, or intrauterine. Angular pregnancies may have a favorable outcome than the latter and can even reach term (Figs. 22A and B).

OTHER EXTREMELY RARE SITES

Splenic Pregnancy[16]

It is an extremely uncommon scenario, with only a very few previously documented cases reported. Patient usually presents with complaints of amenorrhea and upper left-sided abdominal pain.

This type of pregnancy has a high risk of potentially uncontrollable, torrential, and life-threatening intraperitoneal bleeding which has a high risk of mortality.

Previously, preoperative diagnosis of this entity was near to impossible and often required emergency surgical intervention and splenectomy. With the help of modern diagnostic imaging technologies such as ultrasonography and MRI,[17] it is now possible to make an accurate diagnosis at a very early stage without any invasive methods.

- The spleen is very favorable for implantation as it is a flat-shaped organ, very rich in blood flow, and easily approachable in the supine position by the fertilized ovum.
- However, the spleen cannot accommodate placental attachment or a growing embryo, therefore, rupture in the 1st trimester itself followed by a massive hemorrhage which is very likely, if active intervention is not done immediately once diagnosed. (Figs. 23 and 24).

Hepatic Pregnancy[18]

It is an uncommon presentation of abdominal pregnancy. Patients present with a H/O amenorrhea, abdominal pain which is localized to the right hypochondria (right upper quadrant, right flank), signs of shock, and the presence of hemoperitoneum on admission. These signs (apart from that of amenorrhea) often mislead the diagnosis toward digestive and hepatobiliary pathologies.

Abdominal ultrasound is the first-line medical imaging modality that helps in the diagnosis of ectopic pregnancy, however the accuracy is far better with magnetic resonance imaging (MRI),[17] as it helps in accurately

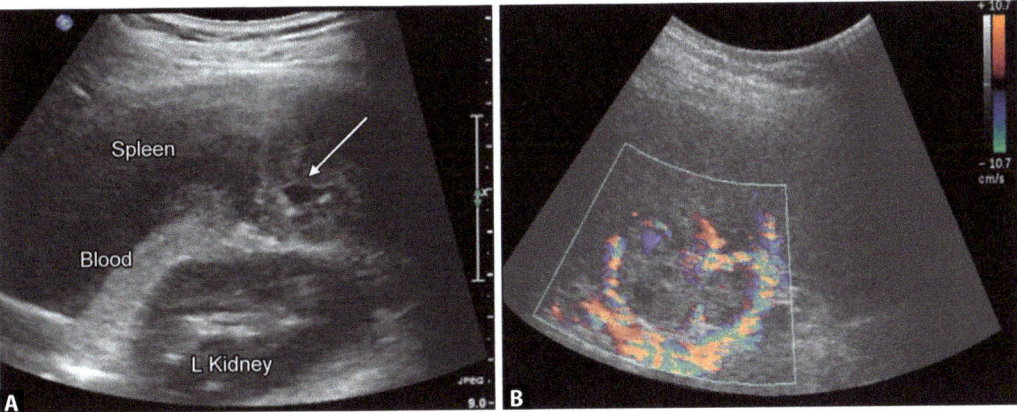

Figs. 23A and B: (A) Splenic pregnancy; (B) Color Doppler sonogram showing a vascular rim surrounding the sac.
Source: Python JL, Wakefield BW, Kondo KL, et al. Ultrasound-Guided Percutaneous Management of Splenic Ectopic Pregnancy. J Minim Invasive Gynecol.2016;23(6):997-1002.
https://encrypted-tbn0.gstatic.com/images?q=tbn:ANd9GcTnekoWo2P3jx6SrTmmt-oBHQY_dpsejv9Nt3ck32pM62YK-LuF-g

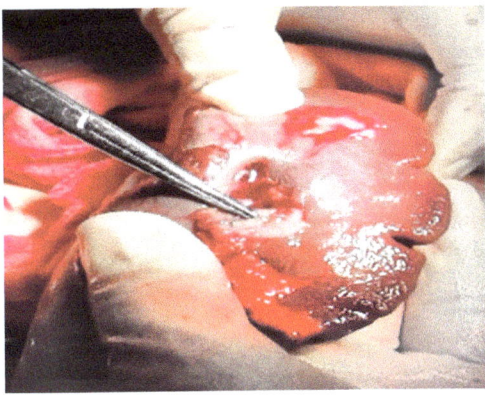

Fig. 24: Splenic ectopic pregnancy.
Source: Jhang Y, Kang D, Jhang B, et al. Ectopic pregnancy causing splenic rupture. Am J Emerg Med. 2016;34(6):1184.e1-2.
https://ai2-s2-public.s3.amazonaws.com/Figureures/2017-08-08/969dd169a00051d5e70f4e976659937b576785dc/2-Figureure2-1.png

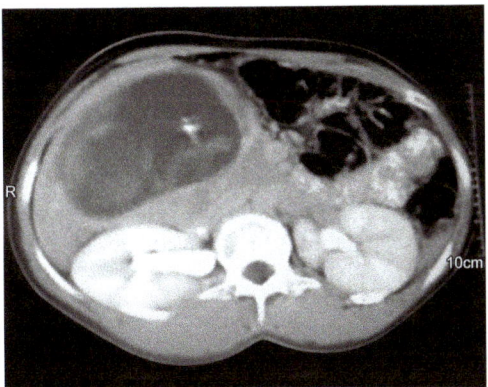

Fig. 25: MRI of a hepatic pregnancy with an 18-week fetus within.
Source: https://www.jamesedwardhughes.com/uploads/3/6/0/3/3603475/2228871.png?340

describing the regional anatomy, location of the placenta, and its attachments to the neighboring structures. The implantation site that is mostly described in the literature is under the right lobe of the liver (Fig. 25).

The management of hepatic pregnancies: Surgical Intervention—laparotomy or laparoscopy (depending on the size of the pregnancy). The main challenge is the torrential hemorrhage that can occur during the surgical intervention. The common surgical interventions are that of partial lobectomy, hepatic artery ligation, devascularization,

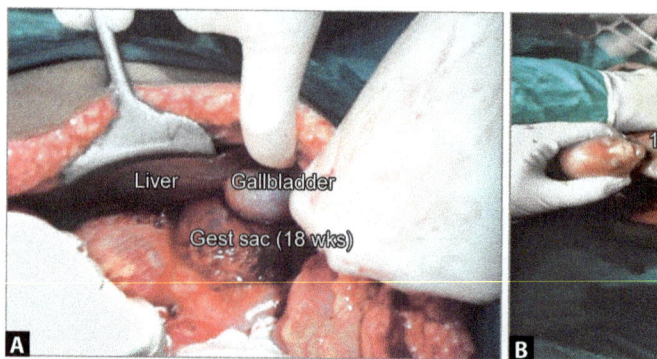
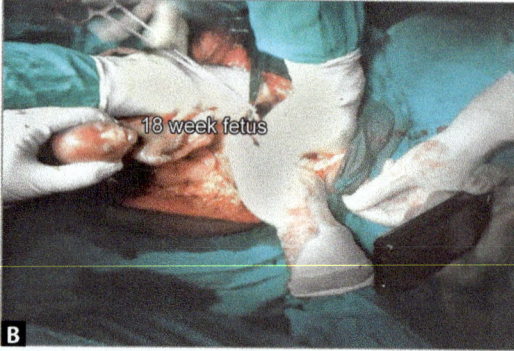

Figs. 26A and B: (A) Shows the relation of the gestational sac with the liver and gallbladder and (B) shows an 18-week fetus being delivered out. Due to torrential bleeding from the placental site on the liver it led to maternal mortality.
Source: Yadav R, Raghunandan C, Agarwal S, et al. Primary Hepatic Pregnancy. J of Emerg Trauma Shock. 2012;5(4):367-9.

omental transplantation, and liver packing to aid hemostasis (Figs. 26A and B).

Methotrexate is administered during surgical intervention such as a diagnostic laparotomy or a combination of preoperative arterial embolization and laparoscopic extraction of the fetus. Postoperative administration of methotrexate is implied for the placenta left *in situ*. These patients should be counseled and β-hCG surveillance should be done.

Omental Pregnancy[19]

This rare type of pregnancy poses difficulties in differentiating primary from secondary omental ectopic pregnancies. Maternal mortality from abdominal pregnancies is reported to be 7.7 times higher than that of tubal ectopic pregnancies and 90 times of a normal intrauterine pregnancy.

The clinical literature suggests there is much difficulty in diagnosing these pregnancies clinically and a laparoscopic approach is normally required, if it fails to find the site of the omental pregnancy, a laparotomy should be carried out. During a laparoscopy/laparotomy, it is essential to exclude this

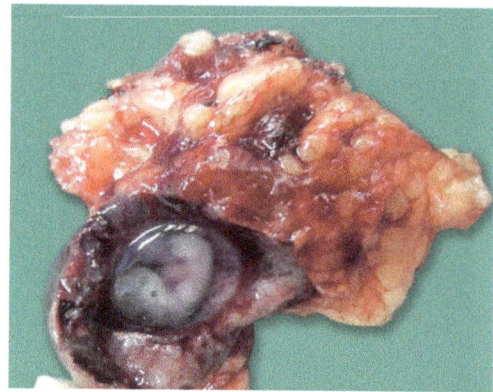

Fig. 27: Omentum containing an intact gestational sac with fetal pole.
Source: Razi ZRM, Lim PS, Tan GC, et al. Primary Omental Ectopic Pregnancy: A Rare Disease Not to be Missed Introduction. J Women Health Gynecol. 2014;1:1-3.

rare entity of abdominal pregnancy, hence the abdominal cavity should be patiently examined, hence reducing morbidity and also litigation. Once the site is localized, a partial omentectomy containing the gestational sac is done and care is taken to remove the products of conception completely.

Pathological diagnosis helps in confirmation of omental pregnancy and its surrounding connecting structures (Fig. 27).

Diaphragmatic Ectopic Pregnancy[20]

Implantation that occurs at the diaphragm is an extremely rare and serious presentation. Due to the close proximity to the vital organs like heart, and lungs, placental separation can lead to torrential bleeding hence has a high risk of morbidity and mortality. A cardiothoracic surgeon should be involved in the management of such cases. MRI[17] is the best and accurate investigation in order to identify the site, size, and extension of pregnancy to the neighboring structures.

An awareness of this condition is vital in cases where the location of the pregnancy cannot be found in the entire abdominal cavity. The patient's symptoms of pain should be scaled hourly and if it continues to persist or increase and if her condition deteriorates with time, diaphragmatic ectopic pregnancy should be considered. Early diagnosis in such cases can be managed with a laparoscopic intervention and hydrodissection of the ectopic pregnancy is implemented to minimize trauma and manipulation at this dangerous site. The patient should be counseled and β-hCG follow-up should be monitored (Fig. 28).

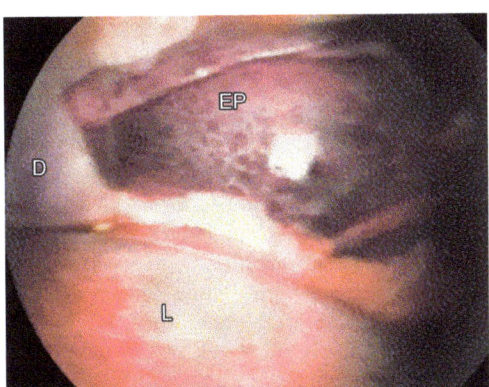

Fig. 28: Ectopic pregnancy (EP) situated in the diaphragm (D) above the liver [L]
Source: Dennert IM, van Dongen H, Jansen FW. Ectopic Pregnancy: a heart beating case. J Minim Invasive Gynecol. 2008;15(3):377-9.

CONCLUSION

In the past 20 years, the incidence of ectopic pregnancy has significantly increased. Clinical findings still represent reliable but imperfect clues that aids in the diagnosis of an ectopic pregnancy. It is the advent of newer diagnostic techniques such as serial serum β-hCG testing, imaging techniques, and laparoscopy that has allowed for the earlier diagnosis of ectopic pregnancy.

Today 85% of ectopic pregnancies are diagnosed as unruptured and 15% as ruptured, which has reduced the morbidity and mortality rates as well. Medical therapy remains to be a boon for the patients who fall in the criteria required for therapy. The diagnosis of several small, uncomplicated, and unruptured ectopic pregnancies has led to an increase in conservative reconstructive surgery.

Rare presentations of ectopic pregnancy should always be kept in mind, as their presentations are not typical but due to the associated high rate of morbidity and mortality, early diagnosis and immediate intervention is essential.

KEY POINTS

- Think "ectopic pregnancy" when a woman presents with atypical features and presents with the TRIAD (amenorrhea + abdominal bleeding and pain) in early pregnancy.
- Tubal pregnancy is the most common of all ectopic pregnancies and the risk and etiological factors are well defined.
- An early unruptured ectopic pregnancy is detected with the aid of ultrasound and β-hCG levels. Laparoscopy is used for diagnosis only if required.
- Acute ectopic pregnancies are life threatening and require immediate surgical intervention.
- Subacute and chronic ectopic pregnancies require investigations to confirm diagnosis

and then appropriate management is followed
- Medical management and conservative surgery can salvage the tube for future fertility, however 15% do develop recurrent ectopic pregnancy.
- With successful assisted reproductive technology, the incidence of heterotopic pregnancy has increased over the last decade.
- Cesarean scar ectopic pregnancy incidence has also risen over the past decade, due to the increase in the rate of cesarean sections.
- Cervical, ovarian, and abdominal pregnancies are very rare.
- Recurrent ectopic pregnancy remains a threat and needs follow-up. The patient needs good counseling and monitoring in future pregnancies.
- Early diagnosis and prompt treatment (medical/surgical) decreases the morbidity and mortality rates in any ectopic pregnancy.

REFERENCES

1. Cunningham FG. Ectopic Pregnancy. Williams Obstetrics, 23rd edition. New York: McGraw-Hill Education; 2000.
2. Padubidri VG. Ectopic Pregnancy. Howkins and Bourne Shaw's textbook of Gynaecology, 15th edition. India: Elsevier India;2010.
3. Hoffman BL, O Schorge J, Bradshaw KD, et al. Ectopic pregnancy. Williams Gynaecology, 3rd edition. New York: McGraw-Hill Education; 2016.
4. Konar H. Ectopic pregnancy. DC Dutta's Textbook of Obstetrics, 8th edition. India: Jaypee Brothers Medical Publishers (P) Ltd; 2018.
5. Virkud A. Ectopic pregnancy. Modern Obstetrics, 2nd edition. India:The National Book Depot; 2013.
6. Cole LA, Butler SA. Human Chorionic Gonadotropin (hGC), 2nd edition. USA: Elseiver; 2014.
7. Hajenius PJ, Mol F, Mol BW, et al. Cochrane Database Syst Rev. 2007;(1): CD000324.
8. Mol F, Mol BW, Ankum WM, et al. Current evidence on surgery, systemic methotrexate and expectant management in the treatment of tubal ectopic pregnancy: a systematic review and meta-analysis. Hum Reprod Update. 2008; 14(4):309-19.
9. Jazayeri A. (2015) Surgical Management of Ectopic Pregnancy.[online] available from https://emedicine.medscape.com/article/267384-overview. [Last accessed September, 2019]
10. Damario MA, Rock JA. Ectopic Pregnancy. Te Linde's Operative Gynecology, 10th edition. Philadelphia: Lippincott Williams & Wilkins; 2011.
11. Roy G, Luciano A, Pasic R, et al. Ectopic Pregnancy Practical Manual of Laparoscopy: A clinical cookbook. United Kingdom: Informa Pvt Ltd. 2007. pp.157-71.
12. Timor-Tritsch IE, Monteagudo A, Santos R, et al. The diagnosis, treatment, and follow-up of cesarean scar pregnancy. Am J Obstet Gynecol. 2012;207:44.e1-13.
13. Sagiv R, Debby A, Feit H, et al. The optimal cutoff serum level of human chorionic gonadotropin for efficacy of methotrexate treatment in women with extrauterine pregnancy. Int J Gynecol Obstet. 2012;116 (2):101-4.
14. Singh S. Diagnosis and management of cervical ectopic pregnancy. J Hum Reprod Sci. 2013;6(4):273-6.
15. Walid MS, Heaton RL. Diagnosis and laparoscopic treatment of cornual ectopic pregnancy. Ger Med Sci. 2010;8:Doc16.
16. Yael Y, Beck-Razi N, Amit A, et al. Splenic pregnancy: The role of abdominal imaging. J Ultrasound Med. 2007; 26:1629-32.
17. Parker RA, Yano M, AW, et al. MR Imaging Findings of Ectopic Pregnancy: A Pictorial Review. Radiographics. 2012;32(5):31.
18. Yadav R, Raghunandan C, Agarwal S, et al. Primary hepatic pregnancy. J Emerg Trauma Shock. 2012;5(4):367-9.
19. Razi ZMR, Ng BK, et al. Primary Omental Ectopic Pregnancy: A Rare Disease Not to be Missed. J Womens Health Gynecol. 2014;1:1-3.
20. Dennert IM, van Dongen H, Jansen FW. Ectopic Pregnancy: a heart beating case. Journal of Minimally Invasive Gynecology. 2008;15(3):377-9.

CHAPTER 5

Retroverted Gravid Uterus

CS Sushma Madhuprakash

CLINICAL ANATOMY OF THE UTERUS

The dimensions and weight of the uterine vary considerably and are dependent on the status of parity and hormonal milieu. The uterus is a hollow pear-shaped fibromuscular organ that can be divided into three main parts the fundus and the body of the uterine corpus which is muscular and the lower fibrous cervix, and the lower fibrous cervix partly extends into the vagina, and the part of the uterus above the level of the fallopian tubes is called the fundus. The narrow region between the body of uterus and cervix is known as isthmus and it marks the level of the internal os of the cervix and the course of the uterine artery. The endometrial cavity lies within the body of the uterus and is enclosed by a thick muscular wall.

The uterine position is described based on the relative location of the fundus. The uterine position is of considerable interest but of much less importance in practice. The most common position of the uterus in a nulligravid female is in moderate anteflexion or tipped slightly anteriorly, and the uterus is completely inclined toward the symphysis in anteversion against the bladder, changing its position as the adjacent organs distend or empty. In a variable number of women, the uterus is retroverted or tipped posteriorly or retroflexed toward the sacrum. Quite a few symptoms were attributed to these "malposition's" in the past including dysmenorrhea, functional uterine bleeding, backache, dyspareunia, and leucorrhea. Some normal uteri are in mid position, with the axis of the uterus being almost parallel to the spine (Figs. 1A and B).

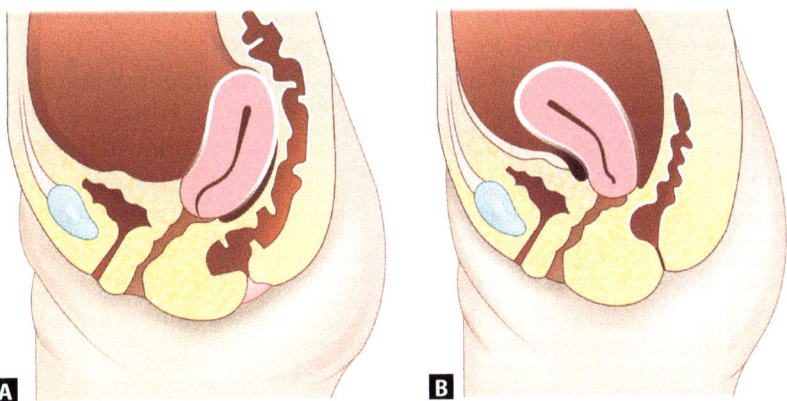

Figs. 1A and B: Position of uterus. (A) Retroverted uterus; (B) Anteverted uterus.

RETROVERTED UTERUS AND PREGNANCY

In most cases, the position of the uterus is of least significance in pregnancy as it does not interfere with pregnancy. In several studies during first trimester, uterine retroversion has been reported to occur in 6%, 11%, or 15% of pregnancies and spontaneous anteversion nearly always occurs after the first trimester (14–15 weeks), the growing uterus lifts out of the pelvis and, for the remaining part of the pregnancy, assumes the typical forward-tipped position.

1:3000 mid trimester pregnancies will have persistent retroversion of the uterus. This condition is known as "incarcerated uterus" and this can cause overflow incontinence or retention of urine. Continuous urinary bladder drainage will encourage the uterus in spontaneous correction to anteversion.

Several techniques have been described for dealing with cases of persistent retroversion of the uterus in pregnancy, including vaginal manipulation with constant upward pressure on the fundus or gentle upward displacement of the uterus at laparotomy.

Causes for a Retroverted Uterus

- *Natural variation*: Generally, the uterus moves into a forward tilt as the female matures. Sometimes, this does not happen and the uterus remains tilted backward.
- *Endometriosis*: Endometriosis is the presence of active endometrial cells outside the uterine cavity. Endometriosis especially of the pouch of Douglas or on uterosacral ligament leading on to adhesion or scaring can lead on to retroverted uterus.
- *Adhesions*: Pelvic surgeries, pelvic infections can cause adhesion. Adhesions between the fundus of uterus and pouch of Douglas can then pull the uterus into a backward tilt position.
- *Fibroids*: These small uterine lumps can make the uterus susceptible to retroversion.
  - Anterior wall fibroid at the junction of the body of the uterus and isthmus may cause persistent uterine retroversion as there is a hindrance by the fibroid for normal anteversion.
  - Posterior wall fundal fibroid can also facilitate retroversion, especially in a pregnant uterus.

  It is important that urinary retention does not occur in such patients, and the patient should be instructed to visit the hospital if there is a premature rupture of membranes or if there is any uterine activity.
- *Pregnancy*: The uterus is in its anatomical position by bands of connective tissue around it. During pregnancy under the influence of hormones, these connective tissue and ligaments relax and allow the uterus to tip backward. The majority of cases, the uterus returns to its normal anteversion after delivery, but sometimes parous uterus remains retroverted.

Fate of Retroverted Gravid Uterus

- *Spontaneous correction*:
  - It is seen in a vast number of patients by the end of the first trimester.
- *Incarceration*:
  - It is a complication seen usually in early second trimester where the gravid uterus continues to grow retroflexed into the pelvis and its uterine fundus lies below the sacral promontory
  - *Causes for incarceration are*:
    - Prominent sacral promontory
    - Adhesions in the pouch of Douglas (Fig. 2)
    - Large low anterior wall subserious fibroid.

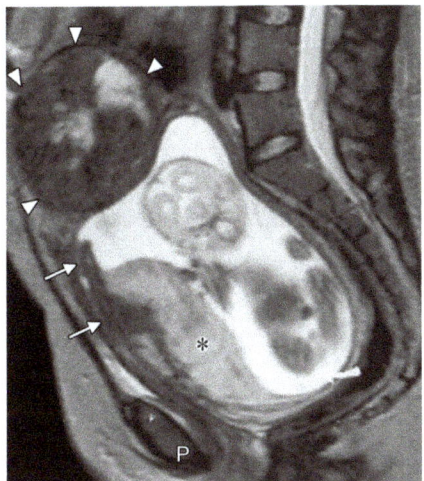

Fig. 2: Sagittal view of T2-weighted fast spin magnetic resonance image at 20 weeks of pregnancy showing uterine fundus containing the breech (curved arrow) in the Pouch of Douglas. The placenta (*) is in the posterior uterine wall with a large intramural myoma (arrowheads) superiorly on the lower portion of the anterior wall, with the cervix (arrows) just below, above the level of the symphysis pubis (P).

- *Abortion*:
  - May occur in the early second trimester (14–16 weeks) due to:
    - Increase blood flow to the gravid uterus
    - Elongating of the isthmus, as the body of the uterus is impinged below the sacral promontory and is unable to accommodate the growing fetus.
- *Anterior sacculation*:
  - It is the consequence of neglected incarceration, where the anterior part of the lower uterine segment distends to accommodate the growing pregnancy. This may lead to thinning of the lower uterine segment and later rupture of the uterus.

Clinical Picture of Incarceration

Symptoms:
- *Urinary symptoms* increase the frequency of micturition followed by difficulty in micturition followed by acute retention of urine due to compression and elongation of the urethra
- *Pain* may be due to:
  - Abortion
  - Bladder distension due to the retention of urine
  - Pressure on pelvic organs
  - Pelvic congestion symptoms.

Signs:
- *Abdominally*: The distended bladder may be felt.
- *Vaginally*:
  - The cervix is directed anteriorly and high on examination
  - The fundus of the gravid uterus is palpable in the pouch of Douglas as a soft mass.

Differential diagnosis:
- Pelvic hematocele
- Pregnancy with a tubo-ovarian mass
- Posterior wall fibroid with pregnancy.

Management:
Prophylactic:
- Frequent prone position
- Avoid over distension of the bladder, frequent emptying of the urinary bladder
- Examine the patient during the early second trimester (14–18 weeks), if a spontaneous correction has not occurred, then manual correction is advised (Fig 3).

Curative: Slow emptying of the bladder and leaving Foley's catheter in situ for continuous bladder drainage. Place the patient in Sims' position or Knee-chest position. These usually succeed to correct the retroversion by the help of gravity, if it fails then decide on manual correction with or without anesthesia.

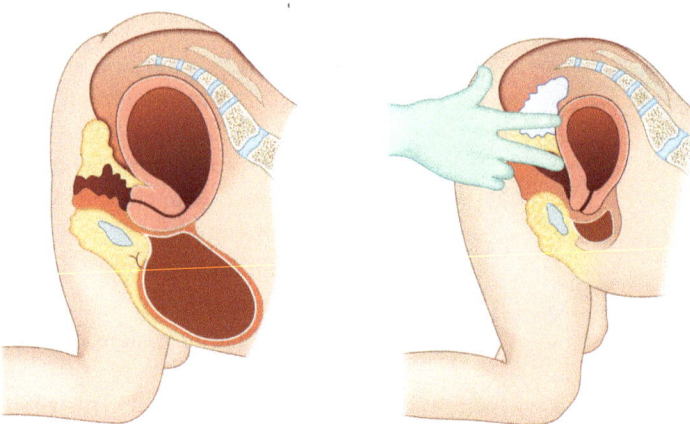

Fig. 3: Manual correction of retroverted gravid uterus.

In extremely rare cases, laparotomy may be needed to free the adhesions if retroversion is due to adhesions.

Management of Anterior Sacculations

- *In early pregnancy*: Manual correction is attempted and if fails, do laparotomy to free the uterus from adhesions.
- *In late pregnancy*: Deliver the fetus by cesarean section.

Predisposing factors:
- Lax abdominal wall of grand multipara
- Exaggerated lumbar lordosis
- Contracted pelvis.

Complications:
- Uneasiness to the patient
- Preterm premature rupture of membranes
- Umbilical cord prolapse
- Malpresentations and nonengagement
- Protracted labor
- Obstructed labor and uterine rupture.

Management:
Antepartum:
- Advice abdominal binder in case of the lax abdominal wall
- Pessary—a plastic device or a small silicone pessary can be placed either temporarily or permanently to help keep the uterus in proper anteverted position. However, pessaries have increased chances of infection and inflammation.

Intrapartum:
- Exclude cephalic pelvic disproportion and maintain the dorsal position during labor. Instrumental delivery is advised in cases of prolonged labor to facilitate the presenting part in the pelvis
- In case of disproportion or any other obstetric indication, plan elective lower segment cesarean section.

Take home message:
- The pessary should be advised with caution, though they are easy to use, pessary use has increased chances of infection, the patient needs to be explained about its care.
- Conservative management is usually opted, the rule in conservative management for retroverted uterus is continuous bladder drainage/frequent emptying of bladder.

6

Hydatidiform Mole

Nisha Singh

BACKGROUND

Gestational trophoblastic disease (GTD) describes a group of tumors characterized by abnormal trophoblast proliferation. Trophoblast produces human chorionic gonadotropin (hCG), thus the measurement of this peptide hormone in serum is essential for GTD diagnosis, management, and surveillance.

The histological classification of GTDs includes:
- *Hydatidiform moles*, which are characterized by the presence of villi
- *Nonmolar trophoblastic malignant neoplasms,* which lack villi.

Hydatidiform mole is a premalignant form of gestational trophoblastic neoplasia. It is synonym for vesicular mole.[1]

The classification of GTDs mainly includes a spectrum of cellular proliferation arising from placental villous trophoblast. This mainly consists of:
- *Hydatidiform mole* (complete and partial)
- Invasive mole
- Choriocarcinoma
- Placental site trophoblastic tumor (Fig. 1).

The latter three conditions can be collectively grouped into gestational trophoblastic neoplasia, which can progress, invade, metastasize, and lead to death if left untreated. These malignancies develop weeks or years following any type of pregnancy, but frequently follow a hydatidiform mole.[1]

DEFINITION

Hydatidiform moles are excessively edematous immature placenta,[2] where there are partly degenerative and partly proliferative changes in the young chorionic villi.[3] These result into formation of clusters of cysts of various sizes. Because of its superficial resemblance to hydatid cyst, it is termed as hydatidiform mole.[1]

Hydatidiform mole can be divided into complete or partial moles based on gross morphology, genetic, and histopathological features (Table 1). However, unless specified, molar pregnancy relates one with complete mole.[4]

RISK FACTORS

The cause cannot be ascertained definitively but it appears to be related to the ovular defect as it sometimes affects one ovum of a twin pregnancy. The strongest risk factors are age and a prior hydatidiform mole.
- *Age*: Women at both extremes of reproductive age are most vulnerable. Those older than 40 have an almost 10-fold risk.[5.]
- *Previous molar pregnancy*: With a prior complete mole, the risk of another mole is 0.9%, and with a previous partial mole, the rate is 0.3%. After two prior complete moles, approximately 20% of women have a third mole.[6]
- *Diet/nutrition*: Molar pregnancies are associated with low levels of carotene and vitamin A in a person's diet.

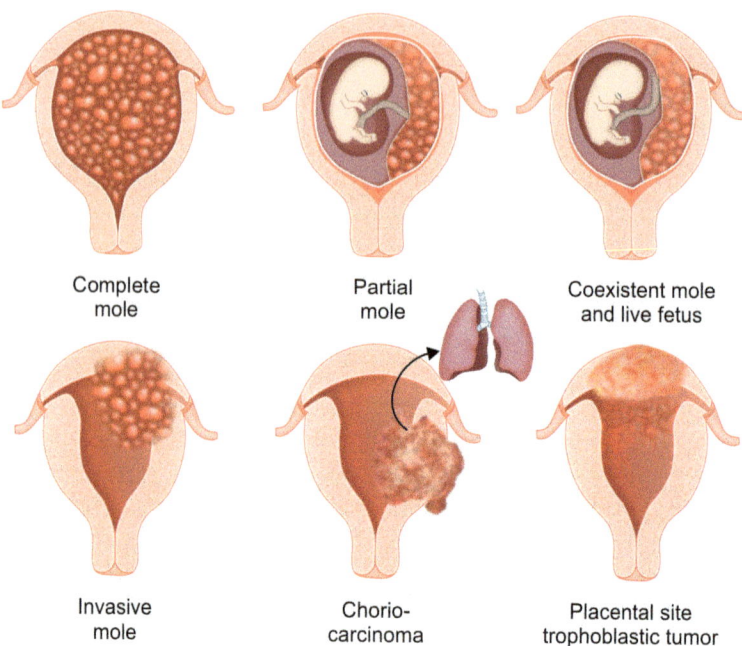

Fig. 1: Classification of gestational trophoblastic disease.

TABLE 1: Features of partial and complete hydatidiform moles.		
Features	Complete mole	Partial mole
Karyotype	46XX (mainly), 46XY	Triploid (90%) (69XXY, 69XYY, and 69XXX) Diploid (10%)
Presentation		
Preliminary diagnosis	Molar gestation	Missed abortion
Classic clinical symptoms	Common	Rare
Beta-hCG	High (>1,00,000 mIU/mL)	Slight elevation (<100,000 mIU/mL)
Uterine size	More than date	Less than date
Theca lutein cyst	Common	Uncommon
Risk of persistent GTD	20%	<5%
Pathology		
Embryo/fetus	Absent	Present
Hydronic degeneration of villi	Pronounced and diffused	Variable and focal
Trophoblast hyperplasia	Diffuse	Focal
(hCG: human chorionic gonadotropin; GTD: gestational trophoblastic disease)		

- *Blood group*: AB blood group shows highest association.[1]
- *Race and ethnicity*: There is wide range of geographical and ethnic variation of the prevalence of this condition. Highest prevalence in Philippines of 1 in 80. The incidence in India is 1 in 400.[1]

PATHOGENESIS

Molar pregnancies arise from chromosomally abnormal fertilizations. When a 23, X-bearing haploid sperm fertilizes a 23,X-containing haploid egg whose genes have been "inactivated" a 46,XX complete mole may be formed. Paternal chromosomes then duplicate to create a 46,XX embryo after meiosis. Since both the set of chromosomes have paternal origin, it is termed as androgenesis.

Less commonly, the chromosomal pattern may be 46,XY or 46,XX and due to fertilization by two sperm, that is, dispermic fertilization or dispermy.[7,8]

A partial mole may be formed if two sperm—either 23,X- or 23,Y-bearing both fertilize (dispermy) a 23,X-containing haploid egg whose genes have not been inactivated. The resulting fertilized egg is triploid with two chromosome sets being donated by the father. This paternal contribution is termed diandry. So, partial moles have triploid karyotype 69XXY, 69XX, or rarely 69XYY (Figs. 2A and B).

Rarely, in some twin pregnancies, one chromosomally normal fetus is paired with a complete diploid molar pregnancy. Importantly, these cases must be distinguished from a single partial molar pregnancy with its associated abnormal fetus. Amniocentesis and fetal karyotyping aid confirmation.

These triploid zygotes of a partial molar pregnancy result in some embryonic development, however, it ultimately is a lethal fetal condition.[9] Fetuses that reach advanced ages have severe growth restriction, multiple congenital anomalies, or both.

However in twin pregnancies, where a chromosomally normal fetus exists with a complete molar pregnancy, survival depends on the comorbidities associated with molar

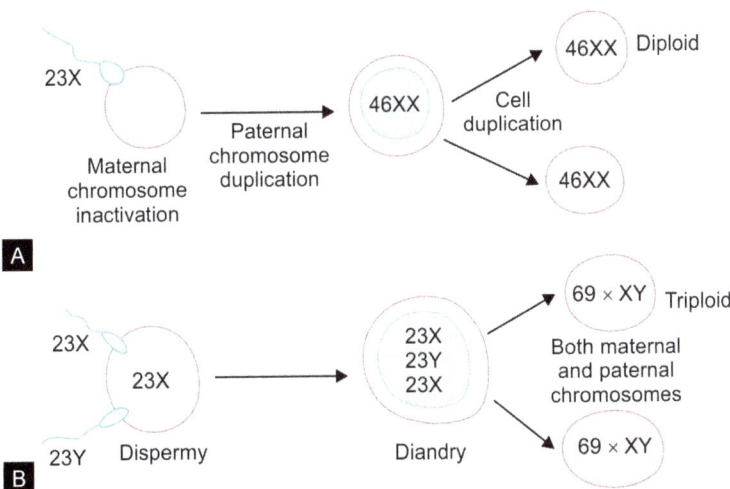

Figs. 2A and B: (A) A 46,XX complete mole may be formed if a 23,X-bearing haploid sperm fertilizes a 23,X-containing haploid egg whose genes have been "inactivated"; (B) A partial mole may be formed, if two sperm—either 23,X- or 23,Y-bearing both fertilize (dispermy) a 23,X-containing haploid egg whose genes have not been inactivated hence triploidy (69XXY).

component. Most common are preeclampsia and hemorrhage necessitating preterm delivery. Also there is risk of developing subsequent gestational trophoblastic neoplasia. Although postnatal surveillance remains same.[10,11]

PATHOLOGY[1,12]

It is principally disease of chorion. The secretion from the hyperplastic cells and transferred substances from the maternal blood accumulate in the stroma of the villi which are devoid of blood vessels. This results in distension of the villi to form small vesicles. The distension may also be due to edema and liquefaction of the stroma.

Naked Eye Appearance

- No trace of embryo or amniotic sac.
- Mass filling the uterus consists of clusters of cysts of varying size.

Microscopic Appearance

The basic findings are:
- There is marked proliferation of the syncytial and cytotrophoblastic epithelium.
- Marked thinning of the stromal tissue due to hydropic degeneration.
- There is absence of blood vessels in the villi, which seems primary rather than due to pressure atrophy.
- The villous pattern is distinctly maintained.

CLINICAL PRESENTATION

The presentation of women with a molar pregnancy has changed remarkably over the past several decades because of the advancements in seeking prenatal care much earlier where sonography favors early detection. Several studies have shown a reduction in mean gestational age at detection when diagnosis is made through ultrasound.[13] As a result, it leads to detection of most molar pregnancies before complications ensue.[14]

As gestation advances symptoms tend to be more pronounced with complete moles. Common presentations are:[3]

- *Profuse uterine bleeding*: Most common presentation (90%) in more advanced moles with considerable concealed uterine hemorrhage, moderate iron-deficiency anemia develops.
- *Excessive vomiting*: Vomiting may be exacerbated to the extent of hyperemesis (15%).
- *Varying degree of lower abdominal pain*:
  - *Expulsion of grape like vesicles per vaginum* is diagnostic of vesicular mole. Actually, in approximately 50% of cases, the mole is not suspected until it is expelled in part or whole.
  - *Thyroid storm:* The thyrotropin-like activity of hCG stimulates thyroid-stimulating hormone (TSH) receptor which causes serum free thyroxine (fT4) levels to be elevated and TSH levels to be decreased. Despite this, clinically apparent thyrotoxicosis is unusual. Tremors and tachycardia in approximately 2% of cases.[15]
  - *Severe preeclampsia, eclampsia, and intrauterine growth restriction (IUGR):* Common with advanced molar gestation. Although the incidence is rare due to early diagnosis. But may present in twin gestation with one normal fetus along with complete mole. Features of early onset preeclampsia.
  - *Breathlessness:* Due to pulmonary embolization of the trophoblastic cells (2%). But rare presentation.

CLINICAL SIGNS

Clinical signs of molar pregnancies are shown in Table 2 and Figure 3.

TABLE 2: Clinical signs of molar pregnancies.

General examination	Per abdomen	Per vulval: Finding of vesicles is pathognomic (Fig. 3)
Looks more ill than symptoms	*Inspection*: Uterus>dates (50%)	*Per vaginal*
Pallor	*Palpation*: Doughy uterus, fetal parts not felt, no external ballottement	No internal ballottement
Edema	*Auscultation*: Absence of fatal heart sounds	*Adnexa*: Enlarged ovary may not be palpable due to enlarged uterus
Hypertension		*Theca lutein cyst*: May be palpable in 25–50% of cases

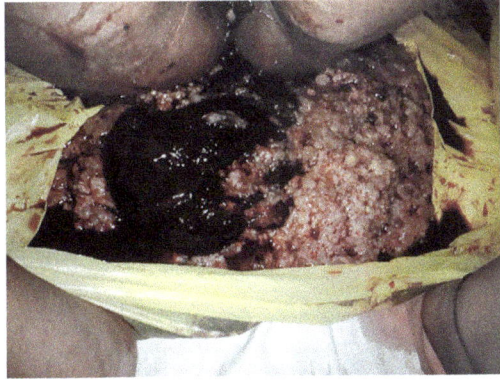

Fig. 3: Expulsion of vesicles per vaginam—suggestive of molar pregnancy.

DIAGNOSIS[16]

With the increasing availability of rapid and accurate tests for the detection of hCG to diagnose pregnancy and the use of early ultrasound examination, molar pregnancy is now typically discovered in the first trimester before the classic clinical signs and symptoms develop.[17,18]

Human Chorionic Gonadotropin

Estimation of hCG levels may be of value in diagnosing molar pregnancies—hCG levels greater than two multiples of the median may help in complete molar pregnancies with approximately 50% of patients having hCG levels > 100,000 mIU/mL.

Rapidly increasing value of serum hCG (hCG > 100,000 mIU/mL), is usual with molar pregnancies. With more advanced moles, values of beta-hCG in millions are not unusual. Sometimes despite these high values, there could be falsely low reading. At serum levels of hCG above 5,00,000 mIU/mL, a *"hook effect"* can occur,[19] resulting in an artificially low or negative value when using the current commercially available immunometric hCG assays.

Human chorionic gonadotropin is tested using a two-site noncompetitive immunometric assays, also known as "sandwich" assays. When hCG is present, it is immobilized or captured by the capture antibody and then labeled by a tracer or signal antibody. As a result, hCG molecules link up both immobilized (capture) and tracer (signal) antibody to form a sandwich (immobilized-hCG-tracer antibody). After washing away excess material, the amount of now immobilized label is measured and is directly proportional to the amount of hCG joining the sandwiches together. The hCG level in the sample is then obtained by comparing the amount of tracer signal in the sample to a standard hCG concentration curve.

In molar pregnancies with hCG levels >500,000 mIU/mL, both the capture and detection antibody used in sandwich immunometric assay are saturated with

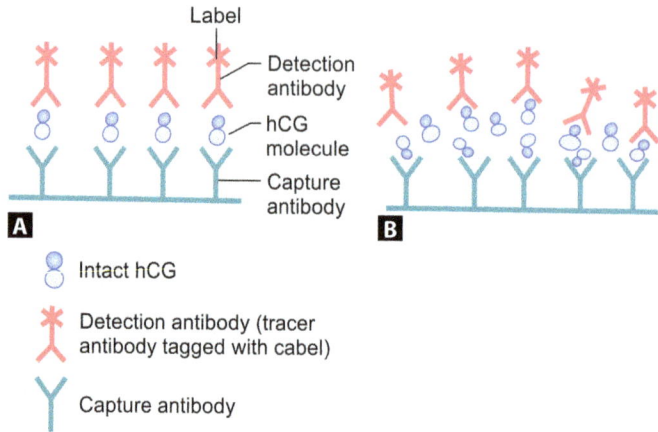

Figs. 4A and B: (A) Sandwich assay where hCG is immobilized between capture and detection antibody; (B) A false negative value depicting hook effect, where excess hCG molecules saturate both antibodies and prevent sandwich formation.

high levels of hCG, preventing sandwich formation (Figs. 4A and B). Since the non-sandwiched tracer antibodies are washed away with the excess material, the hCG test will be negative.[20,21] The sensitivity of most hCG assays is set to the normal pregnancy hCG range at 8–11 weeks of about 25,000–250,000 mIU/mL.[22] When suspecting GTD associated with higher beta-hCG levels, hCG assay should be performed after dilution of sample and multiplied later by diluting factor to get correct reading.

Ultrasound

Although this is the mainstay of trophoblastic disease diagnosis, not all cases are confirmed initially. Ultrasound helps us in pre-evacuation diagnosis.

In Complete Moles

Sonographically, a complete mole appears as an echogenic uterine mass with numerous anechoic cystic spaces but without a fetus or amnionic sac. The appearance is often described as a "*snowstorm*".[23] Also many times histologically proven complete moles may present early as anembryonic pregnancy and ultrasound favors early detection (Fig. 5).

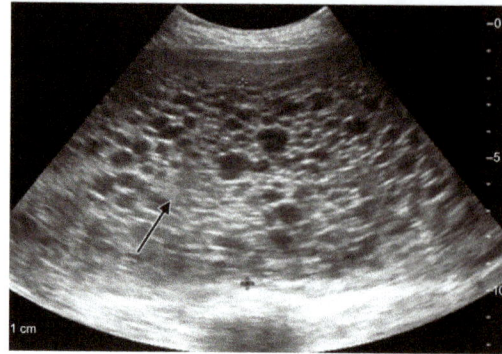

Fig. 5: Complete mole.

In Partial Moles

A partial mole has features that include a thickened, multicystic placenta along with a fetus, or at least fetal tissue. However, in early pregnancy, these sonographic characteristics are seen in fewer than half of hydatidiform moles.

The ultrasound diagnosis of a partial molar pregnancy is more complex; the finding of multiple soft markers, including both cystic spaces in the placenta and a ratio of transverse to anterioposterior dimension of the gestation sac of greater than 1.5, is required for the reliable diagnosis of a partial molar pregnancy.[24]

Sometimes confusion arises with missed abortion or uterine leiomyoma with cystic degeneration or multiple pregnancy.

In the largest series of more than 1,000 patients with molar pregnancy, the reported sensitivity and specificity of sonography were 44% and 74%, respectively.[25]

X-ray Abdomen

Straight X-ray chest may be helpful for evidence of pulmonary embolization even in benign moles.

Computed Tomography Scan and Magnetic Resonance Imaging

Routine use of computed tomography/magnetic resonance imaging (CT/MRI) is not required for diagnosis.

Histopathology

Histological examination of the products of conception gives the definitive diagnosis.

Histopathologic evaluation can be enhanced by immunohistochemical staining for p57 expression and by molecular genotyping.[26]

p57^{KIP2} is a nuclear protein whose gene is paternally imprinted and maternally expressed. This means that the gene product is produced only in tissues containing a maternal allele.[27]

In complete moles, tissue does not pick this stain since they contain only paternal genes and hence immunostaining with p57^{KIP2} helps in differential diagnosis of complete moles.

For distinction of a partial mole from a nonmolar hydropic abortus, both of which express p57, molecular genotyping can be used. Molecular genotyping determines the parental source of alleles. Thereby, it can distinguish among a diploid diandric genome (complete mole), a triploid diandric-monogynic genome (partial mole), or biparental diploidy (nonmolar abortus).

■ MANAGEMENT[3]

Early diagnosis, timely evacuation, and vigilant postevacuation surveillance for gestational trophoblastic neoplasia (GTN) have reduced maternal mortality from molar pregnancies (Flowchart 1).

Preoperative[3]

Patient may present with:
- Massive bleeding, in process of expulsion
- Or diagnosed on ultrasound with inert uterus.

Regardless of uterine size, molar evacuation by suction curettage is usually the preferred treatment.

Patient is to be admitted and managed as a high-risk pregnancy.
- Wide bore intravenous (IV) cannula to be inserted.
- Intravenous infusion with Ringer lactate to be started.
- Laboratory investigations in the form of complete blood count, ABO-Rh, liver function test (LFT), renal function test (RFT), beta-hCG, TSH levels, and free T4 levels should be sent. Preoperative evaluation attempts to identify known potential complications such as preeclampsia, hyperthyroidism, anemia, electrolyte depletions from hyperemesis, and metastatic disease.[17.]
- High-risk consent should be taken for surgical evacuation.
- Blood is kept reserved during the evacuation as there is risk of hemorrhage.
- *Chest X-ray*: Most recommend chest radiography, whereas CT and MRI are not routinely done unless a chest radiograph shows lung lesions or unless other extrauterine disease is suspected.

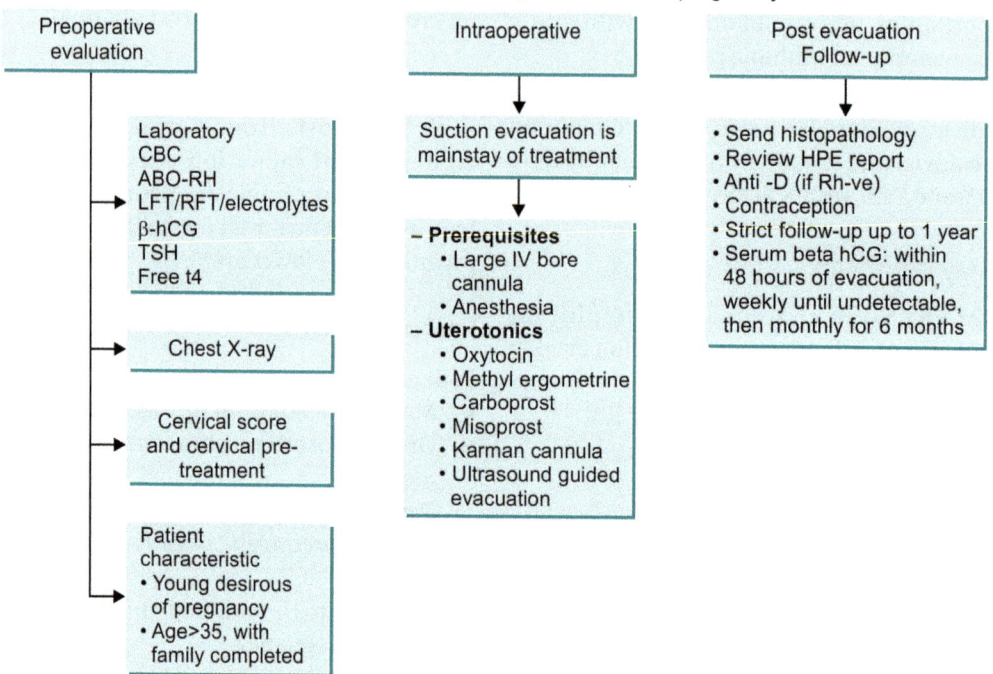

Flowchart 1: Summary of management of molar pregnancy.

(CBC: complete blood count; hCG: human chorionic gonadotropin; HPE: histopathological examination; IV: intravenous; LFT: liver function test; RFT: renal function test; TSH: thyroid-stimulating hormone)

- *Cervical pretreatment*:
  - Cervix should be assessed—whether it is *favorable* or whether *tubular and closed*.
  - Grade D recommendation from Royal College of Obstetricians and Gynaecologists (RCOG)[16] states that preparation of cervix immediately prior to evacuation is regarded safe, although prolonged cervical preparation especially with prostaglandins should be avoided in order to prevent risk of embolization.
  - Preoperative cervical dilatation with an osmotic dilator is recommended if the cervix is minimally dilated. The cervix is mechanically dilated to preferably allow insertion of a larger suction curette.

- *Deciding treatment strategy*:[1]
  - Young patient, desirous of pregnancy: Suction evacuation is the main stay of management. Hysterectomy may be advised in cases of *uncontrolled hemorrhage or perforation during surgical evacuation*.
  - Patient with age >35 years, or with completed family irrespective of age: Hysterectomy is indicated.

Surgical Evacuation

Intraoperative bleeding can be greater with molar pregnancy than with a comparably sized uterus containing nonmolar products. Thus with large moles, adequate anesthesia, sufficient IV access, and blood-banking support are imperative (Flowchart 2).

Flowchart 2: Management of molar pregnancies.

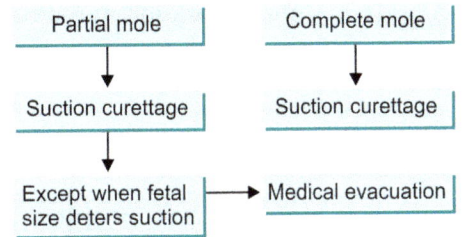

Complete Molar Pregnancy

- Regardless of uterine size, molar evacuation by suction curettage is usually the preferred treatment in complete molar pregnancies, since complete molar pregnancies are not associated with fetal parts.
- The procedure can be performed under diazepam sedation or general anesthesia.
- Medical evacuation of complete molar pregnancies should be avoided, since there is theoretical concern over use of oxytocic agents which can cause trophoblastic tissues to embolize and also increase the sensitivity of uterus to prostaglandins.[16]
- During evacuation procedure, patient should ideally be monitored by pulse oximeter (oxygen saturation). 500 mL Ringer's solution IV infusion is set up. Risk of hemorrhage is high especially when the uterus is large. Senior surgeon should be present during the SE procedure.
- Depending on uterine size, a 10–14-mm diameter Karman cannula is typically used.
- Intraoperative sonography is often recommended to help ensure complete uterine cavity emptying.

Role of oxytocic agents[16]

- The use of oxytocic infusions prior to evacuation is not advisable.[28,29] Although, if a molar pregnancy is associated with significant hemorrhage, then the need of oxytocic infusion should be carefully calculated as up against the risk of tumor embolization.
- However if there is vigorous bleeding per vaginum prior to evacuation, then surgical evacuation should be expedited and oxytocin agents use is permissible owing to greater benefits in use than avoidance.
  - As evacuation is begun, oxytocin is infused to limit bleeding. Oxytocin is started as 20 units in 1 liter of ringerlactate (RL) as continuous infusion.
- When the myometrium has contracted, a thorough but gentle curettage with a sharp large-loop Sims curette is performed.
- Digital exploration and removal of the mole by ovum forceps under general anesthesia may also be an alternative procedure
- If bleeding continues despite oxytocin infusion and uterine evacuation then other uterotonic agents in the form of following may be used:
  1. *Methylergometrine*: 0.2 mg/mL 1 ampoule intramuscular every 2 hours
  2. *Carboprost [prostaglandin F2 alpha (PGF2α)*: 250 μg = 1 mL = 1 ampule IM every 15–90 min.
  3. *Misoprostol*: 200 mg tablets for rectal administration, 800–1,000 mg once.
- In cases of profuse hemorrhage, pelvic artery embolization or hysterectomy may be required.

Partial Molar Pregnancy[16]

- Suction evacuation is the treatment of choice in partial molar pregnancy except when the size of fetal parts deters suction curettage, then medical methods can be used. Although data from use of mifepristone and misoprostol is very limited.

Complications of vaginal evacuation: Apart from the injury to the uterus, hemorrhage,

and shock, there are two more rare but fatal complications:
1. *Acute pulmonary insufficiency*: Due to pulmonary embolization of the trophoblastic cells. Symptoms of acute chest pain, tachycardia, tachypnea, and dyspnea develop about 4–6 hours following evacuation. Medical induction (oxytocin infusion) before evacuation may increase the risk of pulmonary insufficiency (RCOG). Arterial PO_2 is monitored. Patient may need ventilatory assistance and intensive care unit management.[29]
2. *Thyroid storm*: In presence of hyperthyroid state when evacuation is done under general anesthesia, the acute features such as hyperthermia, delirium, convulsions, coma, and cardiovascular collapse develop. The condition can be managed by administration of beta-adrenergic blocking agents.

Other Methods of Management

Hysterectomy

Methods other than suction curettage can be considered for select cases. Hysterectomy with ovarian preservation may be preferable for women with complete moles who have finished childbearing. Of women aged 40–49 years, 30–50% will subsequently develop GTN, and hysterectomy markedly reduces this likelihood.[30] It should be remembered that following hysterectomy, persistent GTD is observed in 3–5% cases. As such, it does not eliminate the necessity of follow-up.

Theca-lutein cysts seen at the time of hysterectomy do not require removal, and they spontaneously regress following molar termination.

Hysterotomy

Hysterotomy is rarely performed these days, the only existing indications are:

- Profuse vaginal bleeding
- Cervix is unfavorable for immediate vaginal evacuation and
- Accidental perforation of the uterus during surgical evacuation.

Postoperative Management

Histopathology of Product of Conception

- Grade D recommendation from RCOG emphasizes on histological assessment of material obtained from medical and surgical management of all failing pregnancies to exclude gestational trophoblastic neoplasia.
- In view of the difficulty in making a diagnosis of a molar pregnancy before evacuation, it is recommended that, in failed pregnancies, products of conception are examined histologically.
- But once the fetal parts have been identified on prior ultrasound examination, there is no need to routinely send products of conception for histological examination following therapeutic termination of pregnancy (RCOG).[16]
- A urine pregnancy test should be performed 3 weeks later after medical management of failed pregnancy, if products of conception have not been sent to histopathological examination.

Anti-D Administration[31]

- Following curettage, anti-D immunoglobulin (RhoGAM) is given to Rh D-negative women because fetal tissues with a partial mole may include red cells with D- antigen.
- Because of poor vascularization of the chorionic villi and absence of the anti-D antigen in complete moles, anti-D prophylaxis is not required. It is, however, required for partial moles.
- Confirmation of the diagnosis of complete molar pregnancy may not occur

for some time after evacuation and so administration of anti-D could be delayed when required, within an appropriate timeframe.
- Any woman who develops persistent or irregular vaginal bleeding postpregnancy event is at risk of having GTN. GTN can occur after any GTD event, even when separated by a normal pregnancy.

Contraception

- *The patient is advised not to be pregnant for at least 1 year.*[32]
- A rise in hCG titers might cause confusion between a fresh pregnancy or persistent GTD. However, with vaginal probe ultrasound scan, pregnancy can be diagnosed even as early as 5-6 weeks.
- *Thus, if the patient so desires, she may be pregnant after a minimum of 6 months, following the negative hCG titer.* But pregnancy is delayed at least up to 1 year for GTN and up to 2 years, if there is metastasis.
- *The risk of a recurrent molar pregnancy is low (1/80)*: More than 98% of women who become pregnant following a molar pregnancy will not have a further molar pregnancy nor are they at increased risk of obstetric complications. If a further molar pregnancy does occur, in 68–80% of cases it will be of the same histological type (RCOG).[16]
- Women should be counseled for barrier method of contraception till hCG levels come to normal.
- Once hCG levels are normalized, the combined oral contraceptive (OCP) pill may be used. There is no evidence as to whether single-agent progestogens have any effect on GTN
- But in case, OCPs are started before the diagnosis of GTD, they should be continued but she should be advised that there is a potential but low increased risk of developing GTN.
- Intrauterine contraceptive device (IUCD) are contraindicated until hCG turns normal because of risk of perforation owing to soft uterus and also because of its frequent association of irregular bleeding—a feature often coexists with choriocarcinoma.
- *Surgical sterilization* is another alternative when she has completed her family.

Follow-up

- Close biochemical surveillance (hCG) for persistent gestational neoplasia follows each hydatidiform mole evacuation.[33]
- The prime objective is to diagnose persistent trophoblastic disease (20–30%) that is considered malignant.

Beta-hCG surveillance:
- Initial beta-hCG is obtained 48 hours after evacuation, to get baseline hCG values, then weekly once till hCG gets normalized. *This usually happens by 4-8 weeks*. Once negative within 56 days, the patient is followed up at every 1 month interval for 6 months.
- *The median time for such resolution is 7 weeks for partial moles and 9 weeks for complete moles*. Once β-hCG is undetectable, this is confirmed with monthly determinations for another 6 months.[34]
- As a glycoprotein, hCG shows structural heterogeneity and exists in different isoforms. Thus for surveillance, an hCG assay that can detect all forms of hCG should be used.[35]
- Follow-up after GTD is increasingly individualized depends on the days, it takes for hCG to return to normal (Flowchart 3).
- Importantly, during β-hCG level surveillance, either increasing or persistently plateaued levels mandate evaluation for trophoblastic neoplasia.

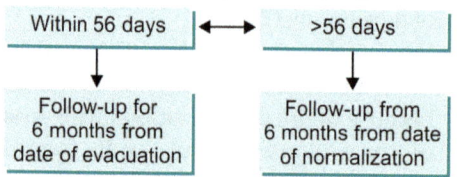

Flowchart 3: Follow-up of molar pregnancies.

- Risk factors which predispose a patient after molar evacuation to GTN are:[3]
  - *Type of mole*: Complete moles have a 15–20% incidence of malignant sequelae, compared with 1–5% following partial moles.
  - *Age*: Both extremes, >40 years as well as <20 years.
  - *Uterine size*: >20 weeks
  - *Beta-hCG levels*: >100,000 mIU/mL
  - *Theca lutein cyst*: >6 cm
  - *Slow decline in beta-hCG levels*.

History and clinical examination:
- Patient should be enquired about symptoms like irregular vaginal bleeding, breathlessness, cough, or hemoptysis.
- Abdominovaginal examination to note: (1) involution of the uterus, (2) ovarian size, and (3) malignant deposit if any, in the anterior vaginal wall. The lutein cysts usually regress within 2 months. Pelvic examination is done after 1 week of molar evacuation.

Role of Prophylactic Chemotherapy[36]

Majority of molar pregnancy follow-up undergo spontaneous resolution after evacuation. Also sensitive beta-hCG assays can detect persistence of trophoblastic disease going into neoplasia. There are risks of toxicity due to these drugs and the fear of premature ovarian failure.

PERSISTENT GESTATIONAL TROPHOBLASTIC DISEASE

Definition

Persistent GTD is defined where there is persistence of trophoblastic activity as evidenced by clinical, imaging, pathological, and/or hormonal study following initial treatment. This may be following treatment of hydatidiform mole, invasive mole, choriocarcinoma, or placental site trophoblastic tumor.[37]

About 50% follow hydatidiform mole, 25% follow miscarriage or tubal pregnancy, and rest 25% follow preterm or term gestation.[38]

A postmolar GTD may be benign or malignant. But a GTD after nonmolar pregnancy is always a choriocarcinoma. Overall incidence of persistent GTN after complete hydatidiform moles is 15–20%.

Although these four tumor types are histologically distinct, they are usually diagnosed solely by persistently elevated serum β-hCG levels.

CRITERIA FOR DIAGNOSING PERSISTENT GTN[39]

- Plateau of serum β-hCG level (± 10%) for four measurements during a period of 3 weeks or longer—days 1, 7, 14, and 21
- Rise of serum β-hCG level >10% during three weekly consecutive measurements or longer, during a period of 2 weeks or more—days 1, 7, and 14
- Serum β-hCG level remains detectable for 6 months or more
- Histological criteria for choriocarcinoma.

Clinical Presentation

- *Irregular vaginal bleeding*
- *Uterine subinvolution.*

Diagnosis and Prognostic Scoring

Consideration for the possibility of GTN is the most important factor in its recognition. Unusually, persistent bleeding after any type of pregnancy should prompt.
- Beta hCG levels.
- Assessment of uterine size and local examination of lower genital tract metastases,

which usually appear as bluish vascular masses.[40]
- *Laboratory investigations*: Hemogram, LFT, and RFT.
- *Search for metastasis*: Transvaginal sonography, chest CT scan or radiograph, and brain and abdominopelvic CT scan, or MR imaging. Less commonly, positron-emission tomographic (PET) scanning and cerebrospinal fluid β-hCG level determination are used to identify metastases.

Gestational trophoblastic neoplasia is staged clinically using the system of the International Federation of Gynecology and Obstetrics (FIGO) (2009).[39] This includes a modification of the World Health Organization (WHO) (1983) prognostic index score, with which scores of 0–4 are given for each of the categories (Tables 3 and 4).

Histological Classification

Again, it is stressed that the diagnosis of trophoblastic neoplasias is usually made by persistently elevated serum β-hCG levels without confirmation by tissue study. Clinical staging is assigned without regard to histological findings, even if available. Still, there are distinct histological types.

Invasive Mole

These are the most common trophoblastic neoplasms that follow hydatidiform moles, and almost all invasive moles arise from partial or complete moles. Previously known as chorioadenoma destruens, invasive mole is characterized by extensive tissue invasion by trophoblast and whole villi.

Choriocarcinoma

This is the most common type of trophoblastic neoplasm to follow a term pregnancy or a miscarriage, and only a third of cases follow a molar gestation.[41] Choriocarcinoma is composed of cells reminiscent of early cytotrophoblast and syncytiotrophoblast, however, it contains no villi.

TABLE 3: FIGO anatomical staging.

Stage 1	Disease confined to the uterus
Stage 2	GTN extends outside uterus but limits to the genital structure (adnexa, broad ligament, and vagina)
Stage 3	GTN extends to lungs with/without genital tract involvement
Stage 4	All other metastatic sites

(FIGO: International Federation of Gynecology and Obstetrics; GTN: gestational trophoblastic neoplasia)

TABLE 4: Modified World Health Organization (WHO) prognostic scoring system.

Scores	0	1	2	4
Age	<40	>40		
Antecedent pregnancy	Mole	Abortion	Term	
Interval after index pregnancy	<4	4–6	6–12	>12
Pretreatment beta-hCG	<10^3	10^3–10^4	10^4–10^5	10^5–10^6
Largest tumor size	<3	3–5	>5	
Site of metastasis	—	Spleen, Kidney	GI	Liver, Brain
Number of metastasis	—	1–4	5–8	>8
Previously failed chemotherapy drugs			1	≥2

Low risk: WHO score: 0–6
High risk: score ≥7

Placental Site Trophoblastic Tumor

This rare tumor arises from intermediate trophoblasts at the placental site. These tumors have associated serum β-hCG levels that may be only modestly elevated. However, they produce variant forms of hCG, and identification of a high proportion of free β-hCG is considered diagnostic.

Treatment[3]

The prognosis is excellent with rare exceptions, and patients are routinely cured even in the presence of widespread disease. Chemotherapy alone is usually the primary treatment.

Low Risk/Good Prognosis Metastatic Disease

Single-agent chemotherapy protocols are usually sufficient for nonmetastatic or low-risk metastatic neoplasia.[42] In general, methotrexate is less toxic than actinomycin D,[43] although both are equally effective. Regimens are repeated until serum β-hCG levels are undetectable (Table 5).

High Risk/Poor Prognosis Metastatic Disease

Combination chemotherapy is given for high-risk disease, and reported cure rates approximate 90%.[44] One is EMA-CO, which includes etoposide, methotrexate, actinomycin D, cyclophosphamide, and Oncovin (vincristine). In selected cases, adjuvant surgical and radiotherapy may also be employed.

TABLE 5: Treatment modalities.

Low risk/good prognosis patients	Single agent chemotherapy (MTX or actinomycin)
High risk/poor prognosis	Combination (EMACO regimen)

(EMACO: etoposide, MTX, ACT-D, cyclophosphamide, and vincristine; MTX: methotrexate)

During chemotherapy, following tests have to be done:
- *Daily*: Blood counts, liver function, and renal function.
- *X-ray chest*: To repeat only if hCG level plateau or rises.

Follow-up is mandatory for all patients for at least 2 years, with either low or high-risk disease, once serum β-hCG levels are undetectable. Serum hCG is measured weekly until negative for 3 consecutive weeks, then monthly for 6 months and 6 monthly thereafter for lifetime. During this time, contraception is crucial to avoid any teratogenic effects of chemotherapy to the fetus[45] and to mitigate confusion from rising β-hCG levels caused by superimposed pregnancy.

Subsequent Pregnancy

Women with prior hydatidiform mole generally do not have impaired fertility, and their pregnancy outcomes are usually normal.[46] There is around 2% risk for developing trophoblastic disease in a subsequent pregnancy, sonographic evaluation is recommended in early pregnancy, and subsequently if indicated.

Women who have successfully completed GTN chemotherapy are advised to delay pregnancy for 12 months. Fertility and pregnancy outcomes are typically normal, and congenital anomaly rates are not increased.[18,47,48] One exception is an unexplained higher stillbirth rate of 1.5% compared with a background rate of 0.8%.[49]

After hydatidiform mole or GTN treatment, in subsequent pregnancy, the placenta or products of conception are sent for pathological evaluation at delivery. A serum β-hCG level is measured 6 weeks postpartum.

REFERENCES

1. DC Duttas Textbook of Obstetrics, 8th edition.
2. Benirschke K, Burton GJ, Baergen RN (eds): Molar pregnancies. In: Pathology of the Human

Placenta, 6th edition. New York, Springer, 2012. p. 687.
3. Williams Textbook of Obstetrics, 25th edition, McGraw Hill.
4. American College of Obstetricians and Gynecologists: Diagnosis and treatment of gestational trophoblastic disease. Practice Bulletin No. 53, June 2004, Reairmed 2016.
5. Altman AD, Bently B, Murray S, et al. Maternal age-related rate of gestational trophoblastic disease. Obstet Gynecol. 2008;112:244.
6. Eagles N, Sebire NJ, Short D, et al. Risk of recurrent molar pregnancies following complete and partial hydatidiform moles. Hum Reprod. 2015;30(9):2055.
7. Lawler SD, Fisher RA, Dent J. A prospective genetic study of complete and partial hydatidiform moles. Am J Obstet Gynecol. 1991;164:1270.
8. Lipata F, Parkash V, Talmor M, et al. Precise DNA genotyping diagnosis of hydatidiform mole. Obstet Gynecol. 2010;115(4):784.
9. Joergensen MW, Niemann I, Rasmussen AA, et al. Triploid pregnancies: genetic and clinical features of 158 cases. Am J Obstet Gynecol. 2014;211(4):370.
10. Massardier J, Golfner F, Journet D, et al. Twin pregnancy with complete hydatidiform mole and coexistent fetus obstetrical and oncological outcomes in a series of 14 cases. Eur J Obstet Gynecol Reprod Biol. 2009;143:84.
11. Sebire NJ, Foskett M, Parainas FJ, et al. Outcome of twin pregnancies with complete hydatidiform mole and healthy co-twin. Lancet. 2002b;359:2165.
12. Wells M. The pathology of gestational trophoblastic disease: recent advances. Pathology. 2007;39:88–96.
13. Sebire NJ, Rees H, Paradinas F, et al. The diagnostic implications of routine ultrasound examination in histologically confirmed early molar pregnancies. Ultrasound Obstet Gynecol 2001;18:662-5.
14. Kerkmeijer LG, Massuger LF, Ten Kate-Booij MJ, et al. Earlier diagnosis and serum human chorionic gonadotropin regression in complete hydatidiform moles. Obstet Gynecol. 2009;113:326.
15. Kofinas JD, Kruczek A, Sample J, et al. Thyroid storm-induced multi-organ failure in the setting of gestational trophoblastic disease. J Emerg Med. 2015;48(1):35.
16. RCOG green top guidelines. Management of Gestational Trophoblastic Disease, 2010;38.
17. Lurain J.R. Gestational trophoblastic disease I: epidemiology, pathology, clinical presentation and diagnosis of gestational trophoblastic disease, and management of hydatidiform mole. Am J Obstet Gynecol. 2010;203:531-9.
18. Berkowitz RA, Goldstein DP, Horowitz NS. Management options of gestational trophoblastic disease. Curr Obstet Gynecol Rep. 2014;3:76-83.
19. Winder AD, Mora AS, Berry E, Lurain JR. The "hook effect" causing a negative pregnancy test in a patient with an advanced molar pregnancy. Gynecologic Oncology Reports. 2017;21:34-6.
20. Mori KM, Lurain JR. In: Human Chorionic Gonadotropin: Testing in Pregnancy and Gestational Trophoblastic Disease and Causes of Persistent Low Levels. Goff Barbara., editor. Wolters Kluwer; 2015. UpToDate.
21. Yeung CW, Cheung ANY. Negative pregnancy test in patients with trophoblastic diseases. Curr Obstet Gynecol Rep. 2014;3:102-6.
22. Griffey RT, Trent CJ, Bavolek RA, et al. "Hook-like effect" causes false-negative point-of-care urine pregnancy testing in emergency patients. J Emerg Med. 2013;44:155-60.
23. Fine C, Bundy AL, Berkowitz R, et al. Sonographic diagnosis of partial hydatidiform mole. Obstet Gynecol. 1989;73:414-18.
24 Benson CB, Genest DR, Bernstein MR, et al. Sonographic appearance of first trimester complete hydatidiform moles. J Ultrasound Obstet Gynecol. 2000;16:188-91.
25. Fowler DJ, Lindsay I, Seckl MJ, et al. Routine pre-evacuation ultrasound diagnosis of hydatidiform mole: experience of more than 1000 cases from a regional referral center. Ultrasound Obstet Gynecol. 2006;27(1):56.
26. Banet N, DeScipio C, Murphy KM, et al. Characteristics of hydatidiform moles: analysis of a prospective series with p57 immunohistochemistry and molecular genotyping. Mod Pathol. 2014;27(2):238.
27. Merchant SH, Amin MB, Viswanatha DS, et al. p57KIP2 immunohistochemistry in early molar pregnancies: emphasis on its complementary role in the dierential diagnosis of hydropic abortuses. Hum Pathol. 2005;36:180.

28. Flam F, Lundstrom V, Pettersson F. Medical induction prior to surgical evacuation of hydatidiform mole: is there a greater risk of persistent trophoblastic disease? Eur J Obstet Gynaecol Reprod Biol. 1991;42:57-60.
29. Attwood HD, Park WW. Embolism to the lungs by trophoblast. J Obstet Gynaecol Br Commonw. 1961;68:611-17.
30. Bandy LC, Clarke-Pearson DL, Hammond CB. Malignant potential of gestational trophoblastic disease at the extreme ages of reproductive life. Obstet Gynecol. 1984;64(3):395.
31. Hancock BW. Differences in management and treatment: a critical appraisal. In: Hancock BW, Newlands ES, Berkowitz RS, Cole LA, editors. Gestational Trophoblastic Disease, 3rd edition. London: International Society for the Study of Trophoblastic Disease; 2003. p. 447-59 [www.isstd.org/isstd/book.html].
32. Dantas PRS, Maestá I, Filho JR, et al. Does hormonal contraception during molar pregnancy follow-up influence the risk and clinical aggressiveness of gestational trophoblastic neoplasia aer controlling for risk factors? Gynecol Oncol, 2017.
33. Pisal N, Tidy J, Hancock B. Gestational trophoblastic disease: is intensive follow up essential in all women? BJOG. 2004;111:1449-51.
34. Sebire NJ, Foskett M, Short D, et al. Shortened duration of human chorionic gonadotrophin surveillance following complete or partial hydatidiform mole: evidence for revised protocol of a UK regional trophoblastic disease unit. BJOG. 2007;114(6):760.
35. Ngan HY, Seckl MJ, Berkowitz RS, et al. Update on the diagnosis and management of gestational trophoblastic disease. Int J Gynaecol Obstet. 2015;131(Suppl 2):S123.
36. Wang Q, Fu J, Hu L, et al. Prophylactic chemotherapy for hydatidiform mole to prevent gestational trophoblastic neoplasia. Cochrane Database Syst Rev.
37. Sebire NJ, Fisher RA, Foskett M, et al. Risk of recurrent hydatidiform mole and subsequent pregnancy outcome following complete or partial hydatidiform molar pregnancy. BJOG. 2003;110:22-6.
38. Goldstein DP, Berkowitz RS. Current management of gestational trophoblastic neoplasia. Hematol Oncol Clin North Am. 2012;26(1):111.
39. International Federation of Obstetrics and Gynecology Oncology Committee. FIGO staging for gestational trophoblastic neoplasia 2000. Int J Gynecol Obstet. 2002;77:285-7.
40. Cagayan MS. Vaginal metastases complicating gestational trophoblastic neoplasia. J Reprod Med. 2010;55(5-6):229.
41. Soper JT. Gestational trophoblastic disease. Obstet Gynecol. 2006;108:176.
42. Lawrie TA, Alazzam M, Tidy J, et al. First-line chemotherapy in low-risk gestational trophoblastic neoplasia. Cochrane Database Syst Rev, 2016;6:CD007102.
43. Chan KK, Huang Y, Tam KF, et al. Single-dose methotrexate regimen in the treatment of low-risk gestational trophoblastic neoplasia. Am J Obstet Gynecol. 2006;195:1282.
44. Lurain JR. Gestational trophoblastic disease II: classification and management of gestational trophoblastic neoplasia. Am J Obstet Gynecol. 2011;204(1):11.
45. Seckl MJ, Rustin GJS. Late toxicity after therapy for gestational trophoblastic tumours. In: Hancock BW, Newlands ES, Berkowitz RS, Cole LA, (eds). Gestational Trophoblastic Disease. 3rd ed. London: International Society for the Study of Trophoblastic.
46. Subsequent pregnancy outcome in patients with spontaneous resolution of HCG aer evacuation of hydatidiform mole: comparison between complete and partial mole. Hum Reprod. 2011;16(6):1274.
47. Tse KY, Ngan HY. Gestational trophoblastic disease. Best Pract Res Clin Obstet Gynaecol. 2012;26(3):357.
48. Williams J, Short D, Dayal L, et al. Eect of early pregnancy following chemotherapy on disease relapse and fetal outcome in women treated for gestational trophoblastic neoplasia. J Reprod Med. 2014;59(5-6):248-54.
49. Vargas R, Barroilhet LM, Esselen K, et al. Subsequent pregnancy outcomes aer complete and partial molar pregnancy, recurrent molar pregnancy, and gestational trophoblastic neoplasia: an update from the New England Trophoblastic Disease Center. J Reprod Med. 2010;59(5-6):188.

CHAPTER 7

Trauma in Pregnancy

Haritha Mannem

INTRODUCTION

With changed attitudes of women to pregnancy, there is increase in professional, social, and commercial activities during this period, which leads to an increase in the risk of accidents as compared to the nonpregnant women. Increased abdominal size and laxity of pelvic ligaments result in unstable gait, thus increasing the chances of falls with advancing gestational age.[1]

Trauma is the most common etiology of morbidity and mortality due to nonobstetric cause during pregnancy.[2]

Trauma complicates around 6-7% of the pregnancies and around 0.3-0.4% of these affected women need to be hospitalized.[3-5]

The pattern of injury is different in pregnant trauma patients when compared to nonpregnant women. Abdominal trauma is commoner than head and chest injuries. In cases where the injuries are inconsistent with their alleged cause, the possibility of domestic violence must be suspected.[1]

The causes of maternal trauma in decreasing frequency are motor vehicle accidents (MVA's) (55%), assaults (22%), falls (22%), and burns (1%).[6,7]

While the fetal deaths are due to different etiologies—MVA's (82%), maternal deaths (11%), gunshot injuries (6%), and falls (3%).[8]

The major risk factors found associated with maternal trauma include:[9-14]
- Young age (<25 years)
- Addiction to drugs
- Road traffic accident
- Epilepsy
- Obesity
- Working women
- Low socioeconomic status.

The trimester-wise distribution is more or less equal.[14]

ANATOMICAL AND PHYSIOLOGICAL ALTERATIONS IN PREGNANCY IN RELEVANCE WITH TRAUMA

Many anatomic and physiological changes occur during pregnancy involving all organ systems and this makes the management of pregnant patient with trauma complex.

Hematocrit (HCT)

The signs and symptoms may be altered by the changes which are mentioned in Table 1. and also impact the interpretation of general physical examination and laboratory results. So the outlook and the outcome of the pregnant patient to resuscitative measures will be different.[15,16]

As the pregnancy progresses to third trimester, the uterine size increases and its walls become thin, thus making it more prone to injuries [rupture, penetration, and preterm premature rupture of membranes (PROM)] further leading to placental abruption.

TABLE 1: Anatomical and physiological alterations in pregnancy.[1]

Organ system	Changes relevant to trauma
Uterus	*First trimester:* Intrapelvic organ protected by the bony pelvis *Second trimester:* Becomes an abdominal organ; the fetus is cushioned by a relatively large amount of amniotic fluid *Third trimester:* The uterus is large and thin walled
Blood	Increase in plasma volume greater than in RBC results in a decreased HCT
Cardiovascular system	Increase in plasma volume and decrease in vascular resistance of the uterus and placenta cause an increase in cardiac output Increase in the cardiac rate *Second trimester:* Decrease in both systolic and diastolic blood pressure
Respiratory system	Increased tidal volume and minute ventilation Hypocapnia in late pregnancy Decreased residual volume
GI system	Gastric emptying time is prolonged *Third trimester:* The bowel is pushed upward and lies mostly in the upper abdomen
Other systems	Dilatation of the renal calyces, pelvis, and ureters The pituitary gland increases in size The symphysis pubis and the sacroiliac joints widen

Plasma volume peaks by the 34th week of pregnancy. Hematocrit decreases due to a small rise in red blood cells (RBCs). The blood vessels of the placenta are maximally dilated and become over sensitive to catecholamine stimulation. The uterine vascular resistance increases significantly due to an acute decrease in the intravascular volume caused due to any trauma. This could lead to reduced delivery of oxygen to the fetus, even when the maternal vital signs are within normal range.[17,18]

The maternal factors like sympathetic nervous system response, oxygen carrying capacity of blood, and blood pressure determine the tolerance of the fetus to metal hemorrhage. Since the fetus depends on mother's cardiovascular system and exchange of oxygen by placenta, any acute reduction in the maternal intravascular blood volume leads to early fetal acidosis.[19,20]

While assessing the tachycardia due to it should be kept in mind the fact that with progression of gestation there is gradual increase in heart rate with highest rate in third trimester. Both systolic blood pressure and diastolic blood pressure fall in the second trimester of pregnancy. Hypotension could be prevented by tilting the patient to left lateral position. Hypocapnia is common in late pregnancy. In late pregnancy due to elevation of the diaphragm, the residual volume of lung decreases leading to hypocapnia. Further due to increased oxygen consumption during pregnancy maintaining an appropriate arterial oxygenation is required during resuscitation.[16,17]

The condition of the uteroplacental flow may not always be accurately reflected by the maternal hemodynamic measurements. The maternal vitals can be unreliable in predicting fetal loss.[21]

Due to prolonged gastric emptying time in pregnancy, decompression of stomach by early gastric tubing is needed to prevent aspiration. As the uterus enlarges in third trimester, there is upward pushing of the bowel and it lies relatively protected mostly in the upper part of abdomen. Hence, in blunt trauma, there is increased vulnerability to injury.[17]

When managing pregnant patients with trauma to the pelvis, physiologically dilated renal pelvicalyceal system should be considered. Due to increase in the size of the pituitary gland, shock can lead to necrosed anterior pituitary causing insufficiency of the pituitary gland. The widening of the pubic symphysis and the sacroiliac joints should be taken into account when assessing the pelvic radiographs.[1]

Due to increased levels of maternal plasma fibrinogen, as well as factors II, VII, VIII, IX, and X, and a decrease in plasminogen activator levels leading to hypercoagulability, the propensity to develop deep vein thrombosis (DVT) is increased in all the cases of trauma in pregnancy.[1]

The risk of difficult intubation and airway management complications are significant in pregnancy due to increased maternal weight, increased size of the breasts, mucosal edema of the respiratory tract, increased consumption of oxygen, and decrease in the functional residual capacity (FRC).[22,23]

MECHANISMS OF INJURIES AND TRAUMA DURING PREGNANCY

Maternal and fetal outcomes are decided by the severity of the injuries, which also dictates the line of management. Pregnant women with major injuries are required to be hospitalized and managed in a multidisciplinary setup, where surgical as well as obstetric facilities are available. Those who sustain minor injuries must also be strictly observed due to risk of complications like fetomaternal hemorrhage. Serious maternal trauma especially in late pregnancy is usually associated with direct fetal injuries.[1]

Blunt Injury Abdomen

Blunt trauma in pregnancy occurs due to vehicle accidents (40%), injury due to fall (30%), and domestic violence (20%). In early pregnancy, the maternal pelvis and amniotic fluid protect the uterus by decreasing the force of the impact by equal transmission in all directions. Maternal hypotension leading to hypoperfused uterus and placenta is the usual cause for loss of fetus in first trimester.[1]

During second trimester, the amniotic fluid around the fetus acts as shock absorber and this way gives protection to the fetus partially as the enlarging uterus is no more protected by the pelvic bones. The probability of retroperitoneal hemorrhage also increases due to engorgement of the pelvic vessels. In late third trimester, fetal head gets fixed in the maternal pelvis, reducing shock absorbing effect of the amniotic fluid resulting in injury. These injuries result in fractures of the skull with intracranial hemorrhage, which are the most common fetal injuries from blunt trauma.[4,6] Abruptio placenta, maternal shock, and maternal death can also lead to fetal mortality.[5,24]

The causes are MVAs. The close relation between pelvic fractures and abdominopelvic injuries reflects the kinetic energy dissipated due to the impact and hence should be considered a red flag mandating a careful exploration for other occult visceral injuries. The degree of maternal and fetal distress, fetal maturity, severity of injury to mother, associated pelvic fracture, and the final course of labor determines the method of delivery in cases of pelvic fractures. As pelvic and acetabular fractures heal in about 8–12 weeks, in cases of early pregnancy fractures, vaginal delivery is not contraindicated.[1]

Leggon et al. in their recent review, observed that delivery through the vaginal route was successful in about 75% of the patients with pelvic fractures occurring in third trimester.[25]

Falls are common in the second and third trimesters due to:

- Weight gain
- Shift in the center of gravity to accommodate the expanding uterus
- Increased joint mobility experienced during pregnancy.[26]

The incidence of interpersonal violence varies from 5% to 20% and can even be recurrent. In pregnant women, who suffer domestic violence complications like preterm labor, SGA, and substance abuse were commoner. Management is similar to blunt trauma.[27]

The suspicion for battering raises when the patient presents with a vague or inconsistent history of trauma. The abdomen is the most common target for blows, kicks, and other assaults.[28]

Among pregnant trauma victims, most of the deaths occur due to head injury and hemorrhagic shock. Injuries to the spleen, retroperitoneum, and hematomas are common in pregnant women who suffer blunt abdominal trauma because of increase in vascular supply during pregnancy. However, injury to the bowel is less common.[29,30]

Obstetric Consequences of Blunt Trauma

- *Placental abruption*: Placental abruption leads to fetal death in 70% of the cases post blunt abdominal trauma.[17,18]

  Cause: The uterus contains significant amount of elastic fibers, while the placenta does not have elastic fibers. Therefore, the uterus gets deformed on application of external deforming force. But similar deformation does not happen in placenta, instead a shearing effect takes place at the uteroplacental interface.[1]

- *Preterm labor*: Cause—when traumatic injury occurs to the uterus prostaglandin production is initiated due to destabilization of lysosomal enzymes. This mechanism can lead to preterm labor. The other possibility that can happen is PROMs leading to preterm birth.[1] Administration of sustained release progesterone in those pregnant women with onset of uterine contractions post-trauma prevents these events.[31]

- *Uterine rupture*: Occurrence is 0.6%.[29] Any preceding disease which causes hyaline degeneration of muscle fibers is known to increase the probability of rupture.[1]

- *Fetal-maternal hemorrhage (FMH)*: FMH is four to five times more frequent in pregnant women who sustained trauma. In addition, the amount of blood volume which is transfused is also greater.[29,32] FMH leads to complications like rhesus sensitization in the mother, fetal anemia, arrhythmias in the fetus, and fetal loss.[29] FMH can be detected by the Kleihauer–Betke acid elution assay. This is indicated in trauma victims to calculate the Rh-immunoglobulin dose necessary to prevent isoimmunization to in Rh-women who suffered a massive transfusion.[17,18,29]

- *Rupture of membranes (ROM)*: It is due to trauma in pregnancy is usually associated with other concomitant injuries. So always in addition to continuous fetal monitoring, a detailed search for other injuries is indicated. If there is no onset of compromise in maternal or fetal condition usually management is similar to the management of spontaneous ROM.[1]

- *Urinary bladder rupture*: A cystogram with a maximally distended bladder and a postevacuation film, are minimum to be done if bladder rupture is suspected due to clinical findings or by imaging.[1]

- *Rectus sheath hematoma*: Abdominal wall distension in pregnancy leads to inferior epigastric artery elongation. Added to this further distension beyond its elastic modulus will be caused due to blunt trauma to that region making it vulnerable to tears and lacerations.[1]

Penetrating Trauma

The causes for these are usually the gunshot and stab wounds. With the progress in gestation, changes happen in the location of abdominal organs like the enlarging uterus occupies most of the abdomen and the bowel is pushed up. Due to this upper abdomen, penetrating injuries can cause various multiple gastrointestinal injuries. Trauma to the lower quadrants of the abdomen exclusively affects the uterus. As most of the energy of the penetrating object is absorbed by the uterus and amniotic fluid around it, trauma to other organs around is lessened.[33]

Cranial Trauma during Pregnancy

The most common causes of maternal mortality due to trauma are injuries of head and neck, shock due to hypovolemia, and respiratory failure.[6]

The several constraints in the management of such patients are (1) an increased intracranial pressure, (2) association of cervical spine injury, (3) airway difficulties, (4) hypovolemia, (5) alteration in consciousness, (6) full stomach, (7) decreased oxygenation, and (7) pregnancy itself.[23]

Intubation using fiberoptic, if possible should always be preferred over direct laryngoscope in cases of uncertainty about the cervical spine integrity.[33]

Intubation with mechanical ventilation for airway control and control of ICP are required in patients with Glasgow scale of 8 or less.[34]

Burn Injuries

Burns present a unique problem. The great risks associated with burns are fluid loss, hypoxemia, and sepsis. The emergency management goals in pregnant burn patients should be fluid replacement, respiratory support, and initial wound care. The fluid loss occurring from the denuded burns surface can be significant and is usually not correctly estimated in pregnant patients. Burns can occur either due to thermal or electrical cause.

- *Thermal injury*: Incidence is around 5–10% in pregnant women. The percentage of total body surface area (TBSA) involved in burns and thus the severity can be estimated by applying the rule of nine. The large abdominal surface in near term patients counts for a large percentage of TBSA.[35] In cases of term pregnancy, 5% is added in situation where the anterior abdomen is involved.[22] The general physical condition of the woman and the TBSA involved also determine the fetal outcome.[35]
  - In those who are exposed to fire in a closed-space, facial injury, carbonaceous material in the oropharynx, or respiratory symptoms should arise a suspicion of inhalational injury. In these cases, findings of interstitial edema on chest X-ray film, levels of carboxyhemoglobin greater than 10%, or abnormal arterial blood gas levels may be noticed.[36]
  - Fetus is at a relatively hypoxic state placing them at relatively high-risk during smoke inhalation (i.e. normal umbilical vein PaO_2 = 27 mm Hg). Obstruction to maternal ventilation (e.g. upper airway obstruction from edema), increased diffusion distance (e.g. interstitial alveolar edema), and acute functional anemia due to carbon monoxide poisoning can occur because of the inhalation injury.[27]
  - Inhalational injury can lead to clinical features which may not be seen until after few hours postexposure. Major burns can affect the pulmonary functions.[35]

- *Electrical injury*: These kinds of injuries happen because of the effect of the heat generated due to current and also due to the associated trauma. Electrical injury causes violent muscle contraction, falls leading to skeletal fractures, and neurologic damage eventually causing multisystem trauma. Mother is at a lower risk than the fetus as the fetus is surrounded by amniotic fluid, which is an excellent conductor of electricity.[35]

MATERNAL PATHOPHYSIOLOGY IMPACT ON FETUS

Fetal morbidity and mortality are usually due to hypoxia, preterm delivery, placental abnormalities, infection, and also due to drug effects. Fall in maternal hematocrit greater than 50% and a decrease in maternal mean blood pressure of 20% lead to fetal hypoxia and acidosis. The most important surgical risk to the fetus is preterm delivery and is usually due to abruption placentae.[36]

Fetal Injury

Blunt abdominal trauma and cranial injuries are most common. They are more common in cases of maternal pelvic fractures with fetal head engagement.[37,38]

LABORATORY EVALUATION

Laboratory tests in a pregnant trauma victim are directed toward identifying the sequelae of trauma, i.e. anemia due to acute blood loss, disseminated intravascular coagulopathy (DIC), and maternofetal hemorrhage.[39,40]

In cases of major trauma, i.e. internal bleeding or placental abruption, it is judicious to evaluate complete blood count, partial thromboplastin time, prothrombin time, and fibrinogen. In the setting of injury to urinary tract, hematuria may be revealed by urinalysis.[41]

DIAGNOSTIC IMAGING

Imaging of the pregnant trauma patient starts with an obstetric sonography except in victims who are low-risk with nonpenetrating abdominal injury. Flowchart 1 depicts the imaging protocol to be followed for pregnant trauma patients.

Flowchart 1: Imaging protocol for pregnant trauma patients.[42]

Ultrasound/Focused Abdominal Sonography for Trauma

Abdominal sonography is a safe and quick technique to evaluate the pregnant patient with trauma for well-being of fetus and maternal intraperitoneal hemorrhage. Safety regarding the usage of real-time grayscale sonography in pregnancy is well-proven, though there are concerns regarding the mechanical and thermal effects of prolonged Doppler use.[43]

Besides the parameters of fetal well-being, the most important use of sonography for patients with trauma is the assessment of free fluid in the peritoneum. Even though sensitivity of ultrasound for assessing intra-peritoneal hemorrhage is limited to around 61-83%, a high specificity from 94% to 100% has been reported.[42]

If focused abdominal sonography for trauma (FAST) is done relatively early, a large number of false negative results are seen during the process of resuscitation, i.e. at a stage when hemoperitoneum may not have collected in an amount that can be detected.[1]

Ionizing Radiation

It was suggested by Miller et al. that all patients who have sustained blunt abdominal injuries but are vitally stable should undergo a computerized tomography (CT) scan instead of a FAST examination so as to avoid under-diagnosis of intra-abdominal injury.[44]

In case of severe trauma to the mother, fetal risks should be weighed. Carcinogenesis and teratogenesis are the major theoretical apprehensions post in utero exposure to ionizing radiation. The dose which is needed to cause mental retardation or microcephaly is much more than the doses incurred in common clinical usage. In utero dose of ionizing radiation of 50 mGy (5 rad) may be linked with a 2% lifetime attributable risk of malignancy. However, this dose permits most of the common radiologic procedures to be performed safely, including a single-phase CT scanning of the abdomen and pelvis. Even though contrast media can cross the placental barrier, no reports of fetal goiter have thus far been reported.[45]

Magnetic Resonance Imaging

Magnetic resonance imaging (MRI) may be a useful modality in pregnant patients with trauma as it is not associated with any known adverse effects to the fetus. While the US Food and Drug Administration (FDA) considers the safety of MRI to not be recognized, no cases of adverse outcome during the perinatal period have been reported.[42,46]

However, the use of gadolinium is controversial at present. In few cases, it has caused nephrogenic systemic fibrosis in children. Hence, it is recommended to avoid gadolinium agents during pregnancy barring conditions when it is absolutely necessary.[46]

■ ASSESSING FETAL WELL-BEING

The prime objective of fetal monitoring is to detect fetal distress and eventually the fetal loss. Since even trivial injuries lead to abruption of placenta and other bad obstetric outcomes monitoring for fetal well-being is always recommended in cases of maternal trauma.[47]

Obstetric ultrasound scanning should be done to assess fetal viability and fetal wellbeing. Ultrasound can detect placental abruptions but its sensitivity to detect it is around 40% in the setting of trauma. Evaluating fetal extremity movements, fetal respiratory activity, amniotic fluid volume, and fetal heart rate establishes well-being of the fetus.[29,48]

Fetal Doppler studies may have a role in the assessment of fetus postmaternal trauma in some cases. For example, in severe cases of fetal anemia after placental abruption and/or maternofetal hemorrhage, the peak systolic velocity (PSV) of the fetal middle cerebral artery (MCA) show a characteristic increase which reflects brain sparing in the fetus thus aiding in identifying fetal hemorrhage in otherwise uncertain cases.[2,49]

Cardiotocographic (CTG) monitoring is required in all viable fetuses of 24 weeks or more postmaternal trauma including those patients who have no obvious signs and symptoms of abdominal injury. Pearlman et al. have endorsed a minimum of 4 hours of CTG monitoring to detect any intrauterine pathology; however, others recommend 6 hours of observation, extended to 24 hours if during the first 6 hours there is more than one uterine contraction every 15 min, nonreassuring fetal CTG monitoring, uterine tenderness, vaginal bleed, rupture of the membranes, or any other maternal injury.[29]

The uterine contractions may also be helpful in evaluating the risk of placental abruption postminor trauma. Patients without contractions for more than 4 hours of observation after minor trauma may be suitable for discharge. Presence of contractions or signs of fetal distress should initiate extended monitoring.[50,51]

Pertinent Aspects of Patient History[52]

The history taken during the evaluation of a pregnant trauma victim should be focused toward clarifying those aspects that may change initial management of patient like:
- *Mechanism of injury*: Both blunt and penetrating traumas, if intentional, are usually directed toward the abdomen.
- *Medications/allergies*: Young and otherwise healthy women may be taking medications and may develop venous thromboembolic disease, gestational diabetes mellitus, or pregnancy-induced heart failure.
- *Last menstrual period*: If known, can aid to determine fetal viability to guide the appropriateness of fetal interventions.
- *Fetal movement*: This can serve as a proxy for fetal stability until bedside ultrasonography or fetal monitoring by CTG is performed.
- *Contractions*: Uterine irritability post-trauma can cause early labor pains, thus necessitating monitoring of the fetus.
- *Preterm premature rupture of membranes/pain abdomen/vaginal bleeding*: Should prompt more exhaustive consideration of uterine complications after the trauma.

PREHOSPITAL MANAGEMENT

The important step in the survival of both mother and fetus is prehospital management, before transferring the patient to a higher medical center. As per advanced trauma life support (ATLS) guidelines, the following patients should be transferred to level I trauma centers:
- Glasgow coma score <14
- Respiratory rate <10 or >29
- Systolic blood pressure <90 mm Hg
- Revised Trauma score <11
- Anatomy or mechanism of injury
- Pulse >110
- Chest pain
- Loss of consciousness
- Third trimester gestation.

Standard protocols should be followed by the emergency medical team like extrication with spinal immobilization and should perform resuscitative measures as per the ATLS guidelines. The patient should be intubated in the field, if required, irrespective of pregnancy. However, in pregnancy, there is an increase in aspiration risk due to intra-abdominal hypertension and reduced tone of lower esophageal sphincter, which delays the gastric emptying.[1]

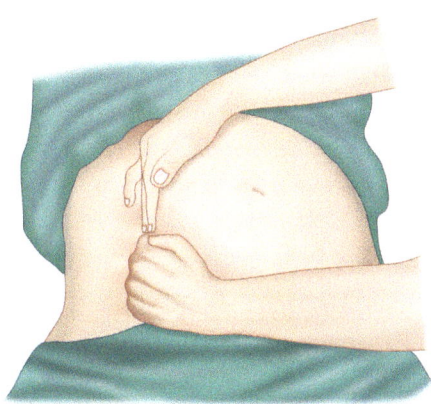

Fig. 1: Manual left lateral tilt.

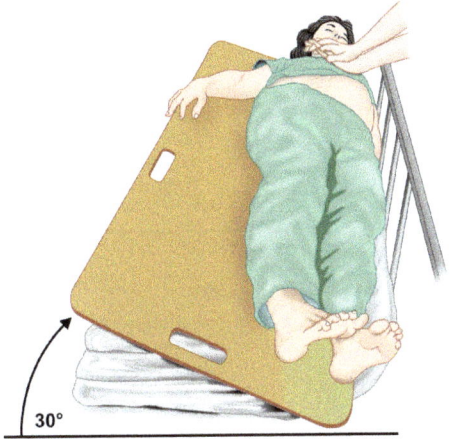

Fig. 2: 30 degrees lateral decubitus tilt.

In pregnant trauma patients, initial resuscitation should always focus on avoiding uterocaval compression. Patients beyond 20 weeks of gestation should be placed with 15° angle to the left. Uterocaval compression leads to considerably decreased cardiac output (approximately 60%), thus leading to increase in acidosis and requirement for vasopressors which further prolongs the resuscitation.[53,54]

For patients less than 24 weeks of gestation manual left lateral tilt might be enough which is demonstrated in Figure 1.

In patients with gestational age more than 24 weeks, a 30° lateral decubitus tilt is suggested. Even though this decreases the efficiency of cardiopulmonary resuscitation (CPR) when compared to the supine position, this slightly decreased effectiveness of chest compressions. Position is demonstrated in Figure 2.[53,55]

Hence, as per Eastern Association for Surgery and Trauma (EAST) guidelines, pregnant patient should be tilted to left lateral position (at least 15°) during initial resuscitation.

Due to increased chances of uterocaval compression, the distribution of intravenous (IV) fluids and medications might be considerably changed, if femoral access is used in pregnant patients. Oxygen should be supplemented by face mask or nasal cannula. In case prehospital blood transfusion is needed, "O" negative blood should be used whenever likely.

Appropriate team should be easily available at the emergency room which should include a trauma surgeon, anesthesiologist, neonatologist, and a sonologist.[1]

Management Post-trauma[56]

The post-trauma management of a pregnant patient is illustrated in Flowchart 2.

Management of the Pregnant Woman after Blunt (Abdominal) Trauma[2,57]

The management of the pregnant woman after blunt (abdominal) trauma is provided in Flowchart 3.

Management of the Pregnant Woman after Penetrating Abdominal Trauma[58]

Management of the pregnant woman after penetrating abdominal trauma is described in Flowchart 4.

Flowchart 2: Post-trauma management of a pregnant patient.

Assess maternal status
Cardiac arrest
Unresponsive
Loss of airway/respiratory arrest
Blood pressure < 80/40 mm Hg or heart rate <50 or >140 bpm
If fetus viable, FHR <110 or >160 bpm

Present →

Advanced cardiac life support

Airway/cervical spine control
Breathing
Circulation
Disability
Exposure
Consultation with trauma team: notify neonatal intensive care unit
Supplemental oxygen
Displace uterus to left if gestational age > 20 weeks
Intravenous access (two peripheral lines)

Laboratory tests: complete blood count; coagulation profile (type and screen); Kleihauer–Betke test if Rh-negative (type and cross)
Viable fetus: continuous FHR monitoring
Previable fetus: FHR via Doppler auscultation or electronic fetal monitoring
Tocodynamometric monitoring if concern for abruption

Absent →

Maternal injury greater than minor bruising, lacerations, or contusions

Present →

Consider trauma team consultation intravenous access
Laboratory tests: complete blood count, coagulation profile (type and screen)
Kleihauer-Betke test if Rh-negative
Viable fetus: FHR monitoring for four hours
Contractions < 6 per hour, consider discharge
Contractions ≥ 6 per hour, consider admission
Previable fetus: FHR via Doppler auscultation or electronic fetal monitoring
Tocodynamometric monitoring if concern for abruption

Absent →

Brief fetal assessment
No laboratory evaluation required
No radiologic imaging required
Patient counseling on signs and symptoms of abruption

Once the patient is stable
Fetal ultrasonography with or without biophysical profile
Consider other laboratory tests: chemistries, urinalysis, urine toxicology screen
Radiologic assessment, peritoneal lavage, focused assessment with ultrasonography for trauma, ultrasonography (if indicated)

Motor vehicle crash	Slips or fails	Burns	Domestic violence/ intimate partner violence	Penetrating trauma	Toxic exposure
Determine whether patient was wearing seat belt	Assess for abdominal trauma and extremities for fractures/ ligament damage	Aggressive fluid resuscitation Consider delivery if burn area > 50%	Assess for depression and suicide risk	Level of entry determines affected organ; gravid uterus may protect from visceral injury	Agent and gestational age at exposure guide maternal therapy and counseling

Trauma in Pregnancy

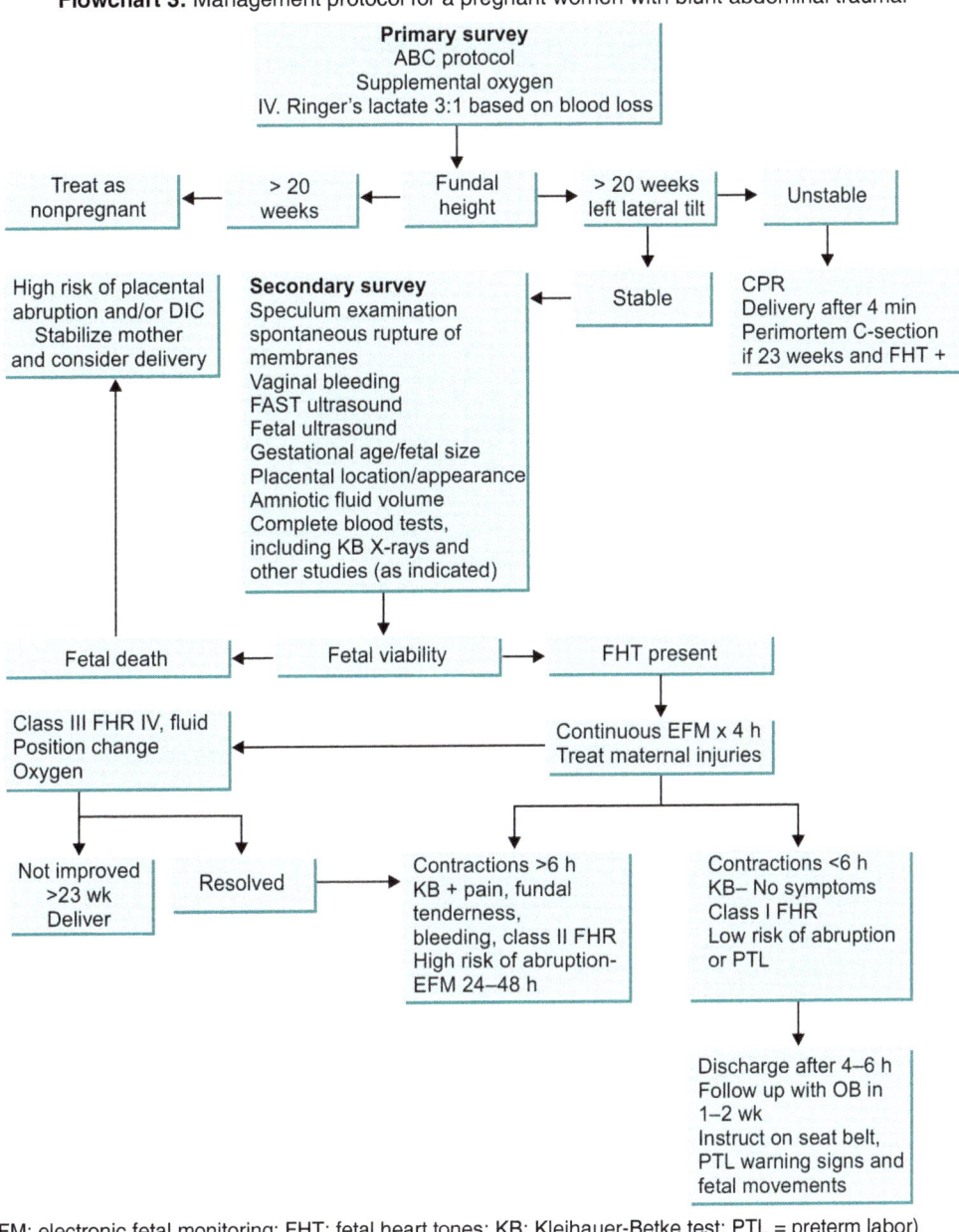

Flowchart 3: Management protocol for a pregnant women with blunt abdominal trauma.

(EFM: electronic fetal monitoring; FHT: fetal heart tones; KB: Kleihauer-Betke test; PTL = preterm labor)

Emergency LSCS and Perimortem Cesarean Section in Trauma[59]

The role of emergency LSCS and perimortem cesarean section in a case of trauma is mentioned in Flowchart 5.

PREVENTION

Prevention is the vital cog essential for the survival of mother and the fetus. MVAs and domestic violence are the etiologies of trauma in which can be prevented.[1]

Obstetric Emergencies

Flowchart 4: Management protocol for a pregnant women with penetrating abdominal trauma.

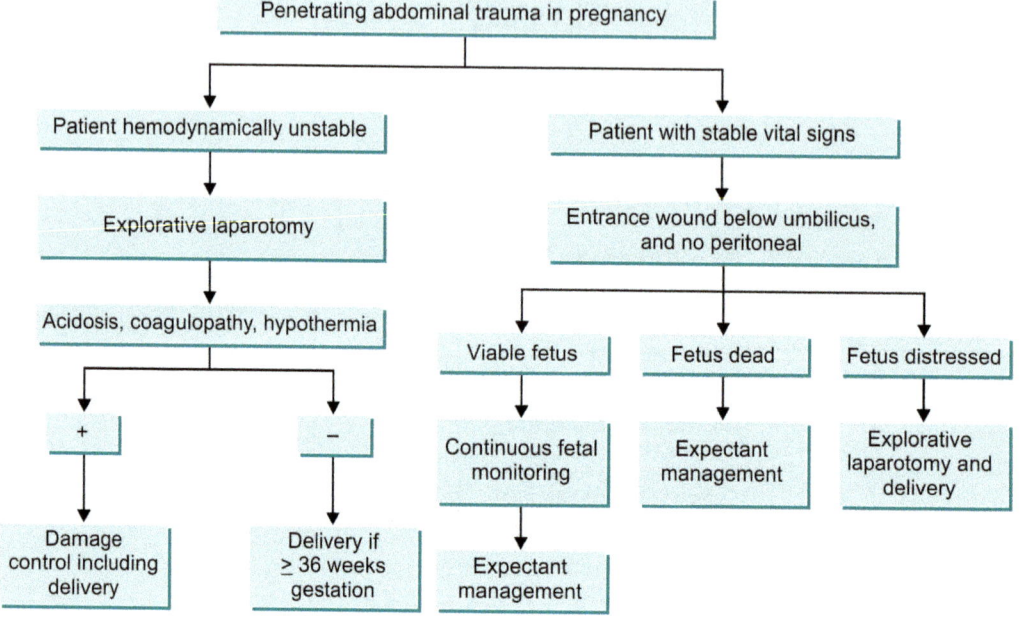

Flowchart 5: Emrgency LSCS and perimortem C section role in a case of trauma.

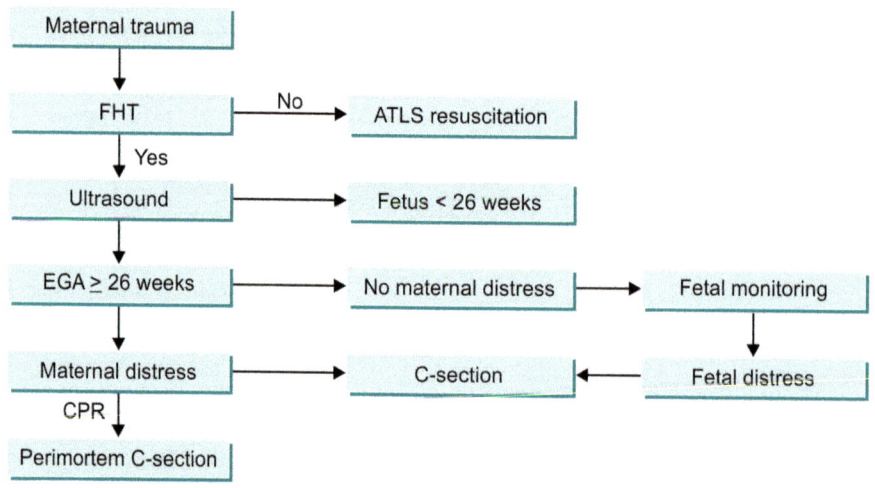

(CPR: cardiopulmonary resuscitation; EGA: estimated gestational age; FHT: fetal heart tone;) If the fetal heart beat is present and estimated gestational age is ≥26 weeks, fetal monitoring is essential. Fetal distress or maternal distress warrants emergency C- section. Perimortem C- section is done if CPR is in progress.[59]

While, MVAs account for grievous maternal injuries and fetal losses due to trauma which can be attributed to decrease use of seat belt use amongst the pregnant women. Thus proper use of seat belt significantly reduces the maternal and fetal injuries postMVAs.[3,51,60-62] The prime reason for decreased seat belt use in pregnancy is the fear that it will hurt the fetus. The most common cause of fetal death in blunt trauma is maternal death.[63]

When the women were appropriately restrained, adverse outcomes in the fetus were noted in 29% of vehicular crashes while on the other hand the women who were inappropriately restrained, adverse fetal outcomes were noted in around 50% of the MVAs.[50]

Right use of the seat belt should be a key issue in prenatal counseling, i.e. the lap belt should be positioned as low as possible, under the protuberant part of maternal abdomen while the shoulder belt should be placed off to the side of the uterus, in between the breasts and above the mid clavicle. Positioning of the lap belt over uterus considerably increases the transmission of pressure on to the uterus and has been linked with substantial injury to the uterus and fetus. Both the restraints, i.e. lap and shoulder belts should be applied snugly and comfortably without excessive slack in each belt as depicted in Figure 3.[64,65]

The deployment of air bags decreases the risk of maternal injury and also cuts the risk of adverse pregnancy outcomes. According to American College of Obstetricians and Gynecologists (ACOG), the pregnant women who travel in motor vehicles should wear shoulder and lap seat belts and should not turn off air bags.[66,67]

Since, younger pregnant women are more prone to MVA's and domestic violence, their screening is of paramount importance.[68]

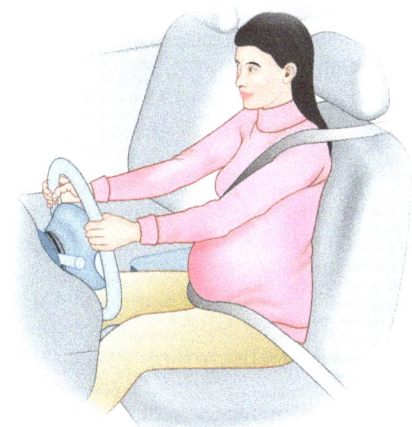

Fig. 3: Correct placement of seat belt for a pregnant woman.

REFERENCES

1. Augustin G. Acute Abdomen during Pregnancy. Switzerland: Springer International Publishing Switzerland; 2014.
2. Michael M, Joseph C. Trauma in pregnancy. Obstet Gynecol Clin N Am. 2007;34(3);555-83.
3. Drost TF, Rosemurgy AS, Sherman HF, et al. Major trauma in pregnant women: maternal/fetal outcome. J Trauma. 1990;30:574-8.
4. Baerga-Varela Y, Zietlow SP, Bannon MP, et al. Trauma in pregnancy. Mayo Clin Proc. 2000;75: 1243-8.
5. Kissinger DP, Rozycki GS, Morris JA Jr, et al. Trauma in pregnancy. Predicting pregnancy outcome. Arch Surg. 1991;126:1079-86.
6. Connolly AM, Katz VL, Bash KL, et al. Trauma and pregnancy. Am J Perinatol. 1997;14:331-6.
7. Lavery JP, Staten-McCormick M. Management of moderate to severe trauma in pregnancy. Obstet Gynecol Clin North Am. 1995;22:69-90.
8. Weiss HB, Songer TJ, Fabio A. Fetal deaths related to maternal injury. J Am Med Assoc. 2001;286:1863-8.
9. Mattox KL, Goetzl L. Trauma in pregnancy. Crit Care Med. 2005;33(10 Suppl):S385-9.
10. Poole Jr GV, Martin JN, Perry KG, et al. Trauma in pregnancy: the role of interpersonal violence. Am J Obstet Gynecol. 1996;174:1873-8.

11. Hoyert DL. Maternal mortality and related concepts. National center for health statistics. Vital Health Stat 3. 2007;33:1-20.
12. Patterson SK, Snider CC, Meyer DS, et al. The consequences of high-risk behavior: trauma during pregnancy. J Trauma Inj Infect Crit Care. 2007;62:1015-20.
13. Schiff MA, Holt VL. Pregnancy outcomes following hospitalization for motor vehicle crashes in Washington state from 1989 to 2001. Am J Epidemiol. 2005;161:503-10.
14. Tinker SC, Reefhuis J, Dellinger AM, et al. Maternal injuries during the periconceptional period and the risk of birth defects, National Birth Defects Prevention Study, 1997–2005. Paediatr Perinat Epidemiol. 2011;25:487-96.
15. Coleman MT, Trianfo VA, Rund DA. Nonobstetric emergencies in pregnancy: trauma and surgical conditions. Am J Obstet Gynecol. 1997;177:497-502.
16. Fisher M, Rivkind AJ. Trauma in pregnancy. Harefuah. 2004;143:733-6..
17. Tsuei BJ. Assessment of the pregnant trauma patient. Injury. 2006;37:367-73.
18. Pearlman MD. Motor vehicle crashes, pregnancy loss and preterm labor. Int J Gynaecol Obstet. 1997;57:127-32.
19. Baker BW. Trauma. In: Chestnut DH (Ed). Obstetric Anesthesia: Principles and Practice. St Louis: Mosby; 1999. pp. 1041-50.
20. Clark SL, Cotton DB, Lee W, et al. Central haemodynamic assessment of normal term pregnancy. Am J Obstet Gynecol. 1989;161(6 Pt 1):1439-42.
21. Hoff WS, D'Amelio LF, Tinkoff GH, et al. Maternal predictors of fetal demise in trauma during pregnancy. Surg Gynecol Obstet. 1991;172:175-80.
22. Kuczkowski KM, Reisner LS, Benumof JL. Airway problems and new solutions for the obstetric patient. J Clin Anesth. 2004;49:214-18.
23. Kuczkowski KM. Trauma in the pregnant patient. Curr Opin. Anaesthesiol. 2004;17: 145-50.
24. Ali J, Yeo A, Gana TJ, et al. Predictors of fetal mortality in pregnant trauma patients. J Trauma. 1997;42:782-5.
25. Leggon RE, Wood GC, Indeck MC. Pelvic fractures in pregnancy: factors influencing maternal and fetal outcomes. J Trauma. 2002; 53:796-804.
26. Cunningham G, Hauth J, Leveno K, et al. Williams' Obstetrics, 22nd edition. New York: McGraw Hill; 2005.
27. Mahoney B, Schwaitzberg SD, Newton ER; Medscape. Trauma and pregnancy. [online] Avaialble from: https://emedicine.medscape.com/article/435224-overview [Last accessed September, 2019].
28. American College of Surgeons. Trauma in pregnancy and intimate partner violence. In: Advanced Trauma Life Support Student Course Manual. 9th ed. Chicago, Ill.: American College of Surgeons; 2012.
29. Pearlman MD, Tintinelli JE, Lorenz PR. A prospective controlled study of the outcome after trauma during pregnancy. Am J Obstet Gynecol. 1990;162:1502-10.
30. Knuppel RA, Hatangadi SB. Acute hypotension related to hemorrhage in the obstetric patient. Obstet Gynecol Clin North Am. 1995;22:111-29.
31. Dodd JM, Flenady V, Cincotta R, et al. Prenatal administration of progesterone for preventing preterm birth. Cochrane Database Syst Rev. 2006;1:CD004947.
32. Goodwin T, Breen M. Pregnancy outcome and fetomaternal hemorrhage after non-catastrophic trauma. Am J Obstet Gynecol. 1990;162:665-71.
33. Stone IK. Trauma in the obstetric patient. Obst and Gynecol Cl N Am. 1999;26:459-67.
34. Kuczkowski KM, Fouhy SA, Greenberg M, et al. Trauma in pregnancy: anaesthetic management of the pregnant trauma victim with unstable cervical spine. Anaesthesia. 2003;58:822-6.
35. Rudra A, Ray A, Chatterjee S. et al. Trauma in pregnancy. Indian J Anaesth. 2007;51:100.
36. Bajwa SK, Jindal R, Bajwa SJ, et al. Management of trauma and injuries during pregnancy: challenges for an obstetrician and the intensivist. Sri Lanka J Obstetr Gynaecol. 2012;34:58-64.
37. Elliott M. Vehicular accidents and pregnancy. Aust N Z J Obstet Gynaecol. 1966;6:279-86.
38. Parkinson EB. Perinatal loss due to external trauma to the uterus. Am J Obstet Gynecol. 1964;90:30-3.
39. Trivedi N, Ylagan M, Moore TR, et al. Predicting adverse outcomes following trauma in pregnancy. J Reprod Med. 2012;57(1-2):3-8.
40. Williams J, Mozurkewich E, Chilimigras J, et al. Critical care in obstetrics: pregnancy-specific conditions. Best Pract Res Clin Obstet Gynaecol. 2008;22(5):825-46.

41. Brown HL. Trauma in pregnancy. Obstet Gynecol. 2009;114(1):147-60.
42. Patel SJ, Reede DL, Katz DS, et al. Imaging the pregnant patient for nonobstetric conditions: algorithms and radiation dose considerations. Radiographics. 2007;27(6):1705-22.
43. Sheiner E, Abramowicz JS. A symposium on obstetrical ultrasound: is all this safe for the fetus? Clin Obstet Gynecol. 2012;55(1):188-98.
44. Miller MT, Pasquale MD, Bromberg WJ, et al. Not so fast. J Trauma. 2003;54:52-60.
45. Lee I, Chew F. Use of IV iodinated and gadolinium contrast media in the pregnant or lactating patient: self-assessment module. AJR Am J Roentgenol. 2009;193(Suppl 6):70-3.
46. Chen MM, Coakley FV, Kaimal A, et al. Guidelines for computed tomography and magnetic resonance imaging use during pregnancy and lactation. Obstet Gynecol. 2008;112(2 Pt 1):333-40.
47. Fischer PE, Zarzaur BL, Fabian TC, et al. Minor trauma is an unrecognized contributor to poor fetal outcomes: a population-based study of 78,552 pregnancies. J Trauma. 2011;71(1):90-3.
48. Williams JK, McClain L, Rosemurgy AS, et al. Evaluation of blunt abdominal trauma in the third trimester of pregnancy: maternal and fetal considerations. Obstet Gynecol. 1990;75(1):33-7.
49. Cosmi E, Rampon M, Saccardi C, et al. Middle cerebral artery peak systolic velocity in the diagnosis of fetomaternal hemorrhage. Int J Gynaecol Obstet. 2012;117(2):128-30.
50. Klinich KD, Flannagan CA, Rupp JD, et al. Fetal outcome in motor-vehicle crashes: effects of crash characteristics and maternal restraint. Am J Obstet Gynecol. 2008;198(4):450.e1-9.
51. Dahmus MA, Sibai BM. Blunt abdominal trauma: are there any predictive factors for abruptio placentae or maternal-fetal distress? Am J Obstet Gynecol. 1993;169(4):1054-9.
52. Raja AS, Zabbo CP. Trauma in pregnancy. Emerg Med Clin N Am. 2012;30:937-48.
53. Rees GA, Willis BA. Resuscitation in late pregnancy. Anaesthesia. 1988;43:347-9.
54. Kasten GW, Martin ST. Resuscitation from bupivacaine-induced cardiovascular toxicity during partial inferior vena cava occlusion. Anesth Analg. 1986;65:341-4.
55. Vanden Hoek TL, Morrison LJ, Shuster M, et al. Part 12: cardiac arrest in special situations: 2010 American Heart Association guidelines for cardiopulmonary resuscitation and emergency cardiovascular care. Circulation. 2010;122(18 Suppl 3):S833-8.
56. Mendez-Figueroa H, Dahlke JD, Vrees RA, et al. Trauma in pregnancy: an updated systematic review. Am J Obstet Gynecol. 2013;209(1):6.
57. Grossman NB. Blunt trauma in pregnancy. Am Fam Physician. 2004;70:1303-10.
58. Rudlof U. Trauma in pregnancy. Arch Gynecol Obstet. 2007;276:101-17.
59. Morris Jr JA, Rosenbower TJ, Jurkovich GJ, et al. Infant survival after cesarean section for trauma. Ann Surg. 1996;223:481-91.
60. Esposito TJ, Gens DR, Smith LG, et al. Trauma during pregnancy. A review of 79 cases. Arch Surg. 1991;126:1073-8.
61. Curet MJ, Schermer CR, Demarest GB, et al. Predictors of outcome in trauma during pregnancy: identification of patients who can be monitored for less than 6 hours. J Trauma. 2000;49:18-25.
62. Scorpio RJ, Esposito TJ, Smith LG, et al. Blunt trauma during pregnancy: factors affecting fetal outcome. J Trauma. 1992;32:213-6.
63. Shah AJ, Kilcline BA. Trauma in pregnancy. Emerg Med Clin North Am. 2003;21(3):615-29.
64. ACOG Educational Bulletin. Obstetric aspects of trauma management. Number 251, September 1998. American College of Obstetricians and Gynecologists. Int J Gynaecol Obstet. 1999;64:87-94.
65. Automobile passenger restraints for children and pregnant women. ACOG Technical Bulletin number 151, January 1991. Int J Gynaecol Obstet. 1992;37:305-8.
66. Schiff MA, Mack CD, Kaufman RP, et al. The effect of air bags on pregnancy outcomes in Washington State: 2002-2005. Obstet Gynecol. 2010;115(1):85-92.
67. American College of Obstetricians and Gynecologists. Car safety for you and your baby. [online] Available from: http://www.acog.org/~/media/For%20Patients/faq018.pdf?dmc=20140703T2121569354 [Last accessed September, 2019].
68. Hedin LW, Janson PO. Domestic violence during pregnancy. The prevalence of physical injuries, substance use, abortions and miscarriages. Acta Obstet Gynecol Scand. 2000;79:625-30.

CHAPTER 8

Shoulder Dystocia

BS Susheela Rani

INTRODUCTION

Described as the obstetrician's nightmare, shoulder dystocia is a difficult situation that is sometimes seen in vaginal delivery which can happen when it is least expected and can be followed by huge risks to the mother and baby. Since it is difficult to predict, shoulder dystocia and therefore to prevent it from happening, shoulder dystocia continues to haunt even the most experienced obstetricians.

DEFINITION

Shoulder dystocia is defined as a difficult situation that is sometimes encountered in vaginal delivery due to impaction of the fetal shoulder in the maternal pelvis after the head is delivered that requires additional obstetric procedures to deliver the fetus after gentle traction has failed.

An objective definition of shoulder dystocia[1] as proposed by Spong and colleagues is "prolonged head-to-body delivery time (e.g. more than 60 seconds) and/or the use of additional obstetric procedures".

Incidence: 0.2–3%. The incidence of shoulder dystocia varies as the definition of shoulder dystocia varies between different studies reporting it.

MECHANISM OF LABOR IN SHOULDER DYSTOCIA

- In a normal delivery, the fetal head is delivered and the fetal shoulders quickly follow. In these situations, the axis of the fetal shoulders enters the pelvis in the oblique diameter of the pelvic brim. This diameter offers the shoulders the most room for their passage.
- In a woman with shoulder dystocia, the shoulders enter the pelvic inlet in the anteroposterior dimension. This dimension is shorter than the oblique diameter of the pelvic inlet.
- The anterior shoulder therefore gets obstructed by the mother's pubic bone.
- Most often, it is the anterior shoulder that is obstructed. Sometimes the posterior shoulder gets caught at the maternal sacrum. This is not very common.
- When the proportions of the fetal shoulders or chest are bigger than those of its head, there can be shoulder dystocia. This is what happens in an especially large baby or a baby of a mother with diabetes.

RISK FACTORS

There are a number of factors associated with an increased risk of shoulder dystocia. However, by themselves, they are not sensitive to predict shoulder dystocia. Their clinical utility in predicting shoulder dystocia is therefore limited.[2] The risk factors for shoulder dystocia can generally be divided into three categories:
1. Preconceptual
2. Antepartum
3. Intrapartum (Box 1).

Box 1: Major risk factors for shoulder dystocia.

Preconceptual:
- History of shoulder dystocia or baby with BPI
- Maternal diabetes
 Maternal obesity
- Increased maternal age
- Multiparity.

Antepartum factors:
- Macrosomia
- Gestational diabetes
 Excessive weight gain
- Postdated pregnancy
- Male baby.

Intrapartum factors:
- Prolonged labor
- Precipitate labor
- Instrumental delivery.

TABLE 1: Fetal weight and shoulder dystocia (Acker et al.).

Estimated fetal weight	Rate of shoulder dystocia	
	Nondiabetic mothers	Diabetic mothers
<4,000 g	1.1	3.7
4,000–4,499 g	10	23.1
>5,000 g	22.6	50

Preconceptual

Shoulder dystocia is seen more commonly in pregnant women, who are older, obese, and multiparous. However, elderly gravida, obesity, and multiparity are only markers for other primary risk factors. In a woman, who has had shoulder dystocia in her previous pregnancy, the risk of recurrence is 10-15%, which is 10 times more than the baseline risk. Hence some obstetricians adduce, "once a shoulder dystocia, always a cesarean".

Antepartum

Macrosomia

- Macrosomia is defined as a fetus large for gestational age (more than 90th centile). A definite cut off weight for defining macrosomia for Indian babies is not available. However, Asian babies are said to be macrosomic when their weight exceeds 4,000 g.
- Risk of shoulder dystocia increases with increasing fetal weight (Table 1).[3]
- Estimation of birth weight of the fetus either clinically or by ultrasound has limitations. A prospective study comparing clinical and ultrasound prediction of macrosomia defined as birth weight 4,000 g found that the sensitivity of clinical estimation was 68% as compared to 58% by ultrasound.
- The accuracy of ultrasound prediction of fetal weight decreased as the birth weight increased.
- Though the risk of shoulder dystocia increases with increasing birth weights, a majority of shoulder dystocia occur in lesser birth weights, 40-60% of shoulder dystocia occur in infants who weigh less than 4,000 g and[4] 70-90% of macrosomic infants (even those >5,000 g) deliver without any sequelae.[5] Even if the birth weight of the infant is over 4,000 g, shoulder dystocia will only complicate 3.3% of the deliveries.[6]

Maternal Diabetes

- Macrosomic infants of diabetic mothers have many of the following features compared to nondiabetic control infants of similar birth weight and length.[7] Their shoulder dimensions are bigger leading to a reduced head-to-shoulder ratio. They have more body fat and thicker skin folds in the upper extremity.
- When maternal diabetes is treated, the risk of macrosomia is reduced. This decreases the risk of shoulder dystocia.[8]

Other Risk Factors

- Maternal weight gain and postdates are secondary risk factors. They increase the

risk of fetal macrosomia and thereby of shoulder dystocia.
- Shoulder dystocia is higher in male babies than female babies. Increased birth weight, increased anthropometric measurements in the male babies compared to the female babies could have contributed to the difference.

Intrapartum Risk Factors

Instrumental Vaginal Delivery

- Operative vaginal delivery significantly increases the risk of shoulder dystocia (OR 4.6–28.0) depending on the station at application and other risk factors.[9]
- The reasons for instrumental delivery in such instances could be—(1) the inability of the mother to push the baby out due to fetal macrosomia. (2) Poor descent due to either an altered distribution of fat between the fetal head, chest, shoulders, and abdomen, or fetal shoulders engaging the A-P diameter of pelvis as opposed to an oblique diameter.

Prolonged Second Stage of Labor

- A prolonged deceleration phase in the first stage of labor is strongly associated with shoulder dystocia and brachial plexus injury (BPI). When the second stage of labor is also prolonged to more than 2 hours, the odds of BPI increase 20-fold.[10]
- However, Lurie (1995)[11] found no correlation between the length of the stages of labor and shoulder dystocia. He showed that there was no difference in (1) the mean rate of dilatation, (2) the percentage of protracted labors, or (3) the mean duration of the second stage of labor in a group of mothers who experienced shoulder dystocia.
It is possible that dysfunctional labors are more common with macrosomic babies.

Shoulder dystocia is more likely to occur in women with dysfunctional labors and macrosomic babies.

TIME TO RESOLVE SHOULDER DYSTOCIA

Hypoxia due to shoulder dystocia results from:
- Compression of the neck leading to central venous congestion
- Compression of the umbilical cord
- Prolonged increased intrauterine pressure causing reduced blood flow within the placental villi and secondary fetal bradycardia.

Prolonged head to delivery intervals is associated with increasing hypoxia although the time required to resolve the shoulder dystocia without causing hypoxic injury is not yet clear. Stallings et al.[12] stated that a threshold interval of 7 or more minutes had a 67% sensitivity and 74% specificity for predicting brain injury.

MANAGEMENT

General Guidelines

Explain the situation quickly to patient and partner and request their cooperation. The following should be undertaken in an attempt to achieve delivery. 30–60 seconds should be spent on each and delivery attempted each time. One labor room staff should document times and maneuvers attempted.

- *Call for help*: Senior obstetric and pediatric staff, anesthetist should be summoned. If the cord is around the neck, clamping and cutting should be avoided.
- Perform an episiotomy, if not already achieved. This allows better access to the fetus to perform certain maneuvers and may prevent further maternal trauma.
- Position patient following McRoberts maneuver (Legs hyper flexed). This leads to

rotation of the symphysis pubis superiorly by a distance of 8 cm. The angle of inclination is reduced from 26° to 10° and which frees the impacted shoulder without changing the pelvic dimensions.
- About 40% cases of shoulder dystocia are resolved by McRoberts maneuver alone.
- Gonik and colleagues[13] demonstrated that McRoberts positioning reduced delivery force up to 37% for endogenous load (maternal force) and up to 47% for exogenous loads (clinician applied), thereby decreasing brachial plexus stretching. Also, McRoberts[14] position almost doubled the intrauterine pressure developed by contractions alone.
- Gentle downward traction applied on the fetal head by the obstetrician is accompanied by suprapubic pressure on the anterior shoulder applied by an assistant. The assistant stands by the side of the mother and with the heel of his hand, applies pressure (similar to CPR) on the posterior aspect of the impacted shoulder in a downward motion. Pressure can be steady and continuous. However, if this not successful, a rocking motion is recommended to dislodge the shoulder from behind the pubic symphysis. This suprapubic pressure is known as Rubin 1 maneuver.
- Two fingers inserted into the vagina apply pressure on the posterior aspect of anterior shoulder and push it into the oblique diameter to disimpact the shoulders, Rubin II maneuver. If this is not helpful, two fingers of the other hand are inserted into the vagina and pressure is applied on the anterior aspect of posterior shoulder. The fingers of the two hands dislodge the impaction by pushing the shoulder into the oblique dimension of the pelvis in a corkscrew manner, the Wood screw maneuver.
- If this fails, the direction of pressure on the shoulders is changed to the opposite direction, reverse Wood screw maneuver.
- If delivery has still not been achieved, the attendant should attempt to remove the posterior arm. This is done by inserting the hand in the posterior vagina over the anterior surface of the fetal chest. The posterior arm is located, the arm is then bent at the elbow, the wrist grasped and the arm swept over the chest. Posterior arm is thus delivered.
- If after exhaustion of the above, delivery is still not achieved, the woman should roll on to her hands and knees where, in reference to the woman, the posterior shoulder is delivered. This is achieved by gentle downward traction on the head accompanied by a finger inserted in the posterior axilla, and gently used to help release the posterior shoulder. The anterior shoulder is then delivered by gentle upward traction on the head. If this proves unsuccessful then the posterior arm may be removed as described earlier.
- If all of the above are unsuccessful then repeat all the maneuvers. If after all these, the shoulders are still not disimpacted, it may be due to bilateral shoulder dystocia or posterior arm shoulder dystocia. The following maneuvers can be tried.[15]
  - *Cleidotomy*: The fetal clavicle is deliberately fractured at its middle by applying digital pressure. This reduces the bisacromial diameter and facilitates delivery of the shoulders. Cleidotomy is also associated with increased injury to the brachial plexus and the major vessels.
  - *Zavanelli maneuver*[16] *(cephalic replacement followed by CD)*: It may be most appropriate for rare bilateral shoulder dystocia. It is associated with a significantly increased risk of

fetal morbidity and mortality and of maternal morbidity.[17]
- *Symphysiotomy*: Deliberate incision of the ligaments of the symphysis pubis, which allows separation of the two pubic bones by about 2 cm facilitating delivery of the fetus. Injury to the bladder and urethra, osteitis pubes are some of the complications.
- *Hysterotomy*: Cesarean section is done and the shoulder is disimpacted through the uterine incision and vaginal delivery of the fetus is completed. Morbidity to the fetus and the mother is very high.

Postpartum Management

Amongst the various causes for medical litigation, shoulder dystocia ranks as the third most common cause.

Following procedures have to be followed.
- Measurement of umbilical cord blood gases
- Details of delivery must be documented by all team members
- Shoulder dystocia form needs to be filled with the following details:
  - Time of delivery of the head
  - Time of noticing shoulder dystocia
  - Who were called for help
  - Which shoulder was anterior
  - Maneuvers performed and their order
  - The force used to deliver the shoulders—mild, moderate, and time of delivery of the baby
  - Condition of the baby
  - Condition of the mother.
- Debriefing with the patient and her family about the delivery and outcome
- Documentation of the debriefing with the patient and her family.

What should not be done?

- *Fundal pressure*: This can further aggravate the impaction of the shoulder at the symphysis pubis and lead to fetal injuries and uterine rupture.
- *Nuchal cord should not be clamped or cut*: Nuchal cord should be untangled over the head. In the face of shoulder dystocia with a nuchal cord, some cord circulation may continue and severing the cord may contribute to fetal hypoxia and hypotension during the time it takes to resolve the dystocia.[18]

COMPLICATIONS IN THE FETUS (BOX 2)

Brachial Plexus Injury[19]

- Traction on the fetal head can cause injury to the brachial plexus.[20]
- Incidence is 2.3–16% of deliveries with shoulder dystocia.
- Only 10% of these result in permanent neurological injury.
- Damage to C5-6 causes Erb's palsy leading to weakness of the shoulder, elbow flexors, and forearm supinators.
- Damage to C8-T1 causes Klumpke's palsy. This leads to weakness of the triceps, forearm pronators, and wrist flexors leading to a "clawlike" hand with good elbow and shoulder function.

Medical litigation pertaining to permanent BPI involves accusation of either not foreseeing BPI or mishandling it.[21]

However, recent reports have shown that BPIs can occur:[22]
- Even when there are no risk factors
- Even when there is no shoulder dystocia

Box 2: Complications due to shoulder dystocia—fetal.

- Fractures
- Brachial plexus injury
- Asphyxia
- Hypoxic ischemic encephalopathy fractures
- Death.

- In the posterior arm of infants, whose anterior shoulder was impacted behind the symphysis pubis
- Where fetuses are delivered by elective cesarean section
- Unrelated to the nature or number of maneuvers used to resolve shoulder dystocia
- In the immediate postpartum period as evidenced by electromyelogram.

Fractures

Though fractures of clavicle or humerus can occur, they are rarely serious and most often heal without long-term effects.

Perinatal Death

Perinatal death due to shoulder dystocia can range from 0 to 2.5. The cause of death is often hypoxia.

COMPLICATIONS IN THE MOTHER (BOX 3)

- Postpartum hemorrhage (PPH) is the most common complication in the mother and is seen in one quarter of the cases with shoulder dystocia. PPH can be both due to uterine atony and maternal injuries.
- Lacerations of the cervix, vagina, and the perineum are common. Third and fourth degree perineal tears are often associated with difficult shoulder deliveries.
- Rupture of the uterus can occur while attempting to resolve shoulder dystocia with various maneuvers.

Box 3: Complications due to shoulder dystocia—maternal.
- Postpartum hemorrhage
- Cervical/vaginal lacerations
- Bladder injury
- Perineal damage
- Uterine rupture.

- Bladder atony can result due to pressure on the bladder by the anterior shoulder against maternal pubic symphysis.
- Rare complications include separation of the symphyseal joint and damage to lateral femoral cutaneous nerve. In an effort to disimpact the shoulders, the maternal legs can be aggressively hyperflexed leading to these complications.

RECURRENCE OF SHOULDER DYSTOCIA

- Recurrence rate of shoulder dystocia ranges from 11.5% to 16.9%.[23]
- Maternal risk factors for recurrence of shoulder dystocia are high prepregnancy weight and excessive weight gain in pregnancy. In the fetus, birth weight greater than the index pregnancy, and birth weight more than 4,000 g are risk factors for recurrence.
- *Management:*[24] The decision regarding the mode of delivery should be undertaken after a thorough discussion with the woman and her family. Birth by cesarean section or vaginal delivery may be appropriate after an informed decision.

PREVENTION OF SHOULDER DYSTOCIA

- It is not possible to prevent shoulder dystocia because it is not possible to predict it in the first place.[25]
- Prophylactic cesarean section in women "likely" to have shoulder dystocia would result in a large number of unnecessary cesareans to prevent a single case of permanent BPI.[26] Elective induction of labor in women suspected to have macrosomic babies has not shown to decrease the number of shoulder dystocia.
  1. Shoulder dystocia drills conducted on regular basis can equip the labor room

personnel in better handling of the cases when it does happen.

> **POINTS TO REMEMBER**
> - Shoulder dystocia is difficult to predict and therefore to prevent
> - Macrosomia and diabetes are important predisposing factors in the woman
> - Though labor abnormalities were thought to be associated with shoulder dystocia, they are more due to macrosomia than being predictive of shoulder dystocia as such
> - It is wiser to be constantly prepared to face shoulder dystocia
> - Awareness and preparedness go a long way in the successful management of shoulder dystocia
> - Good communication and diligent documentation will go a long away even if the case ends up in a law suit.

REFERENCES

1. Spong CY, Beall M, Rodrigues D, et al. An objective definition of shoulder dystocia: prolonged head-to-body delivery intervals and/or the use of ancillary obstetric maneuvers. Obstet Gynecol. 1995;86:433-6.
2. Dodd JM, Catcheside B, Scheil W. Can shoulder dystocia be reliably predicted? Aust N Z J Obstet Gynaecol. 2012;52(3):248-52.
3. Acker D, Sachs B, Friedman E. Risk factors for shoulder dystocia. Obstet Gynecol. 1985;66:762-8.
4. Gherman RB, Goodwin TM, Souter I, et al. The McRoberts' maneuver for the alleviation of shoulder dystocia: how successful is it? Am J Obstet Gynecol. 1997;176:656-61.
5. Gregory KD, Henry OA, Ramicone E, et al. Maternal and infant complications in high and normal weight infants by method of delivery. Obstet Gynecol. 1998;92:507-13.
6. Kolderup LB, Laros RK Jr, Musci TJ. Incidence of persistent birth injury in macrosomic infants: association with mode of delivery. Am J Obstet Gynecol. 1997;177:37-41.
7. McFarland MB, Trylovich CG, Langer O. Anthropometric differences in macrosomic infants of diabetic and nondiabetic mothers. J Maternal Fetal Med. 1998;7:292-5.
8. Balaji V, Balaji MS, Seshiah V, et al. Maternal glycemia and neonates birth weight in Asian Indian Women. Diabetes Res Clin Pract. 2006;73:223-4.
9. Caughey AB, Sandberg PL, Zlatnik MG, et al. Forceps compared with vacuum: rates of neonatal and maternal morbidity. Obstet Gynecol. 2005;106:908-12.
10. Deaver JE, Cohen WR. An approach to the prediction of neonatal Erb palsy. J Perinat Med. 2009;37(2):150-5.
11. Lurie S, Levy R, Ben-Arie A, et al. Shoulder dystocia: Could it be deduced from the labor partogram? Am J Perinatology. 1995;12:61-2.
12. Stallings SP, Edwards RK, Johnson JWC. Correlation of head-to-body delivery intervals in shoulder dystocia and umbilical artery acidosis. Am J Obstet Gynecol. 2001;185:268-74.
13. Gonik B, Zhang N, Grimm M. Prediction of brachial plexus stretching during shoulder dystocia using a computer simulation model. Am J Obstet Gynecol. 2003;189(4):1168-72.
14. Buhimschi CS, Buhimschi IA, Malinow A, et al. Use of McRoberts' position during delivery and increase in pushing efficiency. Lancet. 2001;358:470-1.
15. Gottlirb AG, Galan HL. Shoulder dystocia: an update. Obstet Gynecol Clin N Am. 2007;34:501-31.
16. Vollebergh JH, van Dongen PW. The Zavanelli maneuver in shoulder dystocia. Eur J Obstet Gynecol Reprod Biol. 2000;89(1):81-4.
17. Royal College of Obstetricians and Gynaecologists. (2004). Shoulder Dystocia (RCOG Guideline No. 42. 2005). [online] Available from: https://www.rcog.org.uk/en/guidelines-research-services/guidelines/gtg42/ [Last accessed September, 2019].
18. Iffy L, Varadi V. Cerebral palsy following cutting of the nuchal cord before delivery. Med Law. 1994;13:323-30.
19. Pollack RN, Buchman AS, Yaffe H, et al. Obstetrical brachial plexus palsy: pathogenesis, risk factors, and prevention. Clin Obstet Gynecol. 2000;43:236-46.
20. Mancias P, Slopis JM, Yeakley JW, et al. Combined brachial plexus injury and root avulsion after complicated delivery. Muscle Nerve. 1994;17:1237-8.

21. Lerner HM, Salamon E. Permanent brachial plexus injury following vaginal delivery without physician traction or shoulder dystocia. Am J Obstet Gynecol. 2008;198(3):e7-8.
22. Gurewitsch ED, Johnson E, Hamzehzadeh S, et al. Risk factors for brachial plexus injury with and without shoulder dystocia. Am J Obstet Gynecol. 2006;194:486-92.
23. Lewis DF, Raymond RC, Perkins MP, et al. Recurrence rate of shoulder dystocia. Am J Obstet Gynecol. 1995;172:1369-71.
24. Greentop Guidelines N. 42, 2nd edition, March 2012
25. Gherman RB, Chauhan S, Ouzounian JG, et al. Shoulder dystocia: the unpreventable obstetric emergency with empiric management guidelines. Am J Obstet Gynecol. 2006;195: 657-72.
26. Hankins GD, Clark SM, Munn MB. Cesarean section on request at 39 weeks: impact on shoulder dystocia, fetal trauma, neonatal encephalopathy, and intrauterine fetal demise. Semin Perinatol. 2006;30(5):276-87.

Obstetric Emergencies

Shoulder Dystocia Delivery Note

Name of Patient   Age
Husband's Name   ID Number
Duration of second stage:
Delivery of Head: Spontaneous   ☐
              Instrumental   ☐
              Forceps   ☐
              Vacuum   ☐
Time of delivery of the Head..

Initial Traction:
☐ Gentle attempt at traction, assisted by maternal expulsive forces

The arm under the symphysis: ☐ Right   ☐ Left
Maneuvers used and the order in which they were utilized.

Maneuvers utilized	**In which order (circle)**	**By whom**
☐ McRoberts	1 2 3 4 5 6 7	
☐ Suprapubic pressure	1 2 3 4 5 6 7	
☐ Episiotomy	1 2 3 4 5 6 7	
☐ Posterior arm release	1 2 3 4 5 6 7	
☐ Rubin's maneuver	1 2 3 4 5 6 7	
☐ Woods maneuver	1 2 3 4 5 6 7	
☐ Other (list)	1 2 3 4 5 6 7	

Time body delivered ....

Condition of the Baby   Apgars
                                Injuries
                                Birth weight
                                Any other

Condition of the Mother   PPH
                                Cervical tear
                                Uterine tear
                                Any other
Primary Care Provider   Nurse

Other Care Providers in attendance   1.   2.   3.

Signature ....

CHAPTER 9

Hypertensive Emergencies in Pregnancy and Labor

Sunitha B

INTRODUCTION

Amongst the causes of maternal mortality, hypertensive disorders of pregnancy stands as one of the foremost cause, in both the developed and underdeveloped countries of the world. It is an enigma even today to both the patients and the treating obstetrician and continues to remain as a mystery in obstetrics. It complicates 5–10% of all the pregnancies and is responsible for 10–15% of maternal mortality especially in the third world countries.[1-3]

DEFINITION OF HYPERTENSIVE DISORDERS

- A pregnant mother whose mean reading of systolic blood pressure (SBP) was greater than or equal to 140 mm Hg and/or diastolic blood pressure (DBP) was greater than or equal to 90 mm Hg was the landmark criteria to call a patient to be hypertensive (DBP ≥90 mm Hg and/or SBP ≥140 mm Hg).
- Recording of the blood pressure must be taken appropriately with adequate size of the cuff.
- Korotkoff V sound is used to define diastolic pressure.
- In the previous decade, SBP recording of more than 30 mm Hg or DBP recording of more than 15 mm Hg, than the recording done in the midpregnancy was used as the main criteria to diagnose hypertension in pregnancy, even when the recent blood pressure recording was less than 140/90 mm of Hg. It is suggested that these women should be under more close surveillance because eclampsia can still occur even though the blood pressures have been lower than 140/90 mm Hg.[4]

LATEST CLASSIFICATION OF HYPERTENSIVE DISORDERS OF PREGNANCY

American College of Obstetricians and Gynecologists (2013) Task Force has described four types of hypertensive disease:
1. Preeclampsia and eclampsia syndrome
2. Chronic hypertension of any etiology
3. Preeclampsia superimposed on chronic hypertension
4. Gestational hypertension.

In gestational hypertension, preeclampsia syndrome does not develop and hypertension does not persist beyond 12 weeks postpartum. This has replaced the traditional pregnancy-induced hypertension.

More importantly, this way of classifying hypertensive disorders has helped to differentiate the preeclampsia—eclampsia syndrome from other causes because it is a more dangerous condition with increased morbidity and mortality (Table 1).[5]

INCIDENCE

- *Age of the pregnant woman*: Young women may develop preeclampsia, whereas old

TABLE 1: Essential findings in hypertensive disorders of pregnancy.

Type of hypertension	Diagnostic requirements
Gestational hypertension	Blood pressure ≥ 140/90 mm Hg in a previously normotensive woman after completing 20 weeks of gestation
Preeclampsia	• Blood pressure of ≥ 140/90 mm Hg after 20 weeks of pregnancy in a woman • Proteinuria with excretion ≥ 300 mg of protein in 1L of urine or 500 mg in 24 hours, without urinary tract infection
Eclampsia	Convulsions or seizures occurring in a woman with preeclampsia, with no other causes of seizures
Chronic hypertension	Hypertension is noted before 20th week of pregnancy or remains to be present for longer than 6 weeks postdelivery, or both
Superimposed preeclampsia	If a woman with chronic or essential hypertension is found to become proteinuric, it is called superimposed preeclampsia during pregnancy

women with chronic hypertension can develop superimposed preeclampsia.
- *Maternal race and ethnicity*: In a study conducted by Maternal–Fetal Medicine Units (MFMU) network, it was noticed that the incidence of preeclampsia was about 11% in African-American women, 9% in Hispanic and 5% in white.[6]
- Parity, nulliparity has 3–10% risk and in multiparity, the risk for preeclampsia is 1.4–4%.[7]

RISK PREDICTORS

- Medical conditions like systemic lupus erythematosus, chronic kidney disease, diabetes, and antiphospholipid antibody syndrome increase risk of preeclampsia.[8]
- Increased risk seen in metabolic syndrome and hyperhomocysteinemia.[9]
- *Past obstetric history*: Previous abruption, previous preeclampsia, and prior stillbirth.
- Women conceived with assisted reproductive techniques, multiple pregnancy and obesity during pregnancy are at increased risk to develop hypertension during pregnancy.
- Pregnancies with a male fetus are also at slightly higher risk.[10]
- Smoking can sometimes reduce the risk for hypertension during pregnancy.[11]
- Other factors known to be associated are human immunodeficiency virus (HIV) seropositivity and sleep-disordered breathing.[12]
- *Genetic predisposition*: Numerous candidate genes have been proposed to cause pathological mechanism as a risk factor for preeclampsia.[13]

PATHOPHYSIOLOGY

Hypertensive disorders during pregnancy are seen in women with the following characteristics:
- Predisposition to chorionic villi in the first pregnancy
- Twin pregnancy or hydatidiform mole
- Women having medical conditions such as cardiovascular or kidney disease
- Diabetic women with obesity and women with immunological disorders
- Some women are genetically predetermined to become hypertensive in pregnancy
- The series of events, which culminate in preeclampsia syndrome are:
  - *Stage 1*: Faulty endovascular trophoblastic remodeling
  - *Stage 2*: Systemic inflammatory response, leading to clinical preeclampsia.

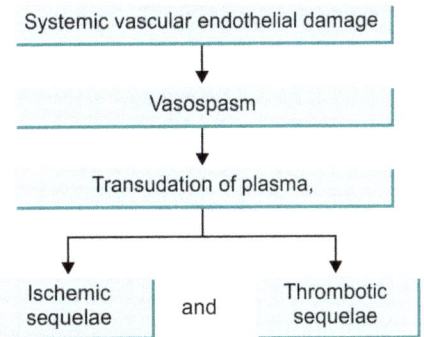

The mechanisms proposed to explain the cause of preeclampsia are:

- *Asynchronous trophoblastic invasion*: In normal placentation, the spiral arterioles undergo changes in the decidua basalis and endovascular trophoblasts invade and remodel the endothelial and muscular lining of the arterioles to enlarge the diameter of the vessel.
  - In preeclampsia, trophoblastic invasion is never complete. It is faulty trophoblastic invasion, which is significantly seen in the biopsy specimens of these placentae. The decidual vessels are lined with endovascular trophoblasts, but remodeling does not happen at the myometrial arterioles and the average external diameter of the vessel is very less, lesser than 50% than that seen in normal placentae.
  - Soluble antiangiogenic growth factors are elevated.
  - There can be lipid accumulation in myointimal cells and macrophages as seen in atherosis.

  Resultant decreased placental blood flow and perfusion results in a low oxygen or a hypoxic environment and there is release of microparticles, which causes systemic inflammatory response (Fig. 1).[14-16]

- *Immunological factors*:
  - There can be acute rejection of the fetus due to loss of maternal immune tolerance to paternally originated placental and fetal antigens. This can cause poor outcome of pregnancy.[17]
  - Blocking antibodies to placental antigenic sites is not formed sufficiently.
  - Antiangiogenic factors, soluble fms-like tyrosine kinase 1 and soluble endoglin levels are elevated in the serum and angiogenic growth factors like placental growth factors are reduced. The gene for sFlt-1 is on chromosome 13.[18]

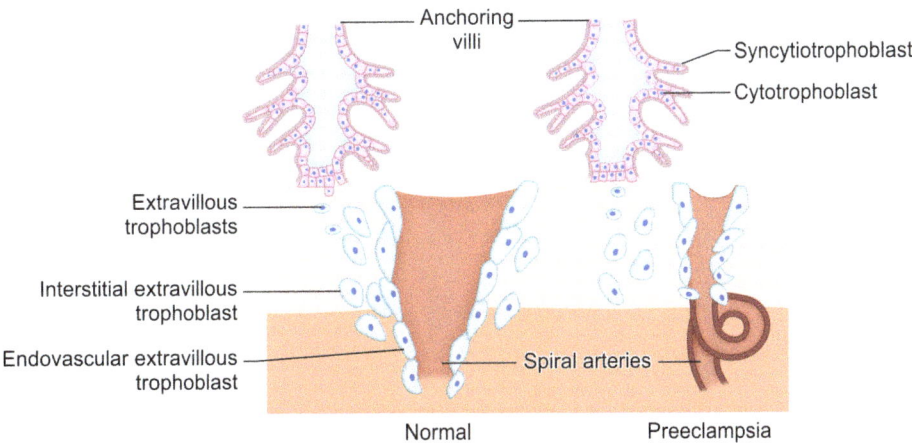

Fig. 1: Trophoblastic invasion.

- There can be reduced expression of immunosuppressive nonclassic human leukocyte antigen G (HLA G).
- Type 2 T helper cells activity, which facilitates humoral immunity, is increased when compared to type 1, which releases inflammatory cytokines. In preeclamptic women, in the early part of second trimester, Th1 action is increased (Figs. 2A and B).
- *Endothelial cell activation (Flowchart 1)*[20,21]
- *Genetic factors*:
  - Preeclampsia appears to be a multi-factorial, polygenic disorder. It involves the inherited genes from both mother and father, which control the enzyme actions and metabolic functions in all the organs of the body.[22]
  - Phenotypic expression may vary among similar genotypes depending on the environmental factor interaction.
  - Fetal genes on chromosome 18 have been linked preeclampsia predisposition (Tables 2 and 3).[23]

SCREENING TESTS

- Tests for increased vascular resistance and decreased placental blood flow (Table 4).
- Tests for endocrine function of the fetal-placental unit:
  - Analysis of β-human chorionic gonadotropin, α-fetoprotein, estriol, pregnancy-associated plasma protein A, inhibin A, etc. has been proposed, but none of these tests are clinically useful predicting development of hypertension.
- *Renal function tests (Table 5).*[35]
- Tests for endothelial dysfunction (Table 6).
- Other markers:
  - Increased and accelerated apoptosis of cytotrophoblastic cells causes release of cell-free DNA (cfDNA) in preeclampsia.[30]
  - Proteomic, metabolomic, and transcriptomic technologies can be used to understand serum and urinary proteins and their cellular metabolites. These may become future useful in prediction of preeclampsia.[31]

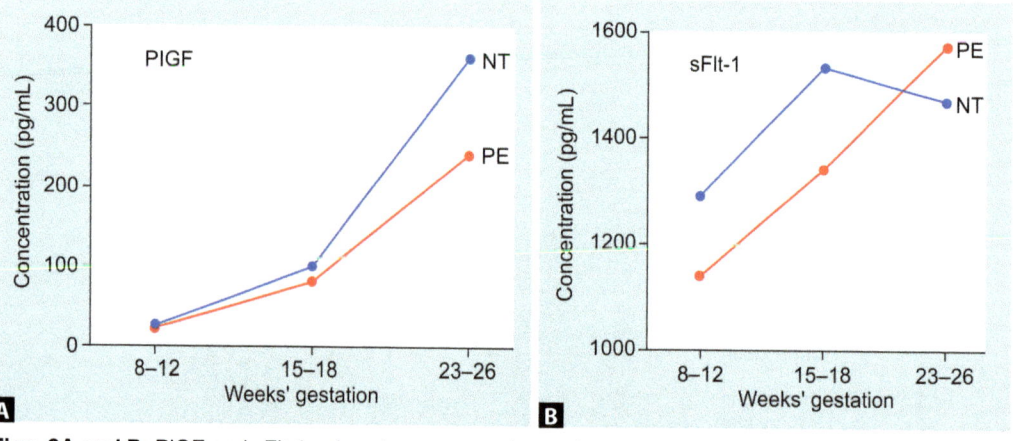

Figs. 2A and B: PlGF and sFlt-1 values in normotension and preeclampsia.
(NT: normotensive; PE: preeclampsia; sFlt: soluble fms-like tyrosine molecule; PlGF: placental growth factor)[19]

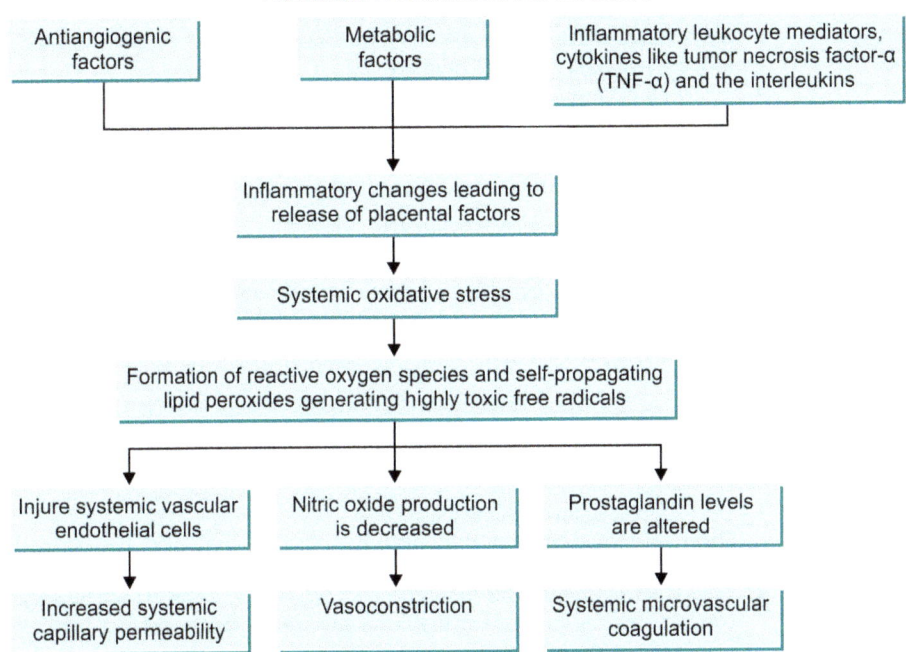

Flowchart 1: Endothelial cell activation.

TABLE 2: Classical features in preeclampsia.	
Vasospasm	• Constriction of blood vessels because of activation of the endothelium • Injury to the basement membrane causes leakage of blood constituents like platelets and fibrinogen, which gets deposited in the subendothelium plane
Endothelial cell injury	There is less nitric oxide and hence more coagulation and increased sensitivity to vasopressors
Increased pressor responses	• Endothelial prostacyclin (PGI2) (which reduces the pressor response) is lower in preeclampsia • Thromboxane A2 levels are increased, and the prostacyclin: thromboxane A2 ratio reduces • Endothelins which cause vasoconstriction are elevated to super normal levels[24]
Angiogenic and antiangiogenic proteins	• Due to hypoxia at the uteroplacental interface, there is imbalance between angiogenic and antiangiogenic factors[25] • Soluble fms-like tyrosine kinase 1 (sFlt-1) causes endothelial dysfunction • Soluble endoglin (sEng) reduces endothelial nitric oxide-dependent vasodilatation

TABLE 3: The summarized changes in organs and various systems.	
Myocardial function	• *Diastolic dysfunction* is seen in 40–45% with this dysfunction, ventricles do not properly relax and cannot fill properly • In chronic hypertension, there is concentric ventricular hypertrophy and diastolic dysfunction which gives rise to cardiogenic pulmonary edema[26]
Blood volume	Hemoconcentration is absolutely seen in eclampsia. Importantly, women with severe hemoconcentration are highly sensitive to even normal blood loss during delivery
Maternal thrombocytopenia	• There is *platelet activation* and *increased clearance* • Count <100,000/µL is more troublesome
Hemolysis	There is rise in serum lactate dehydrogenase levels and fall in haptoglobin levels
HELLP syndrome	Hemolysis, thrombocytopenia with abnormally elevated serum liver transaminase levels that indicated hepatocellular necrosis.[27] Coined by Weinstein (1982)
Endocrine and hormonal alterations	• Renin • Angiotensin II • Aldosterone • Deoxycorticosterone and atrial natriuretic peptide (ANP) are elevated
Fluid and electrolyte alterations	• The extracellular fluid volume is increased • There is reduced plasma oncotic pressure • Intravascular volume is contracted • Lactic acidosis (metabolic acidosis) is seen in eclampsia, serum pH and bicarbonate concentration are lowered and the subsequent respiratory loss of carbon dioxide causes respiratory acidosis
Kidney	• Renal plasma flow and glomerular filtration rate are reduced • The histopathological changes are those of glomerular endotheliosis • Serum creatinine levels increase • *Urine osmolality and urine*: Plasma creatinine ratio is increased • Plasma uric acid concentration is characteristically on the higher side • Acute tubular necrosis which can cause acute kidney injury can be caused by hemorrhage with hypovolemia and hypotension
Proteinuria	• It is defined by 24-hour urinary excretion of protein more than 300 mg • *Urine protein:* Creatinine ratio of more than or equal to 0.3, or • Urine protein values of 30 mg/dL (1+ dipstick) in random urine samples
Liver	• Hepatic lesions in severe preeclampsia and eclampsia are regions of periportal hemorrhage with hepatic infarction and hepatocellular necrosis, in the liver periphery with elevated serum hepatic transaminase levels (Hecht, 2017) • Subcapsular hematoma can be seen which may rupture
Brain	• Intracerebral hemorrhage • There can be cortical and subcortical petechial hemorrhages • Subcortical edema
Cerebrovascular pathophysiology	• Cerebrovascular overregulation can lead to vasospasm resulting in ischemia, edema, and infarction • Sudden increase in systemic blood pressure can cause vasogenic edema
Neurological symptoms	• Headache and scotomata • Convulsions • Confusion and sometimes irreversible coma • Visual symptoms include diplopia, scotomata, and sometimes blindness • Occipital blindness also called as amaurosis (dimming)

PREVENTION

Several methods have been evaluated (Table 7).[32]

PREECLAMPSIA

Proteinuria with hypertension, preeclampsia, is managed based on the clinical condition of the patient and the duration of pregnancy.

The main objectives in the management of preeclampsia are:
- Delivering the mother with reduced morbidity to both the mother and the baby,
- Birth of a healthy baby and
- Restoring the health of the mother.

Surveillance (Tables 8 and 9)

- Possible by increasing outpatient visits by watching out for imminent symptoms.
- Hospitalization in cases of overt hypertension, rapid weight gain, proteinuria, headache, visual symptoms, or when woman experiences epigastric pain.
- When hospitalized:
  - 4th hourly blood pressure readings with an appropriate-size cuff
  - Detailed clinical examination
  - Daily weight measurement
  - *Quantification of proteinuria* or urine *protein*: Creatinine ratio

TABLE 4: Tests which can predict the development of the preeclampsia syndrome.

Tests to see whether the blood pressure increases when exposed to a stimulus	• Done at 28–32 weeks of gestation. Woman first rests in the left lateral decubitus position and if increase in blood pressure is noted when she rolls over to supine position, then the test is said to be positive test • In the angiotensin II infusion test, angiotensin is given intravenously in slow increasing doses, and the blood pressure is quantified Sensitivity Specificity 55–70% 85%[35]
Uterine artery Doppler	• There is increased pulsatility index in uterine artery Doppler in the first two trimesters • There can be exaggerated diastolic notch

TABLE 5: Biochemical predictors: Sensitivity and specificity.

Biochemical test	Sensitivity	Specificity
Hyperuricemia	0–55%	77–95%.
Microalbuminuria	7–90%	29–97%

TABLE 6: Pathophysiological basis of biochemical tests.

Biochemical tests	Pathophysiology
Thrombocytopenia and platelet dysfunction	• Platelet activation • Mean platelet volume increases as there are immature platelets
Imbalance in angiogenic and antiangiogenic factors	• Serum levels of angiogenic factors, VEGF and PlGF reduce • Serum levels of sFlt-1 and sEng (antiangiogenic factors) starts to increase[28] Sensitivity Specificity 30–50% 90%[29]

(PlGF: placenta growth factor; VEGF: vascular endothelial growth factor)

TABLE 7: Preventive methods.

Dietary manipulation	• Low-salt diet, • Calcium or fish oil supplementation
Exercise	Physical activity and stretching
Cardiovascular drugs	Antihypertensive drugs
Antioxidants	Ascorbic acid (vitamin C), α-tocopherol (vitamin E), and vitamin D
Antithrombotic drugs	Low-dose aspirin, aspirin/dipyridamole, aspirin + heparin, and aspirin + ketanserin

TABLE 8: Mild and severe preeclampsia.

Abnormality	Mild	Severe
Diastolic BP	<110 mm of Hg	≥ 110 mm of Hg
Systolic BP	<160 mm of Hg	≥ 160 mm of Hg
Proteinuria	Nil or may be traces	Nil to 4+
Headache	--	+
Visual disturbances	–	+
Upper abdominal pain	–	+
Oliguria	–	+
Convulsion	Within range	+
Serum creatinine	–	Elevated
Thrombocytopenia (<1 lakh/cmm)	Mild	+
Serum transaminase increase	–	Marked
Fetal growth restriction	–	+
Pulmonary edema	Late	+
Gestational age		Early

TABLE 9: Management for mild cases.

< 37 weeks	>37 weeks
• Watchful expectancy • Be guarded about the progress of disease • Increase surveillance and evaluation if necessary	• Wait for spontaneous onset of labor • Or until Bishops score becomes suitable for induction of labor

- Hemoglobin with packed cell volume (PCV)
- Platelet count
- Checking serum creatinine and hepatic transaminase levels
- Serum uric acid and lactate dehydrogenase levels and coagulation studies[33]
- Obstetric examination for growth and well-being
- Ultrasound for estimated fetal weight by fetal biometry, for amniotic fluid volume and Doppler.

TABLE 10: Management for severe cases.

Cervix unfavorable	• Induce labor, cervical ripening with prostaglandins, or osmotic dilator may be required • Cesarean delivery is carried out in cases of failed induction[34]
Cervix favorable and gestational age near term	Induce labor

- Management protocols include:
  - Reduced physical activity
  - Protein rich diet, and sodium and fluid optimal
  - Assess the severity of disorder
  - Formulating plan for timely delivery.

Severe preeclampsia management includes anticonvulsant and more than often antihypertensive therapy which is followed by delivery (Table 10).

Preventive Management Strategies

- *Antioxidants*: No beneficial effects noted.
- Statins can inhibit sFlt-1 release. The MFMU network has designed a randomized control trial to test use of pravastatin for prevention of preeclampsia.[35]
- Metformin reduces sFlt-1 and sEng activity and thus has the potential to prevent preeclampsia.[36]
- *Antithrombotic agents*: Low-molecular-weight heparin for prophylaxis has been studied in several randomized trials. The risk for recurrent preeclampsia, abruption, or fetal-growth restriction was similar in women receiving heparin or placebo.
- Aspirin orally, in low doses of 50–150 mg daily can block platelet thromboxane A2 synthesis but does not interfere with the prostacyclin pathway.[37] The US Preventive Services Task Force has recommended use

of low-dose aspirin prophylaxis for women at high risk for preeclampsia.[38]

Drugs to Reduce Blood Pressure in Mild-to-Moderate Hypertension

Antihypertensive treatment in mild-to-moderate hypertension has been controversial and disappointing. It has a definitive role when severe preeclampsia develops in a woman with fetal viability. It helps to improve neonatal outcome without causing any harm to the mother.

Indications for Delivery in Women with Gestational Age Less than 34 Weeks

Plan emergency delivery after stabilizing the mother and after giving the first dose of corticosteroid for lung maturity in cases of:
- Hypertensive crisis
- Eclampsia
- Pulmonary edema
- Placental abruption
- Disseminated intravascular coagulation
- Fetal compromise
- Fetal demise.

Delivery can be delayed by 48 hours after giving corticosteroid therapy for lung maturity in the following cases:
- Preterm prelabor rupture of membranes
- Thrombocytopenia especially when the value is <100,000/μL
- Hepatic transaminase levels elevated more than two times of the normal
- Fetal-growth restriction
- Oligoamnios
- Umbilical artery Doppler showing reversed end-diastolic flow
- Increasing serum creatinine indicating progressive renal disease.

Experimental Therapies

Therapies have attempted to lower serum levels or mitigate the action of antiangiogenic factors. Some of these include therapeutic apheresis, done to lower sFlt-1 levels.[39]

ECLAMPSIA

- When generalized tonic-clonic convulsions occur in a woman with preeclampsia, it is termed as eclampsia.
- Eclampsia is usually seen in the third trimester.
- The incidence of postpartum eclampsia has reduced in recent past, due to improved pregnancy care, early identification of preeclampsia, and prophylactic use of magnesium sulfate for prevention of eclampsia.[40]

Clinical Features in Eclampsia

- There are generalized tonic clonic convulsions followed by a confused state, wherein the woman is drowsy, but arousable
- The respiratory rate is increased
- There can be respiratory and lactic acidosis with central cyanosis
- High fever can be seen in women with cerebrovascular hemorrhage and the prognosis becomes poor
- Proteinuria—nil to 4+
- Urine output—reduced or woman can become anuric
- Edema—both peripheral and sometimes pulmonary edema
- Rarely, sudden death can occur simultaneously with an eclamptic convulsion, or it may occur later due to massive cerebral hemorrhage
- Hemiplegia can result from cerebral hemorrhage not amounting to death
- Sometimes blindness may occur following a seizure.

Differential diagnosis of convulsions during pregnancy:
- Epilepsy
- Infections resulting in encephalitis and meningitis

- Space occupying lesions like brain tumor and neurocysticercosis
- Immunological causes like amniotic fluid embolism
- Iatrogenic causes like postdural puncture cephalalgia
- Intracerebral hemorrhage due to ruptured cerebral aneurysm in late pregnancy or in the puerperal period.

The prime principles in the management of eclampsia:
- To predict onset of convulsions
- To prevent intracerebral hemorrhage and to prevent injuries to major organs of the body
- To have a healthy mother and to deliver a healthy newborn.

The management objectives are:
- *Control of convulsions*: The drug of choice in eclampsia is magnesium sulfate.
- *Antihypertensives* to reduce blood pressure
- *Judicious use of diuretics*, only in cases of pulmonary edema. Fluid overload to be prevented by reducing intravenous fluid administration and avoiding the use of hypertonic agents
- *Careful timing of delivery of the fetus.*

Dosage Regimen of Magnesium Sulfate in Management of Severe Preeclampsia and Eclampsia

Loading dose consists of administering 4 g of magnesium sulfate intravenously over 20 minutes, and maintenance dose of 2 g/h infusion.[41] Maintenance dose of magnesium sulfate therapy is continued for at least 24 hours postdelivery or after last convulsion whichever is later.
- Monitor urine output and serum creatinine levels
- Patellar reflexes to be checked as it is seen to disappear when the plasma magnesium level reaches 12 mg/dL, most likely due to curariform action. This is a warning sign of impending magnesium toxicity.
- With magnesium toxicity, respiratory rate decreases. Treatment is by giving calcium gluconate or calcium chloride, 1-g intravenously.[42]

Treatment of Severe Hypertension

Severe hypertension can increase maternal and fetal morbidity and mortality as it can cause:
- Cerebrovascular hemorrhage
- Hypertensive encephalopathy
- Eclamptic convulsions in women with preeclampsia
- Abruption placental abruption
- Congestive heart failure.

The working group for the National High Blood Pressure Education Program (NHBPEP) (2000) and the 2013 Task Force recommends that the antihypertensives should be used to reduce SBP to 160 mm of Hg or low, and to reduce diastolic pressure to 110 mm of Hg or low.

The drugs routinely used are *hydralazine, labetalol, and nifedipine* (Table 11).

Other antihypertensive agents which have not been widely used are methyl dopa, verapamil, nitroglycerin, nitroprusside, ketanserin, nicardipine, and nimodipine.[43]

Postpartum Hypertension

- In about 8% of the women, persistent severe hypertension can develop de novo in the postpartum.
- In reversible cerebral vasoconstriction syndrome, which can cause persistent hypertension in the postpartum period, women complain of "thunderclap" headaches and seizures. It is a form of postpartum angiopathy.

TABLE 11: Antihypertensives.

Drug	Hydralazine	Labetalol	Nifedipine
Category of antihypertensive	Vasodilator	Selective α- and nonselective β-blocker	Calcium-channel blocker
Initial dose	5 to 10 mg intravenously	10 mg intravenously single dose	10-mg immediate-release oral dose
Subsequent dose	10 mg doses to be given at 15 to 20 minute intervals until the blood pressure is normalized	20 mg IV If the blood pressure does not reduce in 10 minutes. Next, 40 mg, 80 mg dose can be given, maximum 200 mg	10–20 mg in next 20–30 minutes
Onset of action	10 minutes	10 minutes	20 minutes
Contraindication	Lupus syndrome	Bronchial asthma	Cardiac failure

LONG-TERM CONSEQUENCES

Future Pregnancies

- Hypertensive disorders in the first pregnancy can become markers of preterm labor and fetal-growth restriction in the later pregnancies.[44]

Long-term Morbidity and Mortality

- Preeclampsia syndrome is known to cause subsequent long-term cardiovascular disorders with its resultant sequelae.

CONCLUSION

Hypertension in pregnancy is known to have increased maternal and fetal morbidity and mortality. It is possible to prevent complications by early diagnosis, careful surveillance, and timely intervention. Screening methods are not highly sensitive at present. We need to have a sound screening strategy in order to improve the maternal and fetal outcomes.

REFERENCES

1. Vigil-De Gracia P, Montufar-Rueda C, Ruiz J. Expectant management of severe preeclampsia and preeclampsia superimposed on chronic hypertension between 24 and 34 weeks gestation. Eur J Obstet Gynecol Reprod Biol. 2003;107:24-7.
2. Barron WM, Murphy MB, Lindheimer MD. Hypertension pathophysiology, diagnosis and management. In: Laragh GH, Brenner BM, (Eds). Management of Hypertension during Pregnancy, Vol. 2, 3rd edition. Raven; New York: 1990. pp. 1809-27.
3. Magee LA, Pels A, Helewa M, et al. Diagnosis, evaluation, and management of the hypertensive disorders of pregnancy. Pregnancy Hypertension: An International Journal of Women's Cardiovascular Health. 2014;4(2):105-45.
4. American College of Obstetricians and Gynecologists: Hypertension in pregnancy. Report of the American College of Obstetricians and Gynecologists' Task Force on Hypertension in Pregnancy. Obstet Gynecol. 2013;122:1122.
5. Alexander JM, Cunningham FG. Management. In: Taylor RN, Roberts JM, Cunningham FG (Eds). Chesley's Hypertensive Disorders in Pregnancy, 4th edition. Amsterdam, Academic Press, 2015.
6. Myatt L, Clifton RG, Roberts JM, et al. First-trimester prediction of preeclampsia in nulliparous women at low risk. Obstet Gynecol. 2012;119(6):1234-42.
7. Fisher S, Roberts JM. The placenta in normal pregnancy and preeclampsia. In: Taylor RN, Roberts JM, Cunningham FG (Eds). Chesley's Hypertensive Disorders in Pregnancy, 4th edition. Amsterdam, Academic Press, 2015.

8. Bartsch E, Medcalf KE, Park AL, et al. Clinical risk factors for preeclampsia determined in early pregnancy: systematic review and meta-analysis of large cohort studies. BMJ. 2016;353:i1753.
9. Karumanchi SA, Granger JP. Preeclampsia and pregnancy-related hypertensive disorders. Hypertension. 2016;67:238-42.
10. Jaskolka D, Retnakaran R, Zinman B, et al. Fetal sex and maternal risk of pre-eclampsia/eclampsia:a systematic review and meta-analysis. BJOG. 2017;124(4):553-60.
11. Bainbridge SA, Sidle EH, Smith GN. Direct placental effects of cigarette smoke protect women from pre-eclampsia: the specific roles of carbon monoxide and antioxidant systems in the placenta. Med Hypotheses. 2005;64(1):17-27.
12. Facco FL, Parker CB, Reddy UM, et al. Association between sleep-disordered breathing and hypertensive disorders of pregnancy and gestational diabetes mellitus. Obstet Gynecol. 2017;129(1):31-41.
13. Buurma AJ, Turner RJ, Driessen JH, et al. Genetic variants in pre-eclampsia: a meta-analysis. Hum Reprod Update. 2013;19(3):289-303.
14. Phillips JK, Janowiak M, Badger GJ, et al. Evidence for distinct preterm and term phenotypes of preeclampsia. J Matern Fetal Neonatal Med. 2010;23(7):622-6.
15. Redman CW, Sargent IL, Taylor RN. Immunology of abnormal pregnancy and preeclampsia. In: Taylor RN, Roberts JM, Cunningham FG (Eds). Chesley's Hypertensive Disorders in Pregnancy, 4th edition. Amsterdam, Academic Press, 2015.
16. Brosens I, Pijnenborg R, Vercruysse L, et al. The "Great Obstetrical Syndromes" are associated with disorders of deep placentation. Am J Obstet Gynecol. 2011;204(3):193-201.
17. Hertig AT. Vascular pathology in the hypertensive albuminuric toxemias of pregnancy. Clinics. 1945;4:602-14.
18. Zhou Y, Damsky CH, Fisher SJ. Preeclampsia is associated with failure of human cytotrophoblasts to mimic a vascular adhesion phenotype. J Clin Invest. 1997;99(9):2152-64.
19. Erlebacher A. Immunology of the maternal-fetal interface. Annu Rev Immunol. 2013;31: 387-411.
20. Evans CS, Gooch L, Flotta D, et al. Cardiovascular system during the postpartum state in women with a history of preeclampsia. Hypertension. 2011;58(1):57-62.
21. Bdolah Y, Palomaki GE, Yaron Y, et al. Circulating angiogenic proteins in trisomy 13. Am J Obstet Gynecol. 2006;194(1):239-45.
22. Myatt L, Clifton R, Roberts J, et al. Can changes in angiogenic biomarkers between the first and second trimesters of pregnancy predict development of pre-eclampsia in a low-risk nulliparous patient population? BJOG. 2013;120(10):1183-91.
23. Manten GT, van der Hoek YY, Marko Sikkema J, et al. The role of lipoprotein (a) in pregnancies complicated by pre-eclampsia. Med Hypotheses. 2005;64(1):162-9
24. Triche EW, Uzun A, DeWan AT, et al. Bioinformatic approach to the genetics of preeclampsia. Obstet Gynecol. 2014;123(6): 1155-61.
25. Majander KK, Villa PM, Kivinen K, et al. A follow-up linkage study of Finnish pre-eclampsia families identifies a new fetal susceptibility locus on chromosome 18. Eur J Hum Genet. 2013;21(9):1024-6.
26. Suzuki Y, Yamamoto T, Mabuchi Y, et al. Ultrastructural changes in omental resistance artery in women with preeclampsia. Am J Obstet Gynecol. 2003;189(1):216-21.
27. Myers JE, Hart S, Armstrong S, et al. Evidence for multiple circulating factor in preeclampsia. Am J Obstet Gynecol. 2007;196(3):266. e1-6
28. Spitz B, Magness RR, Cox SM. Low-dose aspirin. I. Effect on angiotensin II pressor responses and blood prostaglandin concentrations in pregnant women sensitive to angiotensin II. Am J Obstet Gynecol. 1988;159(5):1035.
29. Davidge S, de Groot C, Taylor RN. Endothelial cell dysfunction and oxidative stress. In: Taylor RN, Roberts JM, Cunningham FG (Eds). Chesley's Hypertensive Disorders in Pregnancy, 4th edition. Amsterdam, Academic Press, 2015.
30. Ajne G, Wolff K, Fyhrquist F, et al. Endothelin converting enzyme (ECE) activity in normal pregnancy and preeclampsia. Hypertens Pregnancy. 2003;22(3):215-24.
31. Karumanchi SA. Angiogenic factors in preeclampsia from diagnosis to therapy. Hypertension. 2016;67(6):1072-9.

32. Wardhana MP, Dachlan EG, Dekker G. Pulmonary edema in preeclampsia: an Indonesian case-control study. J Matern Fetal Neonatal Med. 2018;31(6):689-95.
33. Chesley LC, Williams LO. Renal glomerular and tubular function in relation to the hyperuricemia of preeclampsia and eclampsia. Am J Obstet Gynecol. 1945;50:367.
34. Handor H, Daoudi R. Images in clinical medicine. Hypertensive retinopathy associated with preeclampsia. N Engl J Med. 2014;370(8):752.
35. Conde-Agudelo A, Romero R, Roberts JM. Tests to predict preeclampsia. In: Taylor RN, Roberts JM, Cunningham FG (Eds). Chesley's Hypertensive Disorders in Pregnancy, 4th edition. Amsterdam, Academic Press, 2015.
36. DiFederico E, Genbacev O, Fisher SJ. Preeclampsia is associated with widespread apoptosis of placental cytotrophoblasts within the uterine wall. Am J Pathol. 1999; 155:293-301.
37. Bahado-Singh RO, Akolekar R, Mandal R, et al. First-trimester metabolomic detection of late-onset preeclampsia. Am J Obstet Gynecol. 2013;208(1):58.e1-7.
38. Staff AC, Sibai BM, Cunningham FG. Prevention of preeclampsia and eclampsia. In: Taylor RN, Roberts JM, Cunningham FG (Eds). Chesley's Hypertensive Disorders in Pregnancy, 4th edition. Amsterdam, Academic Press, 2015.
39. Thangaratinam S, Ismail KMK, Sharp S, et al. Accuracy of serum uric acid in predicting complications of pre-eclampsia: a systematic review. BJOG. 2006;113: 369-78.
40. Alexander JM, Bloom SL, McIntire DD, et al. Severe preeclampsia and the very low-birthweight infant: is induction of labor harmful? Obstet Gynecol. 1999;93:485-8.
41. Cleary KL, Roney K, Costantine M. Challenges of studying drugs in pregnancy for off-label indications: pravastatin for preeclampsia prevention. Semin Perinatol. 2014;38:523-7.
42. Brownfoot FC, Hastie R, Hannan NJ, et al. Metformin as a prevention and treatment for preeclampsia: effects on soluble fms-like tyrosine kinase 1 and soluble endoglin secretion and endothelial dysfunction. Am J Obstet Gynecol. 2016;214(3):356.e1-356.
43. Wallenburg HC, Makovitz JW, Dekker GA, et al. Low-dose aspirin prevents pregnancy-induced hypertension and preeclampsia in angiotensin-sensitive primigravidae. Lancet.1986;327:1-7.
44. Askie LM, Henderson-Smart DJ, Stewart LA. Antiplatelet agents for the prevention of preeclampsia: a meta-analysis of individual data. Lancet. 2007;369(9575):1791-8.

CHAPTER 10

Cardiac Failure in Pregnancy

Shalini MA

DEFINITION

Heart failure (HF) is a clinical syndrome characterized by typical symptoms and signs caused by a structural and/or functional cardiac abnormality, resulting in a reduced cardiac output and/or elevated intracardiac pressures at rest or during stress.[1]

TERMINOLOGY OF VARIOUS TYPES OF HEART FAILURE

- Relevant to ejection fraction (Table 1).[1]
- *Relevant to the onset of heart failure:*[1]
    - *Asymptomatic left ventricular (LV) systolic dysfunction*: Patient with no typical symptoms and/or signs of HF and with reduced LV ejection fraction.
    - *Chronic HF*: Patient with previous history of HF for some time
    - *Stable HF*: In this condition, symptoms and signs of HF remain persistent for at least 1 month following treatment.
    - *Decompensated HF*: Worsening of the condition in a previous chronic stable patient of HF.
    - *New-onset (de-novo)*: Patients presenting with acute onset of HF.
- *Relevant to functional severity of heart failure [New York Heart Association (NYHA) classification]:*[1]

TABLE 1: Types of heart failure based on ejection fraction.

Types of heart failure	Heart failure with reduced ejection fraction	Heart failure with mid-range ejection fraction	Heart failure with preserved ejection fraction (HFpEF)
1	Symptoms +/− Signs[a]	Symptoms +/− signs[a]	Symptoms +/− Signs[a]
2	LVEF < 40%	LVEF 40–49%	LVEF >50%
3	–	• Natriuretic peptides levels are elevated[b] • Either one of additional criteria: – Related structural cardiac condition (LVH and/or LAE) – Diastolic dysfunction	• Natriuretic peptides levels are elevated[b] • Either one of additional criteria: – Related structural cardiac condition (LVH and/or LAE) – Diastolic dysfunction

(BNP: B-type natriuretic peptide; NT-proBNP: N-terminal pro-B type natriuretic peptide; LVH: left ventricular hypertrophy; LAE: left atrial enlargement; LVEF: left ventricular ejection fraction).
[a]Signs may be absent in early stages of HF (especially in HFpEF) and also in individuals treated with diuretics.
[b]BNP >35 pg/mL and /or NT-proBNP >125 pg/mL.

- *Class I*: No symptoms and no limitation in ordinary physical activity (e.g. fatigue, palpitations, shortness of breath when walking, climbing stairs, etc.).
- *Class II*: Mild symptoms (fatigue, palpitations, mild shortness of breath and/or angina) and slight limitation during ordinary activity.
- *Class III*: Marked limitation in ordinary physical activity due to symptoms, even during less-than ordinary activity (e.g. fatigue, palpitations, and shortness of breath when walking short distance; 20–100 m).
- *Class IV*: Severe limitation. Experiences symptoms even at rest.

MAGNITUDE OF HEART FAILURE

Pregnancy associated with cardiac disease is considered as an unintended cause of maternal death. As such the condition itself is irrelevant to any adverse outcome in pregnancy. Globally, indirect causes contribute about 25% of deaths disclosed in industrialized countries and even more so in sub-Saharan Africa and southern Asia; 28.6 and 29.3, respectively.[2]

Medical and surgical disorders account for 8.8% of deaths under indirect causes, marking this as a fourth most-leading cause of maternal death. In the subset of "medical and surgical disorders", significant deaths are due to cardiac disorders (more than half of deaths are due to ventricular failure; 36.5%).[2]

Hemodynamic Changes in Pregnancy[2]

Hemodynamic changes in pregnancy are given in Figure 1.

ETIOLOGY OF HEART FAILURE IN PREGNANCY[2]

- *Increased vascular resistance*:
  - Preeclampsia
  - Hypertensive cardiomyopathy
  - Pulmonary hypertension and right HF.
- Diseases affecting the aortic root
- Cardiac disease—ventricular failure:
  - Peripartum cardiomyopathy
  - Hereditary cardiomyopathies
  - Drug-induced cardiomyopathy
  - Autoimmune and infective cardiomyopathies
  - Amniotic fluid embolism
  - Ischemic heart disease.
- Cardiac disease—Valvular lesions.
- Cardiac disease—congenital abnormalities of heart and proximal vasculature.

SYMPTOMS AND SIGNS

Symptoms and signs of HF are discussed in Table 2.

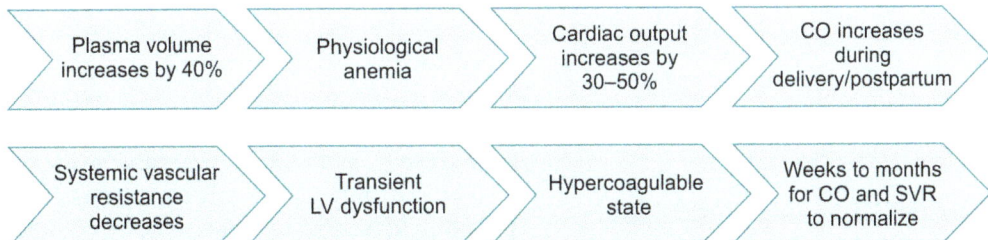

Fig. 1: Physiological changes occurring during pregnancy.
(CO: cardiac output; LV: left ventricle; SVR: systemic vascular resistance)

TABLE 2: Symptoms and signs typical of heart failure.[1]

Symptoms	Signs
Typical	*More specific*
• Breathlessness • Paroxysmal nocturnal dyspnea • Orthopnea • Ankle swelling • Fatigue, tiredness, and increased time to recover after exercise • Reduced exercise tolerance	• Third heart sound (gallop rhythm) • Elevated jugular venous pressure • Laterally displaced apical impulse • Hepatojugular reflux
Less typical	*Less specific*
• Wheezing • Nocturnal • Loss of appetite • Bloated feeling • Palpitations • Syncope • Depression • Confusion (especially in elderly) • Dizziness	• Tissue wasting (cachexia) • Weight gain (>2 kg/week) • Weight loss (in advanced HF) • Peripheral edema (ankle, sacral) • Cardiac murmur • Tachycardia • Irregular pulse • Tachypnea • Narrow pulse pressure • Pulmonary crepitations • Reduced air entry and dullness to percussion at lung bases (pleural effusion) • Cheyne–Stokes respiration • Ascites • Hepatomegaly • Oliguria • Cold extremities

DIAGNOSIS OF NONACUTE ONSET OF HEART FAILURE[1]

Refer to Flowchart 1.

DRUG THERAPY

The pharmacological management of cardiac condition in pregnant women involves the evaluation and treatment of HF and its effect on the fetus.

Diuretics

Diuretics are the first drug of choice in management of heart failure complicating pregnancy as it reduces preload. Hyperdynamic circulation which develops in pregnancy is due to the increased preload. Women with normal ventricular function respond to this change by increasing cardiac output. This mechanism does not happen when there is abnormal ventricular contractility. Interstitial fluid resorption occurs due to decreased pulmonary capillary pressures and filling pressures on left side, when preload is reduced.

Limitations

It slightly overthrows or limits the physiological changes of pregnancy, leading to limitation of essential rise of perfusion in both uterus and placenta. Intrauterine growth restriction is more often seen in the fetus of women with cardiac failure due to the low cardiac output in ventricular failure, which discerns the effects of treatment. There is no evidence, which suggests diuretic as any independent risk factor for fetal growth restriction.[2]

Preeclampsia when presented as an acute severe disease, it causes some degree of elevated ventricular diastolic dysfunction on the left side and vascular resistance. In such cases, management with parenteral vasodilators causing afterload reduction is preferred, as the fall of vascular resistance leads to increase in stroke volume in left ventricle leading to increased cardiac output with diminished filling pressures in the left side, secondarily. In contrast, the diuretic

Flowchart 1: Algorithmic approach for diagnosis of heart failure of nonacute onset.

```
Patient with suspected heart failure (nonacute onset)
                          ↓
ASSESSMENT OF HEART FAILURE PROBABILITY
I. Clinical history:
 • History of coronary artery disease
   (Myocardial infarction, revascularization)
 • History of arterial hypertension
 • Exposition to cardiotoxic drug/radiation
 • Use of diuretics
 • Orthopnea/paroxysmal nocturnal dyspnea
II. Physical examination:
 • Rales
 • Bilateral
 • Heart murmur
 • Jugular venous dilatation
 • Laterally displayed /broadened apical beat.
III. ECG: Any abnormality
```

- Assessment of natriuretic peptides not routinely done in clinical practice

≥ 1 present → **Natriuretic peptides**
- NT-proBNP ≥ 125 pg/mL
- BNP ≥ 35 pg/mL

All absent → **HF unlikely:** Consider other diagnosis

No → HF unlikely
Yes → Echocardiography → Normal → HF unlikely

On confirmation of heart failure: start appropriate treatment once aetiology is established

---

therapy causes pulmonary edema by depleting the already reduced intravascular volume and without any reduction in systemic vascular resistance.[2]

In acutely ill pregnant women, admitted in ICU due to preeclampsia with simultaneous LV failure and renal failure, nitroglycerine plays a major role as a combined arterial and venous vasodilator. With such context, reducing venous capacitance is beneficial.[2]

ACE Inhibitors

Angiotensin receptor blockers (ARB) and angiotensin-converting enzyme inhibitors (ACE) are included in this class of drugs. These drugs reduce the intravascular volume and vasodilation by intercepting angiotensin-aldosterone axis leading to natriuresis. Pregnancy is a state of physiological hyper-reninism, therefore these drugs are relatively contraindicated.[2]

Women treated with ACE inhibitors during their pregnancy, has risk of neonatal renal failure in the fetus and therefore, it is contraindicated during pregnancy. Breastfeeding women can safely use ACE inhibitors.[2]

Beta-blockers

Beta-blockers lower the heart rate and grant pronounced filling during diastole.

These are more useful in patients with systolic dysfunction and ejection fraction <40%. During pregnancy, data shows the correlation between escalated perinatal mortality, intrauterine growth restriction, and beta-blocker use in pregnancy. Beta-blockers can be used in cases where the mother's life is at risk, without considering the drug as contraindication in pregnancy.[2]

Spironolactone

It acts as a mild diuretic and is a potent potassium-sparing aldosterone antagonist. When given with other diuretics, spironolactone has synergistic action. Combined treatment with spironolactone, remarkably decreases the mortality rate in women with heart failure complicating the pregnancy. There is evidence of teratogenesis in rat models when spironolactone is used due to the anti-androgenic effect; therefore this drug should not be used in pregnancy. Less than one percent of the drug passes through breast milk to the child.[2]

MANAGING ARRHYTHMIAS

Up to 50% deaths in a population of heart failure, is due to sudden death. Atrial fibrillation is the most common type of arrhythmia in HF, which requires usage of beta-blockers and if necessary digoxin. When implantable devices are used for continuous monitoring, sustained ventricular tachyarrhythmia may be diagnosed better. It mandates the use of implantable cardioverter defibrillators and amiodarone.[2]

ASSIST DEVICES AND INOTROPIC SUPPORT

Inotropic support may be required to women with severely impaired ventricular function. Assist devices are a possible add on in treatment of intractable HF. It acts as a tie between access to cardiac transplantation services from the time of initial presentation to the hospital but evidence is limited.[2]

TREATING REVERSIBLE FACTORS

Anemia, overt or occult infection, and hyperthyroidism may exasperate the heart failure by elevating the heart rate. In puerperium, hyperthyroidism may be under diagnosed in relation to pregnancy. Postpartum thyroiditis affects about 5% of the women in the first year after delivery.[2]

During pregnancy, urinary infection is a common form of sepsis and following delivery, they are at risk of developing genital tract sepsis. Early recognition and treatment are required in these cases.

SUPPORTIVE MEASURES IN DECOMPENSATED HEART FAILURE DURING PREGNANCY[2]

- Early diagnosis and immediate management
- Maintenance and monitoring of oxygenation
- Thromboprophylaxis (low molecular weight heparin 40 mg S/C)
- Obstetric management
    - Assessing the risks of continuing the pregnancy and degree to which pregnancy is contributing to the development of HF.
    - Consequences of preterm delivery to be explained
    - Perspective of both partners in obtaining the decision regarding continuation or termination of the pregnancy
    - In preeclamptic mothers, development of pulmonary edema acts as an warning in pregnancy for pregnancy termination due to its high fatality rate.

MODE OF DELIVERY

The hemodynamic consequences of labor:
- Pain-mediated catecholamines
- Left ventricular workload increases.

The above changes cause intravascular blood volume to rise abruptly at the time of delivery. So these women require pain management and to cut short the second stage of labor using either forceps or a vacuum extractor.

Cesarean delivery can be either emergency or elective procedure which is associated with hemorrhage, anesthesia, and complication in the postoperative period. Decision for mode of delivery should be individualized, considering the parity, other comorbid conditions in pregnancy, and the severity of the cardiac condition.[2]

THE PUERPERIUM AND LONG-TERM MANAGEMENT[1,2]

- In the immediate puerperium, attention to be directed toward avoiding fluid overload.
- Women with failing ventricles and severe stenosed valves may benefit from intravenous diuretic therapy.
- Oxytocic drugs should be cautiously used as it has vasoactive properties (bolus dose of oxytocin causes vasodilatation and reflex tachycardia and ergometrine has vasoconstrictor effect on peripheral circulation).
- Prevention of infection by prophylactic antibiotics to limit the risk of endocarditis.
- The use of intrauterine device is recommended since hormonal contraceptives may interact with heart failure medications.[3]
- Breastfeeding in peripartum cardiomyopathy is still a question, up until now.

REFERENCES

1. Ponikowski P, Adriaan A, Stefan D. 2016 ESC Guidelines for the diagnosis and treatment of acute and chronic heart failure. Eur Heart J. 2016;37:2129-200.
2. Anthony J, Sliwa K. Decompensated Heart Failure. Card Fail Rev. 2015;1(2):20-6.
3. Hilfiker-Kleiner D, Haghikia A, Nonhoff J, et al. Peripartum cardiomyopathy: current management and future perspectives. Eur Heart J. 2015;36:1090-7.

CHAPTER 11

Acute Fatty Liver and Jaundice in Pregnancy

Chandana C

INTRODUCTION

Acute fatty liver of pregnancy (AFLP) is an uncommon, unique, disorder of pregnancy that occurs in the third trimester and early postpartum period. AFLP has incidence in the range of 1 in 7,000 to 1 in 15,000.[1-4] AFLP is distinguished by microvesicular liver steatosis, fulminant hepatic failure, and hepatic encephalopathy. AFLP is an obstetric emergency, with maternal and perinatal mortality as high has 75% and 85%, respectively in the past. In recent years with prompt early diagnosis and advances in intensive obstetric care, maternal and perinatal mortalities have been reduced to 18 and 23%, respectively.[5-7]

PATHOPHYSIOLOGY

Defect in fatty acid β-oxidation is a recognized cause of AFLP. The AFLP occurs, if the fetus has a defect in the enzymes required in the fatty acid β-oxidation. These defects are autosomal recessive and the fetus may be homozygous or heterozygous for these defects. The mutation in the long-chain 3-hydroxyacyl CoA dehydrogenase (LCHAD) enzyme is the most commonly identified defect in AFLP.

Newborns of AFLP mothers have shown to have LCHAD gene mutation, which leads to deficient LCHAD enzyme deficiency, this causes defect in fatty acid oxidation leading to accumulation of fetal fatty acids, which is transferred to the mother through the placenta. These fatty acids are deposited in the maternal liver and causes AFLP.[8,9]

The risk factors for AFLP are multigravida, male fetus, multiple gestation, low body mass index (BMI), previous episode of AFLP, and other coexisting liver disease of pregnancy [hemolysis, elevated liver enzymes, low platelets (HELLP) and preeclampsia].[10-13]

CLINICAL FEATURES

The AFLP occurs in the last trimester and immediate postpartum period. Usually, patients present with nonspecific symptoms include anorexia, nausea, vomiting, fatigue, malaise, pain abdomen in the epigastric/right upper quadrant, polydipsia/polyuria, and Jaundice. The disease may progress very quickly to acute hepatic failure with complications like coagulopathy, hypoglycemia, hepatic encephalopathy, and renal failure.[14,15] The laboratory findings of AFLP are leukocytosis, hemolysis, thrombocytopenia, elevated bilirubin, elevated serum aminotransferase, elevated alkaline phosphatase, prolongation of prothrombin and partial thromboplastin times, decreased levels of fibrinogen and antithrombin III, and positive for fibrin split products. The elevated aminotransferase can be related with elevated serum ammonia, uric acid, amino acid, hypoglycemia, and metabolic acidosis. Complicated cases may have elevated blood urea and creatinine.

The ultrasound imaging can show bright echotexture of the liver with fatty hepatic infiltration and ascites. Liver biopsy findings include diffuse or perivenular microvesicular steatosis, are gold standard for diagnosis of AFLP.[16,17] The Swansea criteria are used for diagnosis of AFLP (Box 1).[1,3] AFLP is diagnosed if at least 6 or more out of 15 criteria are satisfied, in the absence of other etiology of liver dysfunction. The AFLP condition is closely related and difficult to differentiate from HELLP, preeclampsia/eclampsia, intrahepatic cholestasis of pregnancy, and viral hepatitis. The characteristics and the management of common liver diseases in pregnancy are described in Table 1.

MANAGEMENT

Increased maternal and fetal mortality is associated with AFLP, hence, early recognition and diagnosis are important. Early recognition, prompt delivery, and multidisciplinary intensive care are the main stay in the treatment of AFLP (Flowchart 1). Monitoring and treatment of patients in intensive care unit are advised. Prior to delivery, maternal condition should be stabilized as follows:

- Assessment/management of airway and breathing
- Management of hypertension
- Aggressive management of hypoglycemia with 50% intravenous dextrose
- Aggressive management of coagulopathy with cryoprecipitate, fresh frozen plasma (FFP), and platelets
- Frequent maternal vital signs assessment and fetal well-being assessment
- Expedite delivery once mother is stabilized.

Cesarean section is indicated, if successful vaginal birth within 24 hours of induction of labor is unlikely or if there is rapid deterioration in maternal or fetal condition. In the presence of coagulopathy, delivery should be undertaken with perioperative administration of blood products. Mode of anesthesia has to be tailored based on the condition of the patient. Regional anesthesia has risk of spinal hematoma in presence of coagulopathy. General anesthesia has a negative impact on hepatic encephalopathy.

After delivery, patients of AFLP have increased risk of postpartum hemorrhage. The patient's coagulation profile and liver function test are monitored to assess for the evolving, or overt coagulopathy and hepatic encephalopathy. Liver transplantation to be considered in women with hepatic encephalopathy, worsening coagulopathy, or severe metabolic acidosis.[18]

The liver function and coagulation profile show improvement in 3–4 days after delivery. The AFLP can recur in subsequent pregnancy. Hence, these women should be advised, counseled, and investigated with

Box 1: Swansea diagnostic criteria for AFLP.

6 or more of criteria below in the absence of alternate etiology

Symptoms and signs:
- Pain abdomen
- Vomiting
- Polydipsia and polyuria
- Hepatic encephalopathy

Laboratory parameters:
- Raised bilirubin levels (> 14 µmol/L)
- Raised aminotransferase (ALT or AST > 42 IU/L)
- Increased total leukocyte count (>11 x 10^9/L)
- Hypoglycemia (<4 µmol/L)
- Hyperuricemia (>340/µmol/L)
- Hyperammonemia (>47 µmol/L)
- Impaired coagulation profile (PT > 14 s or APTT > 34 s)
- Deranged kidney function (serum creatinine > 150 µmol/L)

Imaging and histology:
- Bright liver or ascites on ultrasound
- Live biopsy showing microvesicular steatosis

Adapted from reference 1 and 3
(AST: aspartate transaminase; ALT: alanine transaminase; APTT: activated partial thromboplastin time; PT: prothrombin time)

TABLE 1: Characteristic features and management of different liver diseases in pregnancy.

	Clinical features	Laboratory findings	Management
AFLP	• Pain abdomen • Nausea and vomiting • Jaundice • Hypoglycemia • Coagulopathy	• Hyperbilirubinemia—Elevated aminotransferase • Leukocytosis • Hypoglycemia • Hyperuricemia • Hyperammonemia • Coagulopathy • Deranged renal function	• Urgent delivery • Aggressive management of coagulopathy and hypoglycemia • Liver transplantation
Preeclampsia/eclampsia	• Edema • Hypertension • Nausea and vomiting • Visual disturbance • Headache • Abdominal/Epigastric pain • Jaundice	• Thrombocytopenia • Proteinuria • DIC	• Blood pressure control • Magnesium sulfate • Early delivery
HELLP syndrome	• Abdominal pain • Nausea and vomiting • Hypertension • Hematuria • Jaundice	• Hemolysis • Thrombocytopenia • Elevated liver enzymes • Elevated LDH • DIC	• Prompt delivery • Management of coagulopathy
Viral Hepatitis	• Nausea and vomiting • Fever • Jaundice	• Hyperbilirubinemia • Elevated liver enzymes • Positive serology test for hepatitis	Supportive management
Intrahepatic cholestasis of pregnancy	• Pruritis • Steatorrhea • Jaundice	• ALP and GGT markedly elevated • Elevated bile acids	• Ursodeoxycholic acid • Consider delivery at 37 weeks of gestation

(AFLP: acute fatty liver of pregnancy; ALP: alkaline phosphatase; DIC: disseminated intravascular coagulation; GGT: gamma glutamyl transpeptidase; HELLP: Hemolysis, elevated liver enzymes, low platelets; LDH: lactic acid dehydrogenase).

their newborns for LCHAD deficiency. In subsequent pregnancies, these women should be monitored closely for early symptoms and signs of acute fatty liver.

CONCLUSION

In summary, AFLP is an obstetric emergency with high maternal and fetal mortality. In recent years with early diagnosis, prompt delivery and multidisciplinary intensive care, have greatly improved maternal and fetal outcome. The Swansea criteria are useful in diagnosing AFLP. These patients usually have complete recovery without any risk of chronic liver disease. AFLP may recur in subsequent pregnancies, so all women with AFLP and babies born to them should be investigated for defects in fatty acid oxidation.

Flowchart 1: Algorithm for jaundice workup in late pregnancy.

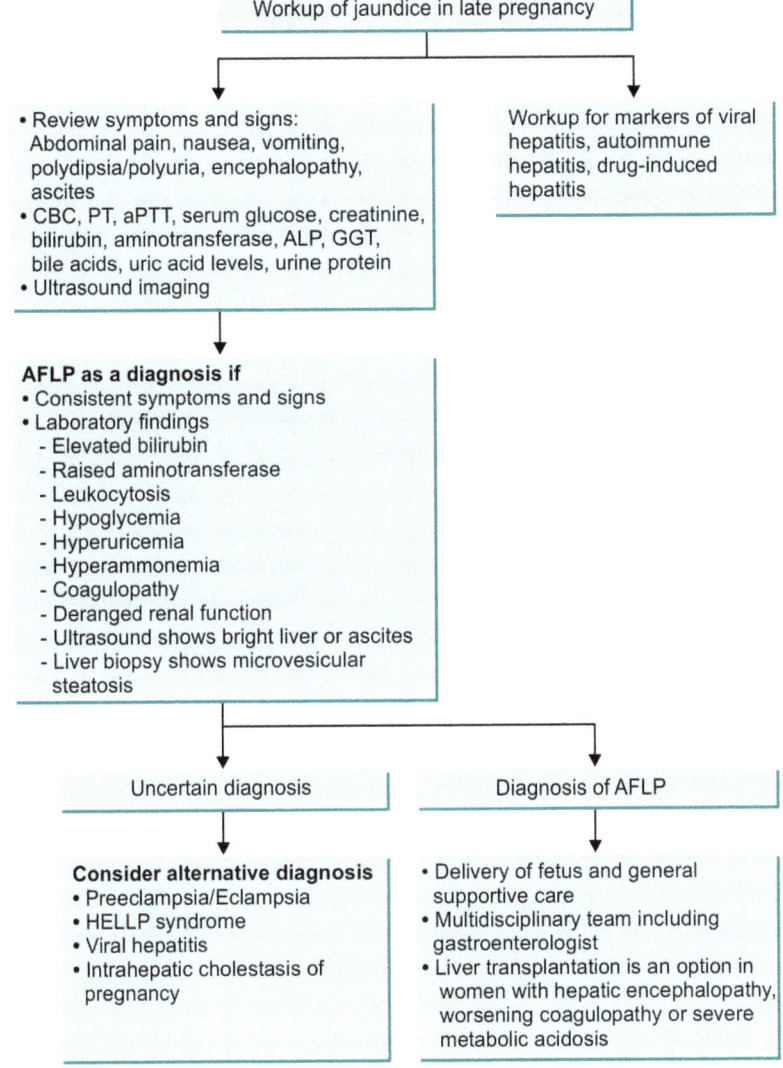

(AFLP: acute fatty liver of pregnancy; ALP: alkaline phosphatase; aPTT: activated partial thromboplastin time; CBC: complete blood count; GGT: gamma glutamyl transpeptidase; HELLP: hemolysis, elevated liver enzymes, low platelets; LDH: lactic acid dehydrogenase; PT: prothrombin time)

REFERENCES

1. Knight M, Nelson-Piercy C, Kurinczuk JJ, et al. A prospective national study of acute fatty liver of pregnancy in the UK. Gut. 2008;57:951-6.
2. Nelson DB, Yost NP, Cunningham FG. Acute fatty liver of pregnancy: clinical outcomes and expected duration of recovery. Am J Obstet Gynecol. 2013;209:456.e1-7.
3. Ch'ng CL, Morgan M, Hainsworth I, et al. Prospective study of liver dysfunction in pregnancy in Southwest Wales. Gut. 2002;51: 876-80.
4. Allen AM, Kim WR, Larson JJ, et al. The epidemiology of liver diseases unique to pregnancy in a US community: a population-based study. Clin Gastroenterol Hepatol. 2016;14:287-94.

5. Sheehan HL. The pathology of acute yellow atrophy and delayed chloroform poisoning. J Obstet Gynaecol Br Emp. 1940;47:49-62.
6. Kaplan MM. Acute fatty liver of pregnancy. N Engl J Med. 1985;313:367-70.
7. Knox TA, Olans LB. Liver disease in pregnancy. N Engl J Med. 1996;335:569-76.
8. Ibdah JA, Bennett MJ, Rinaldo P, et al. A fetal fatty-acid oxidation disorder as a cause of liver disease in pregnant women. N Engl J Med. 1999;340:1723-31.
9. Yang Z, Yamada J, Zhao Y, et al. Prospective screening for pediatric mitochondrial trifunctional protein defects in pregnancies complicated by liver disease. JAMA. 2002;288:2163-6.
10. Meng J, Wang S, Gu Y, et al. Prenatal predictors in postpartum recovery for acute fatty liver of pregnancy: experiences at a tertiary referral center. Arch Gynecol Obstet. 2015;293:1185-91.
11. Davidson KM, Simpson LL, Knox TA, et al. Acute fatty liver of pregnancy in triplet gestation. Obstet Gynecol. 1998;91:806-8.
12. Homer L, Hebert T, Nousbaum JB, et al. Comment confirmer le diagnostic de stéatose hépatique aiguë gravidique en urgence? [how to confirm the presence of acute fatty liver of pregnancy in an emergency] . Gynécol Obstét Fertil. 2008;37:245-61.
13. Bacq Y. Liver diseases unique to pregnancy: a 2010 update. Clin Res Hepatol Gastroenterol. 2011;35:182-93.
14. Vigil-De Gracia P. Acute fatty liver and HELLP syndrome: two distinct pregnancy disorders. Int J Gynaecol Obstet. 2001;73:215-20.
15. Reyes H, Sandoval L, Wainstein A, et al. Acute fatty liver of pregnancy: a clinical study of 12 episodes in 11 patients. Gut. 1994;35:101-6.
16. Natarajan SK, Eapen CE, Pullimood AB, et al. Oxidative stress in experimental liver microvesicular steatosis: role of mitochondria and peroxisomes. J Gastroenterol Hepatol. 2006;21:1240-9.
17. Joshi D, James A, Quaglia A, et al. Liver disease in pregnancy. Lancet. 2010;375:594-605.
18. Pereira SP, O'Donohue J, Wendon J, et al. Maternal and perinatal outcome in severe pregnancy-related liver disease. Hepatology. 1997;26:1258-62.

CHAPTER 12

Infections in Pregnancy

Deepa Patil, Shravya Tallapureddy

INTRODUCTION

Infections are an important cause of maternal and neonatal morbidity and mortality. They influence mother and fetus. This can be explained by three mechanisms.
1. Pregnancy-induced immunological changes in mother affect the disease course, severity, and obstetric outcome.
2. Fetomaternal interface is unique, wherein two scenarios are possible—either:
   i. It acts as a barrier, protecting the fetus, or
   ii. It acts as a conduit to transmitting infections.
3. Drugs used to treat the infections can cause teratogenic effects.

Classification of Infections in Pregnancy

- Viral infections
- Bacterial infections
- Parasitic infections
- Other infectious conditions

A few of the infections are described here in detail.

GROUP B STREPTOCOCCUS

Group B *Streptococcus* (GBS) especially *Streptococcus agalactiae* colonizes genitourinary and gastrointestinal tract of around 20–30% women at some point during gestation.[1] The colonization may be transient, intermittent or chronic and the rate of colonization does not vary with gestational age.

The important determinant of susceptibility to invasive infection after colonization may be maternal antibodies directed against the capsular polysaccharide antigens of GBS. This antibody, which has some broad reactivity to all group B streptococcal types, is an IgG that readily crosses the placenta. Baker and associates demonstrated that 73% of 45 GBS colonized mothers with healthy neonates had high serum levels of type 3 antibody in contrast to only 19% of 32 GBS colonized mothers whose neonates developed early onset septicemia or meningitis.[2]

Maternal and Fetal Risks

Group B *Streptococcus* is an important pathogen for maternal intrapartum, postpartum, and occasionally prenatal infections. Data from an earlier report suggest puerperal septicemia due to GBS occurs with an incidence of approximately 1 to 2 per 1,000 deliveries and accounts for up to 15% of positive blood cultures from postpartum patients. GBS has also been associated with premature rupture of membranes and with preterm deliveries prior to 32 gestational weeks in some.[3]

Early neonatal infection is presumed to result from vertical transmission of GBS from a colonized mother. There is a direct relationship between neonatal attack rates and the size of the inoculum and number of colonized neonatal sites.[4]

Spectrum of neonatal infection may vary from early-onset neonatal sepsis to late-onset disease manifesting as meningitis.

Diagnosis

Group B streptococci is grown on selective or nonselective media. GBS can be recovered from overnight growth on nonselective media like blood agar. The use of a selective broth medium such as Todd-Hewitt broth or Lim broth greatly enhances the isolation rates of GBS from any culture site.[5,6]

Management

Prepregnancy

Treatment of GBS carrier before pregnancy has no benefit. Immunization strategies currently are being evaluated.

Prenatal, Labor, and Delivery (Flowcharts 1 and 2)[7,8]

- Universal screening-based approach is recommended:
  - Intrapartum antibiotic prophylaxis (IAP) must be recommended for all women with positive culture unless delivery by cesarean section prior to rupture of membranes and onset of labor is required.
  - If culture status is unknown at times of delivery, IAP is administered for gestation <37 weeks, rupture of membranes ≥ 18 hours, or intrapartum temperature ≥ 38.0°C
- *Suggested management of threatened preterm delivery:*[7]
  - *No culture done*: Cultures must be obtained and IAP is initiated for 48 hours until results are obtained, or delivery occurs.
  - *Culture positive prior to or during labor*: IAP for 48 hours or until delivery occurs.
- *Culture negative prior to labor or after 48 hours*:
  - No IAP (or stop IAP).
- Recommended GBS prophylaxis regimens: Table 1 describes the recommended regimens.[9-12]

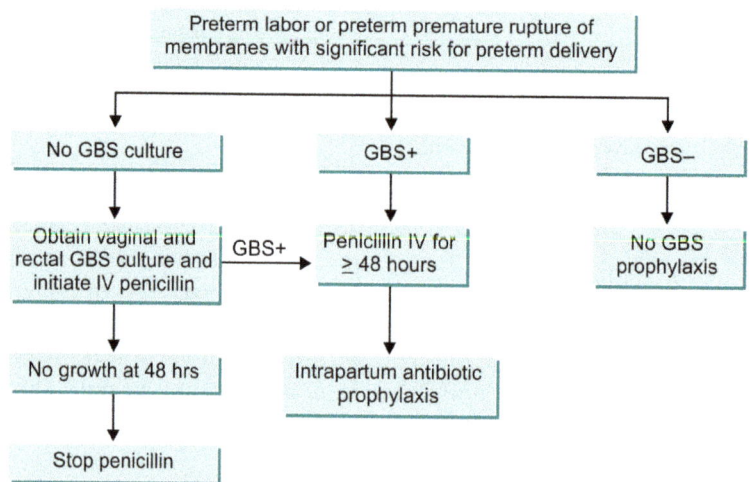

Flowchart 1: Algorithm for management of threatened preterm labor—Group B *Streptococcus* (GBS) prophylaxis.

Flowchart 2: Indications for intrapartum antibiotic prophylaxis to prevent perinatal Group B *Streptococcus* (GBS).

Cultures at 35–37 weeks gestation for GBS screening (vaginal and rectal swabs) in all pregnant women (exceptions—H/O GBS bacteriuria during present pregnancy or a history of previous neonate with invasive GBS disease)

Intrapartum prophylaxis indicate in–
- Previous baby with invasive GBS disease
- GBS bacteriuria in current pregnancy
- Positive GBS culture during current pregnancy
- Unknown GBS status (culture results unknown, incomplete or not done) and any of the following:
  - Delivery at ≤37 weeks gestation
  - Rupture of membrane ≥18 hours
  - Intrapartum temperature ≥100.4°F (≥38.0.°C)

Intrapartum prophylaxis not indicate–
- Previous pregnancy with a positive GBS screen (unless a culture was positive during the current pregnancy as well)
- Planned cesarean delivery performed in the absence of labor or rupture of membranes (regardless of present maternal GBS culture results)
- Negative vaginal and rectal GBS culture

Source: Adapted from Centers for Disease Control and Prevention. Prevention of perinatal group B streptococci disease. Revised guidelines from the CDC. MMWR. 2010;59(10):1.

TABLE 1: Recommended GBS prophylaxis regimens.

	Regimen
Primary option	Penicillin G 5 million U IV followed by 2.5 million U IV every 4 hours until delivery
Alternative	Ampicillin 2 g IV initially followed by 1 g IV 4 hours until delivery
Penicillin allergic	
• Not at high anaphylactic risk	• Cefazolin 2 g IV initial dose followed by 1 g IV every 8 hours until delivery
• High anaphylactic risk • Resistant to clindamycin	• Clindamycin 900 mg IV every 8 hours till delivery • Vancomycin 1 g IV every 12 hours till delivery

HEPATITIS VIRUS INFECTIONS

Hepatitis A

Diagnosis

Nonspecific initial clinical symptoms—fever, fatigue, nausea, malaise, and anorexia. Pregnant woman may present with significant weight loss. Liver function test abnormalities, typically elevations in ALT higher than AST, peaking prior to jaundice.[13]

Serological marker for acute infection is hepatitis A virus (HAV)-specific immunoglobulin M (IgM) and it can be identified with an automated ELISA. HAV-specific immunoglobulin G (IgG) however, will persist for many years after an acute infection.[14]

Maternal and Fetal Effects

Hepatitis A virus is a self-limited infection. Poor maternal nutritional status is associated with adverse obstetric outcomes. Perinatal transmission of HAV is rare.[15,16]

Management

- *Prenatal:* Supportive care.
- *Intrapartum/neonatal:* Immunoglobulin to newborn if acute maternal infection occurs proximate to delivery[17]
- *Prevention:*
  - Hepatitis A vaccine is available; not contraindicated in pregnancy.[18]
  - Women travelling to endemic areas should be vaccinated.[19]

Hepatitis B

Hepatitis infection is a global health problem because 5–10% of infected individuals become chronic hepatitis B carriers and a mortality of 25–30% is seen in carriers due to hepatitis B virus (HBV)-related disease.

Transmission is through exposure to blood and blood products, body fluids or sexual transmission or perinatal transmission.

Diagnosis

Three antigens are found in hepatitis B virus—surface, core, and e antigen. Hepatitis B surface antigen test—hepatitis B surface antigen (HbsAg) appears approximately 4 weeks before clinical manifestations.[20]

Hepatitis B surface antibody test—absence of hepatitis B carrier state is defined by this test. Antibody titers gradually increase during the recovery period and may rise till 10–12 months after HBsAg is no longer detected.[21]

Hepatitis B core antibody test—appears 3 to 5 weeks after HBsAg. HBcAb may drop in the first 2 years after infection.[22]

Hepatitis B e antigen appearance parallels that of HBsAg. HBeAb is seen shortly after HBeAg disappears.[23]

Maternal and Fetal Risks

During pregnancy, acute HBV infection is usually mild with only 30% women having clinical manifestations. During acute maternal infection, rate of vertical transmission depends on weeks of gestation. In case of maternal infection during the first trimester, up to 10% of neonates may be infected. In contrast, maternal infection during the third trimester, 80–90% of neonates may be HBsAg-positive. Universal screening is advocated for prenatal patients by several groups.[24,25]

Management

- *Prenatal*: Supportive care
- *Intrapartum/Neonatal*: Newborns of chronic carriers should receive HBV immunoglobulins (HBIg) within 12 hours of birth and HBV vaccine 72 hours of birth.[26]
- *Prevention*:
  - Universal screening of pregnant women (HBsAg).[27]
  - No contraindications to HBV vaccine during pregnancy.[27]

Hepatitis C Virus

Blood and other products transfusion and use of intravenous drugs are the principal risk factors for hepatitis C virus (HCV) transmission.[28]

Diagnosis

Initial screening with ELISA for anti-HCV antibodies is advised. Polymerase chain reaction (PCR) is used to detect small amounts of HCV-RNA in serum. Currently quantitative and qualitative tests are available commercially.[29]

Maternal and Fetal Risks

Antibody positive women were more likely to undergo cesarean section, pointing toward an increased risk of coexisting obstetric complications in them. Although reported rates of perinatal transmission have been variable, it is encouraging that most studies show the risk under 5%.[30]

The interaction between maternal and fetal, humoral and immunologic factors is a critical contributor to the occurrence and persistence of perinatally acquired neonatal HCV infection.[31]

Management Options

Prenatal: Primary source currently illicit drug use. Most cases asymptomatic, supportive care for clinical illness.
- *Intrapartum/neonatal*: No need to alter delivery route for maternal HCV infection. Risk of neonatal transmission is up to 10%,

if mother is viremic. No neonatal measures are available to lower risk of transmission. Breastfeeding is not contraindicated.[32-34]
- *Prevention*:
  - Screen pregnant women only if in high risk groups.
  - No vaccine or passive (Ig) prevention available.
  - Blood products screening has lowered risk of infection.[35]

TOXOPLASMOSIS

Toxoplasmosis is caused by the obligate intracellular parasite *Toxoplasma gondii*. Infections in immunocompetent individuals are frequently subclinical and innocuous unless the individual is pregnant, during which time vertical transfer can occur and lead to significant disease and possibly death in the fetus or neonate.[36]

Transmission

Outbreaks of toxoplasmosis in humans have been attributed to ingestion of raw or undercooked ground beef, lamb, pork, unpasteurized goat's milk and aerosolized soil exposure.[36]

Diagnosis

The diagnosis may be established by serological tests, amplification of specific nucleic acid sequences (using PCR), histological demonstration of the parasite and/or its antigens (immunoperoxidase stain), or isolation of the organism.
- *Serological tests*: Demonstration of specific antibody to *T. gondii* in maternal blood by serological tests is the initial method of diagnosis. IgG antibodies appear within 1-2 weeks, peak within 1-2 months, decline later but persist throughout life.[37] Sabin–Feldman dye test, ELISA, immunofluorescence assay (IFA), and modified direct agglutination test are the common tests used to measure IgG titers. IgG avidity testing is used to identify chronic infection. Higher IgG avidity points toward a more long-standing infection and is useful when other tests are inconclusive.
- *PCR test* in amniotic fluid can be used to diagnose intrauterine infection with high sensitivity.
- *Isolation of T. gondii* establishes the infection as acute and mouse inoculation with amniotic fluid PCR analysis has a sensitivity of 91–94%.[38,39]
- *Serial ultrasound* will give an identification of signs of fetal infection.[39,40] Ventricular dilation, intracranial calcifications, hepatic enlargement, ascites, and increased placental thickness may be seen in over one-third of cases of fetal infection and may be useful in evaluation.

Maternal and Fetal Risks

Maternal risk of toxoplasmosis is negligible and around 90% of infections are asymptomatic and self-limiting.

Fetal risks vary widely depending on the trimester of acquisition and presence and absence of treatment for mother.[41] Maternal infection occurring before 5 weeks of gestation has almost no risk of fetal infection, whereas infection late in pregnancy (third trimester) is associated with increased risk of transmission to fetus and congenital infections are seen in up to 60% of newborns.[42]

Management

Confirmed acute maternal infection—spiramycin 3 g/day.

Documented fetal infection—addition of pyrimethamine/sulfadiazine is required.[43,44] However, pyrimethamine should be avoided in first trimester.

SEXUALLY TRANSMITTED DISEASES

Gonorrhea

Gonorrhea is a common sexually transmitted disease caused by *Neisseria gonorrhoeae*, a gram-negative *Diplococcus*. Risk factors for gonococcal infections include multiple sexual partners, young age, and low socioeconomic status.[45]

Maternal and Fetal Risks

The rate of pharyngeal gonococcal infection increases during pregnancy, possibly as a result of altered sexual practices.[46] In pregnancy, gonococcal cervicitis has been associated with premature rupture of membranes, premature delivery, chorioamnionitis and both post abortion and postpartum endometritis. In addition, gonococcal ophthalmia neonatorum may develop in up to 40% of newborns exposed to maternal infection.[47,48]

Diagnosis

Diagnosis depends upon the demonstration of gram-negative intracellular diplococcic within leukocytes of a smear obtained from an exudate. Cultures should be inoculated immediately after collection onto a selective medium such as Thayer–Martin.

Management[49]

- *Uncomplicated gonorrhea in pregnancy*:
  - Inj. ceftriaxone 250 mg IM single dose *plus* azithromycin 1 g orally single dose
- *Disseminated gonococcal infection*:
  - Inj. ceftriaxone 1 g intramuscularly or intravenously (IV) every 24 hours.
  - After 24–48 hours of improvement, therapy changed to oral drug till 1 week.

In pregnancy, prompt recognition and treatment usually result in favorable outcomes.

Chlamydia trachomatis

Chlamydiae are obligate intracellular organisms. *Chlamydia trachomatis* may be differentiated into 15 serotypes. Risk factors for cervical infection include young age, multiple sexual partners, and previous history of sexually transmitted disease.[50]

Maternal and Fetal Risks

Several studies have found an association between maternal cervical infection and preterm delivery, premature rupture of membranes, low birth weight, perinatal death and late-onset postpartum endometritis.[51,52] Maternal chlamydial also poses significant risk to the neonate. The most common manifestations of neonatal infection are inclusion conjunctivitis and pneumonia.[53]

Diagnosis

The diagnosis of *Chlamydia* infections is based upon isolation of the organism, or culture-independent detection by immunoassay, DNA detection by PCR, and serologic testing.

Management[49]

Azithromycin 1 g oral, single dose or amoxicillin 500 mg orally three times daily for 7 days.[54]

Alternatives:
- Erythromycin 500 mg orally four times daily for 7 days.
- Erythromycin 250 mg orally four times daily for 14 days.

ZIKA VIRUS

Zika viral disease is a mosquito-borne viral disease first identified in African monkeys. Sporadic cases of infection in humans have been reported since 1950s across Africa, Asia, the Americas, and the Pacific.

The first outbreak of Zika viral disease was recorded in 2007 followed by a larger outbreak in 2013 in the Pacific. Brazil had reported an outbreak of febrile illness with rash which was identified as Zika viral infection in 2015, and it was later known to be associated with Guillain–Barré syndrome.[55]

Further in October 2015, an association between Zika virus infection in pregnancy and microcephaly in fetus was identified.[56]

Transmission

It is primarily transmitted by the bite of an infected *Aedes aegypti* mosquito. Zika virus is also transmitted from mother to fetus during pregnancy, through sexual contact, transfusion of blood and blood products, and organ transplantation.

Maternal Risks

Many are asymptomatic. Acute onset of fever with maculopapular rash and arthralgia are the characteristic findings. Conjunctivitis, myalgia, and headache are the other commonly reported symptoms. Symptoms are mild in many patients. Severe disease needing hospitalization is not common.[55]

Fetal Risks[57]

Congenital Zika syndrome: Mother to fetus transmission during pregnancy can result in microcephaly and other congenital malformations in the fetus, collectively referred to as congenital Zika syndrome.

Abnormal brain development or loss of brain tissue causes microcephaly. Infant outcomes vary depending on the extent of brain damage.

Other malformations include eye abnormalities, hearing loss, high muscle tone, and limb contractures. Following zika virus infection in pregnancy, the risk of congenital malformations remains unknown. Congenital malformations might occur following both asymptomatic and symptomatic infection.

Diagnosis and Management[55]

No specific antiviral treatment is available. However, the infection is usually mild, short-lived, and requires no treatment. Symptomatic pregnant woman should be advised rest, adequate hydration, and should be offered pain and fever relief with regular paracetamol and other cooling measures. In the rare possibility of symptoms becoming severe, patient should seek medical advice.

Prevention[57,58]

Currently no vaccine or drug is available to prevent Zika virus infection. Prevention of mosquito breeding and personal protection measures are advised.

Measures to Avoid Sexual Transmission

In areas with active Zika virus transmission:
- Pregnant women are advised to practice barrier contraception or avoid sexual activity for at least the entire duration of the pregnancy.
- Pregnant women advised not to travel to areas with ongoing Zika virus outbreaks.

In regions with NO active Zika virus transmission:
- Couples returning from areas with transmission of Zika virus are advised safer sex practices or abstinence for at least a period of 6 months upon return.
- Couples are advised to wait at least 6 months before trying to conceive to ensure that possible Zika virus infection has cleared.

CONCLUSION

The complexity of pregnancy and the immunologic changes associated with the acceptance of the fetus makes it challenging to treat infections in pregnancy. Vaccination during pregnancy is a strategy that has proven safe and effective for a number of infectious agents. Its beneficial effects may not be limited to the mother, but, by reducing fetal and placental inflammation, may have potential long-term benefits for the infant. Education of pregnant women about prevention of infections and the early identification and appropriate treatment of infectious diseases during pregnancy remain important strategies for protecting maternal and infant health.

REFERENCES

1. Regan JA, Klebanoff MA, Nugent RP, et al. Colonization with group B streptococci in pregnancy and adverse outcome. VIP Study Group. Am J Obstet Gynecol. 1996;174(4):1354-60.
2. Baker CJ, Edwards MS, Kasper DL. Role of antibody to native type 3 polysaccharide of group B streptococcus in infant infection. Pediatrics. 1981;68(4):544-9.
3. Blanco JD, Gibbs RS, Castaneda YS. Bacteremia in obstertrics: clinical course. Obstet Gynecol. 1981;58(5):621-5.
4. Schrag SJ, Zywicki S, Farley MM, et al. Group B streptococcal disease in the era of intrapartum antibiotic prophylaxis. N Engl J Med. 2000;342(1):15-20.
5. Yancey MK, Armer T, Clark P, et al. Assessment of rapid identification tests for genital carriage of group B streptococci. Obstet Gynecol. 1992;80(6):1038-47.
6. Walker CK, Crombleholme WR, Ohm-Smith MJ, et al. Comparison of rapid tests for detection of group B streptococcal colonization. Am J Perinatol. 1992;9(4):304-8.
7. Centers for Disease control and Prevention. Prevention of perinatal group B streptococcal disease: a public health perspective. MMWR. 1996;45(RR-7):1-24.
8. Schrag SJ, Zell ER, Lynfield R, et al. A population based comparison of strategies to prevent early-onset group B streptococcal disease in neonates. N Engl J Med. 2002;347(22):233-9.
9. Centers for Disease Control and Prevention. Prevention of perinatal group B streptococci disease. Revised guidelines from the CDC. MMWR. 2010;59(10):1.
10. Allen UD, Navas L, King SM. Effectiveness of intrapartum penicillin prophylaxis in preventing early onset group B streptococcal infection: result of meta-analysis. Can Med Assoc J. 1993;149(11):1659-65.
11. de Cueto m, Sanchez MJ, Sampedro A, et al. Timing of intrapartum ampicillin and prevention of vertical transmission of group B Streptococcus. Obstet Gynecol. 1998;91(1):112-4.
12. Lin FY, Brenner RA, Johnson YR, et al. The effectiveness of risk-based intrapartum chemoprophylaxis for the prevention of early onset neonatal group B streptococcal disease. Am J Obstet Gynecol. 2001;184(6):1204-10.
13. Gust ID. The epidemiology of viral hepatitis. In: Vyas GN, Dienstag JL, Hoofnagle JH (Eds). Viral Hepatitis and Liver Disease. Orlando, FL: Grune & Stratton; 1984. pp. 415-8.
14. Duermeyer W, Wielaard F, van der Veen J. A new principle for the detection of specific IgM antibodies applied in an ELISA for hepatitis A. J Med Virol. 1979;4(1):25-32.
15. Tong MJ, Thursby M, Rakela J, et al. Studies on the maternal-infant transmission of the viruses which cause acute hepatitis. Gastroenterology. 1981;80:999-1004.
16. Zhang RL, Zeng JS, Zhang HZ. Survey of 34 pregnant women with hepatitis A and their neonates. Chin Med J (Engl). 1990;103(7):552-5.
17. Papaevangelou V, Pollack H, Rochford G, et al. Increased transmission of vertical hepatitis C virus (HCV) infection to human immunodeficiency virus (HIV)-infected infants of HIV- and HCV-coinfected women. J Infect Dis. 1998;178:1047-52.
18. ACOG educational bulletin. Viral hepatitis in pregnancy. Number 248, July 1998 (replaces No. 174, November 1992). American College of Obstetricians and Gynecologists. Int J Gynaecol Obstet. 1998;63(2):195-202.
19. ACOG Committee Opinion: Guidelines for hepatitis B virus screening and vaccination during pregnancy. Washington DC: American College of Obstetricians and Gynecologists; 1990.

20. Beasley RP, Hwang LY. Epidemiology of hepatocellular carcinoma. In: Vyas GN, Dienstag JL, Hoofnagle JH (Eds). Viral Hepatitis and Liver Disease. Proceedings of the 1984 International Symposium on Viral Hepatitis. Orlando: Grune & Stratton; 1984. pp. 209-24.
21. Shulman RN. Hepatitis-associated antigen. Am J Med. 1971;49:669.
22. Krugman S, Overby LR, Mushahwar IK, et al. Viral hepatitis, type B: studies on natural history and prevention re-examined. N Engl J Med. 1979;300(3):101.
23. Aldershvile J, Skinhoj P, Frosner GG, et al. The expression pattern of hepatitis B e antigen and antibody in different ethnic and clinical groups of hepatitis B surface antigen carriers. J Infect Dis. 1980;142(1):18.
24. Hieber JB, Dalton D, Shorey J, et al. Hepatitis and pregnancy. J Pediatr. 1977;91(4):545-9.
25. Towers CV, Keegan KA. The many forms of viral hepatitis. Contemp Ob/Gyn. 1987;8:39.
26. Totos G, Gizaris V, Papaevangelou G. Hepatitis A vaccine: persistence of antibodies 5 years after the first vaccination. Vaccine. 1997;15:1252-3.
27. Beasley RP, Hwang LY, Lee GC, et al. Prevention of perinatally transmitted hepatitis B virus infections with hepatitis B immune globin and hepatitis B vaccine. Lancet. 1983;2(8359):1099-102.
28. Japanese Red Cross Non-A, Non-B Hepatitis Research Group: Effect of screening for hepatitis C virus antibody and hepatitis B virus core antibody on incidence of post-transfusion hepatitis. Lancet. 1991;338(8774):1040.
29. Inchauspe G, Abe K, Zebedee S, et al. Use of conserved sequences from hepatitis C virus for the detection of viral RNA in infected sera by polymerase chain reaction. Hepatology. 1991;14(4):595-600.
30. Silverman NS, Snyder M, Hodinka RL, et al. Detection of hepatitis C virus ribonucleic acid sequence in cord bloods from a heterogeneous prenatal population. Am J Obstet Gynecol. 1995;173(5):1396.
31. Lin HH, Hsu HY Chang MH, et al. Low prevalence of hepatitis C virus and infrequent perinatal or spouse infection in pregnant women in Taiwan. J Med Virol. 1991;35(4):237-40.
32. ACOG Committee Opinion: Guidelines for hepatitis B virus screening and vaccination during pregnancy. Washington DC: American College Of Obstetricians and Gynecologists; 1990.
33. Wejstal R, Widell A, Mansson AS, et al. Mother-to-infant transmission of hepatitis C virus. Ann intern Med. 1992;117:887.
34. Silverman NS, Jaffee FN, Hodinka RL. Hepatitis C virus infection in pregnancy: is maternal viral burden related to vertical transmission? Infect Dis Obstet Gynecol. 1996;4:357.
35. Kumar RM, Shahul S. Role of breast feeding in transmission of hepatitis C virus to infants of HCV-infected mothers. J Hepatol. 1998;29:191-7.
36. Donahue JG, Munoz A, Ness PM, et al. The declining risk of post-transfusion hepatitis C virus infection. N Engl J Med. 1992;327(6):369-73.
37. Dubey JP. Toxoplasmosis. J Am Vet Med Assoc. 1994;205:1593-8.
38. Montoya J. Laboratory diagnosis of Toxoplasma gondii infection and toxoplasmosis. J Infect Dis. 2002;185:S73-S82.
39. Foulon W, Pinon JM, Stray-Pederson B, et al. Prenatal diagnosis of congenital toxoplasmosis: a multicentre evaluation of different diagnostic parameters. Am J Obstet Gynecol. 1999;181(4):843-8.
40. Foulon W, Villena I, Stray-Pedersen B, et al. Treatment of toxoplasmosis during pregnancy: a multicenter study of impact on fetal transmission and children's sequelae at age 1 year. Am J Obstet Gynecol. 1999;180:410-5.
41. Antsaklis A, Daskalakis G, Papantoniou N, et al. Prenatal diagnosis of congenital toxoplasmosis. Prenat Diagn. 2002;22(12):1107-11.
42. Hohlfeld P, Daffos F, Thulliez P, et al. Fetal toxoplasmosis: outcome of pregnancy and infant followup after in utero treatment. J Pediatr. 1989;115(5):765-9.
43. Forestier F, Daffos F, Hohlfeld P, et al. Infectious fetal diseases. Prevention, prenatal diagnosis, practical matters. Presse Medicale. 1991;20(30):1448-54.
44. Daffos f, Forestier F, Capella-Pavlovsky M, et al. Prenatal management of 746 pregnancies at risk for congenital toxoplasmosis. N Engl J Med. 1988;318(5):271-5.
45. Gay-Andrieu F, Marty P, Pialat J, et al. Fetal toxoplasmosis and negative amniocnetesis. Necessity of an ultrasound follow-up. Prenat Diagn. 2003;23(7):558-60.

46. Charles AG, Cohen S, Kass MB, et al. Asymtomatic gonorrhea on prenatal patients. Am J Obstet Gynecol. 1970;108:595-9.
47. Corman LC, Levison ME, Knight R, et al. The high frequency of pharyngeal gonococcal infection in a prenatal clinic population. JAMA. 1974;230:568-70.
48. Edwards LE, Barrada MI, Hamann AA, et al. Gonorrhea in pregnancy. Am J Obstet Gynecol. 1978;132(6):637-41.
49. Crombleholme WR, Schachter J, Grossman M, et al. Amoxicillin therapy for chlamydia trachomatis in pregnancy. Obstet Gynecol. 1990;75(5):752-6.
50. Burkman RT, Tonascia JA, Atienza MF, et al. Untreated endocervical gonorrhoea and endometritis following elective abortion. Am J Obstet Gynecol. 1976;126:648-51.
51. Centres for Disease Control and Prevention. Ten leading nationally notifiable infectious diseases-United states. MMWR. 1996;45(41): 883-4.
52. Martin DH, Koutsky L, Eschenbach DA, et al. Prematurity and perinatal mortality in pregnancies complicated by maternal Chlamydia trachomatis infections. JAMA. 1982;247(11):1585-8.
53. Wager GP, Martin DH, Koutsky L, et al. Puerperal infectious morbidity: Relationship to route of delivery and to antepartum *Chlamydia trachomatis* infection. Am J Obstet Gynecol. 1980;138(7):1028-33.
54. Schachter J, Grossman M, Sweet RL, et al. Prospective study of prenatal transmission of Chlamydia trachomatis. JAMA. 1986;255(24): 3374-7.
55. Workowski KA, Berman S; Centers for Disease Control and Prevention (CDC). Sexually transmitted disease treatment guidelines, 2010. MMWR Recomm Rep. 2010;59(RR-12):1-110.
56. World Health Organization. (2017). Zika virus and complications: Questions and answers. [Online] Available from: https://www.who.int/features/qa/zika/en/ [Last accessed October, 2019].
57. Mlakar J, Korva M, Tul N, et al. Zika Virus Associated with Microcephaly. N Engl J Med. 2016;374(10):951-8.
58. Possible Association Between Zika Virus Infection and Microcephaly - Brazil, 2015. Centres for Disease Control and Prevention Morbidity and Mortality Weekly Report. 2016;65(3):59-62.

CHAPTER 13

Deep Vein Thrombosis in Pregnancy

Rinke S Tiwari

INTRODUCTION

Deep vein thrombosis (DVT) is a serious medical condition in which blood clot forms in a deep vein. This generally tends to occur in the leg, thigh, or pelvis.

Although DVT is not a common medical condition during pregnancy, but if it does occur, it can happen anytime during the 9 months and even 6 weeks postpartum. Pregnant women have a greater likelihood of getting DVT than nonpregnant ones of the same age group.[1-3]

INCIDENCE

For every 1,000 pregnancies, the incidence of DVT is 0.13–0.61 for lower extremities during pregnancy.[4]

The risk of antenatal venous thromboembolism (VTE) is four to five times higher in pregnant women than in nonpregnant women of the same age.[5,6]

Although the incidence of DVT is relatively low, it is important to be cautious as DVT is likely to cause pulmonary embolism (PE), which is a primary cause of maximum number of maternal deaths in both developing and developed nations.

Research indicates that the frequency of VTE is almost equal in all trimesters.[7]

PATHOGENESIS OF DVT

Pregnancy is a state that may be defined as prothrombotic.[8] It also exhibits all constituents of Virchow's Triad, which include the following:

Venous Stasis

- In pregnancy, enlarging uterus causes venous obstruction. Also, hormonally-induced decrease in venous tone will be there during pregnancy.
- Both of these result in venous stasis.
- By 25–28 weeks, the velocity of venous flow in the legs goes down to almost 50%. This may last until 6 weeks postpartum.
- The most common site for DVT in pregnant and postpartum women is left lower extremity[7,9] (left common iliac vein is compressed by the right common iliac artery, and heightened by the enlarging uterus).

Endothelial Damage

Venous hypertension or any damage of pelvis vein during delivery can lead to endothelial injury in pelvic veins.

Hypercoagulability

Pregnancy is the hypercoagulable state. This is a critical factor DVT in pregnancy.

Certain changes in coagulating factors take place while a woman's body prepares for the critical challenge of giving birth.

Some of these changes include:
- Increased fibrin leads to decreased fibrinolytic activity.

- Surge in coagulation factors II, VII, VIII, and X.[1,10]
- Progressive decline in levels of Protein S.
- Body resisting activated Protein C.[1,10]

SYMPTOMS OF DVT IN PREGNANCY

The most common symptom observed in 88% of pregnant patients (nearly 88%) and postpartum patients (about 79%) is swelling of the affected limb. Other symptoms are:
- Extremity discomfort
- Difficult in walking
- Along with pain in abdomen, inflammation in the leg, and pain in the back isolated iliac vein thrombosis may be noticed.

Physiological swelling and discomfort of pregnancy can mask these symptoms of DVT. Therefore, in pregnancy, identifying DVT becomes all the more challenging.

DIAGNOSIS OF DVT

Clinical diagnosis of DVT during pregnancy and thromboembolism is highly unreliable.

Physiological changes that occur during the natural course of pregnancy can make analysis of the patient's medical background, actual findings, and diagnostic reports more complex.

For instance, edema in lower extremity and pain in the leg may be a result of lymphatic obstruction and surge in intravascular blood volume and not due to DVT.[11]

Objective testing is critical for any woman with symptoms of VTE. Unless treatment is strongly contraindicated, treatment with LMWH needs to start until diagnosis is excluded.[12,13]

Venography has been the standard test to check for DVT in both pregnant and nonpregnant patients.

But in the last decade, numerous noninvasive diagnostic tests have come up to help with diagnosis of DVT. Some of them include:

Compression Duplex Ultrasound

This is the chief investigative test for diagnosing this disorder.[14,15]

This is the most preferred test for pregnant women with suspected DVT. Compression duplex ultrasound has a sensitivity of 97% and specificity of 94% for the diagnosis of symptomatic femoropopliteal DVT in general population.

It is, however, less accurate for pelvic vein thrombosis due to deep location of pelvic vein. Imaging becomes difficult with the enlarging size of uterus in the second half of pregnancy. Furthermore, performing compression in the pelvis area of a pregnant woman is quite difficult.
- If the diagnosis is confirmed by ultrasound, anticoagulant therapy needs to be continued.
- In case, the result is negative and clinical suspicion is negligible, anticoagulant therapy may be stopped.
- If result is negative and clinical risk seems to be high, anticoagulant therapy may be withdrawn. Nonetheless, ultrasound has to be repeated on day 3 and day 7.[16]
- If repetition-testing results also indicate absence of DVT, additional treatment is not necessary.
- If results indicate DVT, anticoagulant therapy has to be recommended and continued.

Impedance Plethysmography

Impedance plethysmography (IPG) is used extra-corporally to measure perfusion, the arterial pulse wave, and venous occlusion. A pregnant woman with negative results, even after continuous IPG, can safely be withheld from anticoagulant therapy.

Magnetic Resonance Imaging

Magnetic resonance imaging (MRI) should be taken into consideration in women when there is negative compression ultrasonography (USG) and still clinical suspicion is present. An MRI has a high sensitivity for pelvic vein thrombosis and is also a reliable method to diagnose both pelvic and lower extremity venous thrombosis. Its accuracy almost matches that of venography in case of proximal thrombosis in the lower limb.

D-dimer

The value of D-dimer steadily increases throughout pregnancy. The universally acceptable normal range of D-dimer is not yet established. However, D-dimer value at the lower end would be helpful in ruling out the possibility of DVT. In pregnancy, a positive result is common and almost always.

Still low D-dimer value may be helpful in ruling out DVT, a positive D-dimer result will be common during pregnancy and always requires confirmatory testing.

Venography

It is an invasive test. Venography is the definite diagnostic test for DVT. It may also be used in cases where empiric anticoagulation is contraindicated, noninvasive tests are ambiguous and high level clinical suspicion exists. This diagnostic method is considered more reliable in comparison to noninvasive tests. However, this method has a few side effects:
- Swelling in the leg
- Chemical phlebitis
- Pain in the leg
- Skin necrosis.

Risks involved in venography include:
- Contrast reaction
- Provoking thrombosis.

Computed Tomography

Multidetector computed tomography (CT) is the preferred diagnostic test in cases where D-dimer and compression USG results are equivocal.

Computed tomography pulmonary angiography (CTPA) is more readily available. Also, in case of CTPA, the fetal exposure to radiation is much less compare to V/Q scanning. In CTPA, nonionic contrast exposure is safer for fetus.

Computed tomography pulmonary angiography can also help in diagnosis of:
- Pneumonia
- Pulmonary edema
- Aortic dissection (in some cases).[17,18]

V/Q Scanning

V/Q scanning may be a good alternative when CTPA is unavailable. It is the preferred choice of test in case of women with a family history of breast cancer as spiral CT poses a risk of exposure to greater radiation.[19,20]

MANAGEMENT OF DVT

Objective testing is advisable for women who present with thromboembolism symptoms.

In case of a woman presenting symptoms and/or signs of thromboembolism, treatment with low-molecular-weight heparin (LMWH) has to be recommended unless:
- Contraindication of treatment
- Objective testing excludes diagnosis.[12,13]

Hospitals need to have an acceptable protocol in place to objectively diagnose suspected VTE in pregnancy.

Performing a compression duplex ultrasound is advised if the doctors are suspicious of DVT in a patient:
- In case of a negative result and low clinical suspicion, anticoagulant treatment needs not be continued.

- In case of a negative result and high clinical suspicion, anticoagulant must be continued. In this case, ultrasound should be repeated on day-3 and day-7.[16]

Nearly 15–24% of patients are likely to develop PE, if DVT remains untreated. During pregnancy, PE is considered to be fatal in nearly 15% of the cases.[12,13]

Patients with any symptoms of acute PE are recommended to go for an electrocardiography (ECG) and a chest X-ray.

Testing through D-dimer plays no role in VTE in pregnancy.

Initial Anticoagulant Therapy

- Prior to starting the anticoagulant therapy, a patient has to be checked for complete blood picture (CBP), urea, coagulation screen, electrolytes, and liver function test (LFT).[21]
- No recommendation for performing thrombophilia profile before starting the LMWH.[21]
- Low-molecular-weight heparin needs to be commenced immediately in case of clinical suspicion of DVT or PE, unless treatment is strongly contraindicated.
- The doses of LMWH have to be continuously monitored and adjusted against patient's weight during early pregnancy. There has not been enough proof to suggest if doses need to be given once or twice a day (RCOG Greentop guidelines 2015).

MONITORING

- Other than in patients with a body weight of below 50 kg and above 90 kg or other kinds of complications (such as recurring VTE or renal impairment), regular monitoring of peak anti-Xa activity for women on LMWH for treatment of acute VTE in pregnancy or postpartum is not advisable.[22-24]
- It is not advisable to measure count of platelets on a regular basis.
- However, in obstetric cases, where the patient is receiving heparin that is unfractionated after surgery, monitoring the platelets once every 2–3 days between day 4 and day 14 is advisable (RCOG Greentop guidelines 2015).

Initial dose of different LMWH are given in Tables 1 and 2 and Box 1 (RCOG Greentop guidelines 2015).

Maintenance Treatment of VTE

- For the remaining part of pregnancy, continue with treatment of LMHW (subcutaneous).[25-32]
- Women patients can be treated on outpatient basis until delivery. Safe disposal of needles and syringes have to be ensured.
- Women on LMWH require monitoring in cases of extreme bodyweight (below 50 kg or above 90 kg) or kidney damage. After 3 hours of having injected 0.5–1.2 µ/mL peak anti-Xa activity has to be achieved.
- In cases where the patient cannot tolerate heparin, generally due to skin allergies

TABLE 1: Determination of initial dose of enoxaparin.

Weight during early pregnancy	Enoxaparin: Initial dose
Less than 50 kg	40 mg two times a day or 60 mg once a day
Between 59 and 69 kg	60 mg two times a day or 90 mg once a day
Between 70 and 89 kg	80 mg two times a day or 120 mg once a day
Between 90 and 109 kg	100 mg two times a day or 150 mg once a day
Between 110 and 125 kg	120 mg two times a day or 180 mg once a day
More than 125 kg	Consult a hematologist

TABLE 2: Determination of initial dose of dalteparin.

Weight during early pregnancy	Dalteparin
Less than 50 kg	5,000 IU two times a day or 10,000 IU once a day
Between 50 and 69 kg	6,000 IU two times a day or 12,000 IU once a day
Between 70 and 89 kg	8,000 IU two times a day or 16,000 IU once a day
Between 90 and 109 kg	10,000 IU two times a day or 20,000 IU once a day
Between 110 and 125 kg	12,000 IU two times a day or 24,000 IU once a day
More than 125 kg	Consult a hematologist.

Box 1: Determination of initial dose of tinzaparin.

Tinzaparin: Initial dose (on the basis of weight during early pregnancy) 175 units per kilo

with no indication of heparin-induced thrombocytopenia (HIT), another LMWH may be recommended. If problem persists, or there is evidence of HIT, use of a low molecular weight heparinoid known as danaparoid may be prescribed.

Vitamin-K Antagonist

During pregnancy, do not use vitamin-K antagonist (for example warfarin) as it readily crosses the placenta and may lead to complications including:
- Miscarriage
- Prematurity
- Neurological development issues
- Low birth weight (LBW)
- Fetal and neonatal bleeding.

During the first trimester, associated characteristic embryopathy may be noticed following the fetal exposure.[33,34]

Anticoagulant Therapy during Labor and Delivery

The risk of recurrent thrombosis escalates in case of discontinuation of anticoagulant therapy to allow for a C-section or a planned induction of labor. Intravenous unfractionated heparin may be considered as it can be easily manipulated.[35]

Patients on LMWH for maintenance therapy have to be instructed to not inject any heparin, once she is in labor.

Maintenance dose of LMWH has to be halted at least a day in advance, in case of elective delivery by C-section or planned induction.

Reassurance has to be given to women, who go into labor soon after a dose of LMWH that risk of bleeding is highly unlikely. In case of unplanned labor in patients taking subcutaneous heparin that is unfractionated, careful monitoring of APTT is necessary.

Anesthesia can be given only after a day of having taken the dose of heparin. In case of a woman undergoing VTE treatment, epidural anesthesia can be administered only after consultation with a senior consultant anesthetist.

Until after 4 hours of spinal anesthesia or removal of epidural catheter, LMWH should not be administered. Furthermore, the catheter cannot be removed until after 12 hours of the recent dose.[36]

Cesarean Delivery

It is best to avoid the dose of LMWH for 24 hours prior to the elective C-Section. A thromboprophylactic dose should be administered 4 hours postsurgery and the treatment dose to be given only 8–12 hours later.

To allow drainage of hematoma, wound drains need to be considered and skin incisions should be closed with sutures in case of patients under a therapeutic dose of LMWH.

Postnatal Anticoagulation

- Therapeutic anticoagulant therapy should be continued for at least 6 weeks after the birth of the baby and a minimum of 90 days of treatment has been administered to the patient in total.[37]
- Risk assessment of thrombosis needs to be done before stopping the treatment.
- Especially during the first 10 days after delivery, the patient needs to be given a choice of LMWH or oral anticoagulant based on the need for regular blood tests to check warfarin.
- Warfarin should not be administered at least for 5 days after delivery.
- In case of patients with high risk of PPH, warfarin needs to be avoided for over 5 days.
- Unfractionated heparin or LMWH or warfarin is not contraindicated in breastfeeding.

Post-thrombotic Syndrome

It is characterized by:
- Persistent and chronic pain in the leg
- Leg swelling
- Heaviness
- Pigmentation for prolonged period
- Dependent cyanosis
- Telangiectasis
- Eczema
- Varicose veins
- Venous ulceration (in severe cases).

The risk of getting post-thromobotic syndrome is almost nil with 12 weeks of heparin.

This syndrome may or may not be prevented with the help of compression stockings. The link as such has not yet been established. However, after diagnosis of DVT, patient is to be advised to wear graduated elastic compression stockings to subside swelling and pain.

Breastfeeding

Low-molecular-weight heparin or unfractionated heparin and even warfarin are not contraindicated during breastfeeding. Since neither unfractionated heparin nor LMWH is orally active so there is no chance of clinical affects in the infant. Even in case of warfarin, there is no evidence that it passes into breast milk to any quantifiable degree.[38,39]

VENOUS THROMBOEMBOLISM DURING PREGNANCY AND THE PUERPERIUM: RISK FACTORS

Pre-existing	
	• Previous VTE
	• *Thrombophilia:*
	– Heritable
	▪ Antithrombin deficiency
	▪ Protein C deficiency
	▪ Protein S deficiency
	▪ Factor V Leiden
	▪ Prothrombin gene mutation
	– Acquired:
	▪ Antiphospholipid antibodies
	▪ Persistent lupus anticoagulant and/or persistent moderate/high titer anticardiolipin antibodies and/or beta 2-glycoprotein 1 antibodies

Contd...

Contd...

	• Medical comorbidities, e.g. cancer, heart failure, active SLE, nephrotic syndrome, type-1 DM with nephropathy, and sickle cell disease. • Age >35 years • Obesity—(BMI more than or equal to 30 kg/m²) either prepregnancy or in early pregnancy • Parity equal or more than 3 • Smoking • Gross varicose veins • Paraplegia
Obstetrics risk N Factors	• Multiple pregnancy • Current preeclampsia • C-section • Extended labor time (>24 hours) • Mid-cavity or rotational operative delivery • Stillbirth • Preterm birth • Postpartum hemorrhage (>1 liter/requiring transfusion)
New onset/transient	• Any surgical procedure in pregnancy or puerperium except immediate repair of the perineum e.g. appendectomy, postpartum sterilization. • Bone fracture • Hyperemesis, dehydration • Ovarian hyperstimulation syndrome (first trimester only) • Admission or immobility (3 or more days rest) e.g. pelvic girdle restricting mobility • Long distance travel (>4 hours) • Current systemic infection (requiring intravenous antibiotics or hospital admission) e.g. pneumonia, pyelonephritis, postpartum wound infection.

Refer to trust-nominated thrombosis in pregnancy expert/team in Appendix 1.

At least 6 weeks' postnatal prophylactic LMWH.

RISK ASSESSMENT FOR VENOUS THROMBOEMBOLISM

- In cases, where the total score is more than or equal to four before delivery, recommend thromboprophylaxis from trimester 1
- In cases, where the total score is equal to three before delivery, consider thromboprophylaxis from 28 weeks onward.
- In cases, where the total score is less than or equal to 2 after delivery, thromboprophylaxis needs to be administered for a minimum of 10 days
- Thromboprophylaxis should be recommended if patient is admitted during pregnancy before delivery.
- In case of where the patient is admitted for 3 or more days or is readmitted to the hospital within the puerperium, thromboprophylaxis is advised.

Obstetric Emergencies

Appendix 1: Obstetric thromboprophylaxis risk assessment and management.

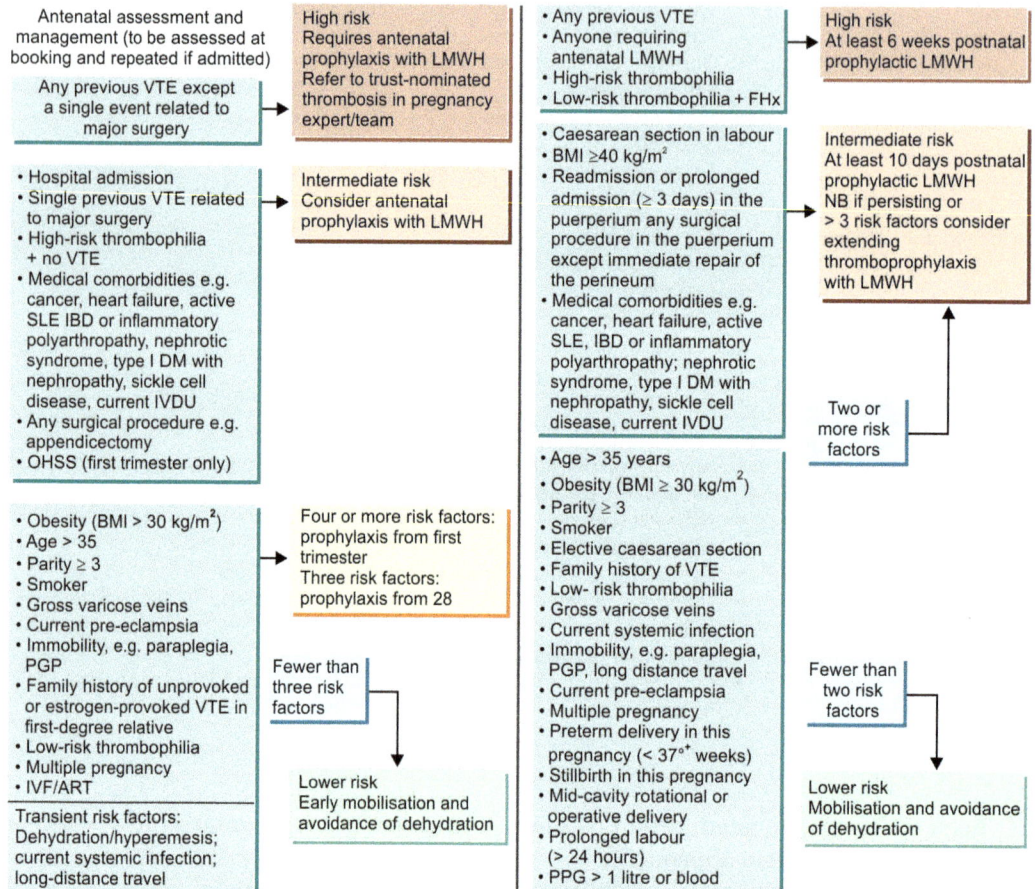

APL: antiphospholipid antibodies (lupus anticoagulant, anticardiolipin antibodies, β_2-glycoprotein 1 antibodies); ART: assisted reproductive technology; BMI based on booking weight; DM: diabetes mellitus; FHx: family history; gross varicose veins: symptomatic, above knee or associated with phlebitis/edema/skin changes; high-risk thrombophilia: antithrombin deficiency, protein C or S deficiency, compound or homozygous for low-risk thrombophilias, IBD. inflammatory bowel disease; immobility: ≥3 days; IVDU: intravenous drug user; IVF: in vitro fertilization; LMWH: low-molecular-weight heparin; long-distance travel: > 4 hours; low-risk thrombophilia: heterozygous for factor V Leiden or prothrombin $G_{20210}A$ mutations; OHSS: ovarian hyperstimulation syndrome; PGP: pelvic girdle pain with reduced mobility; PPH: postpartum haemorrhage; thrombophilia: inherited or acquired; VTE: venous thromboembolism

Antenatal and postnatal prophylactic dose of LMWH
Weight < 50 kg = 20 mg enoxaparin/2500 units dalteparin/3500 units tinzaparin daily
Weight 50–90 kg = 40 mg enoxaparin/5000 units dalteparin/4500 units tinzaparin daily
Weight 91–130 kg = 60 mg enoxaparin/75000 units dalteparin/7000 units tinzaparin daily
Weight 131–170 kg = 80 mg enoxaparin/10000 units dalteparin/9000 units tinzaparin daily
Weight 170 kg = 0.6 mg/kg/day enoxaparin/75 u/kg/day dalteparin/75 u/k/day tinzaparin

Deep Vein Thrombosis in Pregnancy

Risk factors: Pre-existing	
Previous VTE provoked by major surgery	3
Established case of high-risk thrombophilia	3
Medical comorbidities such as: • Heart failure • Inflammatory bowel disease • Active systemic lupus erythematosus • Cancer • Inflammatory polyarthropathy • Type 1 diabetes mellitus with nephropathy • Nephrotic syndrome • Current intravenous drug user • Sickle cell disease	3
Patient has a family history of or estrogen-related or even unprovoked VTE in a first-degree relative	1
Established case of low-risk thrombophilia (without VTE)	1[a]
Age of 35 years or more	1
Obesity	1 or 2[b]
Parity ≥ 3	1
Smoker	1
Risk factors: Obstetric	
Preeclampsia in current pregnancy	1
ART/IVF (antenatal only)	1
Multiple pregnancy	1
Cesarean section in labor	2
Elective cesarean section	1
Mid-cavity or rotational operative delivery	1
Prolonged labor (24 hours)	1
PPH (1 liter or transfusion)	1
Preterm birth 37^{+0} weeks in current pregnancy Stillbirth in current pregnancy	1
Risk factors: Transient	
Surgery during pregnancy or 6 months after delivery (except a case of immediate repair of perineum), for instance—appendicectomy and sterilization	3
Hyperemesis	3
Current systemic infection	1
Immobility and dehydration	1

a: If the known low risk thrombophilia is in a woman with the family history of VTE in a first degree relative, postpartum thrombopropylaxis should be continued for 6 weeks.

b: BMI ≥ 30 = 1, BMI ≥ 40 = 2

RISK ASSESSMENT AND MANAGEMENT: OBSTETRIC THROMBOPROPHYLAXIS: (RCOG GREEN-TOP GUIDELINE NO-37A)

- Antenatal assessment and management (to be assessed at booking and repeated on admission):

History of VTE except related to major surgical procedure	*High risk:* • Requires antenatal prophylaxis with LMWH • Refer to an expert in nominated thrombosis
Admitted in hospital: • Previous VTE related to a major surgical procedure • High-risk thrombophilia but no VTE • Comorbidities such as cancer, heart failure, active SLE, IBD, or inflammatory polyarthropathy, sickle cell disease, type -1 Diabetes with renal disorder, nephrotic syndrome, and current IVDU • Any surgical procedure e.g. appendicectomy • OHSS (first trimester only) • Obesity (BMI >30 kg/m²) • Age above 35 • Parity greater than 3 • Smoker • Gross varicose vein • Immobility (for instance, paraplegia) • Current preeclampsia • Patient with a history of estrogen or unprovoked VTE in an immediate relative • Low-risk thrombophilia • Pregnant with twins • IVF/ART	*Intermediate* Antenatal prophylaxis with LMWH should be considered *Four or more risk factor:* Prophylaxis from first trimester *Three risk factor:* Prophylaxis from 28 weeks *Less than 3 risk factors—lower risk:* Mobilizing and avoiding dehydration

Transient factors:
Dehydration, traveling long distance, any infection.

- Postnatal assessment and management (to be assessed on delivery suite)

• Any previous H/O VTE • High-risk thrombophilia • Anyone requiring antenatal LMWH • Low-risk thrombophilia + FHx	*High risk:* At least 6 weeks postnatal prophylactic LMWH
• Cesarean section in labor • BMI more than or equal to 40 kg/m² • Readmission or prolonged admission (3 days or more) in the postpartum • Surgical interventions during postpartum except immediate repair of the perineum • Other comorbidities such as active SLE, cancer, nephrotic syndrome, sickle cell disease, and inflammatory bowel disease	*Intermediate risk:* • At least 10 days postnatal prophylactic LMWH • NB if persisting or >3 risk factors, extending thrombo-prophylaxis with LWMH should be considered
• Age > 35 years • Obesity (BMI > or equal to 30 kg/m²) • Parity > or equal to 3 • Smoker • Elective cesarean section • Family history of VTE • Low-risk thrombophilia • Gross varicose veins • Current systemic infection • Immobility, e.g. paraplegia, PGP, long distance travel • Current preeclampsia • Preterm delivery in this pregnancy (< 37 weeks) • Stillbirth in this pregnancy • Mid-cavity rotational or operative delivery • Prolonged labor (> 24 hours) • PPH> 1 liter or blood transfusion	Lower risk Early mobilization and adequate hydration Fewer than two risk factors Manage as per intermediate Risk Two or more risk factors

CONTRAINDICATION FOR LMWH

- Established bleeding disorder such as:
  - Hemophilia
  - Acquired coagulopathy.

- Women with antenatal or postpartum bleeding, with an augmented risk of major hemorrhage:
  - Placenta previa, for instance
- Thrombocytopenia (platelet count 75 × 10^9/L)
- Patient who has had an acute stroke 4 weeks prior:
  - Hemorrhagic or ischemic
- Serious renal disorder with a GFR (Glomerular Filtration Rate) of 30 mL/min/1.73 m^2)
- Liver disease with a prothrombin time well above normal range or known varices
- Excessive hypertension (200/120 mm Hg)

REFERENCES

1. Kujovich JL. Hormones and pregnancy: thromboembolic risks for women. BR J Haematol. 2004;126:443.
2. Simpson EL, Lawrenson RA, Nightingale AL, et al. Venous Thromboembolism in pregnancy and the puerperium: incidence and additional risk factors from a London perinatal database. BJOG. 2001;108:56-60.
3. James AH, Tapson VF, Goldberg SZ. Thrombosis during pregnancy and the postpartum period. Am J Obstet Gynecol. 2005;193:216-9.
4. Kieregaard A. Incidence and diagnosis of deep vein thrombosis associated with pregnancy. Acta Obstet Gynecol Scand. 1983;62(3):239-43.
5. Heit JA, Kobbervig CE, James AH, et al. Trends in the incidence of venous thromboembolism during pregnancy or postpartum: a 30-year population-based study. Ann Intern Med. 2005;143:697-706.
6. Pomp ER, Lenselink AM, Rosendaal FR, et al. Pregnancy, the postpartum period and prothrombotic defects: risk of venous thrombosis in the MEGA study. J Thromb Haemost. 2008;6:632-7.
7. Ginsberg JS, Brill-Edwards P, Burrows RF, et al. Venous thrombosis during pregnancy: leg and trimester of presentation. Thromb Haemost. 1992;67(5):519-20.
8. Marik PE, Plante LA. Venous thromboembolic disease in pregnancy. N Engl J Med. 2008;359:2025.
9. Bergqvist A, Bergqvist D, Hallbook J. Deep vein thrombosis during pregnancy. A prospective study. Acta Obstet Gynaecol Scand. 1983;62:443-8.
10. Eichinger S. D-dimer testing in pregnancy. Semin Vasc Med. 2005;5:375-8.
11. Toglia MR, Weg JG. Venous thromboembolism during pregnancy. N Engl J Med. 1996;335(2):108-14.
12. Rutherford SE, Phelan JP. Deep venous thrombosis and pulmonary embolism in pregnancy. Obstet Gynecol Clin North Am. 1991;18:345-70.
13. Gherman RB, Goodwin TM, Leung B, et al. Incidence, clinical characteristics, and timing of objectively diagnosed venous thromboembolism during pregnancy. Obstet Gynecol. 1999;94:730-4.
14. Bates SM, Jaeschke R, Stevens SM, et al.; American College of Chest Physicians. Diagnosis of DVT: Antithrombotic Therapy and Prevention of Thrombosis, 9th edition: American College of Chest Physicians Evidence-Based Clinical Practice Guidelines. Chest. 2012;141(2 Suppl):e351S-418S.
15. Le Gal G, Kercret G, Ben Yahmed K, et al. Diagnostic value of single complete compression ultrasonography in pregnant and postpartum women with suspected deep vein thrombosis: prospective study. BMJ. 2012;344:e2635.
16. Chan WS, Spencer FA, Lee AY, et al. Safety of withholding anticoagulation in pregnant women with suspected deep vein thrombosis following negative serial compression ultrasound and iliac vein imaging. CMAJ. 2013;185:E194-200.
17. Shahir K, Goodman LR, Tali A, et al. Pulmonary embolism in pregnancy: CT pulmonary angiography versus perfusion scanning. AJR Am J Roentgenol. 2010;195:W214-20.
18. Revel MP, Cohen S, Sanchez O, et al. Pulmonary embolism during pregnancy: diagnosis with lung scintigraphy or CT angiography? Radiology. 2011;258:590-8.
19. Leung AN, Bull TM, Jaeschke R, et al. An official American Thoracic Society/Society of Thoracic Radiology clinical practice guideline: evaluation of suspected pulmonary embolism in pregnancy. Am J Respir Crit Care Med. 2011;184:1200-8.

20. McLintock C, Brighton T, Chunilal S, et al. Recommendations for the diagnosis and treatment of deep venous thrombosis and pulmonary embolism in pregnancy and the postpartum period. Aust N Z J Obstet Gynaecol. 2012;52:14-22.
21. Scottish Intercollegiate Guidelines Network (SIGN). Prevention and management of venous thromboembolism. SIGN publication no. 122. Edinburgh: SIGN; 2010.
22. Kitchen S, Iampietro R, Woolley AM, et al. Anti Xa monitoring during treatment with low molecular weight heparin or danaparoid: inter-assay variability. Thromb Haemost. 1999;82:1289-93.
23. Greer I, Hunt BJ. Low molecular weight heparin in pregnancy: current issues. Br J Haematol. 2005;128:593-601.
24. Nutescu EA, Spinler SA, Wittkowsky A, et al. Low-molecular-weight heparins in renal impairment and obesity: available evidence and clinical practice recommendations across medical and surgical settings. Ann Pharmacother. 2009;43:1064-83.
25. Dolovich L, Ginsberg JS. Low molecular weight heparin in the treatment of venous thromboembolism: an updated meta-analysis. Vessels 1997;3:4-11.
26. Gould MK, Dembitzer AD, Doyle RL, et al. Low-molecular-weight heparins compared with unfractionated heparin for treatment of acute deep venous thrombosis. A meta-analysis of randomized, controlled trials. Ann Intern Med. 1999;130:800-9.
27. Quinlan DJ, McQuillan A, Eikelboom JW. Low-molecular- weight heparin compared with intravenous unfractionated heparin for treatment of pulmonary embolism: a meta-analysis of randomized, controlled trials. Ann Intern Med. 2004;140:175-83.
28. Bates SM, Greer IA, Middeldorp S, et al. VTE, thrombophilia, antithrombotic therapy, and pregnancy: Antithrombotic Therapy and Prevention of Thrombosis, 9th ed: American College of Chest Physicians Evidence-based Clinical Practice Guidelines. Chest. 2012;141(2 Suppl):e691S-736S.
29. Sanson BJ, Lensing AW, Prins MH, et al. Safety of low-molecular-weight heparin in pregnancy: a systematic review. Thromb Haemost. 1999;81:668-72.
30. Greer IA, Nelson-Piercy C. Low-molecular-weight heparins for thromboprophylaxis and treatment of venous thromboembolism in pregnancy: a systematic review of safety and efficacy. Blood. 2005;106:401-7.
31. Nelson-Piercy C, Powrie R, Borg JY, et al. Tinzaparin use in pregnancy: an international, retrospective study of the safety and efficacy profile. Eur J Obstet Gynecol Reprod Biol. 2011;159:293-9.
32. Galambosi PJ, Kaaja RJ, Stefanovic V, et al. Safety of low-molecular-weight heparin during pregnancy: a retrospective controlled cohort study. Eur J Obstet Gynecol Reprod Biol. 2012;163:154-9.
33. Tang AW, Greer I. A systematic review on the use of new anticoagulants in pregnancy. Obstet Med. 2013;6:64-71.
34. Ciurzynski M, Jankowski K, Pietrzak B, et al. Use of fondaparinux in a pregnant woman with pulmonary embolism and heparin-induced thrombocytopenia. Med Sci Monit. 2011;17:CS56-9.
35. Romualdi E, Dentali F, Rancan E, et al. Anticoagulant therapy for venous thrombo-embolism during pregnancy: a systematic review and a meta-analysis of the literature. J Thromb Haemost. 2013;11:270-81.
36. Gogarten W, Vandermeulen E, Van Aken H, et al. Regional anaesthesia and antithrombotic agents: recommendations of the European Society of Anaesthesiology. Eur J Anaesthesiol. 2010;27:999-1015.
37. Bates SM. Pregnancy-associated venous thromboembolism: prevention and treatment. Semin Hematol. 2011;48:271-84.
38. Clark SL, Porter TF, West FG. Coumarin derivatives and breast-feeding. Obstet Gynecol. 2000;95:938-40.
39. Orme ML, Lewis PJ, de Swiet M, et al. May mothers given warfarin breast-feed their infants? Br Med J. 1977;1:1564-5.

CHAPTER 14

Preterm Labor

Shravya Tallapureddy

INTRODUCTION

Preterm labor is defined as the onset of labor before 37 completed weeks of gestation. Preterm birth is the leading cause of neonatal death and the second most common cause of childhood death below 5 years of age.[1]
Preterm labor may be due to:
- Spontaneous onset with intact membranes
- Secondary to preterm premature rupture of membranes (PROM)
- Iatrogenic-induced labor for maternal or fetal indications.

RISK FACTORS

Many risk factors affect the frequency of preterm labor and have been elucidated in Box 1.

Despite all the factors stated in Box 1, no known antecedent risk factor is identified in up to 50% of women who deliver prematurely.

PATHOPHYSIOLOGY[2]

Similar clinical events are involved in preterm labor and labor at term.[2] These include:
- Uterine component associated with:
  - Increased uterine contractility
  - Cervical changes
  - Chorioamniotic membrane rupture.
- Fetal component—changes in the concentrations of corticotropin-releasing hormone (CRH) and thereby cortisol levels.

These events represent the common pathway of labor, activated physiologically in case of normal labor whereas associated with disease process in case of preterm labor.

Box 1: Risk factors for preterm labor.
- Young or advanced maternal age
- Vaginal bleeding in any trimester
- Previous history of preterm birth
- Uterine overdistention due to multiple gestation or polyhydramnios
- Cervical incompetence
- Uterine abnormalities
- Fetal anomalies
- Infection—chorioamnionitis/urinary tract infection (UTI)/bacterial vaginosis/periodontal disease
- Systemic maternal illness like infections, hypertension or autoimmune diseases
- Lifestyle factors
  - Inadequate maternal weight gain [low body mass index (BMI)] or overweight
  - Low socioeconomic class
  - Cigarette smoking
  - Illicit drug use
  - Domestic violence
  - Psychological factors like stress and anxiety

Increased Uterine Contractility

Change from uterine quiescence to contractile state is associated with a shift in signaling from anti-inflammatory to proinflammatory pathways. Increase in chemokines (IL-8), cytokines (IL-1 and IL-6), and contraction-associated proteins (oxytocin receptor, connexin 43, prostaglandin receptor) is noted. Progesterone represses the expression of these genes and thereby maintains uterine quiescence. Increased expression of the microRNA-200 family near term promotes progesterone catabolism and activates these genes.[3]

Cervical Changes

Cervical ripening is brought about by:[4]
- Changes in extracellular matrix proteins which include:
    - Loss of collagen crosslinking
    - Increase in glycosaminoglycans.
- Changes in the epithelial barrier and immune properties.

Decidual or Membrane Activation

It refers to:
- Anatomical and biochemical events involved in withdrawal of decidual support for pregnancy
- Separation of chorioamniotic membranes from decidua and finally membrane rupture.

These are brought about by:[5,6]
- Increased expression of inflammatory cytokines and chemokines
- Increased protease activity [matrix metalloproteinase (MMP)-8, MMP-9]
- Dissolution of extracellular matrix components such as fibronectin and apoptosis.

The basic pathophysiologic process involved in preterm labor therefore is inflammation. Romero et al. have proposed the term preterm parturition syndrome to elucidate the complex nature of preterm labor and the pathological processes implicated in it. They include:
- Infection
- Excessive uterine distention
- Cervical incompetence
- Uteroplacental ischemia
- Hormone metabolism disorders
- Fetus as an allograft
- Allergy.

Infection

Infection is the only pathological process for which a firm causal role has been established in preterm labor. Microbial invasion of amniotic cavity (MIAC) is defined as the presence of bacteria in amniotic fluid.[2] Most of the infections are subclinical in nature and are detected only on analysis of amniotic fluid. But adverse perinatal outcomes have been noted in women with preterm labor and MIAC than in women with sterile amniotic fluid.[7]

Microbiology

Common organisms involved are *Mycoplasma* species especially, *Ureaplasma urealyticum*, *Streptococcus agalactiae*, *Escherichia coli*, *Fusobacterium* species and *Gardnerella vaginalis*.[8]

Routes of Infection

- Ascending pathway from genital tract (most common)
- Hematogenous dissemination (transplacental spread)
- From peritoneal cavity through fallopian tube
- Direct infection due to invasive procedures like amniocentesis, chorionic villus sampling (CVS) or fetal blood sampling.

Inflammatory mediators that trigger labor at term are similar those that help in defense against infection. The onset of preterm labor in response to infection therefore could be defense mechanism of the host.

Fetal infection is the most advanced stage of intrauterine infection. This may elicit a systemic inflammatory response, the fetal inflammatory response syndrome (FIRS). Higher rates of neonatal complications like sepsis, bronchopulmonary dysplasia, neurodevelopmental delay, necrotizing enterocolitis (NEC) are noted in fetuses with FIRS.[9]

Gene-environment Interactions[10]

Gene-environment interactions elaborate a concept where—the risk of a disease when an individual exposed to both a specific genotype and an environmental factor is greater or lower than the risk of exposure to either conditions alone. This has been reported for bacterial vaginosis, allele 2 of tumor necrosis factor-alpha (TNF-α) and preterm delivery. Therefore, treatment of maternal bacterial vaginosis, a known risk factor for preterm delivery, does not reliably prevent preterm labor.

Uteroplacental Ischemia/ Decidual Hemorrhage[2]

Preterm labor can be precipitated by maternal and fetal vascular lesions due to uteroplacental ischemia. The mechanism involved has not yet been determined but role of renin-angiotensin system has been proposed. Decidual hemorrhage activates preterm labor by production of thrombin, which in turn stimulates myometrial contractility.

Uterine Overdistention and Cervical Insufficiency

Increased risk of preterm labor has been noted in women with polyhydramnios, multiple gestation and uterine abnormalities. Mechanical stress-induced activation of various receptors (integrin receptors, G-proteins, calcium channels) and enzymes synthesizing prostaglandins and nitric oxide have been proposed as the mechanisms for preterm labor.

Allograft Rejection[2]

The fetoplacental unit has been considered the nature's most successful semiallograft. Disruption in maternal immune tolerance has been proposed as a mechanism for preterm labor.

Endocrine Disorders[2]

Progesterone plays a central role in maintaining uterine quiescence and inhibition of cervical ripening. A total of three progesterone receptors have been described. Increased relative expression of progesterone receptor A (PR-A) over progesterone receptor B (PR-B) and activation of nuclear factor kappa B (κB) in amnion is associated with functional progesterone withdrawal. This functional progesterone withdrawal has been proposed as the mechanism behind labor process.

■ DIAGNOSIS

The diagnosis of preterm labor encompasses clinical assessment and diagnostic tests. Clinical assessment includes history and physical examination.

History

Establishing accurate gestational age is one of the important prerequisites before diagnosing preterm labor. Once the dates are confirmed, symptoms are assessed. One of the common presenting symptoms is painful uterine contractions. This must be differentiated from false labor. Braxton Hicks contractions are irregular, nonrhythmical, either painful or painless whereas true labor pains are regular, gradually increase in duration and frequency and are often associated with cervical changes. Apart from uterine contractions, pelvic pressure, low backache and vaginal discharge are often associated with preterm labor.

Physical Examination

Vital signs to be assessed. Abdominal examination for uterine activity and cervical assessment should be done. According to the National Institute for Health and Care Excellence (NICE) guidelines, a sterile speculum examination followed by digital examination is advised if cervical dilatation could not be assessed.

Predictive Tests

- *Cervical length assessment*: Cervical length assessment has been traditionally used to assess the risk as well as to confirm the diagnosis of preterm labor. Transvaginal sonography is the preferred route. Optimal cutoff values varied between individual studies and ranged between 25 and 35 in asymptomatic women at 20-24 weeks of gestation. At these cutoff values, sensitivity rates ranged between 33% and 54%, and specificity rates between 73% and 91%, respectively.[11]
- *Fetal fibronectin (fFN)*:[12] Fetal fibronectin is an extracellular glycoprotein secreted at the maternal-fetal interface by the cytotrophoblast. It is normally present in cervicovaginal secretions, placenta, amniotic fluid till 20-22 weeks of gestation. Presence of fFN after membrane fusion at 22 weeks in cervicovaginal secretions is seen only when the cervix dilates or the membranes rupture. Enzyme-linked immunosorbent assay (ELISA) with FDC-6 monoclonal antibody is the commonly used assay and the threshold of 50 ng/mL is used as a cutoff.
- *Other markers*: Salivary estriol, maternal plasma CRH levels, maternal serum collagenase, serum ferritin, placental alkaline phosphatase and many cytokines are being studied.

Diagnostic accuracy is improved by using a combination of transvaginal cervical length (TVCL) and fFN measurement.

MANAGEMENT

Management depends upon gestational age and stage of preterm labor.

Algorithm for the management of preterm labor is depicted in Flowchart 1.

Threatened Preterm Labor

Women with threatened preterm labor present with uterine contractions and minimal

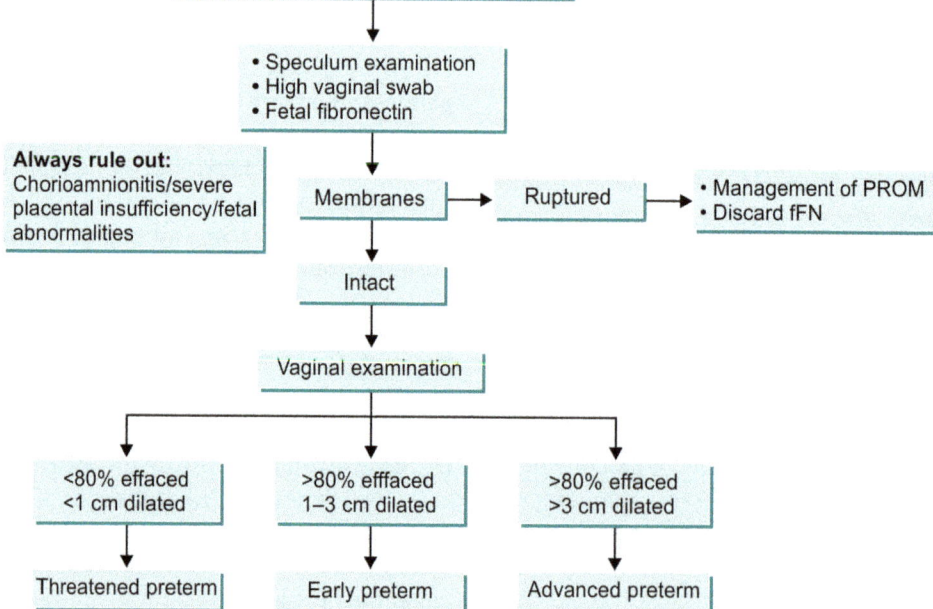

Flowchart 1: Management of preterm labor.

(PROM: premature rupture of membranes; fFn: fetal fibronectin)

or no cervical changes on digital cervical examination. The initial step is to exclude false labor. TVCL is commonly used to confirm the diagnosis. Flowchart 2 gives a brief overview of management in threatened preterm.[13]

Early Preterm Labor

Maternal and fetal well-being is to be assessed in women presenting with early preterm labor initially. While prolongation of pregnancy in women with advanced preterm labor is uncommon beyond 1 week, women in early preterm labor usually respond to tocolytics. Hence, the management encompasses steroids and tocolytics.

Antenatal Steroids

Glucocorticoids cross the placenta and induce enzymes to accelerate fetal pulmonary maturity. They reduce the incidence of respiratory distress syndrome and intraventricular hemorrhage.[14]

Steroid options:
- Betamethasone 12 mg intramuscular injection 24 hours apart for two doses.
- Dexamethasone 6 mg intramuscular injection 12 hours apart for four doses.

Caution:
- Rule out chorioamnionitis
- Where immediate delivery is indicated, do not wait for steroid effect
- Maternal blood sugar levels to be monitored.

Current American College of Obstetricians and Gynecologists (ACOG) recommendations:[15]
- For pregnant women between 24 weeks and 34 weeks of gestation at risk of preterm

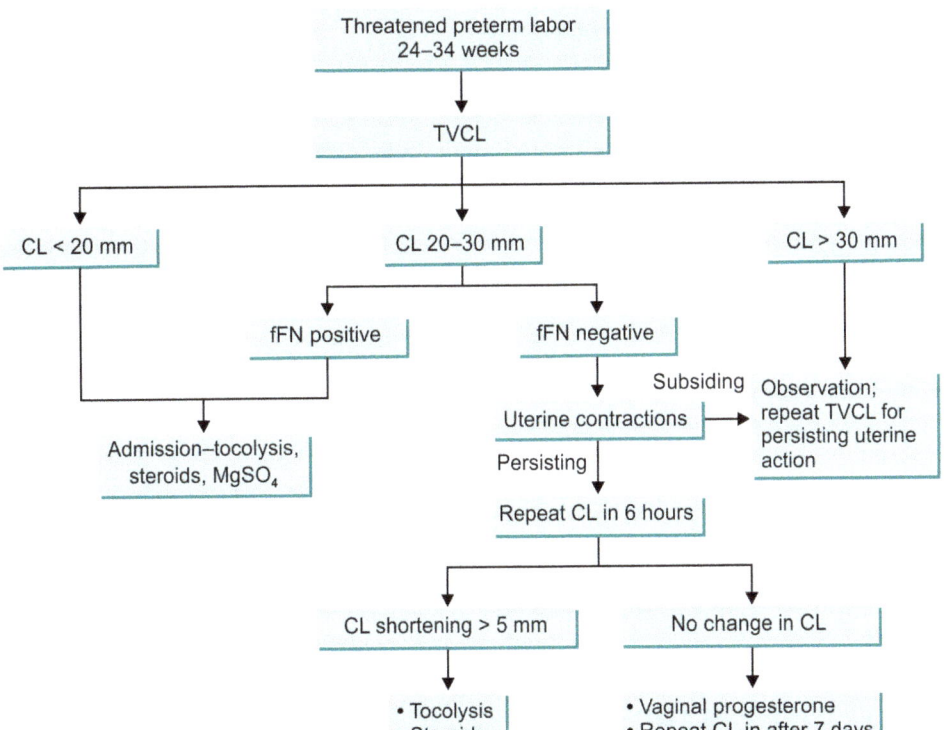

Flowchart 2: Management of threatened preterm labor.

(TVCL: transvaginal cervical length; CL: cervical length; fFN: fetal fibronectin)

labor, a single course of corticosteroids is recommended.
- For pregnant women between 34 weeks and 37 weeks of gestation and at risk of delivery within 7 days, a single course of steroids to be given if they have not received a prior dose.
- *Rescue dose of steroids*: For women at less than 34 weeks of gestation, at risk of delivery within the next 7 days and prior steroid administration was more than 14 days ago, a single repeat course should be considered.

Tocolysis

The word tocolytic was coined by Mosler from the Greek words tokos, contraction and lytic, capable of dissolving.[16] Tocolytic agents are effective up to 48 hours and may prolong pregnancy up to 7 days.

Indications: The main indication for administration of tocolytics is to facilitate administration of corticosteroids and to allow for transfer of patient to a tertiary care center.

Contraindications:
- Severe pre-eclampsia or eclampsia
- Abruptio placentae
- Chorioamnionitis or sepsis
- Advanced cervical dilatation
- Fetal distress
- Intrauterine fetal demise
- Lethal fetal anomaly
- Development of serious side effects to tocolytics.

Therapy should be discontinued if labor progresses despite treatment.

Mechanism of action of tocolytics: Site of action of commonly used tocolytics is illustrated in Figure 1.

The advantages, maternal-fetal side effects and contraindications of tocolytics have been shown in Table 1.

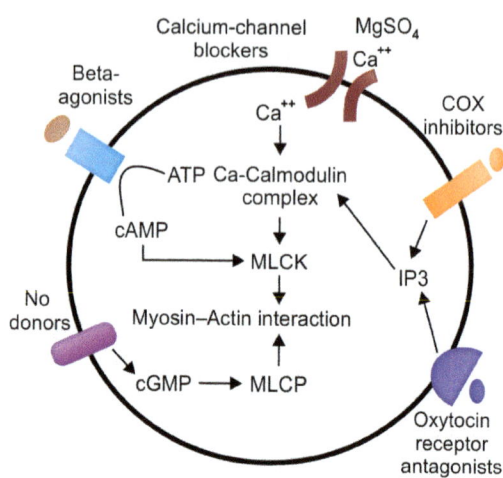

Fig. 1: Mechanism of action of tocolytics.

A brief review of dosages and current recommendations is summarized here:
- *Calcium-channel blockers*:[17] Nifedipine is the most commonly used dihydropyridine calcium-channel blocker. It is the preferred first-line tocolytic agent.
  Dose: Loading dose of 10–30 mg, repeated every 15–20 minutes for first hour if contractions continue followed by 10–20 mg orally every 4–8 hours.
- *Magnesium sulfate*:[18] Two mechanisms of action have been proposed for magnesium sulfate. One is competitive inhibition of calcium at motor end plate prevents release of acetylcholine into the synaptic cleft and the other mechanism is obstruction of calcium at plasma membrane voltage-gated channels.
  Dose: 4–6 g in 10–20% solution over 30 minutes followed by continuous infusion of 2 g/hour.
  Magnesium sulfate use has seen a resurgence due to its neuroprotective effect.
- *Betamimetics*:[19,20] Drugs in this class include ritodrine, terbutaline. They are β2-agonists. However, the concentration of β2-receptors gradually decrease during

TABLE 1: Advantages, maternal-fetal side effects and contraindications of tocolytics.

S. no.	Tocolytics	Advantages	Maternal side effects	Fetal side effects	Contraindications
1.	Calcium-channel blocker—nifedipine	• Oral administration • Low cost • Effective in delaying delivery up to 7 days	Dizziness, flushing, headache, hypotension, elevation of liver enzymes	No known adverse effects	• Relative indication—concurrent use of magnesium sulfate and beta-agonists (risk of hypotension) • Used with caution in cardiovascular disease (risk of cardiac failure)
2.	Magnesium sulfate	Neuroprotective for fetus	Flushing, diaphoresis, loss of deep tendon reflexes, respiratory depression, cardiac arrest	Neonatal depression	Concomitant use with calcium-channel blockers, myasthenia gravis, renal dysfunction
3.	Beta adrenergic receptor agonists—terbutaline, isoxsuprine		Tachycardia, hypotension, palpitations, chest pain, hyperglycemia, hypokalemia, pulmonary edema	Fetal tachycardia, neonatal hypoglycemia, hypocalcemia and ileus	Uncontrolled diabetes mellitus, heart disease
4.	Cyclooxygenase inhibitors (NSAIDs)—indomethacin		Gastritis, esophageal reflux	Premature constriction of ductus arteriosus, oligohydramnios, bronchopulmonary dysplasia, necrotizing enterocolitis	Bleeding disorder or platelet dysfunction, hepatic dysfunction, renal dysfunction, asthma, gastrointestinal ulcerative disease
5.	No donors—nitroglycerin		Flushing, dizziness, hypotension		Cardiac diseases (preload-dependent conditions)
6.	Oxytocin receptor antagonists—atosiban		Hypersensitivity and injection site-related reactions		

their use leading to desensitization and thereby a short duration of action. Although ritodrine was the most extensively studied and the only US Food and Drug Administration (FDA) approved drug in this class, it is no longer marketed. Terbutaline administered subcutaneously, is commonly used. According to the FDA, it is contraindicated by oral route for preterm labor. FDA also gave a "black box" warning for long-term use recently.
Dose: 0.25 mg, can be repeated every 4 hours.

Precaution: Maternal infusion to be discontinued at least 2 hours or more before delivery.
- *Prostaglandin inhibitors*:[21]
  Dose: Orally 50 mg loading dose followed by 25–50 mg orally every 6 hours for up to 48 hours.
  Its use is restricted to cases of preterm labor at less than 32 weeks of gestation to avoid the risk of premature closure of ductus arteriosus.
- *Nitrates*: Nitroglycerin or glyceryl trinitrate belongs to the NO donors group. It can be administered either transdermally or as an intravenous injection. Transdermal patch is the preferred way of administration. Use is currently limited to research trials.
- *Oxytocin receptor antagonists*:[22]
  Dose: Atosiban, an intravenous agent is administered as a bolus of 6.75 mg over 1 minute followed by a continuous infusion at 18 mg/hour for a period of 3 hours and then 6 mg/hour up to 45 hours. Studies have shown atosiban to be superior to placebo but have failed to demonstrate superiority over other tocolytics in terms of tocolytic efficacy or infant outcomes. More studies are needed to validate the use of atosiban.

Tocolysis as maintenance therapy: Long-standing maintenance therapy with tocolytics is neither effective in preventing preterm birth nor in improving neonatal outcomes and therefore not recommended. Studies involving commonly used tocolytics and placebo have not shown any improvement in maternal or neonatal outcomes with maintenance therapy. Atosiban is the only tocolytic which demonstrated significant difference in prolonging pregnancy duration when compared with placebo.[23]

Magnesium Sulfate for Neuroprotection

Current evidence suggests that the use of magnesium sulfate reduces the severity and risk of cerebral palsy in cases with preterm labor at less than 32 weeks of gestation.[24] NICE guidelines advocate a regimen of 4 g intravenous bolus of magnesium sulfate over 15 minutes followed by an intravenous infusion of 1 g/hour until birth or for 24 hours (whichever is earlier).[25]

Antibiotics in Preterm Labor[24]

As per ACOG guidelines, antibiotic use in the absence of documented infection is not recommended in women with preterm labor and intact membranes. This is however not applicable in cases with preterm PROM and group B streptococci carrier status.

Advanced Preterm Labor

Women in advanced preterm labor are at high risk of preterm delivery. Initially, conditions like chorioamnionitis, severe placental insufficiency and fetal abnormalities are to be excluded. After excluding the above conditions, a short trial of tocolytics may be given along with steroid administration. But if labor progresses, fetal monitoring is to be done and delivery to be planned. Preterm neonates are at increased risk of hypoxia, acidosis and intraventricular hemorrhage.

■ PREVENTION

Prevention of preterm birth may be aimed at three levels:
1. *Primary prevention—reduction of risk in the population*: The strategies for primary prevention of preterm birth include lifestyle changes, public awareness programs and changes in professional policies.
2. *Secondary prevention—identification of risk factors and their management*: Many interventions like bed rest, limited activity, screening and treatment of women with bacterial vaginosis have been proposed, but there is little evidence supporting

their role in prevention of preterm labor. The two strategies with favorable evidence are progesterone supplementation and cervical encerclage.

i. *Progesterone supplementation*:[26] Several randomized control trials have shown that progesterone either as weekly intramuscular 17α-hydroxyprogesterone caproate or daily vaginal suppositories reduced the rate of preterm birth in women with history of prior preterm labor and/or short cervix.

ii. *Cervical encerclage*:[27] Cervical encerclage is not universally advocated in women with short cervix. Although, cervical cerclage is beneficial in women with short cervix (<15–25 mm) and a previous history of preterm labor, it has not been shown to reduce preterm risk in women without a history of preterm birth.

Flowchart 3 is for prevention of preterm birth in singleton pregnancies.[25,27]

3. *Tertiary prevention*: Treatment initiated after preterm labor process has begun to limit perinatal morbidity and mortality. This encompasses all the interventions described in management preterm labor.

PREMATURE RUPTURE OF MEMBRANES

Definitions

Premature or prelabor rupture of membranes is defined as rupture of chorioamniotic membranes before the onset of labor. Preterm PROM is defined as the rupture of membranes before 37 weeks of gestation. Preterm PROM is seen in one-third of all preterm births.[28] Preterm PROM is further divided into:
- Previable PROM—at gestational age less than 24 weeks

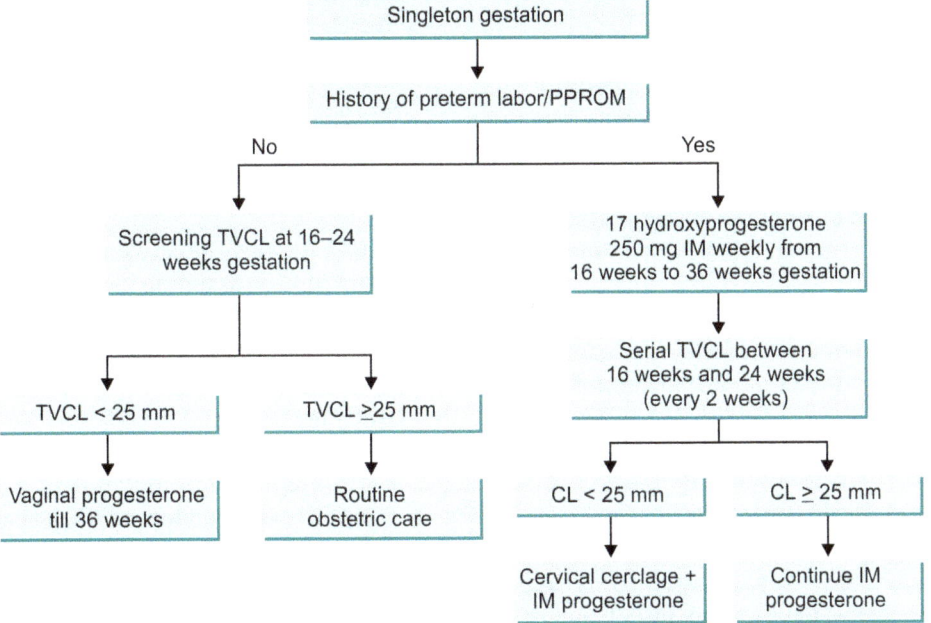

Flowchart 3: Prevention of preterm birth in singleton pregnancies.

(PPROM: preterm premature rupture of membranes; TVCL: transvaginal cervical length; CL: cervical length; IM: intramuscular)

- Preterm PROM remote from term—from 24 weeks to 31 weeks of gestation—associated with significant perinatal morbidity and mortality
- Preterm PROM near term—from 32 weeks to 37 weeks of gestation.

Etiology

Although preterm PROM often occurs without any obvious cause, intra-amniotic infection is one of the common causes. The other risk factors for PROM at any gestational age are similar to those of preterm labor. History of preterm PROM in previous pregnancy is a major risk factor for preterm PROM in present pregnancy.[29] Apart from the common risk factors, procedures that may result in preterm PROM include: cervical cerclage and amniocentesis.

Complications

Common maternal and fetal complications are listed in Table 2.

Diagnosis

Initial evaluation of PROM includes history and physical examination. Common presenting symptoms are continued, uncontrolled fluid leakage from vagina, intermittent leakage or an isolated loss of fluid. Other symptoms like pelvic pressure and lower abdominal pain to be elicited.

Physical examination along with vital data to be recorded to exclude chorioamnionitis. Signs of chorioamnionitis are enumerated in Box 2.

Tests to Confirm the Diagnosis of PROM

- Sterile speculum examination and visualization of fluid leakage
- *Nitrazine test*: Phenaphthazine, i.e. nitrazine paper turns blue from yellow on exposure to alkaline amniotic fluid (pH >7.0). False-positive test is seen in cases of blood/semen contamination, alkaline antiseptics and bacterial vaginosis.
- Ferning pattern on microscopic examination
- Other methods:
  - Ultrasound-guided amniocentesis with injection of indigo carmine dye and observation for vaginal leakage
  - Oligohydramnios on ultrasound
  - Nile blue sulfate staining of vaginal smears
  - Vaginal alpha-fetoprotein screening.

TABLE 2: Common maternal and fetal complications.

Maternal	Fetal
Maternal infection: • Chorioamnionitis • Sepsis	Fetal or neonatal infection
Increased operative delivery	Preterm birth: • Respiratory distress syndrome • Sepsis • Intraventricular hemorrhage • Necrotizing enterocolitis • Neurodevelopmental impairment[30]
Abruptio placentae	Umbilical cord compression or prolapse
	With early and severe oligoamnios: • Pulmonary hypoplasia • Fetal deformations—Potter's sequence

Box 2: Signs of chorioamnionitis.

- Temperature >100.4°F
- Maternal tachycardia
- Hypotension
- Uterine tenderness
- Foul smelling discharge
- Fetal tachycardia
- Laboratory tests—elevated white blood cell (WBC) count/C-reactive protein (CRP)

At speculum examination, cervical swab for gonococcal and chlamydial infection and also vaginal/perianal swab for group B streptococcal infection is taken.

Management

Management of PROM depends on the gestational age at presentation as the frequency of perinatal complications decreases with increasing gestational age. The interval between the rupture of membranes and the onset of labor is called as the latent period. The duration of the latent period varies inversely with age.

- *Premature rupture of membranes at term*: At term, majority of women proceed to spontaneous labor within 24 hours of membrane rupture. In case, patient does not proceed into spontaneous labor at presentation, labor is usually induced with oxytocin infusion, after excluding any maternal or fetal contraindications for normal delivery.
- *Preterm premature rupture of membranes*:[31] Management should be based on assessment of maternal and fetal well-being and predicted neonatal risks with either expectant management or expeditious delivery.

Algorithm for management of preterm PROM has been shown in Flowchart 4.

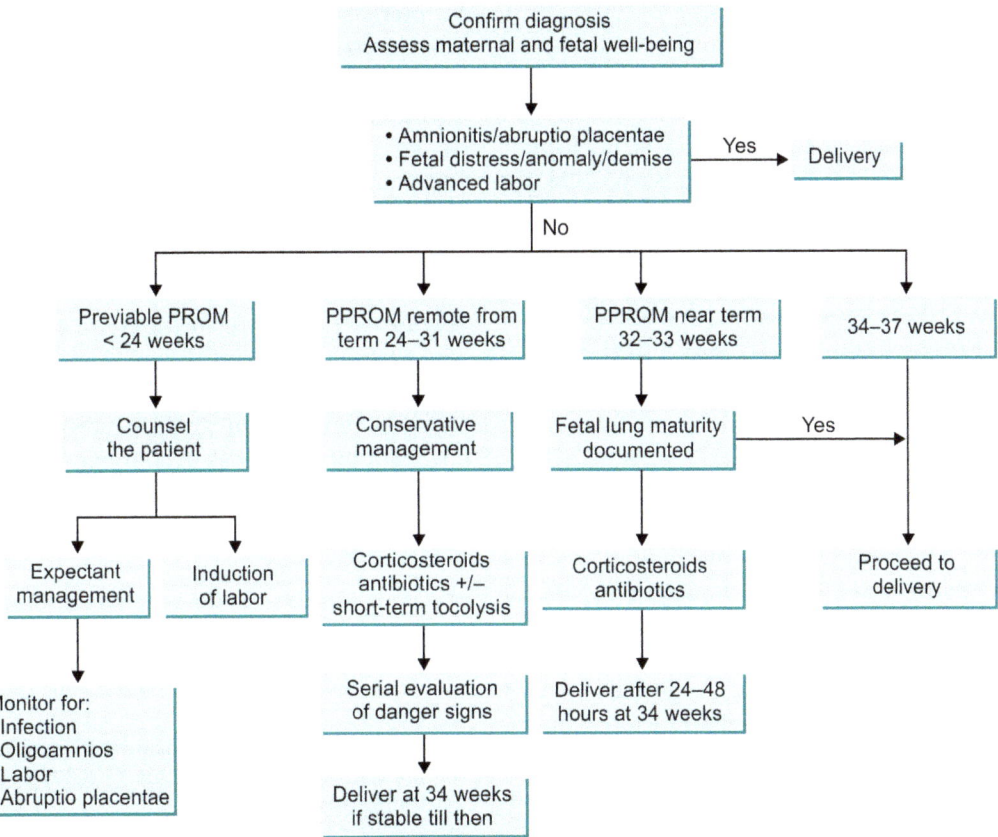

Flowchart 4: Management of preterm premature rupture of membranes.

(PROM: premature rupture of membranes; PPROM: preterm PROM)

Assessment of fetal well-being:
- Maternal perception of fetal activity
- Fetal heart rate monitoring (by NST)
- Biophysical profile and USG Doppler.

Fetal lung maturity (FLM) assessment: In cases with ruptured membranes, amniotic fluid from vaginal pool can be used to assess FLM. The sample obtained by amniocentesis is the most accurate specimen as contaminating substances like gross blood, meconium or urine in vaginal pool specimens may cause interference with the tests. The tests are divided into biochemical and biophysical tests:
- Biochemical tests
    - Lecithin/sphingomyelin ratio
    - Phosphatidylglycerol measurement
- Biophysical tests
    - Surfactant/albumin ratio
    - Lamellar body counts.

The use of FLM testing is no longer recommend by ACOG as a positive FLM test is not predictive of the overall maturity of the neonate and does not lead to improved neonatal outcomes. Also the clinical utility of FLM testing is limited with advances care of neonates by antenatal steroid supplementation and surfactant replacement therapy.[32]

Antibiotic prophylaxis:[33] Antibiotic prophylaxis has been associated with prolongation of pregnancy and improvement in short-term neonatal morbidities in cases with preterm PROM. Although no significant reduction in perinatal mortality and long-term benefit is noted, routine use of antibiotics is recommended. There is no specific choice of antibiotic but co-amoxiclav is avoided due to the risk of NEC in neonates.

The regimen used in the National Institute of Child Health and Human Development Trial[34] is a combination of:

- Intravenous 2 g ampicillin and 250 mg erythromycin 6th hourly for 48 hours followed by—Oral 250 mg amoxicillin and 333 mg (base) of erythromycin 8th hourly for 5 days.

Other commonly used regimens—combination of beta-lactam antibiotics with gram-negative organism coverage with macrolides.

For women who are group B *Streptococcus* carriers, it is better to administer antibiotics for prophylaxis even if they received a course of antibiotics previously.

Prophylactic steroids:[35] Use of antenatal corticosteroids has been associated with reduction in neonatal mortality, RDS, intraventricular hemorrhage and NEC. No increased risk of maternal or neonatal infection has been noted with steroid use in cases with preterm PROM. Therefore, ACOG recommends a single course of prophylactic steroids in women with rupture of membranes between 24 weeks and 34 weeks of gestation. There is sufficient evidence regarding repeat courses of steroids in cases with ruptured membranes.

Tocolysis:[36] Short-term tocolytic therapy may prolong the latent period in cases with ruptured membranes but there is no beneficial effect on neonatal outcomes. However, there is a slight increased risk of chorioamnionitis. Long-term tocolysis is not recommended.

REFERENCES

1. Liu L, Johnson HL, Cousens S, et al. Global, regional, and national causes of child mortality: an updated systematic analysis for 2010 with time trends since 2000. Lancet. 2012;379: 2151-61.
2. Romero R, Espinoza J, Kusanovic JP, et al. The preterm parturition syndrome. BJOG. 2006;113 (Suppl 3):17-42.
3. Renthal NE, Williams KC, Mendelson CR. MicroRNAs—mediators of myometrial

contractility during pregnancy and labour. Nat Rev Endocrinol. 2013;9:391-401.
4. Mahendroo M. Cervical remodeling in term and preterm birth: insights from an animal model. Reproduction. 2012;143(4):429-38.
5. Menon R, Fortunato SJ. Infection and the role of inflammation in preterm premature rupture of the membranes. Best Pract Res Clin Obstet Gynaecol. 2007;21:467-78.
6. Moore RM, Mansour JM, Redline RW, et al. The physiology of fetal membrane rupture: insight gained from the determination of physical properties. Placenta. 2006;27:1037-51.
7. Romero R, Espinoza J, Chaiworapongsa T, et al. Infection and prematurity and the role of preventive strategies. Semin Neonatol. 2002;7:259-74.
8. Romero R, Sirtori M, Oyarzun E, et al. Infection and labor. V. Prevalence, microbiology, and clinical significance of intra-amniotic infection in women with preterm labor and intact membranes. Am J Obstet Gynecol. 1989;161:817-24.
9. Gomez R, Romero R, Ghezzi F, et al. The fetal inflammatory response syndrome. Am J Obstet Gynecol. 1998;179:194-202.
10. Romero R, Chaiworapongsa T, Kuivaniemi H, et al. Bacterial vaginosis, the inflammatory response and the risk of preterm birth: a role for genetic epidemiology in the prevention of preterm birth. Am J Obstet Gynecol. 2004;190:1509-19.
11. Leitich H, Brunbauer M, Kaider A, et al. Cervical length and dilatation of the internal cervical os detected by vaginal ultrasonography as markers for preterm delivery: a systematic review. Am J Obstet Gynecol. 1999;181:1465-72.
12. Lockwood CJ, Senyei AE, Dische MR, et al. Fetal fibronectin in cervical and vaginal secretions as a predictor of preterm delivery. N Engl J Med. 1991;325:669-74.
13. Gomez R, Romero R, Medina L, et al. Cervicovaginal fibronectin improves the prediction of preterm delivery based on sonographic cervical length in patients with preterm uterine contractions and intact membranes. Am J Obstet Gynecol. 2005;192(2):350-9.
14. Roberts D, Dalziel S. Antenatal corticosteroids for accelerating fetal lung maturation for women at risk of preterm birth. Cochrane Database Syst Rev. 2006;(3):CD004454.
15. Committee on Obstetric Practice. Committee opinion no. 713: antenatal corticosteroid therapy for fetal maturation. Obstet Gynecol. 2017;130:e102-9.
16. Mosler KH. Symposion über Physiologie und Pathologie der Wehentätigkeit. Zentralblatt Für Gynäkologie; 1965.
17. Conde-Agudelo A, Romero R, Kusanovic JP. Nifedipine in the management of preterm labor: a systematic review and meta-analysis. Am J Obstet Gynecol. 2011;204(2):134.e1-20.
18. Elliott JP. Magnesium sulfate as a tocolytic agent. Am J Obstet Gynecol. 1983;147(3):277-84.
19. Creasy RK, Resnik R, Iams JD. Creasy and Resnik's Maternal-Fetal Medicine: Principles and Practice, 6th edition. Philadelphia, PA, USA: Saunders; 2009.
20. US Food and Drug Administration. Terbutaline: Label change—warnings against use for treatment of preterm labor; 2001.
21. Abou-Ghannam G, Usta IM, Nassar AH. Indomethacin in pregnancy: applications and safety. Am J Perinatol. 2012;29(3):175-86.
22. Haas DM, Caldwell DM, Kirkpatrick P, et al. Tocolytic therapy for preterm delivery: systematic review and network meta-analysis. BMJ. 2012;345:e6226.
23. Valenzuela GJ, Sanchez-Ramos L, Romero R, et al. Maintenance treatment of preterm labor with the oxytocin antagonist atosiban. The Atosiban PTL-098 Study Group. Am J Obstet Gynecol. 2000;182:1184-90.
24. American College of Obstetricians and Gynecologists' Committee on Practice Bulletins—Obstetrics. Practice bulletin no. 171: management of preterm labor. Obstet Gynecol. 2016;128:e155-64.
25. National Institute for Health and Care Excellence (NG25). (2015). Preterm labour and birth. NICE guideline (NG25). [online] Available from: https://www.nice.org.uk/guidance/ng25/resources/preterm-labour-and-birth-pdf-1837333576645 [Last accessed September, 2019].
26. Fonseca EB, Celik E, Parra M, et al. Progesterone and the risk of preterm birth among women with a short cervix. N Engl J Med. 2007;357(5):462-9.

27. Berghella V, Odibo AO, To MS, et al. Cerclage for short cervix on ultrasonography: meta-analysis of trials using individual patient-level data. Obstet Gynecol. 2005;106(1):181-9.
28. Mercer B. Premature rupture of the membranes. In: Queenan JT, Hobbins JC, Spong CY (Eds). Protocols for High-Risk Pregnancies, 5th edition. West Sussex, UK: Wiley-Blackwell; 2010.
29. Mercer BM, Goldenberg RL, Moawad AH, et al. The preterm prediction study: effect of gestational age and cause of preterm birth on subsequent obstetric outcome. National Institute of Child Health and Human Development Maternal-Fetal Medicine Units Network. Am J Obstet Gynecol. 1999;181:1216-21.
30. Yoon BH, Romero R, Park JS, et al. Fetal exposure to an intra-amniotic inflammation and the development of cerebral palsy at the age of three years. Am J Obstet Gynecol. 2000;182:675-81.
31. Committee on Practice Bulletins-Obstetrics. ACOG practice bulletin no. 188: prelabor rupture of membranes. Obstet Gynecol. 2018;131:e1-14.
32. Halliday HL. Surfactants: past, present and future. J Perinatol. 2008;28(Suppl 1):S47-56.
33. Kenyon S, Boulvain M, Neilson JP. Antibiotics for preterm rupture of membranes. Cochrane Database Syst Rev. 2013;(12):CD001058.
34. Mercer BM, Miodovnik M, Thurnau GR, et al. Antibiotic therapy for reduction of infant morbidity after preterm premature rupture of the membranes. A randomized controlled trial. National Institute of Child Health and Human Development Maternal-Fetal Medicine Units Network. JAMA. 1997;278:989-95.
35. Harding JE, Pang J, Knight DB, et al. Do antenatal corticosteroids help in the setting of preterm rupture of membranes? Am J Obstet Gynecol. 2001;184:131-9.
36. Fontenot T, Lewis DF. Tocolytic therapy with preterm premature rupture of membranes. Clin Perinatol. 2001;28:787-96.

CHAPTER 15

Antepartum Hemorrhage

Chandana C, Srividhya GK

PLACENTAL ABRUPTION

INTRODUCTION

Placental abruption is defined as the premature separation of a normally implanted placenta from the uterine wall before the delivery of fetus. It complicates about one percent of all pregnancies.[1] Placental abruption is one among the major causes of antepartum hemorrhage (APH) accounting for one-third of APH cases. It contributes to significant risk of maternal and perinatal morbidity and mortality. The maternal outcome is dependent on the amount of blood loss. The fetal outcome depends on the period of gestation at which it occurs and the severity of blood loss. Severe hemorrhage is associated complications like disseminated intravascular coagulation (DIC), acute renal failure, couvelaire uterus, postpartum hemorrhage (PPH), and hysterectomy. Majority of fetal mortality is because of intrauterine death (IUD) before hospital admission. Although fetal outcome has improved due to advanced neonatal care, most of the perinatal deaths are because of extreme preterm babies. Surviving neonates are at significant risk of neurodevelopmental delay and cerebral palsy.

RISK FACTORS

The exact etiology of placental abruption is not known. There are many factors, which increases the risk of placental abruption. The risk factors are divided into three groups:

1. *Health history*:
   - History of placental abruption in previous pregnancies. Rate of recurrence is 11% after first episode, after second episode rises up to 25%.[2]
   - Maternal age >35 years.
   - Known case of hypertension.
   - Cocaine/vasoconstrictive medications reducing uteroplacental blood supply.
   - Cigarette smoking containing nicotine results in decidual necrosis, chorionic villi hemorrhage, and thrombosis.[3,4]
2. *Factors specific to current pregnancies*:
   - Pre-eclampsia
   - Thrombophilias[5,6]
   - Multiple pregnancies
   - Polyhydramnios
   - Premature and prelabor rupture of membranes
   - Chorioamnionitis.
3. *Trauma to the abdomen*:[7]
   - Motor vehicle road accident
   - Physical abuse/domestic violence
   - During external cephalic version.

PATHOPHYSIOLOGY

The exact pathogenesis that causes placental abruption is not known in majority of patients. It occurs as a result of hemorrhage at the decidual placental interface. Acute vasoconstriction of placental vascular bed may be the preceding event which results in hemorrhage and thrombosis of decidual vasculature leading to decidual necrosis.[8] As the hematoma increases there is progressive detachment and further compression of intervillous area causing an organized blood clot on the maternal side of the placenta.

Shearing forces resulting from trauma and acute uterine decompression occurring after rupture of membranes in cases of hydramnios or after first twin delivery can result in sudden placental separation.[9]

Acute placental detachment deprives the fetus of nutrients and oxygen resulting in fetal hypoxia and intrauterine fetal death. The coagulation pathway is initiated with utilization of coagulation factors leading to DIC. Further bleeding due to DIC increases the consumption of coagulation cascade factors resulting in a vicious cycle. Hemorrhage can extend to the myometrium reaching up to the serosal surface, causing blotchy blue areas in the uterus which denotes couvelaire uterus. The hematoma in the retroplacental space may extend between decidua and placental membranes then pass down the cervix and leading to vaginal bleeding. There are two types of placental abruption; namely:

1. *Concealed variety (20%)*: When hemorrhage confined within the uterine cavity. The quantity of blood loss is often underestimated and presents as severe form of placental abruption.
2. *Revealed variety (80%)*: When the bleeding drains in to the vagina.

CLINICAL FEATURES

Placental abruption is a clinical diagnosis where patients present with vaginal bleeding and pain abdomen (most of the time continuous pain). In severe cases they may present with shock or fetal demise. The severity of placental abruption poorly correlates with the quantity of vaginal bleeding. Clinical implications of placental abruption vary based on the extent and location of the separation. On clinical examination a tender and tense uterus with a hard feel suggest significant abruption. Depending on the quantity of hemorrhage, mother may present with obstetric shock and fetus may be hypoxic or demised. Fetal hypoxia will lead to nonreassuring fetal heart rate pattern on cardiotocograph. Sonographic examination may be helpful in certain cases to exclude placenta previa. Ultrasonography is not reliable in diagnosing abruption, as it is difficult to differentiate blood clot from the placenta. Since DIC is a common complication, coagulation profile should be done. Depending on the following clinical findings placental abruption is classified as:

- *Class 0: Asymptomatic*
  - Clinical features may be absent.
  - Presence of a blood clot on the maternal surface of a delivered placenta.
  - Diagnosis is made after delivery.
- *Class 1: Mild*
  - No sign of vaginal bleeding or vaginal bleeding is slight.
  - Uterine tenderness may be minimal or absent.
  - Maternal and fetal status normal.
- *Class 2: Moderate*
  - Vaginal bleeding mild to moderate in amount.
  - Uterine tenderness significant with tetanic contractions.
  - Maternal tachycardia and hypotension.
  - Evidence of fetal distress.
  - Hypofibrinogenemia.
- *Class 3: Severe*
  - Vaginal bleeding moderate to severe or may be absent in concealed abruption.
  - Woody feel of uterus with severe uterine tenderness.
  - Maternal shock present.
  - Fetal demise.
  - Hypofibrinogenemia and coagulopathy.

MANAGEMENT

Treatment of placental abruption is based on clinical presentation, period of gestation at the time of presentation, and the extent of maternal and fetal compromise (Flowchart 1). In severe cases, mother should be resuscitated and stabilized with ABCD approach of resuscitation as follows:

- *Assessment of airway and breathing*: Need for oxygen supply.
- *Assessment of circulation*:
  - Securing intravenous line for fluid and blood resuscitation. Send patients blood for complete blood count, coagulation profile, Kleihauer–Betke test, and crossmatch four units of blood.
  - Position the patient in left lateral position and maintain normothermia.
  - In the presence of severe blood loss infuse up to 1-2 liters of warmed crystalloid solution or colloid solution until the crossmatched blood is available. With on going massive hemorrhage transfuse four units of fresh frozen plasma (FFP) and 10 units of cryoprecipitate while waiting for coagulation profile.

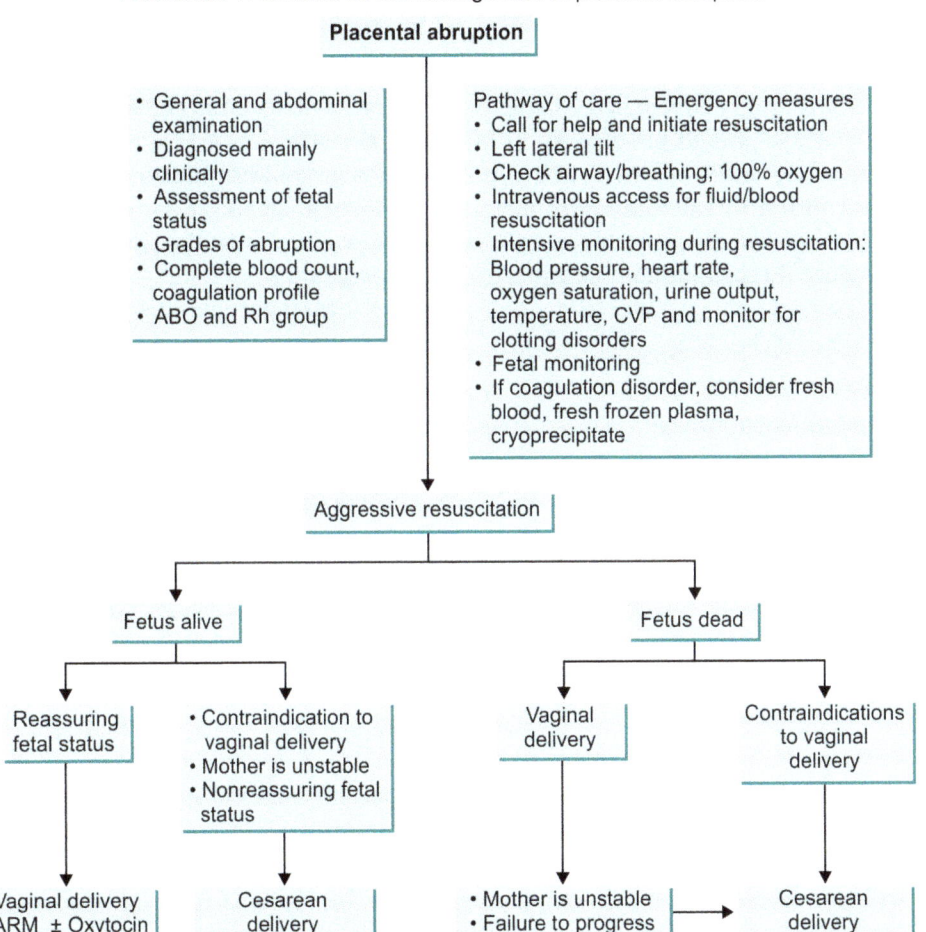

Flowchart 1: Scheme for the management of placental abruption.

- *Assessment of fetal condition and decision for delivery:*
  - Do artificial rupture of membranes if fetus is alive and no fetal distress. Monitor the fetus and in case of fetal distress perform cesarean section.
  - Vaginal delivery is preferred in the presence of a fetal demise, but if there is massive abruption, cesarean section may be considered to control bleeding.
  - If hemorrhage has controlled and not in labor, antenatal steroids can be given to enhance fetal lung maturity and decrease the risk of neonatal respiratory distress syndrome and intraventricular hemorrhage if the gestational age is <34 weeks.
  - Since there is significant amount of fetomaternal hemorrhage, Kleihauer–Betke test should be done for all Rh negative mothers with placental abruption to calculate appropriate dose of anti-D immunoglobulin to reduce rhesus alloimmunization.

COMPLICATIONS

- Hypovolemic shock
- Postpartum hemorrhage
- Disseminated intravascular coagulation
- Renal failure
- Increased risk of amniotic fluid embolism,[10] venous thromboembolism,[11] and sepsis.[12]

Placental abruption is associated with severe hemorrhage, may require blood transfusion and emergency hysterectomy. Placental abruption is associated with significant risk of stillbirth, preterm birth, and perinatal morbidity/mortality.

In subsequent pregnancies there is an increased risk of recurrence, approximately 11% after one episode and raising up to 25% after two episodes.[2] There is also an increased risk of other adverse outcome such as pre-eclampsia, preterm birth, and intrauterine growth restriction (IUGR). Hypertension to be treated prior to pregnancy and during the subsequent pregnancy. Woman with history of smoking or cocaine use should be counseled and encouraged to quit before the next pregnancy.

CONCLUSION

- Placental abruption is an important cause of maternal and fetal morbidity and mortality.
- Placental abruption complicates about 1% of pregnancies and is the major cause of vaginal bleeding in the later half of pregnancy.
- Placental abruption is diagnosed mainly clinically.
- The treatment of placental abruption is based on clinical presentation, gestational age at the time of presentation, and the extent of maternal and fetal compromise.
- Disseminated intravascular coagulation and maternal shock should be treated aggressively.
- Subsequent pregnancies may be associated with increased risk of abruption, pre-eclampsia, IUGR, and preterm birth.

PLACENTA PREVIA

INTRODUCTION

Antepartum hemorrhage is defined as bleeding from the vagina after 20 weeks of pregnancy and before delivery. It complicates around 2-5% of all pregnancies.[13] The most important causes of antepartum hemorrhage are abruption placenta and placenta previa. The other causes are vasa previa, marginal sinus bleeding, cervical erosion, genital trauma, and coagulation defects.

The placenta implanted in the lower segment of the uterus is termed as placenta previa. There is fourfold increased risk of vaginal bleeding during second trimester. Placenta previa has increased risk of adverse maternal and fetal complications.

INCIDENCE

The incidence of placenta previa is around 5/1,000 pregnancies worldwide.[14] However, there is a wide variation in incidence between 2.7 per 1,000 pregnancies and 12.2 per 1,000 pregnancies depending on the region.[15] The Asian studies show high prevalence (12.2/1,000 pregnancies) compared to Africa and North America (2.7/1,000 pregnancies).[14] These racial variations suggest the possibility of genetic predisposition.

ETIOLOGY

The exact mechanism of placental implantation in the lower segment is yet unknown. In majority of the pregnancies, as it advances, the placenta migrates. The process of placental "migration" or relative upward shift of the placenta due to differential growth of the lower segment is continuous into the late third trimester.[16] The migration of the placenta is also said to be due to process of growth known as "trophotropism". The trophoblastic cells seek the areas of higher vascularity towards the fundus leading to migration of the placenta away from the less vascular lower segment.[17] The placental tissue which still remains in the lower segment usually undergo complete atrophy or may persist as succenturiate lobes or may atrophy partially leaving vessels (vasa previa). The probable mechanisms of spontaneous cessation of bleeding are thrombosis of the open sinuses, placental infarction or mechanical pressure by the presenting part.

The placenta previa is most commonly associated with uterine scarring due to uterine instrumentation (such as repeated curettage), previous placenta previa, and previous cesarean section (Box 1).

There is strong likelihood ratio of developing an adherent placenta or invasive placenta, in a case of placenta previa with history of previous cesarean delivery. The adherent placenta includes placenta accreta (placenta penetrates the decidua basalis), placenta increta (placenta penetrates into the myometrium), and placenta percreta (placenta penetrates through the serosa to invade the adjacent organs). The risk of placenta previa and adherent placenta increases with increasing number of cesarean deliveries from baseline of 4.5-5% (no prior cesarean delivery) to 3-24%, 11-47%, 40%, and 61-67% with 1, 2, 3, and ≥4 prior cesarean deliveries, respectively.[18,19]

The diagnosis of placenta previa and accreta before delivery helps in planning a multidisciplinary approach to reduce the potential maternal or neonatal morbidity and mortality.

CLASSIFICATION

The placenta previa was classified based on degree of placental extension into the lower segment into four categories (Fig. 1):
1. *Total placenta previa*: Internal os completely covered by placenta.

Box 1: Risk factors for placenta previa.
- Previous placenta previa
- Previous cesarean sections
- Multiparity
- Advanced maternal age (>40 years)
- Multiple pregnancy
- Smoking
- Deficient endometrium due history of endometritis, manual removal of placenta, curettage, submucous fibroid, and assisted conception.

Obstetric Emergencies

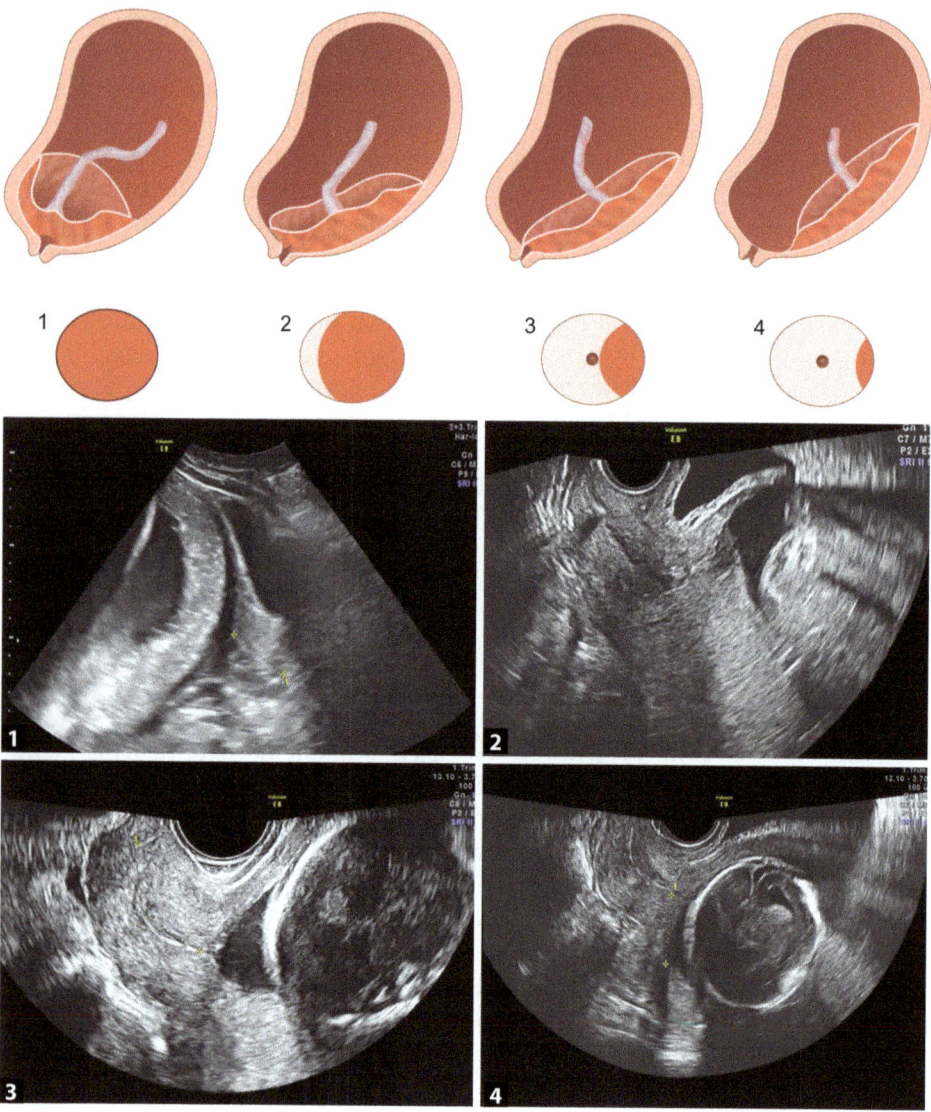

Fig. 1: Classification of placenta previa. (1) Total placenta previa—internal os completely covered by placenta; (2) Partial placenta previa—internal os partly covered by placenta; (3) Marginal placenta previa—placental edge at margin of internal os; (4) Low-lying placenta—placenta implanted in the lower uterine segment.

2. *Partial placenta previa*: Internal os partly covered by placenta.
3. *Marginal placenta previa*: Placental edge at margin of internal os.
4. *Low-lying placenta*: Placenta implanted in the lower uterine segment.

In the recent years, there are various publications on the diagnosis of placenta previa and its outcome based on the localization of the placenta, using transvaginal sonography (TVS) and the distance measured accurately from the placental edge to the internal os. The traditional classification of placenta previa has become obsolete with the increased prognostic value of transvaginal ultrasound diagnosis.

The latest Royal College of Obstetricians and Gynaecologists (RCOG) guidelines on placenta previa and accreta, 2011, have acknowledged the change in the classification of placenta previa.[20-22] The old classification has now been replaced by new classification based on ultrasound findings:
- *Major placenta previa*: When placenta overlaps or covers the internal os.
- *Minor placenta previa*: When the placenta reaches the internal os.

CLINICAL FINDINGS

The most common presentation in placenta previa is painless and recurrent vaginal bleeding, usually in the second trimester or later. Fortunately, the initial bleeding is rarely profuse to prove fatal but subsequent bouts may be heavier. The general condition and anemia are proportionate to the visible blood loss. On examination, the size of the uterus is proportional to the gestational age and uterus is usually relaxed without any tenderness. In majority of the cases, there is persistence of malpresentation or floating head. There is slowing of fetal heart rate on pressing the head into the pelvis in case of placenta previa, especially posterior type. This is known as "Stallworthy's sign". However, it may not be significant always as it can be seen even in normal cases due to head compression. The vaginal examination, especially double setup examination, is obsolete.

DIAGNOSIS

The definitive diagnosis of placenta previa is by ultrasound imaging. In all women with vaginal bleeding (painless or provoked) after 20 weeks of gestation, high presenting part, an abnormal lie, irrespective of previous imaging results usually raise the clinical suspicion of placenta previa.

According to RCOG guidelines, we should screen for placental localization during routine ultrasound scanning at 20 weeks of gestation to identify women whose placenta encroaches on the cervical os. This practice is however not supported by evidence from randomized controlled trials.[22]

Transvaginal sonography is the most accurate and preferred method for the localization of a low-lying placenta. On transabdominal ultrasound, there is poor visualization of the posterior placenta, the fetal head can interfere with the visualization of the lower segment, obesity, and underfilling or overfilling of the bladder interferes the accurate localization of placenta. Hence, transabdominal scan has high-false positive rate for the diagnosis of placenta previa of up to 25%. Whenever the diagnosis of placenta previa is done by abdominal scan at 20 weeks, it should be confirmed by transvaginal scan and all these women require follow-up.[21]

On ultrasound, the distance from the internal os to the placental edge is measured and the following points are noted (Figs. 2A to D):
- When the placenta is 2 cm or more from the os, no follow-up is required.
- When the placenta is <2 cm from the internal os, follow-up at about 32 weeks.
- If the placenta covers the internal os, the distance that it projects beyond the os should be measured.
- Assess the attachment of the umbilical cord to the placenta (vasa previa).
- To exclude adherent placentas—accreta/increta/percreta.

False positives in diagnosis of placenta previa may be due to following reasons: (1) Overfilled bladder compressing lower uterine segment, (2) myometrial contraction (in such cases, repeat scanning is done after an

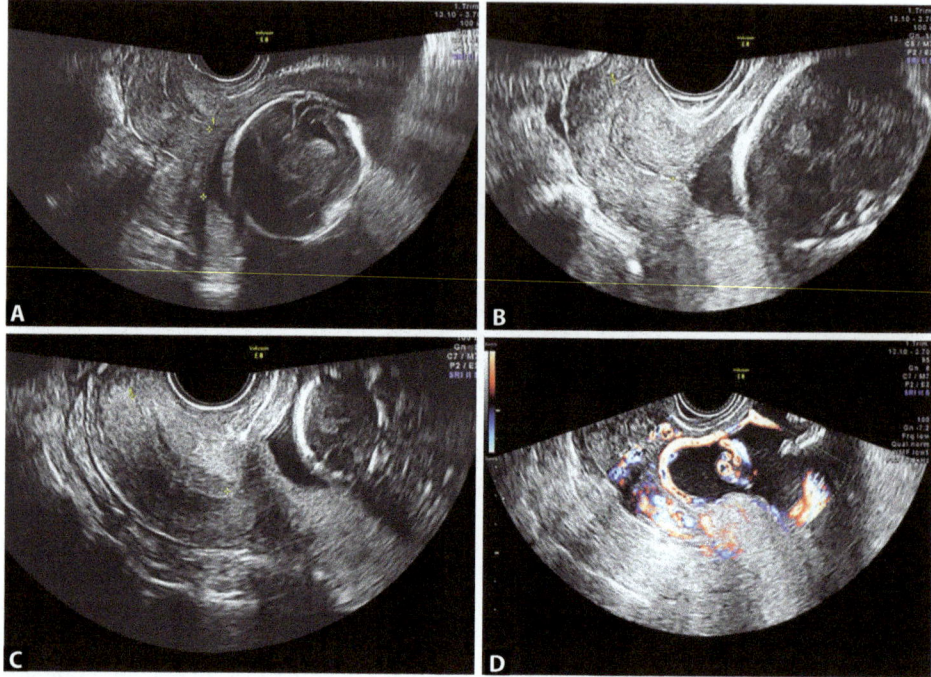

Figs. 2A to D: Ultrasound pictures of low-lying placenta, placental edge thickness, and vasa previa: (A) Distance of the lower edge of the placenta from the os: >2 cm (normal); (B) Distance of the lower edge of the placenta from the os: 1–2 cm; (C) Distance of the lower edge of the placenta from the os: <1 cm; (D) Vasa previa.

interval of 15–30 minutes) or (3) ultrasound in early pregnancy showing low position of the placenta, which in third trimester may be entirely normal due to differential growth of the uterus.

The placenta which is low-lying has an increased chance of being adherent, especially when it is an anterior low-lying placenta in a woman with previous cesarean scar. Diagnosis of a morbidly adherent placenta is very important in order to decrease the maternal morbidity, by choosing the appropriate place for delivery.

Ultrasound Criteria for Diagnosis of Adherent Placenta (Figs. 3A to C)[22]

- Loss of the retroplacental sonolucent space
- Irregular retroplacental space
- Disruption of the uterine serosa and bladder interface
- Presence of focal masses or growth, invading the bladder
- Abnormal placental lacunae.

On Color Doppler

- Diffuse or focal lacunar flow
- Vascular lakes with turbulent flow (peak systolic velocity over 15 cm/s)
- Hypervascularity of serosa-bladder interface
- Markedly dilated vessels over peripheral subplacental zone.

Magnetic resonance imaging (MRI) complements antenatal ultrasound imaging in equivocal cases to distinguish those women at special risk of placenta accreta. The role

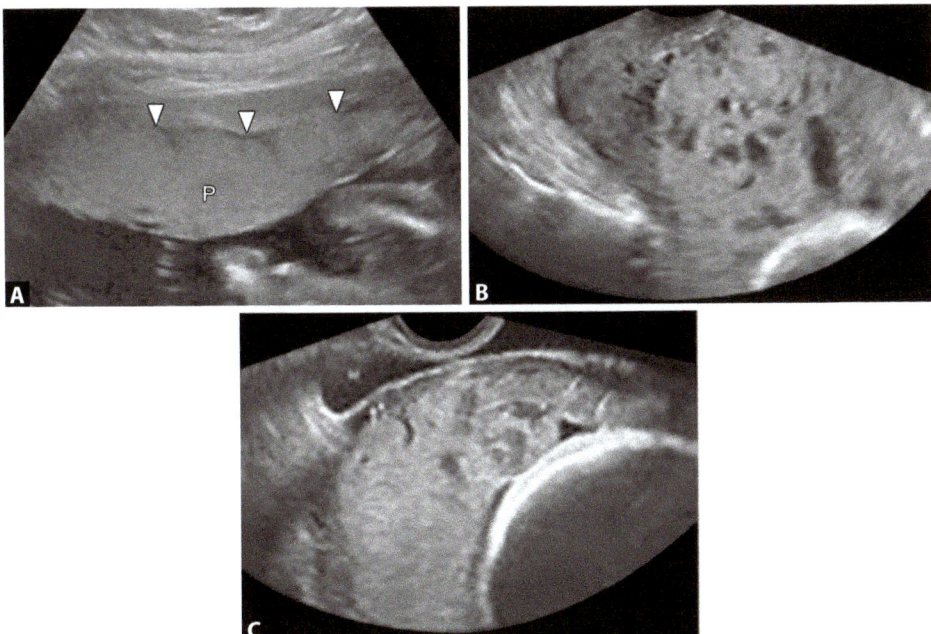

Figs. 3A to C: Adherent placenta: (A) Normal retroplacental space; (B) Abnormal placental lacunae; (C) Loss of retroplacental space.

of MRI in diagnosing placenta accreta is still debated.[22]

PREDICTION OF PLACENTA PREVIA AT DELIVERY

The ultrasound parameters for prediction include:
- Distance between the os and the placental edge (<10 vs. 10–20 mm)
- Placental edge thickness (>1 vs. <1 cm)
- Cervical length.

A low-lying placenta is very common finding during midtrimester scanning, around 15–20% of pregnancies have a low-lying placenta and only 5% remain so at 32 weeks and only a third of these cases are low-lying at 37 weeks.

Low-lying placenta is reported as the distance of the edge from the os, in millimeters. Always a follow-up examination for placental location in the third trimester is recommended. When the placental edge covers the internal os by any distance, it is described as millimeters of overlap. A placental edge reaching up to the internal os is described by a measurement of 0 mm.

When the placenta overlaps more than 20 mm, it is associated with an increased likelihood of placenta previa at term and the need for cesarean delivery. A distance of 20 to 0 mm away from the os is associated with a higher cesarean section rate, although vaginal delivery is still possible depending on the clinical circumstances.

Cervical length and placental edge thickness are considered as predictor of antepartum bleeding and preterm delivery. The cervical length measurements at the third trimester, less than 30 mm is considered as risk for antepartum hemorrhage. Patients with placenta previa with placental edges over the internal os of >1 cm thickness have increased frequency of antepartum hemorrhage, cesarean delivery, and requirement of blood products as compared to those with thin placental edges over the internal os of <1 cm.[23-25]

COMPLICATIONS

Maternal

- Antepartum hemorrhage with varying degree of shock.
- Preterm either spontaneous or induced.
- Postpartum hemorrhage due to either lack of retraction of lower segment of uterus, large placental surface area, increased lower segment vascularity or morbidly adherent placenta.
- Retained placenta due to morbid adhesion.
- Increased risk for puerperal sepsis due to increased operative interference. Coexisting anemia may also precipitate it.
- Subinvolution of uterus.

Fetal

- Low birth weight due to either chronic placental insufficiency causing fetal growth restriction or due to preterm per se.
- Birth asphyxia can be the effect of early placental separation.
- Intrauterine death probably due to increased hemorrhage leading to maternal hypotension and shock.

MANAGEMENT

Patients with placenta previa in the third trimester should be counseled about the risks of preterm delivery and obstetric hemorrhage. Their antenatal care should be tailored to their individual needs. The main goal of the management of an women with placenta previa is to monitor her in the third trimester to determine whether the previa resolves, whether its associated with adherent placenta, to reduce the risk of bleeding and to plan for elective cesarean section.

Asymptomatic Placenta Previa

In asymptomatic women, the placental position is reassessed at 32 weeks of gestation by transvaginal ultrasound and if its more than 2 cm from the os, the placental position is considered as normal and followed up as regular antenatal case. However, if it is less than 2 cm, rescan is done at 36 weeks of gestation to reassess the placenta. If it is over the placenta, cesarean delivery is planned electively. But if it is still less than 2 cm from the os, the risk associated with trial of labor is discussed with patient. However, the possibility of adherent placenta previa (accreta/increta/percreta) should be excluded.

These women are advised to avoid any sexual activity, moderate to strenuous exercise, and heavy lifting to reduce the risk of bleeding. They should also be advised to seek immediate medical attention if pain abdomen or vaginal bleeding occurs.

The pregnancies complicated by placenta previa are at no or minimally increased risk of intrauterine growth restriction. There is no evidence for screening for fetal growth restriction. Asymptomatic women are managed as outpatient basis until vaginal bleeding occurs. It is unclear that hospitalization of these women has any benefit. However, certain patient specific risk factors are also considered like short cervical length, inability to get to hospital promptly in case of an emergency.

The antenatal corticosteroids to asymptomatic women are given 48 hours before a cesarean delivery, if scheduled at less than 37 weeks of gestation. Delivery is planned at 37-38 weeks in uncomplicated asymptomatic placenta previa.[26,27]

Symptomatic Placenta Previa

All cases of antepartum hemorrhage should be considered as placenta previa unless proven otherwise. An actively bleeding placenta previa is considered as an obstetric emergency. The main goal is to maintain maternal hemodynamics and to consider emergency cesarean, if needed. The definitive treatment depends on the extent of the hemorrhage, maternal and fetal status, and the duration of the gestation. These women are admitted for maternal (for signs of hypovolemia like tachypnea, tachycardia, hypotension, and low oxygen saturation) and fetal monitoring (for fetal hypoxemia or anemia).

The estimation of vaginal blood loss is difficult to determine visually. However, it approximately helps us to gauge the amount of bleeding. There is no consensus about the components of routine laboratory assessment of patients with bleeding placenta previa.[28-30] However, we need to assess the complete blood count, send blood for typing and antibody screen, to notify the blood bank in case the need arise.

At admission:
- *Intravenous access and crystalloid*: To achieve or maintain hemodynamic stability and adequate urine output.
- *Transfusion*: Guided by the volume of blood loss over time and changes in hemodynamic parameters, the hemoglobin level.

  Acute hemorrhage may not always be associated with an immediate reduction in either blood pressure or hematocrit in an otherwise healthy young woman. Therefore, a low threshold for transfusion should be maintained in patients with placenta previa. The goal of transfusion is a final hemoglobin value >10 g/dL. If the patient fails to stabilize, a massive transfusion protocol should be initiated. However if delivery is imminent, a preoperative or intraoperative target hemoglobin of 8 g/dL is reasonable.
- *Tocolytic drugs*: Contraindicated in actively bleeding patients.
- Administering anti-D immune globulin to D-negative women who have bleeding from placenta previa.

Indications for delivery:
- Active labor.
- Nonreassuring cardiotocography (CTG) which is unresponsive to resuscitative measures.
- Severe and persistent vaginal bleeding irrespective of the gestational age.
- Significant vaginal bleeding after 34 weeks of gestation.
- Intrauterine fetal death.

Expectant management in symptomatic women is considered in women less than 34 weeks of gestation who are hemodynamically stable and fetus with a normal fetal heart rate pattern. The goal is to prolong pregnancy to enable further fetal growth and maturation, without placing the mother at excessive risk from persistent or recurrent bleeding. A course of antenatal corticosteroid therapy is administered to symptomatic women between 23^{+0} weeks and 37 weeks of gestation to enhance fetal pulmonary maturity. Oral or parenteral iron supplementation may be needed for optimal correction of anemia. If the patient's bleeding stops after the first or second bleeding event, patient can be discharged if she meets the criteria. The criteria are: (1) no active vaginal bleeding, (2) hemoglobin >10 g/dL, (3) less than 37 weeks of gestation, (4) fetal well being assured by ultrasound, (5) patient should stay close to the hospital or should be able to reach the hospital in case of an emergency, (6) patient and her relative understands the risks, and (7) patient is compliant for restricted mobility and regular antenatal follow-up.

A systematic review that attempted to assess the impact of clinical interventions in these pregnancies concluded there were insufficient data upon which to make evidence-based recommendations for clinical practice.

Fetal Assessment

Fetal bleeding can occur if disruption of fetal vessels occurs (due to vasa previa or placental previa). It can be detected by performing a Kleihauer-Betke or flow cytometry test on a specimen of vaginal blood. Fetal middle cerebral artery (MCA) Doppler helps us to identify fetal anemia. The fetus presents as nonreassuring fetal heart rate tracing and rarely fetal death.

Definitive management is by delivery by cesarean section for the major placenta previa. The cesarean section has to be performed in a tertiary center with facilities of blood transfusion and intensive care unit for the mother and the neonate. The problems encountered during the lower uterine cesarean section are: (1) engorged vessels on the lower segment, especially in the anterior placenta previa which may bleed torrentially when cut, (2) chance of fetal exsanguination as the placenta needs to be cut or separated to deliver the baby, (3) the edge of the margins may be friable and vascular leading to difficult closure as the tissues may cut through during closure, (4) placenta accreta, and (5) bleeding sinuses at the placental bed leading to increased blood loss. The associated morbidities include postpartum hemorrhage, abnormal placental adherence, need for cesarean hysterectomy and blood transfusion, septicemia, and thrombophlebitis.

Route of Delivery in Women with Low-lying Placenta

The optimal route for delivery of pregnancies where the distance between the placental edge and internal os is 1–20 mm is unclear. The fetal head may tamponade the adjacent placenta, thus preventing hemorrhage. Recent data support allowing a trial of labor in pregnancies in which the placenta is more than 10 mm from the internal os. If this distance is ≤10 mm, cesarean delivery is indicated.

CONCLUSION

Placenta previa is a serious obstetric issue and should be managed by experienced teams. A prompt diagnosis and good antenatal and fetal surveillance can reduce the maternal and neonatal mortality and morbidity. The emotional distress on the part of the woman involved, arising from episodes of heavy vaginal bleeding, the need for repeated hospitalizations, and concern for her baby's welfare has to be addressed with utmost sensitivity.

REFERENCES

1. Ananth CV, Berkowitz GS, Savitz DA, et al. Placental abruption and adverse perinatal outcomes. JAMA. 1999;282:1646-51.
2. Konje JC, Taylor DJ. Bleeding in late pregnancy. In: James DK, Steer PJ, Weiner CP (Eds). High Risk Pregnancy: Management Options, 3rd edition. Philadelphia: Saunders; 2006. pp. 1259-75.
3. Ananth CV, Savitz DA, Bowes WA Jr, et al. Influence of hypertensive disorders and cigarette smoking on placental abruption and uterine bleeding during pregnancy. Br J Obstet Gynaecol. 1997;104:572-8.
4. Kaminsky LM, Ananth CV, Prasad V, et al. The influence of maternal cigarette smoking on placental pathology in pregnancies complicated by abruption. Am J Obstet Gynecol. 2007;197:275.e1-5.
5. Paidas MJ, Ku D-HW, Arkel YS. Screening and management of inherited thrombophilias in the setting of adverse pregnancy outcome. Clin Perinatol. 2004;31:783-805.
6. Ananth CV, Peltier MR, De Marco C, et al. Associations between 2 polymorphisms in the methylenetetrahydrofolate reductase gene and placental abruption. Am J Obstet Gynecol. 2007;197:385.e1-7.

7. Grossman NB. Blunt trauma in pregnancy. Am Fam Physician. 2004;70:1303-13.
8. Bernischke K, Kaufmann P. Pathology of the Human Placenta, 4th edition. New York (NY): Springer; 2000.
9. ACOG educational bulletin. Obstetric aspects of trauma management. Number 251, September 1998 (replaces Number 151, January 1991, and Number 161, November 1991). American College of Obstetricians and Gynecologists. Int J Gynaecol Obstet. 1999;64:87-94.
10. Spiliopoulos M, Puri I, Jain NJ, et al. Amniotic fluid embolism risk factors, maternal and neonatal outcomes. J Matern Fetal Neonatal Med. 2009;22(5):43944.
11. Jacobsen AF, Skjeldestad FE, Sandset PM. Incidence and risk patterns of venous thromboembolism in pregnancy and puerperium–a register-based case-control study. Am J Obstet Gynecol. 2008;198(2):233.e1-7.
12. Pariente G, Wiznitzer A, Sergienko R, et al. Placental abruption: critical analysis of risk factors and perinatal outcomes. J Matern Fetal Neonatal Med. 2011;24(5):698-702.
13. Sinha P, Kuruba N. Ante-partum haemorrhage: an update. J Obstet Gynaecol. 2008;28(4): 377-81.
14. Cresswell JA, Ronsmans C, Calvert C, et al. Prevalence of placenta praevia by world region: a systematic review and meta-analysis. Trop Med Int Health. 2013;18(6):712-24.
15. Maiti S, Kanrar P, Karmakar C, et al. Maternal and perinatal outcome in rural Indian women with placenta previa. Brit Biomed Bull. 2014;2(4):714-8.
16. Oppenheimer L, Maternal Fetal Medicine Committee. Diagnosis and management of placenta previa. J Obstet Gynaecol Can. 2007;29:261-6.
17. Oyelese Y, Smulian JC. Placenta previa, placenta accreta, and vasa previa. Obstet Gynecol. 2006;107:927-41.
18. Clark SL, Koonings PP, Phelan JP. Placenta previa/accreta and prior cesarean section. Obstet Gynecol. 1985;66:89-92.
19. Silver RM, Landon MB, Rouse DJ, et al. Maternal morbidity associated with multiple repeat cesarean deliveries. Obstet Gynecol. 2006;107:1226-32.
20. Edridge W. Classification, confusion and misclassification. S Afr J Obstet Gynaecol. 2017;23(1):2.
21. Oppenheimer LW, Farine D. A new classification of placenta previa: measuring progress in obstetrics. Am J Obstet Gynecol. 2009;201:227-9.
22. Royal College of Obstetricians and Gynaecologists. (2011). Placenta praevia, placenta praevia accreta and vasa praevia: diagnosis and management (Green-top Guideline No. 27). [online] Available from: https://www.rcog.org.uk/en/guidelines-research-services/guidelines/gtg27/ [Last accessed September, 2019].
23. Zaitoun MM, El Behery MM, El Hameed AAA, et al. Does cervical length and the lower placental edge thickness measurement correlates with clinical outcome in cases of complete placenta previa? Arch Gynecol Obstet. 2011;284:867-73.
24. Ghourab S. Third-trimester transvaginal ultrasonography in placenta previa: does the shape of the lower placental edge predict clinical outcome. Ultrasound Obstet Gynecol. 2001;18:103-8.
25. Vintzileos AM, Ananth CV, Smulian JC. Using ultrasound in the clinical management of placental implantation abnormalities. Am J Obstet Gynecol. 2015;213:S70-7.
26. Lyndon A, Miller S, Huwe V, et al. Blood loss: clinical techniques for ongoing quantitative measurement. California: California Maternal Quality Care Collaborative; 2010.
27. Goodnough LT, Daniels K, Wong AE, et al. How we treat: transfusion medicine support of obstetric services. Transfusion. 2011;51:2540-8.
28. Besinger RE, Moniak CW, Paskiewicz LS, et al. The effect of tocolytic use in the management of symptomatic placenta previa. Am J Obstet Gynecol. 1995;172:1770-5.
29. Sharma A, Suri V, Gupta I. Tocolytic therapy in conservative management of symptomatic placenta previa. Int J Gynaecol Obstet. 2004;84:109-13.
30. Cunningham FG, Leveno KJ, Bloom SL, et al. Williams Obstetrics, 25th edition. New York: McGraw-Hill; 2018.

16

Retained Placenta

Sowparnika SN

DEFINITION

Failure of the placenta and its membranes (separated or unseparated) to expel within 30 minutes of delivery of fetus is called retained placenta (RP).[1] WHO quotes the time as 15 minutes for expulsion of placenta.

INCIDENCE AND THE SCALE OF THE PROBLEM

There are different consensus in defining the RP, hence it is difficult to quote its incidence. On an average, its incidence is 1–3% in India.[1] In the United Kingdom, death due to RP is around 7/100,000 live birth.[2] In Africa, as there is a delay in the intervention leading to 1% of case fatality rate due to RP.[3]

Maternal mortality is one of the dreadful complications, both for the patient and also for the treating physician. Hemorrhage contributes to 30% of maternal mortality ratio (MMR).[4] RP contributes to 10% of postpartum hemorrhage (PPH)[5] and acts as an independent factor contributing for maternal mortality.[6]

TYPES OF RETAINED PLACENTA

Retained placenta is the symptom for which the underlying diagnosis should be established based on the pathogenesis, so that the treatment can be streamlined. RP can be classified into three types as shown in Flowchart 1.

Flowchart 1: Types of retained placenta.

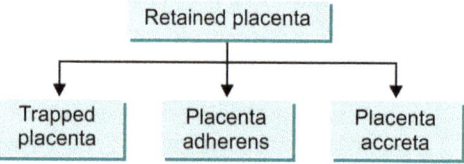

- *Trapped placenta*: Placenta is separated completely, but trapped behind the closed cervix. Hence the name.
- *Placenta adherens*: It occurs due to the failure of the myometrium behind the placental site to contract. The choriodecidual space is maintained; hence the placenta can be easily separated manually.
- *Placenta accreta*: Placenta invades the myometrium obliterating the choriodecidual space. Here the separation of the placenta is difficult and it induces hemorrhage. Hence the management is entirely different in this case. The other two are placenta increta and placenta percreta.

Another classification is:
- *Complete RP*—where whole of the placenta is inside uterus.
- *Partial RP*—where a part of placenta is expelled with a part of it inside. Example: succenturiate lobe of placenta.

The causes are enlisted in Table 1.

TABLE 1: Causes of retained placenta.

Type of retained placenta	Causes	Treatment
Trapped placenta	• Cervical ring • Hourglass contraction of uterus • Rupture uterus—placenta escapes into the abdominal quality	• Uterine relaxation—deepening the plane of anesthesia • Treatment of rupture uterus
Placenta adherens	• Uterine atony • Multiparity • Early preterm labor • Multiple pregnancy • Polyhydramnios • Big baby	• Systemic uterotonics • Umbilical vein injections of uterotonics

Placenta accreta/percreta/increta	• Previous scar uterus—lower segment cesarean section (LSCS), myomectomy, postpartum curettage
	• Uterine infection, ?preterm labor, pre-eclampsia
		• Conservative method
		  – Uterine artery embolization (UAE)
		  – Methotrexate injection for in situ placenta
		• Surgical method
		  – USG-guided removal of bits of placenta
		  – Peripartum hysterectomy

CLINICAL FEATURES

Retained placenta can present in many ways as said here.
- PPH with hemorrhage, or in shock
- Sepsis
- Secondary PPH in partial RP.

In either of these conditions, patient presents with any of the following clinical features:
- PV bleed with or without hemodynamic instability
- Pallor
- Uterus is not well contracted, doughy in consistency.
- Per vaginal examination—active bleed with the umbilical cord in situ. The bleeding may or may not be in proportion with the pallor, as it can be concealed or revealed hemorrhage.
- Examination of the placenta after expulsion to see the completeness of the cotyledons and membranes is very important. If any missing cotyledons with the hemorrhage clinically necessitates the exploration of uterine cavity. In succenturiate lobe of placenta, even when the placental bed is complete, the disruption of the continuity of vessels in the membranes might raise a suspicion of succenturiate lobe in situ.
- The use of ultrasonography (USG) for documentation of RP and differentiation of type the RP through the USG was documented for the first time by Herman et al. But further studies to establish the usefulness of USG have not been done.

TREATMENT

The definitive treatment, till date for the RP is manual removal of placenta. Apart from this, different modality of medical treatment has been tried but with poor success. Before proceeding to the surgical management, Crede's maneuver of placental extraction with active management of third stage of labor (AMTSL) should be tried.

Algorithm for the management of RP has been shown in Flowchart 2.

Flowchart 2: Algorithm for the management of retained placenta.

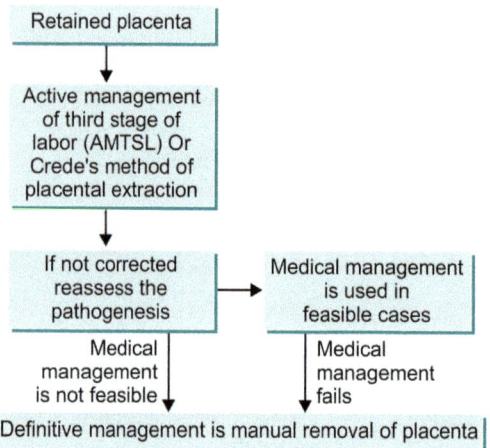

- *Active management of third stage of labor*—goes by the pneumonic "OCM"-WHO 2012:
  - *Oxytocics*: Injection oxytocin 5–10 IU is given intramuscularly after the delivery of the baby.
  - *Control cord traction of placenta (modified Brandt-Andrews method)*: Here one hand is placed above the pubic symphysis pushing the uterus backward and downward, with a gentle pull on the placental cord with the other hand downward and forward to expel the separated placenta. Undue force on the placental cord is not recommended as it might lead to inversion of uterus.
  - *Massage of the uterus*: Contract the myometrium thus helping in the separation of the placenta.
- *Crede's method of placental extraction*:
  - Bladder is emptied
  - Massage of the uterus
  - The hand holds the fundus of the uterus with a thumb behind and the other four fingers in front of the uterus, pushing the fundus downward and backward, thus expelling the placenta out.
- When the above said methods have failed, considering the atony of uterus as a major cause of RP, oxytocics were used for its management. Systemic oxytocics were used, also the umbilical vein infusion of oxytocics.
- *Umbilical vein injection (UVI) of oxytocin*:
  - In 2007, based on a Cochrane review, NICE recommended use of UVI oxytocin for RP, as it reduced the manual removal of placenta significantly[7]
  - In 2014, a contradictory evidence of increase in the PPH with the use of UVI oxytocin made NICE to no longer recommend UVI oxytocin in RP[8]
  - Another large controlled trial, the Release trial showed no extra benefit of using UVI oxytocin in RP. It also guided that IV oxytocin is useful in RP only when the patient has excess bleeding due to uterine atony[9]
- *Umbilical vein injection of prostaglandin*:
  - Meta-analysis and randomized control trials showed a significant reduction in the manual removal of placenta with UVI sulprostone compared with placebo.[10] The sample size of the study was less and also the results were not statistically significant to make it a recommendation.
- *Nitroglycerin (NG)*:
  Sublingual NG has showed decrease in the manual removal of placenta where the cause might be a constriction ring of cervix. Many small studies were conducted where each study showed contradicting evidence to the other.[11,12] A large multicentric trial GOT-IT trial, the results of which are awaited to formulate a recommendation. Medical management becomes detrimental, when the underlining pathogenesis is not well understood. If uterotonics are given when the cause of RP

is constriction ring, it hinders the process rather than helping it. If the uterine relaxants are given when the cause of RP is uterine atony, it further aggravates the PPH. Hence the type of RP placenta should be diagnosed and appropriate medical management needs to be executed.

Yet other cause why the UVI fails to work is, we presume, that the oxytocics we are injecting are directly entering the uterine milieu. But the placental circulation is entirely different.

Placental villi → radical veins in the uterus failing to reach the retroplacental circulation thus the drug is not delivered to the site of interest.

When all these methods fail, the last and the definitive treatment for RP is manual removal of placenta.

Cross-section of the placenta has been shown in Figure 1.

Manual Removal of Placenta

Manual removal of placenta has been depicted in Figure 2.

- The procedure is done under general anesthesia, as it will cause relaxation of the uterus completely, so that the constriction band relaxes.
- The right hand is made into a obstetric cone. It is introduced into the uterus along the direction of umbilical cord, wherein the left hand grasps the fundus of the uterus abdominally.
- The space between the placenta and the uterus is made by to and fro motion side by the side till the fundus of the uterus is reached.
- The whole of the placenta is grasped, Syntocinon drip is started to contract the uterus and the placenta and membranes are removed in toto. The uterus is allowed to contract.
- Left hand will grasp the fundus till the complete delivery of placenta to prevent inversion of uterus.
- Placenta is observed for the completeness, both on maternal and fetal surface.
- Other uterotonics like methylergometrine can be administered after the complete delivery of placenta.

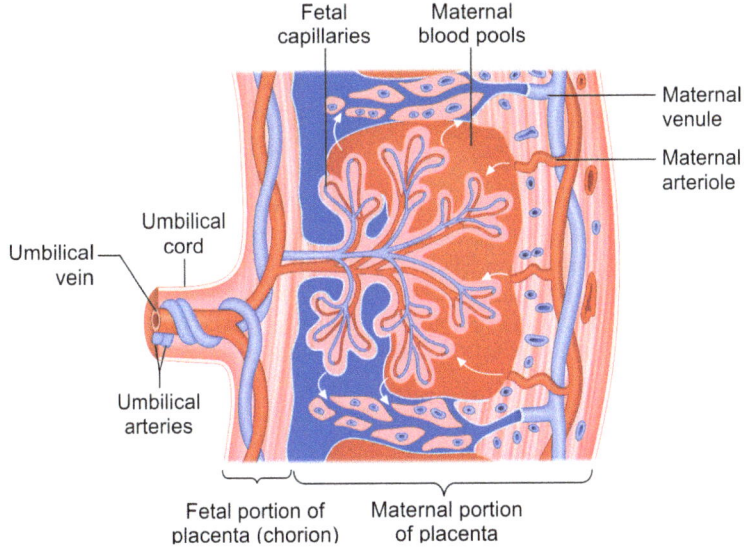

Fig. 1: Cross-section of the placenta.
Source: EmeCeDesigns, 2014

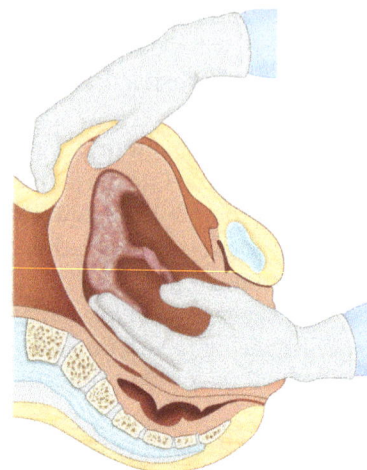

Fig. 2: Manual removal of placenta (MRP).
Source: Posner GD, Jessica DY, Black A, Jones Gd (Eds). Human Labor and Birth, 6th edition. India: McGraw-Hill Education, 2013.

- When the placenta does not separate and with a suspicion of placenta accreta, further investigations should be done. If confirmed, the case needs to be managed as placenta accreta.

CONCLUSION

Retained placenta is one of the leading causes of maternal mortality, if treated at the time of an hour; it will save lives. Finding out the cause and the pathogenesis of the RP and treating accordingly is the key of success.

REFERENCES

1. Coviello EM, Grantz KL, Huang CC, et al. Risk factors for retained placenta. Am J Obstet Gynecol. 2015;213(6):864.e1-864.e11.
2. Kerr RS, Weeks AD. Lessons from 150 years of UK maternal hemorrhage deaths. Acta Obstet Gynecol Scand. 2015;94:664-8.
3. John CO, Orazulike N, Alegbeleye J. An appraisal of retained placenta at the University of Port Harcourt Teaching Hospital: a five-year review. Niger J Med. 2015;24:99-102.
4. Ministry of Health and Family Welfare, Government of India. Estimates of maternal mortality ratios in India and its states: a pilot study. (Online) Available from: www.icmr.nic.in/final/Final%20Pilot%20Report.pdf
5. Louis K, Mahantesh K, Christopher BL. Postpartum hemorrhage: prevention and treatment. J Obstet Gynecol India. 2008;58:392-8.
6. Amanda D, Grace S. (2019). Anesthesiology: Retained placenta, Management. (Online) Available from: https://www.clinicalpainadvisor.com/home/decision-support-in-medicine/anesthesiology/retained-placenta-management.
7. Nardin JM, Weeks A, Carroli G. Umbilical vein injection for management of retained placenta. Cochrane Database Syst Rev. 2011;(5):CD001337.
8. National Institute for Health and Clinical Excellence. Intrapartum care: care of healthy women and their babies during childbirth. NICE clinical guideline 190. London: RCOG Press; 2014.
9. van Beekhuizen HJ, de Groot AN, De Boo T, et al. Sulprostone reduces the need for the manual removal of the placenta in patients with retained placenta: a randomized controlled trial. Am J Obstet Gynecol. 2006;194(2):446-50.
10. Bullarbo M, Tjugum J, Ekerhovd E. Sublingual nitroglycerin for management of retained placenta. Int J Gynaecol Obstet. 2005;91:228-32.
11. Bullarbo M, Bokstrom H, Lilja H, et al. Nitroglycerin for management of retained placenta: a multicenter study. Obstet Gynecol Int. 2012;2012:321207.
12. Visalyaputra S, Prechapanich J, Suwanvichai S, et al. Intravenous nitroglycerin for controlled cord traction in the management of retained placenta. Int J Gynaecol Obstet. 2011;112:103-6.

CHAPTER 17

Intrauterine Growth Restriction

Rekha Viswanath

DEFINITIONS

- *Low birth weight (LBW)*: Birth weight less than 2,500 g, including both preterm and small for gestational age fetuses.
- *Small for gestational age (SGA)*: Fetus whose weight is below 10th percentile for its gestational age; including genetically small fetuses and growth restricted fetuses.
- *Intrauterine growth restriction (IUGR)*: Those fetuses that have failed to attain their genetic growth potential.
- *Genetically small fetus or low profile fetus*: Fetus which is genetically small, but has attained its own growth potential.

The relationship between LBW, SGA and IUGR fetuses has been shown in Figure 1.

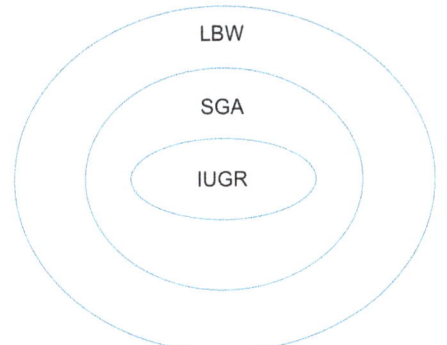

Fig. 1: Showing the relationship between low birth weight (LBW), small for gestational age (SGA), Intrauterine growth restriction (IUGR) fetuses; IUGR is a subset of SGA which in turn is a subset of LBW fetuses.

ETIOLOGY

- Fetal
- Placental
- Maternal (Table 1).

PATHOGENESIS

Normal fetal growth is characterized by hyperplasia and hypertrophy of cells. Hyperplasia or an increase in number of cells predominates during the first half of the pregnancy, hypertrophy and hyperplasia both occur during the second half of the pregnancy.

If an insult happens in the first half of the pregnancy, where hyperplasia of cells predominates, it results in *symmetrical IUGR* where somatic and cerebral growth is equally affected.

If the insult is late, occurring after around 32 weeks of pregnancy, it results in *asymmetrical IUGR*. Uteroplacental insufficiency is the most common cause for asymmetrical IUGR (Table 2).

Formation of Uteroplacental Arteries

- *Stage 1*: Trophoblastic invasion of the decidual segments of spiral arteries which occurs in the first trimester.
- *Stage 2*: Trophoblastic invasion of the intramyometrial segments of spiral arteries which occurs in the second trimester.

These stages convert the spiral arteries into uteroplacental arteries which are like fibrinoid

TABLE 1: Etiology of intrauterine growth restriction.

Fetal causes	Placental causes	Maternal causes
• Chromosomal abnormality • Congenital malformations • Congenital infections, e.g. TORCH	• Pre-eclampsia • Collagen vascular disease • Antiphospholipid antibody syndrome • Inherited thrombophilias • Diabetes with vasculopathy • Placental and cord abnormalities • Multiple pregnancies	• Poor maternal weight gain and undernutrition • Teratogens (smoking, alcohol, cocaine, anticonvulsants) • Chronic maternal disease causing severe hypoxia (severe anemia, congenital cyanotic heart disease)

[TORCH: Toxoplasma gondii, others (including Treponema pallidum, Listeria, varicella, and parvovirus B19), rubella virus, cytomegalovirus (CMV), and herpes simplex virus (HSV)]

TABLE 2: Symmetrical versus asymmetrical intrauterine growth restriction (IUGR).

Symmetrical IUGR	Asymmetrical IUGR
• One-third of cases • Intrinsic fetal pathology • Early onset • Cell number and size affected • Symmetrically small • HC/AC and FL/AC normal • Ponderal index normal • Poor neonatal prognosis	• Two-thirds of cases of IUGR • Uteroplacental insufficiency • Late onset • Cell size is mainly affected • Brain-sparing effect • Head larger than abdomen • HC/AC and FL/AC increased • Ponderal index abnormal • Neonatal prognosis better

(HC: head circumference; AC: abdominal circumference; FL: femur length)

pipes and allow for the increased blood flow to the placenta in normal pregnancy. These vessels are also resistant to the action of vasomotor substances.

Any insult to the stage 2 can result in decrease in uteroplacental blood flow and an asymmetrical IUGR.

What is asymmetrical intrauterine growth restriction?
Type of IUGR where fetal biometric parameters are disproportionately affected and are falling under the 10th percentile.

The parameter commonly affected is the abdominal circumference (AC). The brain growth remains comparatively unaffected (brain-sparing effect). The blood supply to splanchnic organs like the kidneys is reduced. The liver gets affected with reduced glycogen deposition and shrinks in size. Hence there is an increase in brain-to-liver ratio (BLR). The reduction in renal blood flow can result in fetal oliguria with resultant oligoamnios which is characteristic of asymmetrical IUGR.

COMPLICATIONS

- Fetal complications
- Neonatal complications.

Fetal Complications

- Stillbirths due to antepartum hypoxia
- Fetal distress in labor due to intrapartum hypoxia.

Neonatal Complications

- Short-term complications
- Long-term complications (Table 3).

PREDICTION

- Identifying women at risk
- Uterine artery Doppler
- Biochemical tests.

Identifying Women at Risk

Women at high risk for IUGR have been shown in Box 1.

TABLE 3: Neonatal complications of intrauterine growth restriction.

Short-term	Long-term
• Perinatal asphyxia • Meconium aspiration • Persistent pulmonary hypertension • Hypothermia • Hypoglycemia • Hyperglycemia • Hypocalcemia • Polycythemia • Jaundice • Feeding difficulties • Feed intolerance • Necrotizing enterocolitis • Late onset sepsis • Pulmonary hemorrhage	• Poor growth and neurodevelopment • Adult-onset diabetes and metabolic syndrome (thrifty gene/Barkers hypothesis) (Flowchart 1)

Uterine Artery Doppler

Uterine artery Doppler flow study is a major tool for prediction of IUGR. It is known that changes occur in the maternal circulation as early as the first trimester in women who develop pre-eclampsia and IUGR (Zemel et al.). Second trimester pulsatility index (PI) also adds to the prediction process of pre-eclampsia and IUGR.

Abnormal uterine artery Doppler is defined as:
- Persistent diastolic notch in the uterine artery waveform after 24 weeks
- PI >1.45 or/and the presence of bilateral early diastolic notches
- Systolic/diastolic ratio: >2.6
- RI >0.58 after 24 weeks.

Sensitivity: 81.4%, specificity: 89%, negative predictive value: 93.4%.

Although uterine artery Doppler has a high negative predictive value for prediction

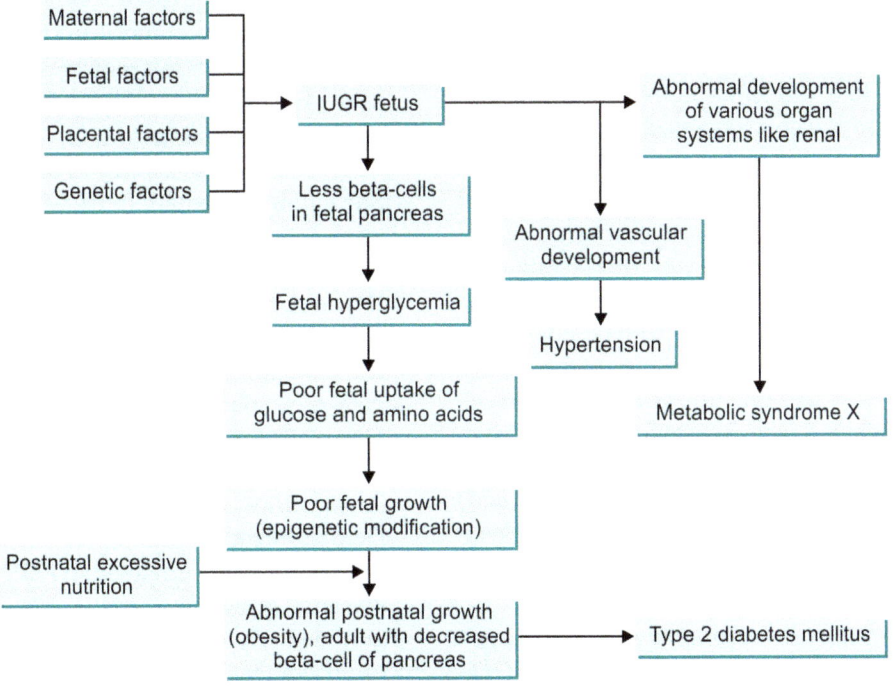

Flowchart 1: Thrifty gene/Barker hypothesis.

Box 1: Women at high risk for intrauterine growth restriction (IUGR).

- Maternal undernutrition
- Previous IUGR
- Previous pre-eclampsia
- *Maternal diseases*: Essential hypertension, renal disease, diabetes with vascular disease, antiphospholipid antibody syndrome, congenital thrombophilias, maternal cardiac disease, sickle cell disease
- Raised maternal serum alpha-fetoprotein with normal fetus
- Smoking and other substance abuse

of adverse perinatal outcomes, the strength of the association between abnormal results and adverse events is not so accurate to make it a screening test. More studies are required in this context.

Biochemical Tests

- Maternal serum analytes were first studied with the aim of screening for aneuploidies during the first and second trimester of pregnancy. However, trophoblastic invasion failure has been found to be the cause of alteration in the serum levels of these placental products.
- In 2008, *Gagnon et al.* studied the obstetrical outcomes seen with abnormal levels of single or multiple maternal serum markers used in the screening for aneuploidy. Pregnancy-associated plasma protein-A (PAPP-A), alpha-fetoprotein, beta-human chorionic gonadotrophin (hCG), estriol, unconjugated estriol, inhibin-A were studied. The conclusion was that: an *unexplained low PAPP-A (0.4 MoM) and/or a low hCG (<0.5 MoM) in the first trimester* was associated with a high frequency of adverse obstetrical outcomes.
- An *increase in maternal serum alpha-fetoprotein* in the absence of fetal anomaly increases the risk of IUGR later in pregnancy by five- to tenfold.
- The recent meta-analysis by *Conde Agudelo et al.* in 2013 which included 53 studies and 39,974 women had evaluated 37 new biomarkers among which the major ones were *angiogenesis-related biomarkers, endothelial function/oxidative stress-related biomarkers, placental proteins/hormone-related biomarkers* and other markers like metabolomics and genetic biomarkers. Overall, none of them showed significant accuracy for prediction of IUGR.

PREVENTION

- Encouraging women to start pregnancy when their body mass index (BMI) is between the accepted limits.
- Avoiding multiple pregnancies especially in assisted reproductive technologies.
- Stabilizing chronic diseases that can influence placental vascularization.
- Stopping smoking as soon as possible.
- Limiting hypoglycemia during pregnancy.
- Monitoring for maternal hypertension throughout pregnancy.
- Women with risk factors for IUGR may be given low-dose aspirin 75 mg daily for prevention, including those women who were detected to be high risk by uterine artery Doppler or biochemical screening. However, there is no role for aspirin in low-risk women.

ASPRE trial[1] *(Rolnik et al. 2017)*: A prospective multicenter study on first trimester screening for preterm pre-eclampsia in 26,941 singleton pregnancies by using an algorithm which combined maternal factors, mean arterial pressures, uterine artery PIs and maternal serum PAPP-A and placental growth factor at 11–13 weeks of gestation. Those women with high risk of pre-eclampsia >1 in 100 participated in a double-blind trial of aspirin (150 mg/day) versus placebo from 11 weeks to 14 weeks until 36 weeks of gestation, and it was concluded that, in the aspirin group, the incidence of pre-eclampsia was reduced by 62%.

DIAGNOSIS

- Identifying high-risk pregnancies.
- *Accurate dating of pregnancy*—from last menstrual period as well as from ultrasonography.
- *Abdominal palpation* has a sensitivity of 30% in detection of SGA babies.
- *Symphyseal-fundal distance* has a sensitivity of 27–86% and specificity of 80–93% for detection of SGA babies.
- *Customized symphyseal-fundal distance charts* based on anthropometric characteristics and ethnicity also improve detection. The growth charts show normal growth and there are curves to indicate the 10th and 90th centiles. Measurements below 10th centile are considered significant.
- *Ultrasound biometry* is the best method for detection of IUGR especially if suspected clinically. After routine anomaly scan at 18–20 weeks, a follow-up scan at 32–34 weeks is suggested for high-risk pregnancies when there is a clinical suspicion of restricted growth. The usual measurements used to assess growth are *biparietal diameter (BPD), head circumference (HC), femur length (FL), abdominal circumference (AC), estimated fetal weight (EFW), HC/AC and FL/AC ratios*. Serial measurements are used to depict a growth lag. The fetus which shows adequate interval growth mostly represents a genetically small fetus. When interval growth is inadequate, IUGR is the most likely diagnosis. The interval between scans should be at least 2 weeks.
- *Abdominal circumference is the most accurate measurement to predict IUGR.* AC below 10th centile is considered significant. AC should increase by at least 10 mm in 2 weeks.
- *Umbilical artery Doppler*: It is used to detect growth restricted fetus at risk of hypoxia. It is used only when a B mode ultrasound picks up an IUGR fetus.
- In a normal pregnancy, the umbilical and uterine arteries have a low resistance and so there will be significant diastolic flow. However, in IUGR pregnancies, there will be reduced diastolic flow. A normal Doppler in an IUGR fetus is reassuring for at least 1 week, and has to be repeated weekly to detect any compromise. Commonly used indices are *systolic/diastolic (S/D) ratio, resistance index, pulsatility index (PI)*. The three different abnormal flow patterns in umbilical artery are as follows:
  - Reduced end-diastolic flow
  - Absent end-diastolic flow
  - Reversal of flow.

  Once the reversal occurs the fetus can die within 1–2 days if not delivered. Once absent end-diastolic flow occurs, on an average the fetus will survive for around a week, even though a period of 26 days has been reported in many studies.
- *Middle cerebral artery Doppler*: In a normal fetus, there is an increased resistance in the middle cerebral artery. When there is a hypoxic stress, the fetus will redistribute the blood flow preferentially to the brain and the heart. This is called brain sparing. This is seen on Doppler as decreased resistance in the middle cerebral artery. As the condition worsens, the flow to the brain will be slowly cut off and the resistance slowly increases. This is a late sign of fetal compromise and is the decompensated state.

- *Venous Doppler*: Alteration in the venous Doppler such as absent or reduced flow in the ductus venosus indicates cardiac failure. Inferior vena caval and umbilical venous pulsations are considered as the terminal sign. Ductus venosus abnormality is the single most important predictor of fetal and neonatal outcome.
- *Amniotic fluid index*: Oligohydramnios is an accompaniment of IUGR. It can also occur as a result of underlying anomalies like renal agenesis. On ultrasound, amniotic fluid index of <5 or single deepest pocket of <2 cm is considered as oligohydramnios.
- *Detection of chromosomal anomalies*: Early-onset IUGR may also be associated with chromosomal anomalies. Normal liquor and normal Doppler make this diagnosis more likely. In such cases, amniocentesis or fetal blood sampling should be planned to karyotype the fetus before planning any intervention.

MANAGEMENT

- The various therapies tried are bed rest, maternal oxygenation, high-protein diet, intravenous glucose and amino acids. None of them are known to be of any definite benefit.
- The only effective management is delivery of fetus as the intrauterine environment is hostile.
- *Antepartum fetal surveillance*:
  Considered when the fetus is too immature to deliver
    - Daily fetal movement count
    - Umbilical artery Doppler
    - Middle cerebral artery Doppler
    - Venous Doppler
    - Amniotic fluid volume
    - Nonstress test
    - Biophysical profile or score (Table 4).

The highest score possible for a fetus is 10. A score of 8–10 is normal, a score of 6 is equivocal and score <4 is abnormal.

- In all cases, delivery is also indicated by an abnormal cardiotocography (CTG), which should ideally be based on the short-term variations, if the fetus is viable according to available neonatal facilities. In cases of absent/reversal of end-diastolic flow, the opinion of fetal medicine specialist should be taken regarding the timing of delivery (Flowchart 2).
- Placenta to be sent for histopathological evaluation, arterial and venous cord pH to be obtained.
- Follow-up appointment to women with IUGR <3rd centile and delivery <34 weeks.
- Review the placental histopathology, consider thrombophilia screening, modification of risk factors, prevention with aspirin/low-molecular-weight heparin (LMWH).

Intrapartum Management

- Delivery should be ideally planned in an institution with good neonatal intensive care unit (ICU) facilities.
- Route of delivery depends on associated medical and obstetrical complications and the state of cervix.
- Cesarean section is indicated in all cases of absent or reversal of flow or an abnormal venous Doppler or an abnormal CTG.
- If cervix is favorable, artificial rupture of membranes and oxytocin is advisable.
- If cervix unfavorable, prostaglandin E2 (PGE2) gel can be used to first ripen the cervix.
- Prolonged labor to be avoided, as these fetuses cannot tolerate hypoxia.
- CTG monitoring during labor is mandatory, and if evidence of compromise, immediate cesarean section is advocated.

TABLE 4: Biophysical profile or score.

Component	Score 2	Score 0
Nonstress test	At least 2 accelerations of >15 bpm for >15 seconds	0 or 1 acceleration
Fetal breathing movements (FBMs)	At least one episode of FBM lasting >30 seconds	<30 seconds of FBM
Fetal movements	At least 3 discrete body or limb movements	<3 discrete movements
Fetal tone	At least one episode of extension of a fetal extremity with return to flexion or opening or closing of hand	No movements or no extension/flexion
Amniotic fluid volume	Single deepest pocket 2 cm or more	Single deepest pocket <2 cm

The Growth Restriction Intervention Trial (GRIT)[2] study- BJOG 2003: A multicenter randomized controlled trial aimed to compare the effect of early delivery versus delaying birth for as long as possible. A total of 588 fetuses between 24 weeks and 36 weeks were randomized to immediate delivery or delayed delivery until the obstetrician was no longer certain. The results of the study showed that there was no difference in outcomes between the early delivery or delayed delivery group (delayed by about 4 days) and although such delay caused some stillbirths, earlier delivery resulted in an almost equal number of additional deaths. Also the follow-up at 2 years of age showed that there were more disabilities in the immediate delivery group. As only 5% of the eligible population was recruited, there are concerns regarding the representativeness of the sample.

The Disproportionate Intrauterine Growth Intervention Trial at Term (DIGITAT)[3,4]—AJOG

Flowchart 2: Timing of delivery.[5]

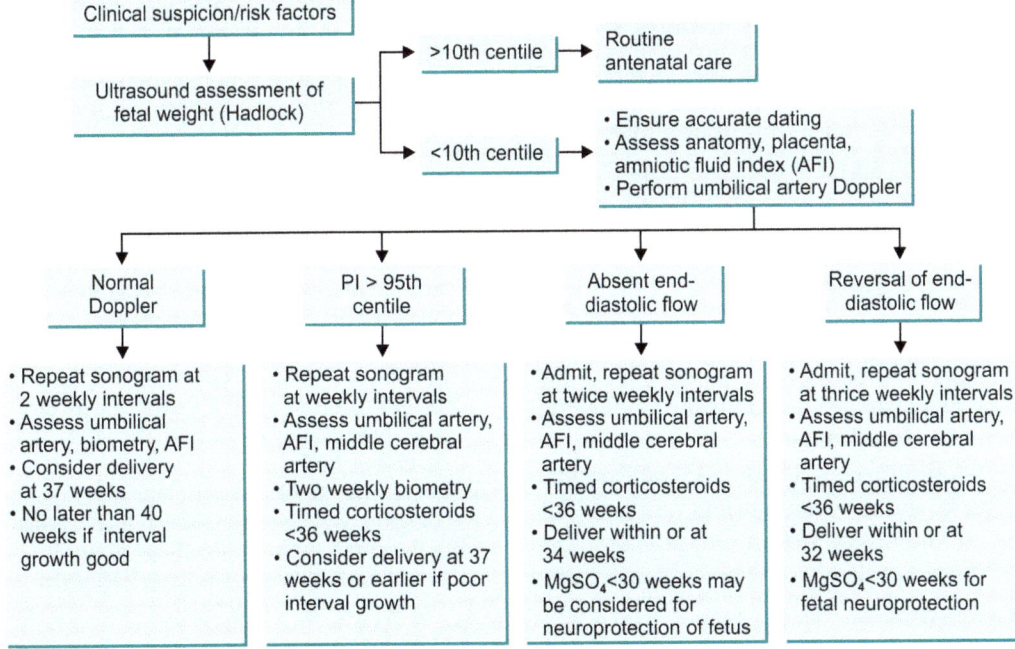

2012 Boers et al: Randomized controlled trial including 650 women, which compared the outcomes of induction of labor or expectant management in women after 37 weeks of gestation with suspected SGA. They found that the differences in peri- and neonatal outcomes between induction of labor and expectant management were negligible. There were no differences in the neurodevelopmental and neurobehavioral assessment, with both the strategies, in the cohort evaluated at 2 years of age. Hence, it was concluded that delivery may be offered after 37 weeks in SGA infants. In the discussion of this study, the authors also concluded that further studies are required to differentiate true IUGR from other causes of SGA not associated with poor perinatal outcome.

Neonatal Care

- A person well trained in neonatal care should be present if there is severe growth restriction or prematurity.
- Early feeding should be instituted.
- Neonatal ICU facilities should be available to immediately deal with all neonatal complications.
- If not, the baby should be immediately referred to a tertiary care center with good neonatal ICU facilities for further management.

CONCLUSION

- Intrauterine growth restriction is a physiological adaptation to various stimuli and is associated with various short- and long-term complications.
- Short-term complications include prematurity and reduced nutrient reserve, while childhood long-term complications are those associated with impaired maturation and abnormal organ development, such as impaired neurodevelopment, adult type 2 diabetes and hypertension.
- Obstetricians should identify those fetuses at risk of developing growth restriction and prepare a comprehensive and institution-based management protocol to carefully decide the time and mode of delivery.
- Intrauterine growth restriction due to placental insufficiency is diagnosed when decreased amniotic fluid volume, abnormal umbilical artery Doppler and reduced interval growth are evident using serial growth scans, provided that chromosomal abnormalities, malformations and infections are ruled out.
- Antenatal surveillance should be based of the severity of the maternal or fetal condition, with Doppler analysis as the most important tool to assess the severity of the fetal disease.

REFERENCES

1. Rolnik DL, Wright D, Poon LC, et al. Aspirin versus placebo in pregnancies at high risk for preterm pre-eclampsia. N Engl J Med. 2017;377(7):613-22.
2. GRIT Study Group. A randomised trial of timed delivery for the compromised preterm fetus: short-term outcomes and Bayesian interpretation. BJOG. 2003;110:27-32.
3. Boers KE, van Wyk L, van der Post JA, et al. Neonatal morbidity after induction vs expectant monitoring in intrauterine growth restriction at term: a subanalysis of the DIGITAT RCT. Am J Obstet Gynecol. 2012;206(4):344.e1-7.
4. Boers KE, Vijgen SM, Bijlenga D, et al. Induction versus expectant monitoring for intrauterine growth restriction at term: randomised equivalence trial (DIGITAT). BMJ. 2010;341:c7087.
5. Royal College of Obstetricians and Gynaecologists. The investigation and management of the small-for-gestational-age fetus. RCOG Green-top Guidelines No. 31. RCOG; 2013.

CHAPTER 18

Management of Amniotic Fluid Emergencies

Arya Rajendran

INTRODUCTION

Physiology of Amniotic Fluid

Amniotic fluid, the liquid that surrounds the fetus, is of paramount importance for maintenance of normal intrauterine homeostasis. It has a number of functions that aid in normal fetal growth and development such as:[1]
- Cushions and protects the fetus from trauma to maternal abdomen.
- Cushions the umbilical cord preventing its compression when fetal part presses on it.
- Source of fluid and nutrients for fetus.
- Permits space for normal development of fetal structures, especially lungs.

Sources of Amniotic Fluid

Sources vary with the period of gestation.

In embryonic life, there are two cavities within the gestational sac—the amniotic cavity bounded by amniotic membrane and the exocoelomic cavity between chorionic and amniotic membranes. When the chorionic and amniotic membranes fuse at around 12-14 weeks, coelomic cavity is obliterated. Composition of coelomic cavity is similar to maternal plasma and is probably sourced from secretion of endometrial glands.[2]

Amniotic fluid production during embryonic life starts from fetal surface of placenta, transmembranous exudation across amniotic membrane, and through fetal surface. As the embryo transforms into a fetus, fetal urination and swallowing start playing the major role in amniotic fluid balance. In late gestation, in addition to fetal urination and swallowing, transmembrane exchange across fetal vessels on fetal placental surface and across fetal skin and umbilical cord as well as fetal lung secretions also contribute to amniotic fluid balance. Specialized water channels called aquaporins are important in this transmembranous exchange of fluid.[3]

Amniotic fluid volume increases till 34–36 weeks of gestation and thereafter it maintains itself or decreases till term. Due to the effective fetal participation in maintenance of its own amniotic fluid volume, amniotic fluid index is a reliable indicator of fetal well-being (Fig. 1).

Methods of Quantifying Amniotic Fluid

Measurement of amniotic fluid is made sonographically, for all practical purposes. Other methods include direct measurement at cesarean section/hysterotomy and indirect measurement during amniocentesis by dye dilution technique.

Methods of sonographic measurement of amniotic fluid:
- *Subjective assessment*: Subjective assessment is an overall overview by the sonographer on the amount of fluid around the fetus. It is the most crude and subjective method of measurement.

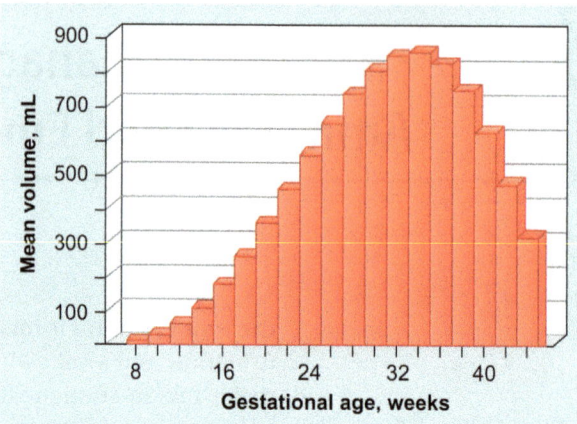

Fig. 1: Mean amniotic fluid volume across normal pregnancy.
These values represent the 50th percentile. These is considerable variability around the mean. The 5th, 50th, and 95th percentiles at 33 weeks of gestation are approximately 300, 800, and 1900 mL, respectively

Source: Brace RA, Wolf EJ. Normal amniotic fluid volume changes throughout pregnancy. Am J Obstet Gynecol. 1989;161(2):382-8.

TABLE 1: Normal values of amniotic estimates

Ultrasound estimate	Olighydramnios	Normal values	Polyhydramnios
AFI	< 5 cm	5–25 cm	> 25 cm
SDP	< 2 cm	2–8 cm	> 8 cm
2 diameter pocket	< 4 cm²	4–50 cm²	> 50 cm²

Sources: Modified from Magann EF. Olighydramnios: Amniotic Fluid and the Clinical Relevance of the Sonographically Estimated Amniotic Fluid Volume, J Ultrasound Med. 2011;30(11):1573-85, and The amniotic fluid index, single deepest pocket, and 2-diameter pocket in normal human pregnancy, Am J Obstet Gynecol. 2000;182(6):1581-8

However, with experience, the sonologist can pick up abnormalities in fluid volume by subjective assessment and follow it up by a more objective measurement to confirm.

- *2 × 2 measurement:* The single largest pocket of amniotic fluid is identified and two perpendicular measurements are multiplied and expressed in centimeter square.
- *Single deepest pocket (SDP):* Largest pocket of fluid is identified by global assessment and the largest vertical depth is measured in centimeters. There should be a minimum horizontal width of 1 cm for the identified fluid pocket.
- *Amniotic fluid index (AFI):* With maternal umbilicus as the central point, the abdomen is divided into four quadrants and largest vertical pocket in each quadrant is measured separately, and added up to get the amniotic fluid index.

Both SDP and AFI are widely practiced and reliable methods of measurement. AFI was found to have a higher sensitivity than SDP in detecting oligohydramnios, at the expense of higher false positivity[4] (Table 1).

MANAGEMENT OF AMNIOTIC FLUID EMERGENCIES

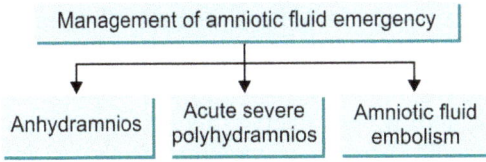

Etiology of Anhydramnios

Fetal causes	Placental causes	Maternal causes
• Chromosomal anomalies • Congenital anomalies • Intrauterine growth retardation • Postterm pregnancy • Premature rupture of membranes (PROM) • Intrauterine fetal demise	• Abruptio placentae • Twin-twin transfusion syndrome	• Severe dehydration • Uteroplacental insufficiency • Hypertensive disorders of pregnancy • Diabetes • Drug induced-ACE inhibitors and indomethacin • Idiopathic

Anhydramnios

Anhydramnios is defined as total lack of amniotic fluid. Any condition that causes severe oligohydramnios can eventually lead to anhydramnios.

Diagnosis of Anhydramnios

Clinical examination:
- Reduced fundal height of abdomen (lesser than period of gestation)
- Palpation of uterus—full of baby, reduced liquor.
- Sterile speculum examination of vagina and cervix for leakage of amniotic fluid.

Ultrasonography (Fig. 2):[5]
- *Absence of fluid pocket around the fetus*
- Fetal growth assessment to rule out Intrauterine growth restriction (IUGR) and color Doppler study of umbilical and uterine arteries for uteroplacental insufficiency
- Fetal structural causes like renal agenesis should also be ruled out.

Management of Severe Oligohydramnios/Anhydramnios

National Institute for Health and Care Excellence (NICE) guidelines, 2016:
- Before term:
  - Referral to a tertiary care center
  - Expectant management till viability is reached with careful antenatal surveillance.
- At term:
  - Deliver—induction of labor after cervical priming
  - Continuous fetal heart rate monitoring during labor.

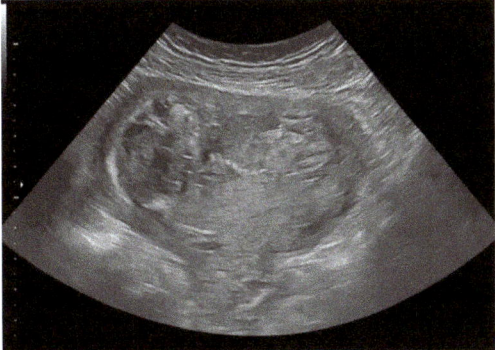

Fig. 2: Rare scenario for anhydramnios—Molar pregnancy.
Source: Szlachetka K, Faske E, Laniewski S, et al. A rare case of two consecutive Breus' molar pregnancies. J Ultrasound Med. 2017;36(6):1279-82.

Role of Amnioinfusion in Pregnancy (When not in Labor) (NICE 2006)

Under ultrasound guidance, isotonic fluid such as normal saline or Ringer's lactate is infused into the amniotic cavity via a needle inserted through the uterine wall to restore the volume of amniotic fluid to normal. The procedure may be repeated on a regular basis if oligohydramnios recurs (serial amnioinfusion).

Key efficacy outcomes include prolongation of gestation, reduced incidence of pulmonary hypoplasia, and improved neonatal survival.

Currently, it is only allowed in a setting of research and audit and not for routine practice.

Role of Vesicoamniotic Shunts (NICE 2006)

When fetal obstructive uropathy is diagnosed as cause of severe oligohydramnios, fetal urine from bladder can be shunted to amniotic cavity via vesicoamniotic shunts. Even though it can reverse oligohydramnios to significant extent, restoration of fetal renal and pulmonary function cannot be guaranteed by vesicoamniotic shunts. NICE guidelines allow the procedure to be undertaken only in a research and audit setting.

Acute Severe Polyhydramnios (Fig. 3)

Acute severe polyhydramnios is defined as a sudden and excessive rise in amniotic fluid volume that causes maternal cardiorespiratory distress. It is uncommon and always has an underlying condition.

Etiology

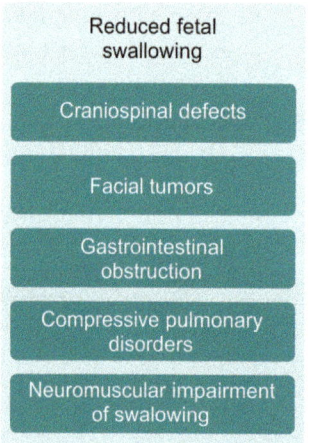
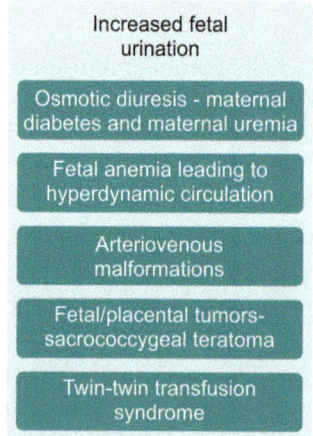

Diagnosis of Acute Polyhydramnios

Clinical examination:
- Fundal height is greater than period of gestation.
- Tense abdomen with fluid thrill.
- Cardiorespiratory compromise—breathless, tachycardia, and palpitations.
- Workup of mother for possible causes such as diabetes and uremia.

Ultrasonogram (Figs. 4 and 5):
- *Single deepest pocket>8 cm, AFI>25*
- Detailed analysis for possible fetal anomalies.
- Middle cerebral arterial (MCA) Doppler study to detect fetal anemia.

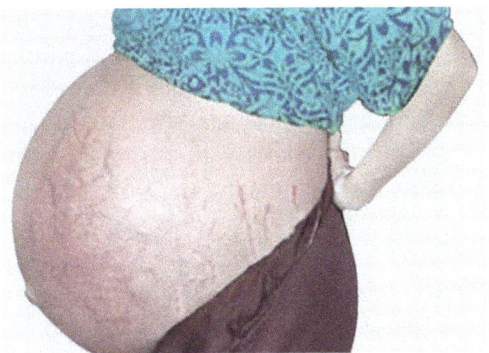

Fig. 3: Larger abdomen with excessive stretch marks— a symptom of polyhydramnios.

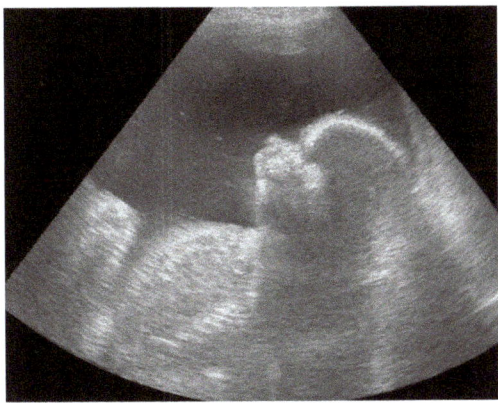

Fig 4: USG—Polyhydramnios.

A case of acute severe polyhydramnios in a G3P2L2 at 41 weeks of gestation that developed over few days and was caused by multiple loops of cord around fetal neck constricting and impairing fetal swallowing (Fig. 5).[6]

Management of Acute Polyhydramnios

Aim of therapy is to relieve the acute maternal distress and to prevent preterm labor.
- *Correction of cause*: Maternal glycemic control, antiarrhythmic medication for fetal hydrops due to dysrhythmias, thoracoamniotic shunts for fetal constricting lung conditions, etc.
- Temporary relief can be brought by indomethacin therapy (at the risk of premature closure of ductus arteriosus), temporary controlled release of amniotic fluid via serial amniocentesis and amnioreduction. There are no guidelines regarding volume of fluid to be aspirated, the speed of aspiration, and prophylaxis with tocolytics or antibiotics.[7] Preterm labor, abruptio placentae, PROM, chorioamnionitis are seen in 1–3% cases following amnioreduction.[8]
- Fetal laser therapy for ablation of arteriovenous malformations and aberrant vessels leading to twin-twin transfusion syndrome.

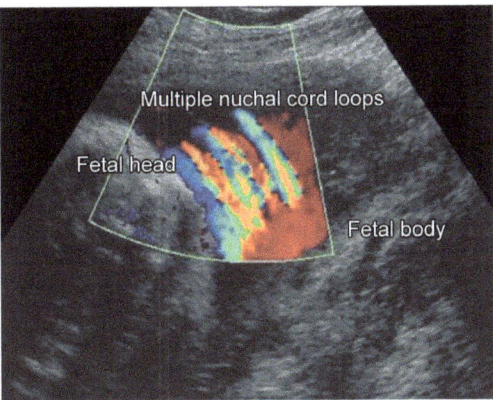

Fig 5: USG image of multiple loops of cord around neck, obstructing fetal swallowing and leading to polyhydramnios.
Source: Y Perlitz, I. Ben-Shlomo et al. Acute polyhydramnios in term pregnancy may be caused by multiple nuchal cord loops. Ultrasound Obstet Gynecol. 2010;35(2):253-4.

- Delivery of a case of polyhydramnios should always be at a tertiary care center due expected complications in labor such as abruptio placentae, abnormal uterine contractions, fetal malpositions, cord prolapse, postpartum hemorrhage, fetal anomalies requiring neonatal intensive care support.

Amniotic Fluid Embolism

Amniotic fluid embolism (AFE) is defined as the phenomenon wherein amniotic fluid breaches fetomaternal barrier and reaches maternal circulation where it causes the triad of hypoxia, hypotension, and coagulopathy, all occurring in relation to labor and delivery.

It is a very rare calamitous event and owing to its rarity and multisystem involvement, most feto-maternal specialists are not experienced in its management.

About 70% of AFE occurs during vaginal delivery, 11% following vaginal delivery, and 19% during cesarean section.[9] Very rarely, it may follow first or second trimester termination of pregnancy or amniocentesis.

Clinical Presentation

- Patient may experience a change in sensorium and mental alertness, a sensation of impending doom, and anxiety.
- Sudden cardiac arrest— could be pulseless electrical activity, asystole, and ventricular fibrillation.
- Fetal cardiac monitor will show absent baseline variability, acute decelerations, and terminal bradycardia.
- Disseminated intravascular coagulation (DIC) will set in after the initial cardiac event and present as bleeding diathesis—venipuncture sites, and vaginal bleeding which might coexist with uterine atony and cause delay in diagnosis[10] (Flowchart 1).

Diagnosis

There is no specific diagnostic test for AFE. It is the diagnosis of exclusion in any woman in labor or postpartum who experiences sudden cardiac collapse, hypoxia, seizure or coagulopathy.

Differential Diagnosis and the Tests to Differentiate

- Myocardial infarction—ECG and cardiac troponins
- Peripartum cardiomyopathy—echocardiography
- Pulmonary embolism— ventilation perfusion scan and CT angiography
- High spinal anesthesia and intravascular injection of local anesthetic
- Air embolism

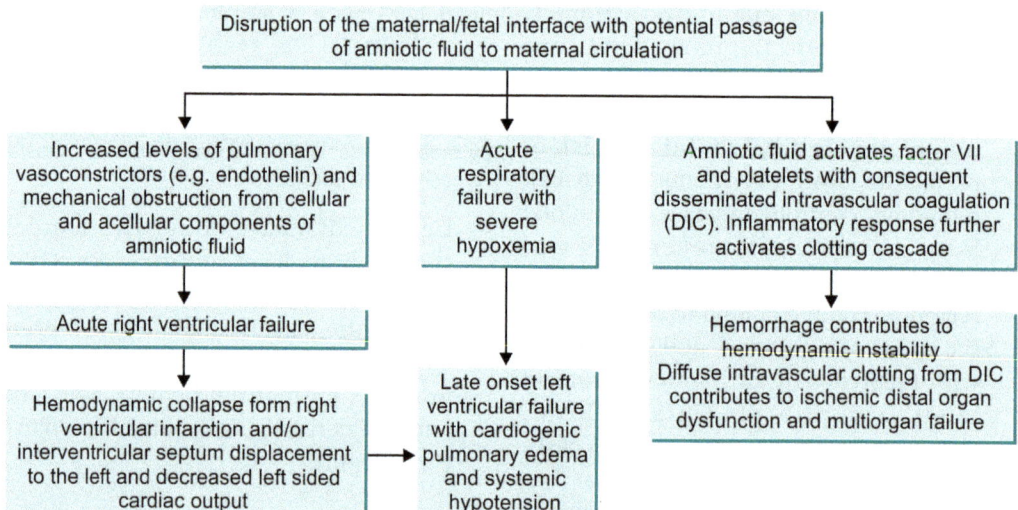

Flowchart 1: Proposed pathophysiology of amniotic fluid embolism.

Source: Society for Maternal-Fetal Medicine (SMFM), Pacheco LD, Saade G et al. Amniotic fluid embolism: diagnosis and management. Am J Obstet Gynecol. 2016;215(2):B16-24.

- Eclampsia
- Transfusion-related acute lung injury
- Anaphylaxis.

Management: Society for Maternal-Fetal Medicine Guidelines (SMFM), 2016 Initial Resuscitation

The diagnosis of amniotic fluid embolism is not necessary to be reached at this stage of management because steps of initial cardiac resuscitation remain the same.
- Chest compressions should precede artificial respiratory efforts
- Chest compressions should achieve a depth of at least 2 inches and should be followed by full recoil
- Left lateral position should be adopted to prevent uterus causing aortocaval compression
- Vasopressors, antiarrhythmic drugs, and defibrillation can be used as in non-pregnant status
- Following initial cardiac resuscitation, all attempts must be directed at expediting delivery of fetus≥23 weeks' gestation. Without delivering the fetus, all attempts at maternal resuscitation will not reach full hemodynamic benefit. If imminent delivery is expected, it should be expedited with operative measures like ventouse/forceps delivery. If delivery is not imminent, emergency cesarean section is indicated as a life-saving measure for the mother, irrespective of fetal viability.

Post-resuscitation management:
- Multi-disciplinary team comprising of obstetrician, intensivist, physician, and respiratory physician is required to care for such a patient.
- Hemodynamic stability will require careful use of intravenous fluids, vasopressors, and inotropes.
- Therapeutic cooling to 32–34°C has been advocated by the American Heart Association to improve the neurological outcome. But this might worsen DIC. So only in patients not showing any features of DIC, therapeutic cooling targeting a temperature of 36°C is advocated.

Management of coagulopathy:
- Disseminated intravascular coagulation must be suspected in this clinical scenario and tested for early detection and management.
- The aim of therapy is to maintain platelet count above 50,000/mm^3 and a normal activated partial thromboplastin time (APTT) and international normalized ratio (INR).
- Hemostatic resuscitation which includes supplementation of blood products in the ratio of 1:1:1 (packed RBCs:fresh frozen plasma:platelets) should be initiated soon upon early diagnosis of DIC.
- Bedside thromboelastography test can help identify those patients who will benefit from use of antifibrinolytics such as epsilon-aminocaproic acid and tranexamic acid.
- Uterine atony often coexists with DIC and needs to be treated with uterotonics (oxytocin, methylergometrine, and prostaglandins), uterine packing, B-Lynch suturing for approximation of uterine walls and hysterectomy, as the situation may demand.

CONCLUSION

Amniotic fluid performs the essential function of maintaining an ideal intrauterine milieu for protecting the fetus from trauma and compression effects, and maintaining fluid and nutrition balance, and allows optimal growth and development.
- There are many methods of assessment of amniotic fluid volume of which SDP and AFI are the most accurate.

- A severe reduction in amniotic fluid volume, anhydramnios is a serious condition compromising on fetal survival. Prior to fetal viability, the aim of management is conservative with identification and correction of causes. After viability, delivery should be expedited. Amnioinfusion and vesicoamniotic shunt placement are advocated only in a research and audit setup.
- Acute polyhydramnios is a sudden accumulation of amniotic fluid to a large extent that causes maternal distress and cardiorespiratory compromise. Such an acute collection of fluid often has an underlying condition, unlike the idiopathic polyhydramnios that develops slowly. Identifying and correcting the cause and serial amnioreduction are the mainstays of management.
- Amniotic fluid embolism is a catastrophic event which is rare and most obstetricians are not familiar with it due to its rarity. High index of suspicion and expertise in acute cardiac resuscitation are vital to patient's survival. Following resuscitation, a multi-disciplinary approach with a team of critical care intensivist, obstetrician, physician, and respiratory medicine expert should be involved.

REFERENCES

1. Brace RA. Physiology of amniotic fluid volume regulation. Clin Obstet Gynecol. 1997;40(2):280-9.
2. Campbell J, Wathen N, Perry G, et al. The coelomic cavity: an important site of materno-fetal nutrient exchange in the first trimester of pregnancy. Br J Obstet Gynecol 1993;100(8):765-7.
3. Abramovich DR. Fetal factors influencing the volume and composition of liquor amnii. J Obstet Gynecol Br Commonw. 1970;77(10):865-77.
4. Nabhan AF, Abdelmoula YA. Amniotic fluid index versus single deepest vertical pocket: a meta-analysis of randomized controlled trials. Int J Gynaecol Obstet 2009;104(2):184-8.
5. Szlachetka K, Faske E, Laniewski S, et al. A rare case of two consecutive Breus' molar pregnancies. J Ultrasound Med. 2017;36(6):1279-82.
6. Y Perlitz, I. Ben-Shlomo et al. Acute poly-hydramnios in term pregnancy may be caused by multiple nuchal cord loops. Ultrasound Obstet Gynecol. 2010;35(2):253-4.
7. Rode L, Bundgaard A, Skibsted L, et al. Acute recurrent polyhydramnios: a combination of amniocenteses and NSAID may be curative rather than palliative. Fetal Diagn Ther. 2007;22(3):186-9.
8. Leung WC, Jouannic JM, Hyett J, et al. Procedure-related complications of rapid amniodrainage in the treatment of poly-hydramnios. Ultrasound Obstet Gynecol. 2004;23:154-8.
9. Clark SL, Hankins GD, Dudley DA, et al. Amniotic fluid embolism: analysis of the national registry. Am J Obstet Gynecol. 1995;172(4Pt1):1158-67;discussion 1167-9.
10. Society for Maternal-Fetal Medicine (SMFM), Pacheco LD, Saade G et al. Amniotic fluid embolism: diagnosis and management. Am J Obstet Gynecol. 2016;215(2):B16-24.

CHAPTER 19

Intrauterine Fetal Death

Mahesh Koregol, Soumya Mahesh Koregol

INTRODUCTION

Intrauterine fetal death (IUFD) is defined as fetal death after 20 weeks of gestation. IUFD can be classified further into early or late IUFD. Early IUFD, if fetal death occurs before 24 weeks of pregnancy and late IUFD, if fetal death after 24 weeks.[1]

United States accounts to almost about one million fetal deaths at any gestational age in the each year, which at 20 weeks of gestation or above amounts to almost 26,000 fetal deaths.[2] The incidence of IUFD is 5–7/1,000 deliveries. On an average, about 20% IUFDs occur at or near term and around 50% occur before 28 weeks of gestation.[3] When the pregnancy reaches gestation of 42 weeks, IUFD chances increase by 2.74 times compared to 39 weeks of gestation.[4] Final diagnosis of IUFD has to be made after ultrasound scan only and not by auscultation using stethoscope, hand-held Doppler or cardiotocography (CTG) monitor.[5]

COMMON CAUSES[6,7]

Conditions in mother	Preeclampsia, sepsis, and diabetes
Conditions in fetus	Genetic and chromosomal disorders, growth restriction, infections, hydrops, and congenital malformations
Complications of umbilical cord and placenta	Infarction and abruption of placenta, abnormal coiling of umbilical cord, and cord having a tight knot
Fetomaternal conditions	Fetomaternal hemorrhage
Miscellaneous conditions	Increased age of mother more than 40 years, substance abuse, increased body mass index (BMI) of mother, physical injury, social deprivation, inadequately treated medical issues like inherited thrombophilia, antiphospholipid antibody (APLA) syndrome, thyroid disease, and cholestasis

Even after performing autopsy and extensive advanced testing, in majority percentage of IUFD cases, it is not possible to identify the exact cause, and cause in these cases remain unknown. In such situations, Cacciature and Collis coined a phrase in year 2000 called as "sudden antenatal death syndrome" or SADS.[8]

Exact cause of fetal death can only be identified in about 40% of autopsied cases, though full-term healthy mother accounts for majority of still births.[9,10]

RECOMMENDED TESTS FOR WOMAN WITH IUFD[3,6,11]

Name of test	Purpose of test (to identify condition)
Hematological and biochemical parameters including C-reactive proteins (CRPs) and bile salts of mother	• Preeclampsia and associated complications • Sepsis or hemorrhage leading to multiorgan failure
Coagulation profile and plasma fibrinogen of mother	DIC (disseminated intravascular coagulation)
Kleihauer count	Fetomaternal hemorrhage Anti-RhD gammaglobulin requirement
Bacterial infection tests in mother: • Vaginal swab • Cervical swab • Blood culture • Urine culture	To check life-threatening infections and choose appropriate antibiotics
Serology tests in mother: • Syphilis • Tropical infections • Viral diseases screening	Unidentified fetomaternal infections
Random blood sugar of mother	Undiagnosed diabetes mellitus
HbA_1c	Gestational diabetes mellitus
Thyroid profile of mother	Thyroid diseases
Thrombophilia screening in mother	Thrombophilia diseases in mother
Serology for anti-red cell antibody	Immune hemolytic disease
Maternal anti-La and anti-Ro antibodies	Autoimmune disease in mother
Alloimmune antiplatelet antibodies in mother	Alloimmune thrombocytopenia
Peripheral karyotyping of parents' blood	• Parental mosaicism • Parental balanced translocation
Karyotyping of fetal and placental tissues	• Aneuploidy • Single gene disorders
Microbiological examination of fetus and placenta: • Fetal swabs • Fetal blood • Placental swabs	Fetal infections
Postmortem examination: • Autopsy • External • Microscopy • X-ray • Placenta and cord	There are less invasive tests which offer no additional information compared to postmortem examination which provides more information. Such important information is extremely important for management of next pregnancy

One of major reasons for cause of IUFD is placental pathologies. Very useful part of autopsy in clinical setting is histopathology of placenta. There is advantage of finding specific placental pathologies in few of these cases which are responsible for high recurrence rates, and can only be identified by microscopic examination of the placenta.[12]

LABOR AND MODE OF DELIVERY

It is important to note previous obstetric history, mother's preferred mode of delivery, and other medical conditions to decide on mode of delivery of IUFD fetus. Immediate delivery is advisable in cases of preeclampsia, sepsis, rupture of membranes or placental abruption. Though in majority women with IUFD, recommended route of delivery is vaginal birth, some women do require to consider cesarean delivery as an alternative mode. Spontaneous labor within 3 weeks of diagnosis is seen in more than 85% of women with an IUFD. The risk of maternal DIC is 10% within 4 weeks from the date of fetal death in these women and the risk increases thereafter. If these women plan to delay the process of going into labor and delivery for more than 48 hours or who plan to go home should be offered and counseled about DIC possibility and testing at least twice a week as they are at higher risk for developing complications associated with DIC.

Most of these women with IUFD achieve successful vaginal birth within 24 hours after induction of labor. First line of treatment and intervention in induction of labor is a combination of mifepristone followed by prostaglandin preparation (vaginal prostaglandin E2 or vaginal misoprostol). Lower cost, lower doses, equivalent efficacy, and safety makes misoprostol superior in preference to prostaglandin E2.[3,13] Probable chance of undergoing cesarean section during initial 48 hours labor induction is about 15.6%.[14]

Adequate postpartum care and suitable lactation suppression needs to be advised after delivery of IUFD.

Before sending the mothers back home, adequate and relevant information about fertility and contraception should be advised. General pre-pregnancy advice needs to be given to these women. They have to take measures to avoid or reduce weight gain, if they are already overweight and consider weight loss before next pregnancy to avoid similar complications.[3,13]

Unidentified or new fetal or maternal complications are found among 29% of patients with history of previous IUFD and have no identifiable fetal or maternal disease in present pregnancy in new follow-up studies. Therefore, these women with previous IUFD who conceive again have to be managed in specialist referral unit with adequate and anticipatory care.[15]

CARE OF MENTAL HEALTH IN IUFD

Compared to women with live birth, women with intrauterine fetal death have increased risk of undergoing depression and anxiety during initial few months. IUFD is a worrying complication of pregnancy that influences women's short-term psychological well-being. The risk of occurrence of post-traumatic stress disorder (PTSD) and depression is prevalent during the next pregnancy, especially when conception occurs earlier after the loss.[16] There is need to provide counseling services to all women and their partners. Other family members, especially existing children and grandparents, should also be considered for counseling. Couple should be counseled and discussed about the advantages of delaying conception until resolution of severe psychological issues.[3]

CONCLUSION

The incidence of IUFD is 5–7/1000 deliveries. Final diagnosis of IUFD has to be made after ultrasound scan only. The causes of IUFD, in a large percentage of cases remain unknown. Immediate delivery is advisable in IUFD cases of preeclampsia, sepsis, rupture of membranes or placental abruption. Vaginal birth can be achieved within 24 hours of induction of labor for IUFD in about 90% of women. More than 85% of women with an IUFD go into labor spontaneously within 3 weeks of diagnosis. Information about fertility and contraception should be offered to mothers before returning home. Counseling should be offered to all women and their partners who have suffered IUFD.

REFERENCES

1. Robinson GE. Pregnancy loss. Best Pract Res Clin Obstet Gynaecol. 2014;28(1):169-78.
2. MacDorman MF, Kirmeyer S. The Challenge of Fetal Mortality. NCHS Data Brief. 2009(16):1.
3. Royal College of Obstetricians and Gynaecologists. (2010). Late Intrauterine Feta Death and Stillbirth (Green-top Guideline No. 55). [Online]. Available from: https://www.rcog.org.uk/en/guidelines-research-services/guidelines/gtg55/. [Last accessed September 2019].
4. Alimena S, Nold C, Herson V, et al. Rates of intrauterine fetal demise and neonatal morbidity at term: determining optimal timing of delivery. J Matern Fetal Neonatal Med. 2017;30(2):181-5.
5. Hywel DDA Univeristy Health Board, NHS Wales. (2017). Management of late intrauterine fetal death and stillbirth Guideline. [online]. Available from: http://www.wisdom.wales.nhs.uk/sitesplus/documents/1183/Management%20of%20Late%20Intrauterine%20Fetal%20Death%20and%20Stillbirth_Hywell%20Dda%20Guideline%202017.pdf [Last accessed September 2019].
6. Hoyert DL, Gregory EC. Cause of Fetal Death: Data from the Fetal Death Report, 2014. Natl Vital Stat Rep. 2016;95(7):1-25.
7. Williams B, Datta S. Previous fetal death. A Textbook of Preconceptional Medicine and Management. UK: Sapiens Publishing Ltd. pp. 241-50.
8. Collins JH. Umbilical cord accidents: human studies. Semin Perinatol. 2002;26(1):79-82.
9. Man J, Hutchinson JC, Heazell AE, et al. Stillbirth and intrauterine fetal death: factors affecting determination of cause of death at autopsy. Ultrasound Obstet Gynecol. 2016;48:566-73.
10. Cacciatore J, Radestad J, Frederik Frøen J. Effects of contact with still born babies on maternal anxiety and depression. Birth. 2008; 35(4):313-20.
11. Intrauterine Fetal Death and Stillbirth: Reproductive care programme at Nova Scotia. Guidelines for Investigation. Maternal_Newborn Clinical Guideline. 2016.
12. Man J, Hutchinson JC, Heazell AE, et al. Stillbirth and intrauterine fetal death: role of routine histopathological placental findings to determine cause of death. Ultrasound Obstet Gynecol. 2016;48:579-84.
13. National institute for health and care excellence (NICE). [(2013)]. Induction of labour in late intrauterine fetal death: vaginal misoprostol (after oral mifepristone). [online]. Available from: https://www.nice.org.uk/advice/esuom11/chapter/Overview-for-healthcare-professionals. [Last accessed September 2019].
14. do Nascimento MI, Cunha Ade A, Oliveira SR. Clinical management of the induction of labor in intrauterine fetal death: evaluation of incidence of cesarean section and related conditions. Rev Bras Epidemiol. 2014;17(1)203-16.
15. Gebhardt S, Oberholzer L. Elective Delivery at Term after a Previous Unexplained Intra-Uterine Fetal Death: Audit of Delivery Outcome at Tygerberg Hospital, South Africa. PLoS One. 2015;10(6):e0130254.
16. Gravensteen IK, Helgadottir LB, Jacobsen EM, et al. Long-term impact of intrauterine fetal death on quality of life and depression: a case-control study. BMC Pregnancy Childbirth. 2012;12:43.

CHAPTER 20

Amniotic Fluid Embolism

Thejaswini J

INTRODUCTION

Amniotic fluid embolism (AFE) is one of the rare and most annihilating obstetric conditions with high mortality and morbidity.

The etiology of the condition is poorly understood hence this condition cannot be prevented nor predicted.

The diagnosis of the condition requires high degrees of suspicion as the development of the clinical features are dramatic and there are no diagnostic tests to determine the condition.

The treatment is mostly supportive and resuscitative, and requires multidisciplinary management.

INCIDENCE

The definition of AFE varies in between the countries and registries throughout the world, hence the real incidence of AFE is debatable, however the incidence rate of 2–8/100,000 live births in various countries is noted.[1,2] The mortality associated with AFE is estimated to be between 5–15% of all maternal deaths with case fatality of 11–80% and perinatal mortality rates between 7% and 44%.

PATHOGENESIS AND PATHOPHYSIOLOGY[1,3,4-6]

Amniotic fluid embolism is clinically identified by acute hypoxia, cardiovascular collapse, and coagulation failure in the absence of any discernible cause. AFE is always a diagnosis of exclusion.

The pathogenesis of AFE is not clear. Initially, AFE was attributed to mechanical obstruction of pulmonary circulation because of fetal tissues. Currently there are two hypotheses which try to explain the development of AFE.

1. *Anaphylactoid reaction hypothesis*: It hypothesizes that amniotic fluid has many vasoactive substances and procoagulant substances that can cause endothelial activation and severe inflammatory response and lead to mast cell degranulation in the pulmonary circulation. In cases of AFE, b-tryptase (a serine protease contained in mast cells) levels are higher in pulmonary circulation.
2. *Complement activation hypothesis*: It is proposed that complement activation could be the reason for AFE as abnormally low level of complement, i.e. C3 and C4 are seen in AFE patients symbolic of complement activation either through classical or alternate pathway (Flowchart 1).[7]

CLINICAL FEATURES (TABLE 1)

Most incidences of AFE (70%) occur during labor, 19% during cesarean section, and 11% following vaginal delivery. It has also been reported during early gestation, second trimester abortions, during amniocentesis, or following closed abdominal injury.[2,3]

The syndrome may develop with non-specific prodromal symptoms like chills, shivering, sweating, and anxiety.

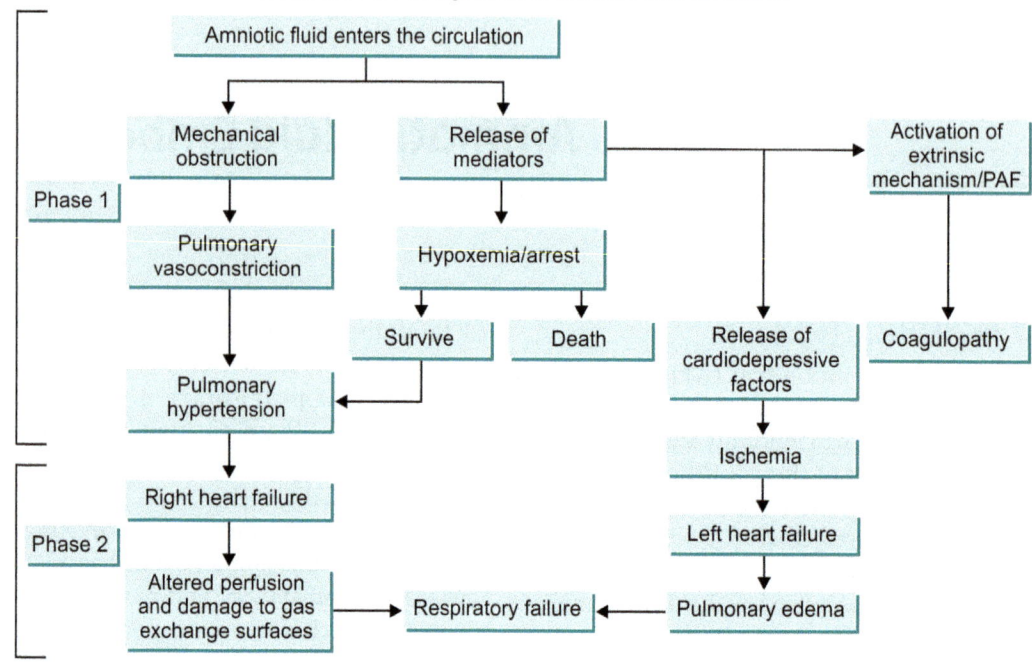

Flowchart 1: Pathogenesis of amniotic fluid embolism.

TABLE 1: Clinical features of amniotic fluid embolism.

Cardiac	Respiratory	Neurological	Coagulopathy	Fetal
Cardiac arrest	Breathlessness	Confusion	Thrombocytopenia	Abnormal cardiotocography (CTG)
Hypotension	Cough	Seizures	Hypofibrinogenemia	Fetal hypoxia
Tachycardia Arrhythmia	Cyanosis	Anxiety	Disseminated intravascular coagulation (DIC)	
	Tachypnea	Coma		
		Headache		

The patient may develop acute dyspnea, hypotension, cardiovascular collapse, fetal distress, confusion, convulsion, and atonic postpartum hemorrhage with disseminated intravascular coagulation.

■ **DIAGNOSIS (TABLE 2)[7,8]**

Amniotic fluid embolism is a diagnosis of exclusion. The diagnosis is mostly made clinically. It should be a differential diagnosis in all cases of abrupt cardiovascular collapse. However Benson et al. and UK obstetric surveillance system (UKOSS) study have set criteria for the diagnosis of AFE.[9] The diagnostic capability of zinc coproporphyrin, sialyl-Tn antigen (component of meconium), tryptase, low levels of C3 and C4 complement, insulin-like growth factor binding protein-1

TABLE 2: Criteria for the diagnosis of AFE.

Benson criteria	UKOSS criteria
Gravid ladies/-+/ up to 48 hours after parturition with one or more of the following symptoms and requiring management	No other clear cause: Abrupt cardiovascular collapse with one or more of the following symptoms
Hypotension/cardiac arrest	Acute fetal compromise
Respiratory difficulty	Cardiac arrest
Disseminated intravascular coagulation	Cardiac arrhythmia
Coma/seizures	Coagulopathy
No other medical cause for the clinical course	Hypotension
	Maternal hemorrhage excluding women with maternal hemorrhage as the first symptom with no evidence of early coagulopathy or cardiorespiratory compromise or in cases of postnatal evidence of fetal squames or hairs in the lung)
	Premonitory symptoms seizures
	Sudden onset of shortness of breath

looks encouraging in detection of AFE, but they are yet to be accepted in conventional clinical diagnosis.[1]

Differential Diagnosis

- Pulmonary embolism
- Peripartum cardiomyopathy
- Myocardial infarction
- Eclampsia
- Acute left heart failure
- Cerebrovascular accidents

MANAGEMENT

The treatment of AFE is majorly supportive and multidisciplinary involving obstetricians, hematologists, intensives, and anesthetist. The basic elements in the treatment are early diagnosis, immediate resuscitation, and quick delivery of the fetus.

General:[10-13]
- Monitor the vitals by using pulse oximeter, noninvasive blood pressure (NIBP), large-bore IV access above the diaphragm, and central line to guide the fluid administration.
- Complete blood count, coagulation studies, electrolytes, and arterial blood gas should be collected and should be repeated frequently to guide the blood component therapy in the initial phase of AFE. Thromboelastogram can be used when available.

Respiratory support:
- Maintain the airway and keep the oxygen saturation above 90% to avoid hypoxic injury. This may often require intubation and advance airway support. Pulmonary vasoconstriction and ventilation perfusion mismatch have been treated with aerosolized prostacyclin and nitric oxide.[14]

Cardiovascular support:
- Treat hypotension with volume resuscitation, inotropes, vasopressors to optimize the preload and contractility and after load. These patients often have pulmonary edema hence volume resuscitation should be guarded. Hemodynamic goals are systolic blood pressure >90 mm Hg PaO_2>60 mm Hg and urinary output>0.5 mL/kg/hour.[15]

Coagulopathy:
- Kanayama and Tamura proposed that about one-third of AFE cases present with atonic bleeding. Atonic postpartum hemorrhage (PPH) has to be delt swiftly with oxytocics, prostaglandins, methergine, Bakri balloon catheter with B-Lynch sutures, hysterectomy, and internal lilac artery ligations as the situation demands. Massive transfusion protocol has to be initiated to combat the uncontrolled hemorrhage. Prevention and treatment of coagulopathy requires early and ongoing transfusion with packed red blood cell (PRBC), fresh frozen plasma (FFP), cryoprecipitate with the guidance of lab coagulation studies, and viscoelastic tests.
- The optimal PRBC to FFP ratio is 1:1–1:5.[16,17] Thrombocytopenia induced by AFE has to be treated with platelet transfusions. Hypofibrinogenemia is noted early in AFE and can be used as marker to assess the severity of obstetric hemorrhage. Cryoprecipitate transfusion to improve the fibrinogen levels have to be undertaken. Antifibrinolytics like tranexamic acid is also useful in combating the hemorrhage.

Delivery of the fetus:
- Delivery of the fetus has to be fast as it improves the maternal cardiac output and reduces the neurologic damage to the fetus. In the setting of cardiac arrest with resuscitation efforts emergency cesarean has to be done to deliver the fetus, but the carrying out of cesarean section in an unstable patient is precarious, hence the treatment has to be individualized.

Novel treatment strategies:[18-26]
- Antithrombin concentrates have been found to be beneficial in patients of AFE with coagulopathy, however heparin is not used due to risk of massive hemorrhage currently.
- Extracorporeal membrane oxygenation
- Cardiopulmonary bypass
- Intra-aortic balloon pump
- Pulmonary artery thromboembolectomy
- Hemofiltration
- Plasma exchange transfusion removes the chemical mediators and cytokines responsible for the anaphylactoid response.
- High-dose corticosteroid treatment is believed to be beneficial as AFE is an inflammatory-mediated anaphylactoid response.
- C1 esterase inhibitors they inhibit complement activation and modulate the coagulation fibrinolytic kallikrein and kinin systems.

PROGNOSIS

About 56% of the patients succumb in the early phase of the disease with patients dying in a median time of 1 hour 42 minutes after the first presentation of AFE.[9,27] The main cause of death are cardiac arrest, acute respiratory distress syndrome (ARDS), disseminated intravascular coagulation (DIC), multiple organ failure.[9] Survivors usually have neurological lacunae.

CONCLUSION

- Amniotic fluid embolism is a rare condition whose onset cannot be predicted nor prevented as the cause of it is not known.
- Early recognition and aggressive treatment of the condition reduces the mortality and morbidity associated with AFE.
- Multi-disciplinary management involving obstetrician, intensivist, anesthetist, and hematologist in ICU gives a better chance of survival for the patient.
- Despite early recognition and aggressive management of the condition mortality and neurological squeal, both in the mother and the child remain high.

REFERENCES

1. Conde-Agudelo A, Romero R. Amniotic fluid embolism: an evidence-based review. Am J Obstet Gynecol. 2009;201(5):445e1-13.
2. Kramer MS, Rouleau J, Liu S, et al. Amniotic fluid embolism: incidence, risk factors and impact on perinatal outcome. BJOG. 2012;119(7):874-9.
3. Clark SL. Amniotic fluid embolism. Clin Obstet Gynecol. 2010;53(2):322-8.
4. Ito F, Akasaka J, Koike N, et al. Incidence, diagnosis and pathophysiology of amniotic fluid embolism. J Obstet Gynaecol. 2014;34(7): 580-4.
5. Tuffnell DJ. United Kingdom amniotic fluid embolism register. BJOG. 2005;112(12):1625-9.
6. Benson MD. Current concepts of immunology and diagnosis in amniotic fluid embolism. Clin Dev Immunol. 2012;2012:946576.
7. Piva I, Scutiero G, Greco P. Amniotic fluid embolism: an update of the evidence. Med Toxicol Clin Forens Med. 2016;2:2.
8. Benson MD. A hypothesis regarding complement activation and amniotic fluid embolism. Med Hypotheses. 2007;68(5):1019-25.
9. Knight M, Tuffnell D, Brocklehurst P, et al. Incidence and risk factors for amniotic-fluid embolism. Obstet Gynecol. 2010;115(5): 910-7.
10. Malhotra P, Agarwal R, Awasthi A, et al. Delayed presentation of amniotic fluid embolism: lessons from a case diagnosed at autopsy. Respirology. 2007;12:148-50.
11. Thongrong C, Kasemsiri P, Hofmann JP, et al. Amniotic fluid embolism. Int J Crit Illn Inj Sci. 2013;3(2):51-7.
12. Sugunadevan M. Amniotic fluid embolism. Sri Lanka J Anaesthesiol. 2009;17:25-7.
13. Gist RS, Stafford IP, Leibowitz AB, et al. Amniotic fluid embolism. Anesth Analg. 2009; 108:1599-602.
14. McDonell NJ, Chan BO, Frengly RW. Rapid reversal of critical hemodynamic compromise with nitric oxide in parturient with amniotic fluid embolism. Int J Obst Anesth. 2007;16(3):269-73.
15. Moore J, Baldisseri MR. Amniotic fluid embolism. Crit Care Med. 2005;33(10 Suppl): S279-85.
16. Kanayama N, Tamura N. Amniotic fluid embolism: pathophysiology and new strategies for management. J Obstet Gynaecol Res 2014; 40:1507-17.
17. Burtelow M, Riley E, Druzin M, et al. How we treat: management of life-threatening primary postpartum hemorrhage with a standardized massive transfusion protocol. Transfusion. 2007;47(9):1564-72.
18. Sharma NS, Wille KM, Bellot SC, et al. Modern use of extracorporeal life support in pregnancy and postpartum. ASAIO J. 2015;61(1):110-4.
19. Stanten RD, Iverson LI, Daugharty TM, et al. Amniotic fluid embolism causing catastrophic pulmonary vasoconstriction: diagnosis by transesophageal echocardiogram and treatment by cardiopulmonary bypass. Obstet Gynecol. 2003;102(3):496-8.
20. Hsieh YY, Chang CC, Li PC, et al. Successful application of extracorporeal membrane oxygenation and intraaortic balloon counterpulsation as lifesaving therapy for a patient with amniotic fluid embolism. Am J Obstet Gynecol. 2000;183(2):496-7.
21. Esposito RA, Grossi EA, Coppa G, et al. Successful treatment of postpartum shock caused by amniotic fluid embolism with cardiopulmonary bypass and pulmonary artery thromboembolectomy. Am J Obstet Gynecol. 1999;163(2):572-4.
22. Weksler N, Ovadia L, Stav A, et al. Continuous arteriovenous hemofiltration in the treatment of amniotic fluid embolism. Int J Obstet Anesth. 1994;3:92-6.
23. Dodgson J, Martin J, Boswell J, et al. Probable amniotic fluid embolism precipitated by amniocentesis and treated by exchange transfusion. Br Med J (Clin Res Ed). 1987; 294(6583):1322-3.
24. Ogihara T, Morimoto K, Kaneko Y. Continuous hemodiafiltration for potential amniotic fluid embolism: dramatic responses observed during a 10-year period report of three cases. Ther Apher Dial. 2012;16(2):195-7.
25. Tamura N, Kimura S, Farhana M, et al. C1 esterase inhibitor activity in amniotic fluid embolism. Crit Care Med. 2014;42(6):1392-6.
26. Todo Y, Tamura N, Itoh H, et al. Therapeutic application of C1 esterase inhibitor concentrate for clinical amniotic fluid embolism: a case report. Clin Case Rep. 2015;3(7):673-5.
27. Fitzpatrick KE, Tuffnell D, Kurinczuk JJ, et al. Incidence, risk factors, management and outcomes of amniotic-fluid embolism: a population-based cohort and nested case-control study. BJOG. 2016;123(1):100-9.

CHAPTER 21

Breech Presentation and its Complications

Ravishankar P

DEFINITION

Breech presentation is defined as the presentation where the fetus is in longitudinal lie and its podalic pole occupies the lower segment of the uterus.[1]

INCIDENCE[2]

- 28 weeks: 20%
- 34 weeks: 5%
- Term: 3%
- One-third are undiagnosed antenatally and discovered in labor.[3]

CLASSIFICATION

As per position of fetus:[2]

Complete breech (25%): Where the hips and knees are flexed and the feet are not below the level of the fetal buttocks. Presenting part consists of the two buttocks, two feet, and the external genitalia. This is common in multipara.

Incomplete breech: It is of three types:
1. *Frank breech* (65%): Where the hips are flexed and the legs are extended. It is common in primigravida.
2. *Footling breech*: Where one or both feet are presenting as the lowermost part of the fetus.
3. *Kneeling*: Where knees are the lowermost part of the fetus (Fig. 1).

As per the maternal condition:[2]
- *Uncomplicated*: When breech presentation is not associated with any obstetrical or medical complications in the mother.
- *Complicated*: When the breech presentation is associated with obstetrical and medical complications in the mother.

Positions of breech presentation:[2] In the breech presentation, the sacrum is considered as the denominator—
- *Left sacroanterior (first position)*: This is the most common. The back is anterior and to the left.
- *Right sacroanterior (second position)*: The back is anterior and to the right.
- *Right sacroposterior (third position)*: The back posterior and to the right.
- *Fourth sacroposterior (fourth position)*: The back posterior and to the left (Fig. 2).

ETIOLOGY

Maternal factors:[4]
- Poly- or oligohydramnios
- Uterine anomalies—septate uterus, bicornuate uterus, etc.
- Space occupying lesions such as fibroids
- Placenta abnormalities like previa or cornufundal attachment
- Multiparity due to the lax abdominal wall
- Contracted pelvis.

Breech Presentation and its Complications

Frank breech (65%)	Complete breech (10%)	Incomplete breech (25%)	
		Footling breech	Kneeling breech
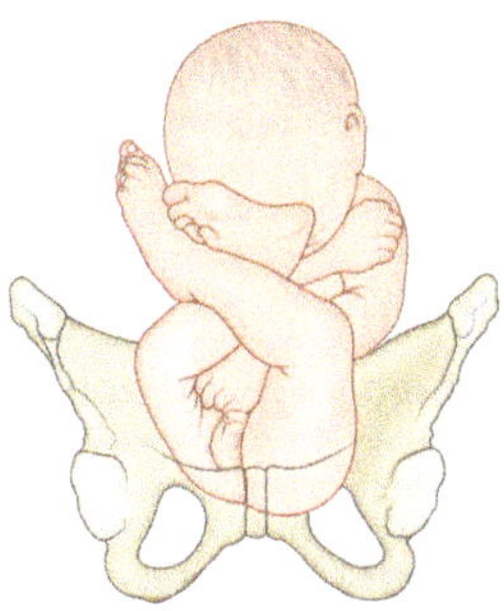 The baby's hip joints are flexed and knee joints are extended	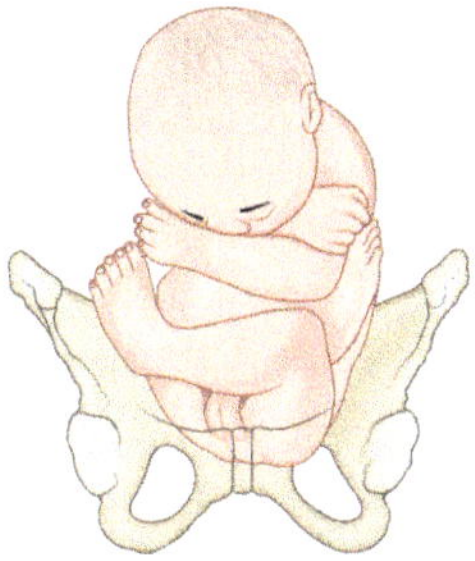 The baby's hip and knee joints are flexed	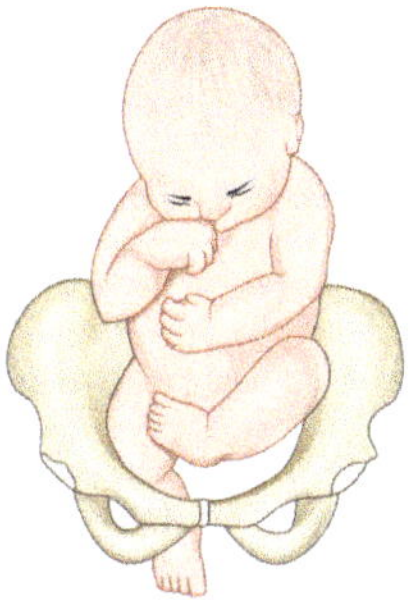 The baby's hip and knee joints are extended on one or both sides	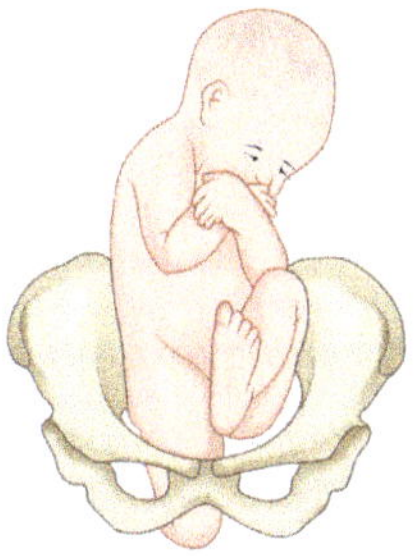 The baby's hip joints are extended and knee joints are flexed on one or both sides

Fig. 1: Incomplete breech positions.

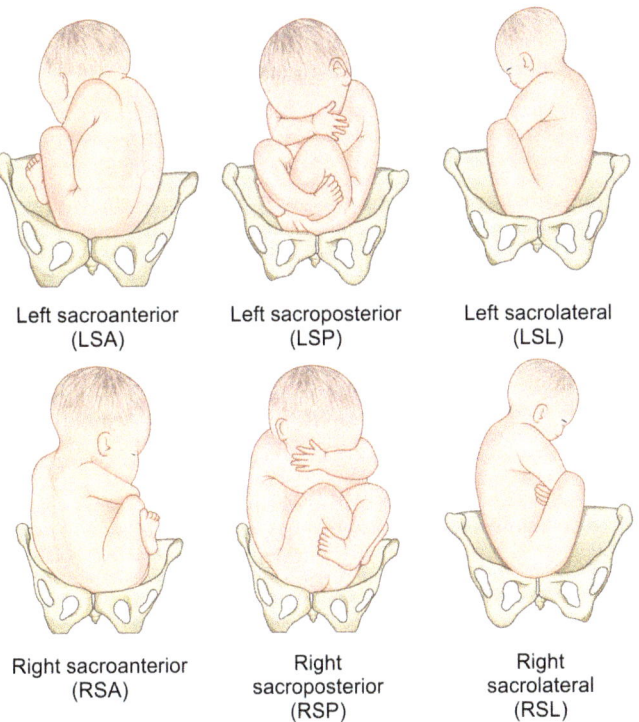

Fig. 2: Positions of breech presentation.

Fetal factors:[4]
- Prematurity
- Fetal anomalies—hydrocephalus and anencephaly
- Multiple pregnancy
- Short umbilical cord.

DIAGNOSIS OF BREECH

Clinical Examination

Abdominal examination: During palpation of the abdomen, the fetal head (hard, globular, and ballotable mass) is felt in the fundal grip and the breech (soft, broad, and irregular, nonballotable mass) is felt in the pelvic grip. Also auscultation reveals that the fetal heart sounds are situated at or just above the umbilicus.[4]

Vaginal examination (in labor):
- Slow dilatation of the cervix.
- Sausage-shaped bag of membranes.
- Breech (two buttocks, anus, and genitalia) can be palpated after rupture of membranes.[4]

Diagnosis of breech is further corroborated by radiological examination (most commonly ultrasound examination) where the position of the fetus is confirmed.[4]

MANAGEMENT OF BREECH PRESENTATION DURING PREGNANCY

If it persists beyond 34 weeks, ultrasound examination is done to exclude any of the causes of breech, such as polyhydramnios, uterine/fetal anomalies, etc. and if by 36 weeks, if there is no spontaneous version, external cephalic version (ECV) may be attempted.[5]

Women with a breech presentation at term should be offered ECV unless there is an absolute contraindication. They should be advised on the risks and benefits of ECV and the implications for mode of delivery.[5]

Procedure:[6]
- External cephalic version is conducted in the labor room, with facilities for emergency lower (uterine) segment cesarean section (LSCS) in place.
- Fetal heart rate is continuously monitored.
- Tocolytic cover may be given.
- Two methods to perform ECV—backward or forward roll.
- One hand firmly grips the fetal head and the other dislodges the breech and mobilizes it.
- Then the fetus is rolled backward or forward until the head is in the lower pole of the uterus.
- Monitor fetal heart rate and perform ultrasound after the procedure.

Success rates of ECV have been reported from many studies ranging from 36% to 85%[6] (Figs. 3A to D).

Risks of ECV:[6]
- Placental abruption
- Premature rupture of membranes
- Cord accidents
- Transplacental hemorrhage (Anti-D to be given in Rh-negative women)
- Fetal bradycardia/hypoxia.

Contraindications of ECV:[6]

Absolute contraindication	Relative contraindication
Congenital anomalies	Rhesus isoimmunization, >2 previous cesarean section (CS)
Placenta previa	Elderly primigravida and morbid obesity
Unexplained antepartum hemorrhage (APH)	Intrauterine growth restriction (IUGR), extended fetal head
Preeclampsia	Oligohydramnios
Multiple pregnancy	Polyhydramnios

Factors affecting the success of ECV:[7]
- Experience of the practitioner
- Maternal weight

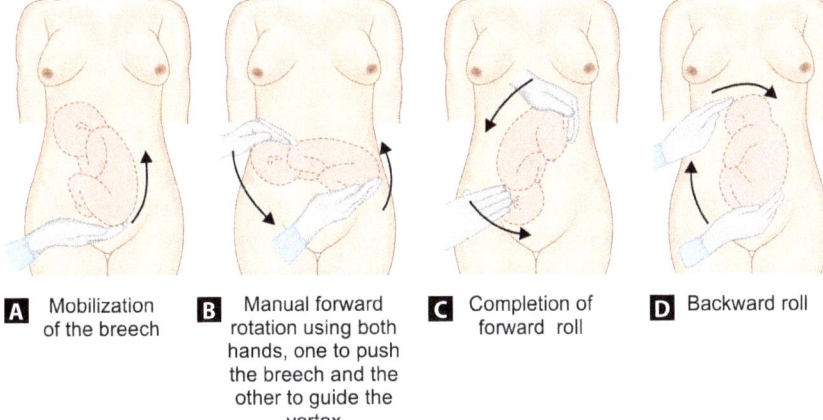

| A | Mobilization of the breech | B | Manual forward rotation using both hands, one to push the breech and the other to guide the vertex | C | Completion of forward roll | D | Backward roll |

Figs. 3A to D: External version of a breech presentation.
Source: World Health Organization (WHO). (2013) Managing complications in pregnancy and childbirth: a guide for doctors and midwives. [online]. Available from: http://www.who.int/reproductive-health/impac/mcpc.pdf. [Last accessed September 2019].

- Palpable fetal head
- Nonengaged breech
- Nonanterior placenta
- Amniotic fluid index (AFI) of 7–10 cm
- Adequate uterine relaxation.

Complications of ECV:[7]
- Intrauterine death
- Rupture of membranes
- Placental abruption
- Stimulation of preterm labor
- Fetal bradycardia.

No good evidence is available to support the use of intravenous (IV) nitroglycerin. A Cochrane review of four small trials showed no efficacy of and also association with significant side effects of sublingual nitroglycerin (Hofmeyr et al. 2004) (Bujold et al. 2003a) (Bujold et al. 2003b).[8-10]

Stop the procedure, if:
- The woman is too uncomfortable.
- If the fetal heart rate (FHR) is nonreassuring.
- Turn the woman to her left lateral position and FHR is monitored every 5 minutes.
- If the FHR does not stabilize within 30 minutes, then deliver by cesarean section.[7]

MECHANISM OF LABOR IN BREECH

Cochrane review of planned cesarean section for term breech delivery in 2003.[10]

In developed countries:

	Planned cesarean section	Planned vaginal birth
Perinatal or neonatal death	0/641 (0%)	4/694 (0.6%)
Serious short-term neonatal morbidity	2/514 (0.4%)	29/511 (5.7%)

Cochrane Review, 2003[10,11]

The reviewed trials indicate that a policy of planned cesarean section compared with planned vaginal birth was associated with a decrease in perinatal or neonatal death and/or neonatal morbidity. Among survivors, there was no significant difference in outcomes at age of 2. As the long-term outcome following perinatal morbidity appeared good, the most relevant outcome is the reduction in perinatal and neonatal death. Based on this meta-analysis of all trials, one death would be prevented for every 112 cesarean sections planned.[10,11]

For the mother, planned cesarean section was associated with a modest increase in short-term maternal morbidity. Outcomes at 2 years were similar between the two groups. The effects of cesarean section on longer-term outcomes, such as risks related to the scarred uterus, have not yet been addressed, nor have the cost implications (Hannah et al, 2000).[10,11]

Women should be informed that planned vaginal breech birth increases the risk of low Apgar scores and serious short-term complications, but has not been shown to increase the risk of long-term morbidity.[12]

The principal movements occur in three places:[13]

1. *Buttocks*:
   i. *Engagement*: Diameter of engagement is one of the oblique diameters of the inlet
   ii. The engaging diameter is the bitrochanteric diameter (10 cm)
   iii. Descent of the buttocks until the anterior buttock touches the pelvic floor
   iv. Internal rotation of the anterior buttock one-eighth of a circle placing it behind the symphysis pubis
   v. Further descent with lateral flexion, anterior hip is released first followed by the posterior hip
   vi. Delivery of lower limbs and trunk takes place
   vii. Restitution—back to the oblique diameter.
2. *Shoulders*:
   i. Engagement of the bisacromial diameter (12 cm) in the oblique diameter
   ii. Descent along with internal rotation
   iii. Delivery of the posterior shoulder followed by anterior shoulder
   iv. Restitution and external rotation
   v. Fetal trunk is now positioned as dorso-anterior.
3. *Head*:
   i. Engagement occurs in the opposite oblique diameter
   ii. Engaging diameter is the suboccipito-frontal (10 cm)
   iii. Descent
   iv. Internal rotation, placing the occiput behind the symphysis pubis
   v. Further descent
   vi. Head is born by flexion.

Zatuchni–Andros breech scoring:[13]

	0 points	1 points	2 points
Parity	0	1	2
Gestational age	39+ weeks	37–38 weeks	<37 weeks
Estimated fetal weight	3.5 kg	3–3.5 kg	<3 kg
Previous breech	0	1	2
Dilatation	2	3	4
Station	−3	−2	−1

If the score is 0–4, cesarean delivery is recommended.[13]

Types of breech delivery:[4]
- Cesarean section
- Vaginal delivery
- Spontaneous breech delivery
- Assisted breech delivery
- Partial or total breech extraction.

Indications for vaginal breech delivery:[14]
- Frank or complete breech presentation
- Estimated fetal weight (EFW) between 1.5 kg and 3.5 kg
- Fetal head must be flexed
- Adequate maternal pelvis
- No other obstetric complications.

MANAGEMENT DURING LABOR[4]

First stage:
- Adequate rest and hydration given
- Repeated vaginal examinations to be avoided
- Vaginal examination to be done in case the membranes rupture to rule out cord prolapse.

Women should be informed that induction of labor is not usually recommended. Augmentation of slow progress with oxytocin should only be considered if the contraction frequency is low in the presence of epidural analgesia.[14]

Second stage:
- Explain the necessity of effective pushing in the second stage of labor
- Ensure adequate analgesia
- Spontaneous descent and expulsion to the umbilicus should occur with maternal pushing only.

DO NOT PULL ON THE BREECH[4]
- Rotation to the sacrum anterior position is desired and may be facilitated.
- Episiotomy may be considered once the anterior buttock and anus are *"crowning"*.
- If the legs do not deliver spontaneously, perform the Pinard maneuver.[1] Do not attempt to extract the legs until the popliteal fossae are visible.

The Pinard maneuver (Figs. 4A and B) in accomplished by inserting two fingers along one extremity to the knee, which is then pushed away from the midline (abducted) at the same time as flexing the leg at the hip. This causes spontaneous flexion of the knee and delivery of the foot.[1]

- Support the baby around the hips and have the woman push until the scapulae are visible. Do not hold the baby by the flank or abdomen, as this may cause kidney or liver damage. Do not pull on the breech or compress the woman's abdomen. Maintain flexion of the fetal head by keeping the body below the horizontal.
- Rotate the body to facilitate delivery of the arms over the chest (Loveset maneuver) (Fig. 5).[1]
- Support the baby to maintain the head in a flexed position. Suprapubic pressure may help. Maternal expulsive efforts should be encouraged.
- The body should be supported in a horizontal position or allowed to hang until the nape of the neck appears at the introitus (vaginal opening) (Fig. 6).[1]
- *Deliver the head*:
  - *Mauriceau–Smellie–Veit maneuver*:[4] Maintain the head in flexion by placing the attendant's fingers over the chin and malar eminences. An assistant may help the delivery by providing suprapubic pressure, as traction is applied by primary healthcare provider (Fig. 7).

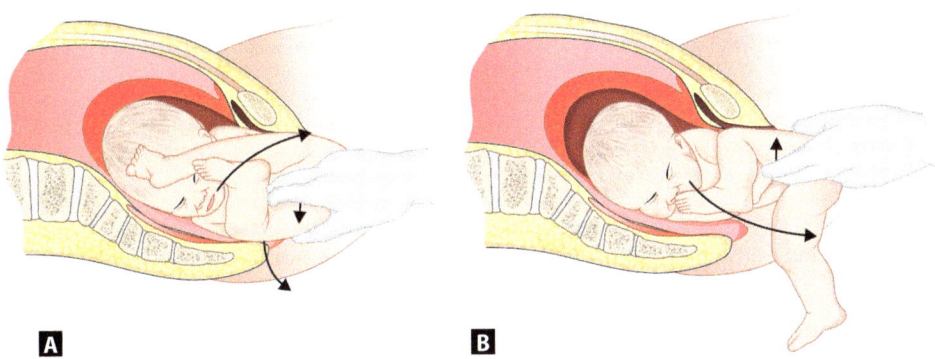

Figs. 4A and B: Pinard maneuver.
Source: Gabbe SG, Niebyl JR, Simpson JL. Obstetrics: Normal and Problem Pregnancies, 2nd edition. New York: Churchill Livingstone; 1991.

204 Obstetric Emergencies

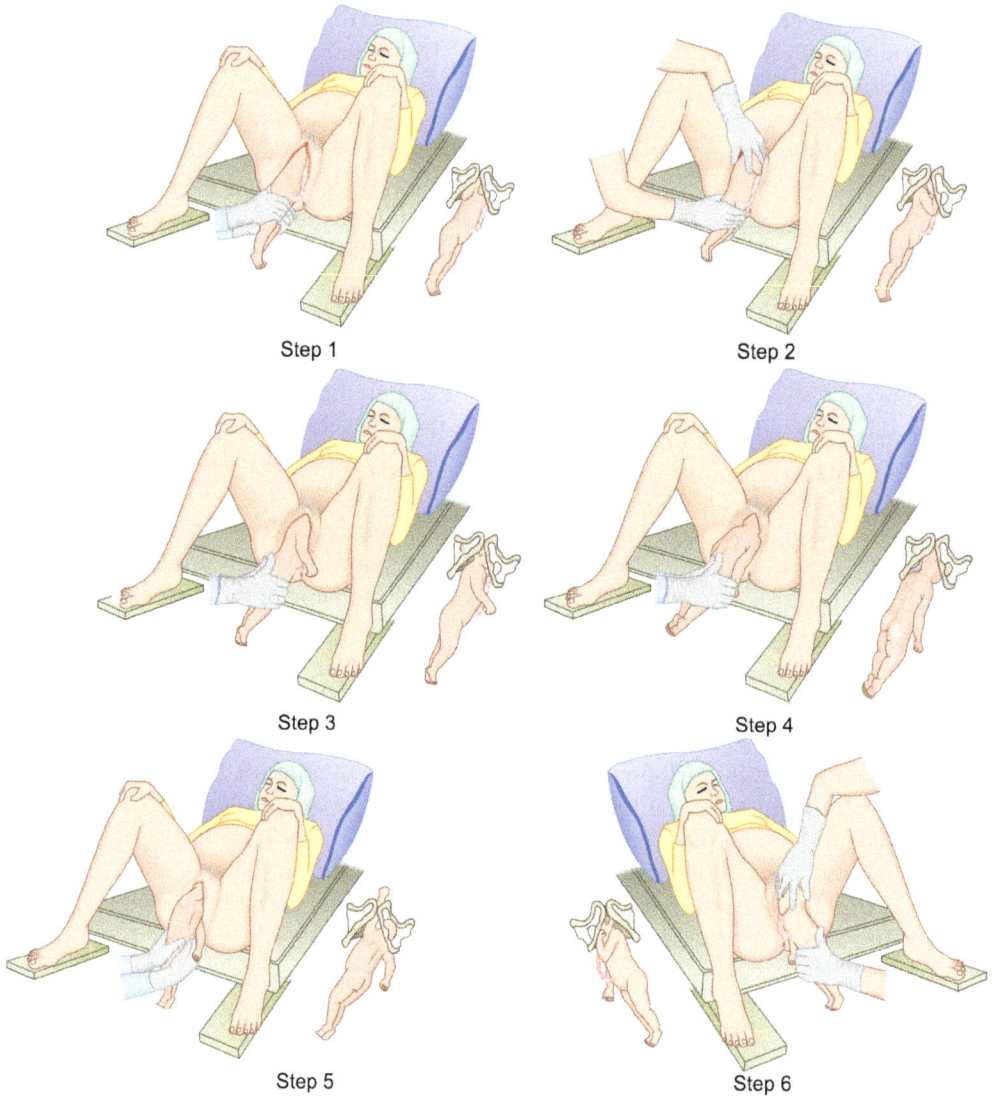

Fig. 5: Loveset maneuver.

- Use forceps, if needed. Piper's forceps were specifically designed for this purpose[4] (Figs. 8A to C).

Third stage:
- Care after breech delivery active management of the third stage of labor (AMTSL)[15]
- Prepare for newborn resuscitation
- Umbilical arterial blood gas analysis, where laboratory facilities exist
- Examination for maternal trauma
- *Examination for neonatal trauma:*[15]
  - Examine the hips of the newborn with care at the time of the initial newborn examination
  - Repeat the examination in the immediate neonatal period and prior to discharge from care.
- Review birth with the family.

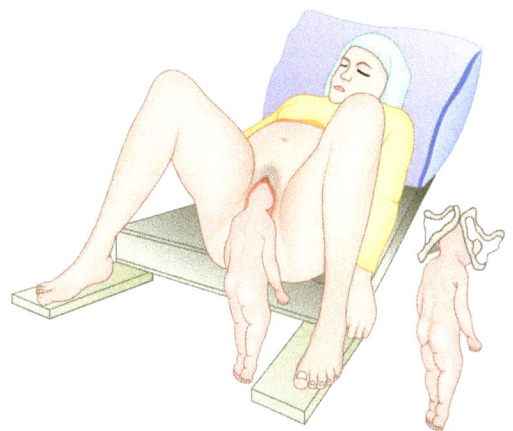

Fig. 6: Allowing the baby to hang until the nape of the neck appears.

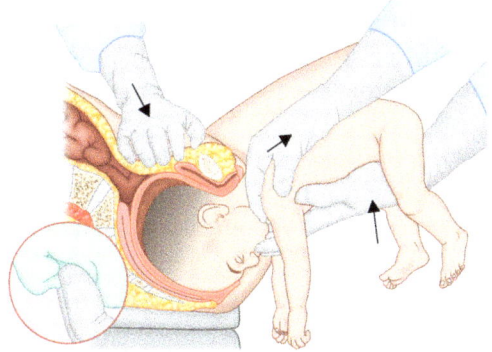

Fig. 7: Delivery of the aftercoming head using Mauriceau maneuver.
Source: Cunningham FG, Leveno KJ, Bloom SL, et al. Breech presentation and delivery. In: Cunningham FG, Hauth JC, Leveno KJ, Gilstrap L, Bloom SL, Wenstrom KD, (Eds) Williams Obstetrics, 22nd edn. New York: McGraw-Hill Medical Publishing Division; 2005. pp. 565-86.

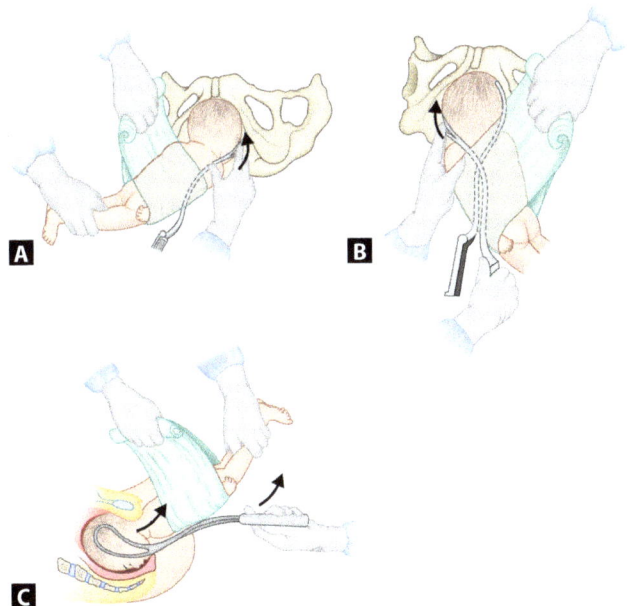

Figs. 8A to C: Piper forceps for delivery of the aftercoming head.
Source: Cunningham FG, Leveno KJ, Bloom SL, et al. Breech presentation and delivery. In: Cunningham FG, Hauth JC, Leveno KJ, Gilstrap L, Bloom SL, Wenstrom KD (Eds). Williams Obstetrics, 22nd edn. New York: McGraw-Hill Medical Publishing Division; 2005. pp. 565-86.

DOCUMENTATION OF BREECH DELIVERY

The indication, complete review of risks and benefits for vaginal delivery, and consent must be clearly and completely documented in all cases.[16]

This is a suggested format for a chart note. Detailed notes should be incorporated into both the woman's and the baby's charts.[16]

- Date and time of birth
- Name of physician or other primary healthcare provider and experience with vaginal breech delivery date and timing of ECV attempts and experience of healthcare provider
- Use of tocolysis, Yes/No drug used:
- Record of informed discussion with the woman of the risks, benefits, and options
- Type of breech at onset of labor assessment of maternal pelvis
- Assessment of the FHR and contractions
- Type of analgesia or anesthesia used (if any)
- Maneuvers performed to deliver baby, use of episiotomy, description, and timing, details of repair, estimated time from birth to umbilicus to birth of head.

Delivery of aftercoming head:
- Mauriceau–Smellie–Veit maneuver Yes/No
- Forceps Yes/No—symphysiotomy Yes/No
- APGAR scores results of cord blood analysis, if done
- Neonatal resuscitation activities, if needed
- Description of maternal and neonatal injuries (if any).

REFERENCES

1. Gabbe SG, Niebyl JR, Simpson JL. Obstetrics: Normal and Problem Pregnancies, 2nd edition. New York: Churchill Livingstone; 1991.
2. Brenner WE, Bruce RD, Hendricks CH. The characteristics and perils of breech presentation. Am J Obstet Gynecol. 1974;118(5):700-12.
3. Cunningham FG, Leveno KJ, Bloom SL, Hauth JC, et al. Williams obstetrics, 22nd edition. New York: McGraw-Hill Medical Publishing Division; 2005.
4. Cunningham FG, Leveno KJ, Bloom SL, et al. Breech presentation and delivery. In: Cunningham FG, Hauth JC, Leveno KJ, Gilstrap L, Bloom SL, Wenstrom KD, (Eds). Williams Obstetrics. 22nd ed. New York: McGraw-Hill Medical Publishing Division; 2005. pp. 565-86.
5. Hofmeyr GJ, Gyte G. Interventions to help external cephalic version for breech presentation at term [Cochrane review]. In: Cochrane Database of Systematic Reviews, Issue 1. Chichester (UK): John Wiley & Sons Ltd; 2004.
6. Hofmeyr GJ, Kulier R. External cephalic version for breech presentation at term [Cochrane review]. In: Cochrane Database of Systematic Reviews 1996 Issue 1. Chichester (UK): John Wiley & Sons, Ltd; 1996.
7. Hutton EK, Kaufman K, Hodnett E, et al. External cephalic version beginning at 34 weeks' gestation versus 37 weeks' gestation: a randomized multicenter trial. Am J Obstet Gynecol. 2003;189(1):245-54.
8. Bujold E, Marquette GP, Ferreira E, et al. Sublingual nitroglycerin versus intravenous ritodrine as tocolytic for external cephalic version: a double-blinded randomized trial. Am J Obstet Gynecol. 2003a;188(6):1454-7.
9. Bujold E, Boucher M, Rinfret D, et al. Sublingual nitroglycerin versus placebo as a tocolytic for external cephalic version: a randomized controlled trial in parous women. Am J Obstet Gynecol. 2003b;189(4):1070-3.
10. Hofmeyr GJ, Hannah ME. Planned caesarean section for term breech delivery [Cochrane review]. In: Cochrane Database of Systematic Reviews 2003, Issue 2. Chichester (UK): John Wiley & Sons, Ltd; 2003.
11. Hannah ME, Hannah WJ, Hewson SA, et al. Planned cesarean section versus planned vaginal birth for breech presentation at term: a randomised multicentre trial. Term Breech Trial Collaborative Group. Lancet. 2000;356(9239):1375-83.
12. Menticoglou SM. Why vaginal breech delivery should still be offered. J Obstet Gynaecol Can. 2006;28(5):380-5.
13. Kish K, Collea JV. Malpresentation and cord prolapse. In: DeCherney AH, Nathan L (Eds).

Current Obstetric & Gynecologic Diagnosis & Treatment, 9th edition. Toronto: McGraw-Hill; 2003.
14. World Health Organization (WHO). (2013) Managing complications in pregnancy and childbirth: a guide for doctors and midwives. [online]. Available from: http://www.who.int/reproductive-health/impac/mcpc.pdf. [Last accessed September 2019].
15. World Health Organization (WHO). (2006). Managing prolonged and obstructed labour: Education material for teachers of midwifery, second edition.. [online]. Available from: https://apps.who.int/iris/handle/10665/44145 [Last accessed September 2019].
16. Royal College of Obstetricians and Gynaecologists. (2017). Management of breech presentation (Greentop guideline number 20b). [online]. Available from: https://www.rcog.org.uk/en/guidelines-research-services/guidelines/gtg20b/. [Last accessed September 2019].

CHAPTER 22

Abnormal Fetal Heart Trace on Cardiotocography

Revathi S Rajan

INTRODUCTION

Cardiotocography (CTG) has now emerged as an essential and important tool aiding clinicians to make appropriate decisions for both maternal and fetal wellbeing especially during the intrapartum period. However, CTG monitoring can only be an adjunct and not replacement for clinical decision making. This chapter aims at discussing abnormalities that could be identified on CTG and the necessary interventions that could be planned to avert adverse perinatal outcomes. A brief about recording a CTG and interpretation of various patterns both normal and abnormal has also been made.

PREREQUISITES FOR CARDIOTOCOGRAPHY RECORDING

Need for Cardiotocography

Cardiotocography monitoring (intrapartum) is considered quintessential in all conditions where fetal hypoxia/acidosis is anticipated. These could include:[1]
- Abnormal fetal growth (antenatally)
- Vaginal hemorrhage
- Probable excessive or exaggerated uterine activity (induced/augmented labor)
- Meconium-stained liquor
- Epidural analgesia.

Continuous CTG monitoring is advised, if there are abnormalities on intermittent auscultation of fetal heart. CTG monitoring interspersed with regular fetal heart rate (FHR) auscultation would add value in monitoring even in low-risk pregnancies avoiding unnecessary interventions.

Recording a Cardiotocography Trace

The essential requirements include:
- *Position*: To position the mother in semi-recumbent and left lateral position to avoid aortocaval compression. *"Wireless telemetry"* is a recent innovation that allows free mobility of the mother simultaneously favoring good trace acquisition of the fetal heart.[2]
- *Paper speed*: Usually, 1 cm/min is preferred. 2 or 3 cm/min may be used in certain countries of the world. A speed of 1 cm/min optimally provides a trace that could furnish details allowing clinical interpretation.

The vertical scale on the trace is usually 20 or 30 bpm/cm. It is imperative that the hospital staff is primed with CTG recording details and its ways of interpretation.

External monitoring of fetal heart rate and maternal uterine contractions is the preferred initial method of fetal monitoring (intrapartum) as it is noninvasive providing adequate clinical information. Probe adjustment to optimize better signal acquisition is preferred intrapartum. Any suspicious recording may warrant a step up evaluation (ultrasound or internal monitoring of FHR). Simultaneous recording of the maternal heart rate especially intrapartum is needed to map fluctuation in maternal and fetal heart rates separately as there could be overlapping changes attributable to rise in maternal heart rate during uterine contractions.

External FHR monitoring is preferred even in twins provided unique and good quality signal acquisition is procured. The tracings should be necessarily labeled with patient name, time of start and end of trace and paper speed to ease better clinical interpretation. These traces should be preserved as part of hospital record or in digital CTG archives.

CARDIOTOCOGRAPHY CHARACTERISTICS: NORMAL VERSUS ABNORMAL

Baseline

Baseline on CTG is considered normal, if it is between 110 bpm and 160 bpm. It represents the mean of the least fluctuating and horizontal FHR tracing usually interpreted in a 10-minute time frame.

- *Tachycardia*: A baseline of more than 160 bpm for at least 10 minute is termed as "*fetal tachycardia*" commonly associated with maternal pyrexia, early stages of fetal distress due to hypoxia, epidural analgesia and administration of beta-agonist drugs like salbutamol and terbutaline and very rarely fetal arrhythmias (Fig. 1).[3,4]
- *Bradycardia*: Baseline less than 110 bpm for more than 10 minutes is termed "*fetal bradycardia*". Most Common causes include beta-blocker administration to the mother and fetal arrhythmias.[5,6]

Variability

Defined as average amplitude of fluctuation of the trace from baseline within a time frame of 1 minute.

- *Increased variability*: Variability exceeding 25 bpm over a period of 30 minutes commonly associated with repetitive decelerations due to hypoxia or acidosis attributable to fetal autonomic instability is termed increased variability.[7]
- *Reduced variability*: When the amplitude of the baseline changes less than 5 bpm over a period of 50 minutes in normal baseline segments or over 3 minutes during decelerations; it is referred to as reduced variability.[8]
  - It could be seen in conditions associated with fetal hypoxia/acidosis leading to decelerations, infections, prior or antecedent cerebral insult, or rarely maternal administration of parasympathetic drugs.
  - Fetal sleep patterns do not show decreased variability of less than 5 bpm. Reduced variability without a

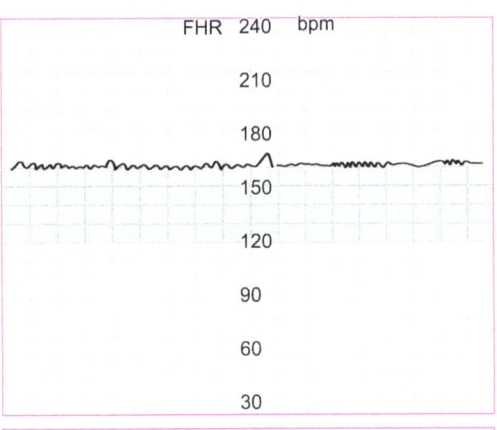
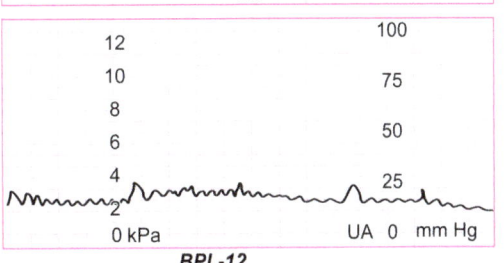

Fig. 1: Fetal tachycardia with absent variability.

preceding deceleration or tachycardia seldom represents fetal distress.

Accelerations

Accelerations are defined as an increase in FHR over the baseline of more than 15 bpm lasting for greater than 15 seconds not exceeding 10 minutes.

Fetal movements trigger accelerations, which are representative of appropriate neurological (autonomic) maturity. Accelerations are well established after 32 weeks of gestation and may not be appreciated during fetal sleep. *Absent accelerations in an otherwise normal CTG trace may not signify hypoxia.* Accelerations coinciding with uterine contractions may be representative of changes of maternal heart rate during labor.

Decelerations

Decelerations are defined as fall in FHR below the baseline exceeding 15 bpm exceeding more than 15 seconds.

- *Early decelerations*: Those decelerations that are short with normal variability associated with uterine contractions usually considered to be associated with uterine contractions. They occur due to fetal head compression.
- *Late decelerations*: Usually, a chemoreceptor-mediated response which occurs gradually with return to the baseline by slightly more than 30 seconds with reduced variability. They usually begin 15–20 seconds after the start of a contraction and return to the baseline after the contraction has ended. This could be a response initiated by fetal hypoxemia (Fig. 2).[9]
    - An amplitude of 10–15 bpm of late decels amidst absent accelerations or variability could indicate fetal distress. They usually occur typically in a "U"-shaped pattern.

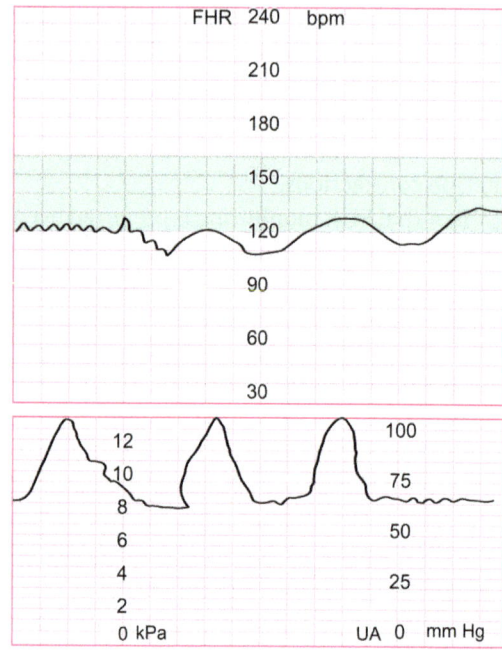

Fig. 2: Late deceleration with absent variability.

- *Variable decelerations*: A sudden dip in baseline with rapid recovery with normal variability without any relation to uterine contractility is defined as a "variable deceleration" which is usually "V" shaped. This is attributable mostly to umbilical cord compression resulting in rise in mean arterial pressure that triggers a baroreceptor response (Figs. 3 and 4).[10]
- *Prolonged deceleration*: This is a chemoreceptor-mediated response with decels lasting for more than 5 minutes with FHR dipping persistently to less than 80 bpm with reduced variability mostly associated with fetal hypoxemia (Fig. 5).[11-13]

■ NAMED PATTERNS AND THEIR RELEVANCE

Saltatory Pattern

Same as trace with increased variability as described previously (Fig. 6).

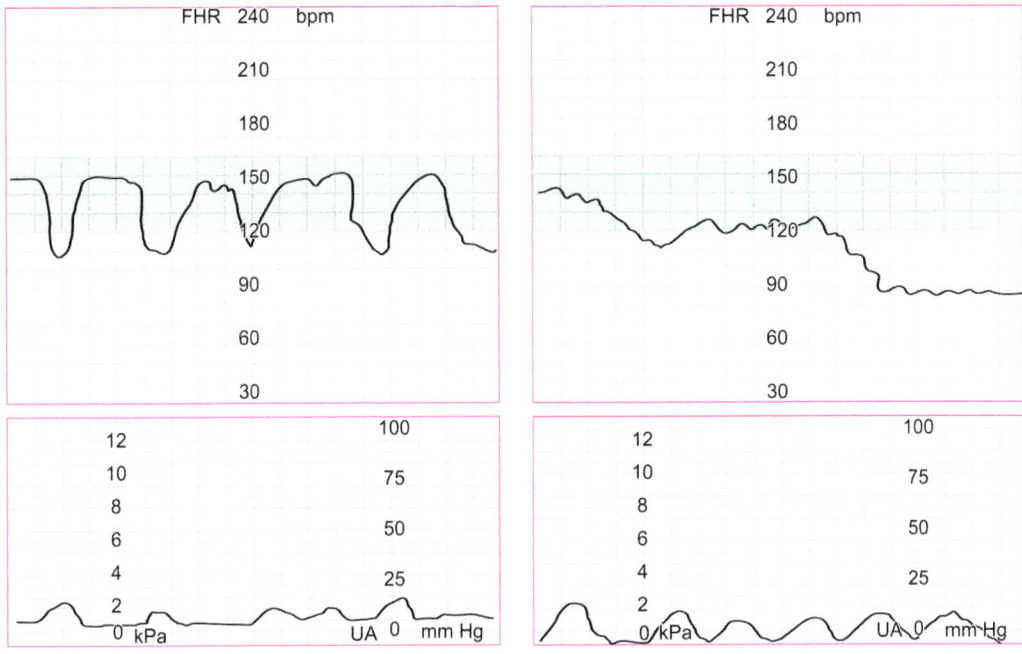

Fig. 3: Several variable decelerations with absent variability.

Fig. 5: Prolonged deceleration with absent variability.

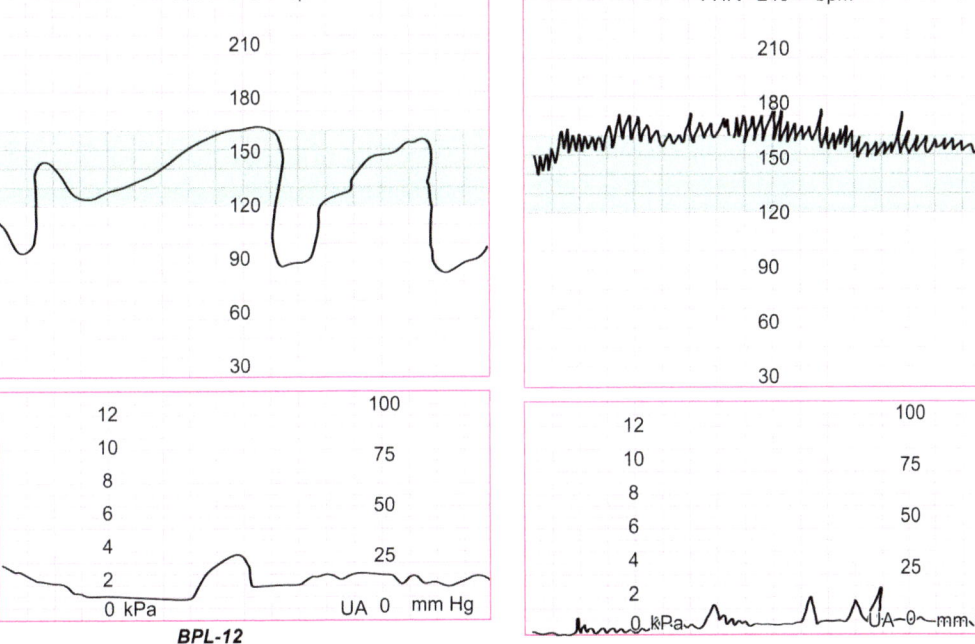

Fig. 4: Mixed variable and late decelerations.

Fig. 6: Saltatory pattern (Increased variability).

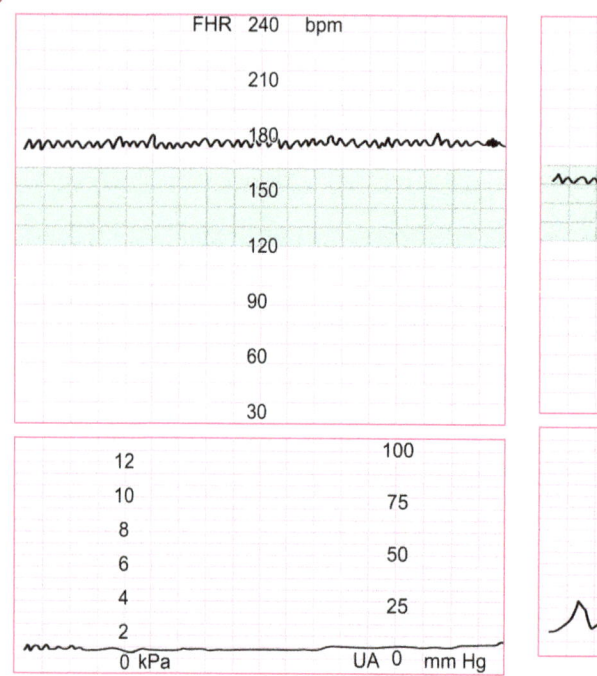

Fig. 7: Sinusoidal pattern in a fetus during intrapartum monitoring.

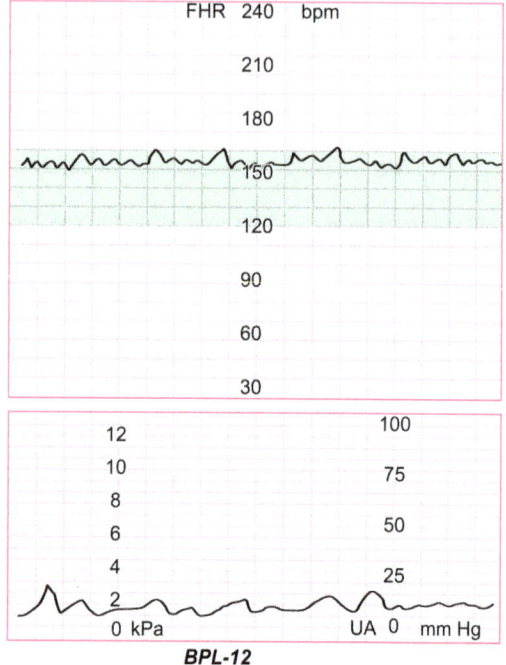

Fig. 8: Sawtooth pattern (pseudo-sinusoidal pattern).

Sinusoidal Pattern

A smooth periodic and oscillatory wave of amplitude 5–15 bpm occurring as 3–5 cycles every minute with the same lasting for 30 minutes without any acceleration is called "*sinusoidal pattern on CTG*". It is commonly associated with acute fetal hypoxia, which could be attributable to infection, structural defects of the fetus like cardiac anomalies, abdominal wall defects, etc. (Fig. 7).[14]

Sawtooth Pattern

This is also called "*pseudo-sinusoidal pattern*". It is typically more jagged, though resembling the sinusoidal type wave except that it does not last for 30 minutes. It is usually interspersed with normal pattern both before and after and may be associated with fetal suckling responses (Fig. 8).[15]

Sleep Pattern

- *Deep sleep*: This can last up to 40–50 minutes. It should not be confused with an abnormal trace pattern as it is represented by a stable baseline with hardly any accelerations and borderline variability.
- *Active sleep*: This is usually associated with rapid eye movements and wakefulness and may be represented on a CTG as slightly reduced number of accelerations but with normal variability.

TRACE CLASSIFICATION AND INTERPRETATION[12]

Normal

A CTG trace is considered *"Normal"* if the baseline is between 110 and 160 bpm with a normal variability of 5–25 bpm (Fig. 9).

Abnormal Fetal Heart Trace on Cardiotocography

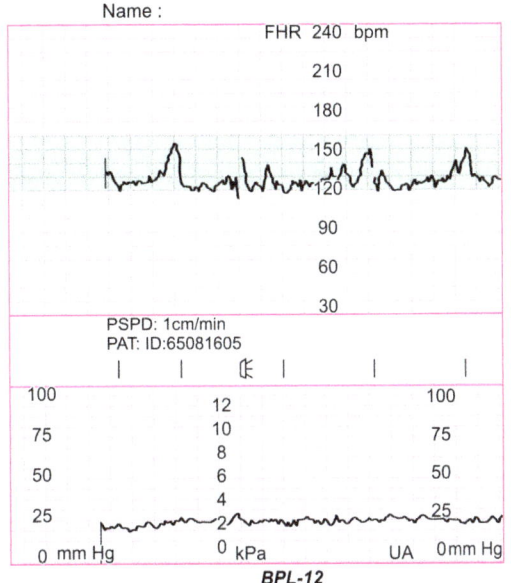

Fig. 9: Normal CTG (34 weeks; singleton gestation).

Suspicious

The trace is called "*suspicious*" if there is at least one component of normalcy lacking (either baseline or variability) but without any pathological features as described further. It is prudent to identify reversible factors contributing to the variation in the trace. This kind of trace may not always suggest fetal hypoxemia.

Pathological

A "*pathological trace*" is one whose baseline is less than 100 bpm with decreased variability for more than 50 minutes or increased variability for more than 30 minutes or if there is a sinusoidal pattern for more than 30 minutes. Serial prolonged or late deceleration occurring for more than 30 minutes or if for 20 minutes, there is no variability or if there is one prolonged deceleration for more than 5 minutes also qualifies for an abnormal or a pathological trace.

"*DR C BRAVADO*" is a popular mnemonic, which helps the clinician to report systematically in a framework aiding comprehensive analysis. The mnemonic reads as below:

DR—define risk—define whether it is a high-risk or a low-risk pregnancy

C—contractions—represented as an upward shift from the baseline recording at the bottom of the CTG trace and reflect the uterine contraction. It has to be reported usually over a period of 10 minutes. The amplitude and duration of each contraction must be reported. The amplitude may not represent the intensity of contraction that needs to be palpated physically over the maternal abdomen.

BRA—baseline fetal heart rate (as described previously)

V—variability (as described previously)

A—accelerations (as described previously)

D—decelerations (as described previously)

O—overall impression (to upset comprehensively as normal, suspicious, or pathological).

INTERVENTIONS IN SUSPECTED FETAL DISTRESS

The following measures need to be implemented, if fetal hypoxemia contributing to fetal distress is suspected.

- Maternal supine position may result in aortocaval compression resulting in compromised placental perfusion or may lead to stimulation of the sacral plexus leading to uterine hyperstimulation. Positioning the mother to one side helps to eliminate these adverse effects and may normalize the trace. Cord compression leading to variable decelerations can also be relieved by changing the maternal position or by amnioinfusion.[16-18]
- Hyperstimulated uterus leading to excessive uterine contractions can lead to fetal hypoxemia. This can be reversed by stopping oxytocin infusion or by removing the vaginally placed prostaglandins or

by administration of beta-adrenergic agonistics (ritodrine/terbutaline), atosiban, etc. for uterine relaxation.[19-22]

- Administration of intravenous fluids rapidly can help correct maternal hypotension triggered by epidural or spinal analgesia, which may sometimes lead to transient fetal hypoxemia.[23]
  - *There is no strong evidence to suggest that oxygen administered to the mother has any beneficial effect on improving a suspicious trace for the better.*

LIMITATIONS OF CARDIOTOCOGRAPHY

These include:
- Cardiotocography interpretation may be subject to inter- and intraobserver variation.
- Cardiotocography has low specificity and low positive predictive value.
- Though there has been a 50% decrease in neonatal seizures and no difference in the incidence of hypoxic ischemic encephalopathy in the new born post-continuous intrapartum monitoring, this evidence has been generated from underpowered trials.
- Use of continuous CTG monitoring in the intrapartum period can lead to an increased risk of operative interventions especially in low pregnant women. Hence in conclusion appropriate implementation of CTG monitoring especially in high-risk pregnancies added to clinical observations will help in the right decision making averting adverse perinatal outcomes.

Training and updating personnel on a periodic basis for proper interpretation of the trace is essential to minimize subjective errors adding value to clinical decision making when encountered with an abnormal FHR trace on CTG.

REFERENCES

1. Ayres-de-Campos D, Spong CY, Chandraharan E, et al. FIGO Consensus Guidelines on Intrapartum Fetal Monitoring: cardiotocography. Int J Gynaecol Obstet. 2015;131(1):13-24.
2. Carbonne B, Benachi A, Leveque ML, et al. Maternal position during labor: effect on fetal oxygen saturation measured by fetal pulse oximetry. Obstet Gynecol. 1996;88:797-800.
3. Segal S. Labor epidural analgesia and maternal fever. Anesth Analg. 2010;111:1467-75.
4. Neilson JP, West HM, Dowswell T. Beta-mimetics for inhibiting preterm labour. Cochrane Database Syst Rev. 2014;2:CD004352.
5. Jadhon ME, Main EK. Fetal bradycardia associated with maternal hypothermia. Obstet Gynecol. 1988;72(3 Pt 2):496-7.
6. Boutrov MJ. Fetal and neonatal effects of the beta-adrenoreceptor blocking agents. Dev Phamacol Ther. 1987;10:224-31.
7. Nunes I, Ayres-de-Campos D, Kwee A, et al. Prolonged saltatory fetal heart rate pattern leading to newborn metabolic acidosis. Clin Exp Obstet Gynecol. 2014;41(5):507-11.
8. Hamilton E, Warrick P, O'Keeffe D. Variable decelerations: do size and shape matter? J Matern Fetal Neonatal Med. 2012;25:648-53.
9. Court DJ, Parer JT. Experimental studies of fetal asphyxia and fetal heart rate interpretation. In: Nathanielsz PW, Parer JT (eds). Research in Perinatal Medicine (I). New York: Perinatalogy Press; 1984. pp. 113-69.
10. Holzmann M, Wretler S, Cnattingius S, et al. Cardiotocography patterns and risk of intrapartum fetal acidemia. J Perinat Med. 2015;43(4):473-9.
11. Westgate JA, Wibbens B, Bennet L, et al. The intrapartum deceleration in center stage: a physiologic approach to the interpretation of fetal heart rate changes in labor. Am J Obstet Gynecol. 2007;197:236.e1-11.
12. Cahill AG, Roehl KA, Odibo AO, et al. Association and prediction of neonatal acidemia. Am J Obstet Gynecol. 2012;207:206.e1-8.
13. Takano Y, Furukawa S, Ohashi M, et al. Fetal heart rate patterns related to neonatal brain damage and neonatal death in placental abruption. J Obstet Gynecol Res. 2013;39:61-6.

14. Modanlou HD, Murata Y. Sinusoidal fetal heart rate pattern: reappraisal of its definition and clinical significance. J Obstet Gynaecol Res. 2004;30:169-80.
15. Graça LM, Cardoso CG, Clode N, et al. An approach to interpretation and classification of sinusoidal fetal heart rate patterns. Eur J Obstet Gynecol Reprod Biol. 1988;27:203-12.
16. Williams EA. Abnormal uterine action during labour. J Obstet Gynaecol Br Emp. 1952;59:635-41.
17. Caldeyro-Barcia R, Noriega-Guerra L, Cibils LA, et al. Effect of position changes on the intensity and frequency of uterine contractions during labor. Am J Obstet Gynecol. 1960;80:284-90.
18. Hofmeyr GJ, Lawrie TA. Amnioinfusion for potential or suspected umbilical cord compression in labour. Cochrane Database Syst Rev. 2012;1:CD000013.
19. Heuser CC, Knight S, Esplin S, et al. Tachysystole in term labor: incidence, risk factors, outcomes, and effect on fetal heart tracings. Am J Obstet Gynecol. 2013:209:32e.1-6.
20. Briozzo L, Martinez A, Nozar M, et al. Tocolysis and delayed delivery versus emergency delivery in cases of non-reassuring fetal status during labor. J Obstet Gynecol Res. 2007;33(3):266-73.
21. Heus R, Mulder EJH, Derks JB, et al. Acute tocolysis for uterine activity reduction in term labor: a review. Obstet Gynecol Surv. 2008;63(6):383-8.
22. Heus R, Mulder EJH, Derks JB, et al. A prospective randomized trial of acute tocolysis in term labour with atosiban or ritodrine. Eur J Obstet Gynecol Reprod Biol. 2008;139:139-45.
23. Simmons SW, Taghizadeh N, Dennis AT, et al. Combined spinal-epidural versus epidural analgesia in labour. Cochrane Database Syst Rev. 2012;10:CD003401.

CHAPTER 23

Anesthetic Complications in Pregnancy and Labor

Swetha, Ravi Kumar IR

■ INTRODUCTION

Obstetrical emergencies are life-threatening medical conditions that occur in pregnancy or during or after labor and delivery.

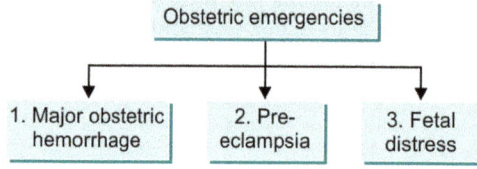

■ MASSIVE OBSTETRIC HEMORRHAGE

Massive obstetric hemorrhage (MOH) is a major cause of maternal death and morbidity. Variably defined as:
- Blood loss >1,500 mL
- Decrease in hemoglobin (Hb) <5g/dL or
- Acute transfusion requirements of more than four units.

The gravid uterus receives up to 12% of cardiac output, thus obstetric hemorrhage can be unexpected and become life-threatening.

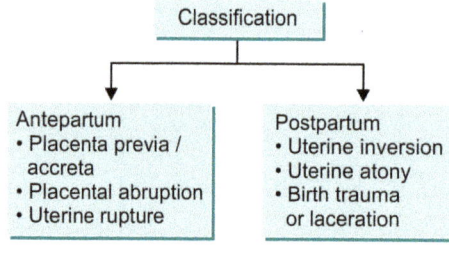

Antepartum Hemorrhage

- Blood loss per vagina after 20 weeks of gestation
- Up to 4% of all pregnancies
- Medical emergency
- Leading cause of maternal morbidity and mortality.

Placenta Previa

It is defined as a placenta implanted in the lower segment of the uterus, presenting ahead of the leading pole of the fetus.

Incidence of placenta previa is 1:200 pregnancies.

- *Total placenta previa*: Completely covers cervical os.
- *Partial placenta previa*: Covers part, but not all of the cervical os.
- *Marginal placenta previa*: Lies close to, but does not cover the cervical os.

Etiology:
- Advancing maternal age
- Multiparity
- Multifetal gestations
- Prior cesarean delivery
- Smoking
- Prior placenta previa.

Clinical features: The most characteristic event in placenta previa is painless hemorrhage.
- Occurs near end or after the second trimester
- The initial bleeding is rarely so profuse as to prove fatal

- Usually ceases spontaneously, only to recur
- Can be associated with placenta accreta, placenta increta or placenta percreta.

Diagnosis:
- Always be suspected in women with uterus bleeding during later half of pregnancy.
- Appropriate evaluation including sonography.
- Examination of cervix is never permissible unless the women are in an operating room with all the preparations for immediate cesarean delivery because even the gentlest examination of this sort can cause torrential hemorrhage.
- Safe method is transabdominal sonography.
- Magnetic resonance imaging (MRI).
- At 18 weeks 5-10% of placentas are low lying. Most "migrate" with development of lower uterine segment.

Obstetric management of placenta previa:
- Vaginal examinations are best avoided
- If needed done under double setups
- Expectant management
- Surgical management.

Anesthetic management:
- For double setup examination:
  - Rarely performed
  - Performed in the operating room
  - Full preparation for cesarean section include:
    - Maternal monitors
    - Insertion of two large gauge intravenous cannulae
    - Administration of a nonparticulate antacid
    - Sterile preparations and draping of the abdomen
    - Two units of packed red blood cells.
- For cesarean section:
  - Choice of anesthetic technique depends on the indication and urgency for cesarean section and the degree of maternal hypovolemia.
  - High risk of intraoperative blood loss due to:
    - Obstetrician may cut into the placenta during uterine incision
    - Lower uterine segment implantation site does not contract well
    - Increased risk for placenta accreta
  - A retrospective study with 350 cases of placenta previa found [60% regional and 40% general anesthesia (GA)]:
    - Decreased estimated blood loss with regional anesthesia versus GA
    - Decreased transfusions needs with regional anesthesia
    - No difference in hypotension.

Preoperative preparation:
- Patient evaluation, resuscitation, and preparation for operative delivery all proceed simultaneously.
- Careful assessment of parturients airway and intravascular volume
- Two large gauge intravenous catheters four units of packed red blood cells (PRBCs)
- Blood administration sets
- Fluid warmer
- Equipment for invasive monitoring.

Fluid therapy and blood product transfusion:
- Crystalloid—up to 2 liters of Hartmann's solution (warm)
- Colloid—up to 1.5 liters until blood arrives (warm)
- Blood cross matched—if cross matched blood still unavailable give uncrossed matched group specific blood or O RhD negative blood
- Fresh frozen plasma (FFP)—four units for every six units of red cells or prothrombin time/activated partial thromboplastin time (PT/aPTT) >1.5 normal (12-15 mL/kg or total 1 liter)
- Platelet concentrate—if platelet count <50,000
- Cryoprecipitate—if fibrinogen <1 g/L (up to 10 U—2 packs).

Main therapeutic goals:
- Hemoglobin >8 g/dL
- Platelet count >75,000
- Prothrombin <1.5 mean control
- Activated PT <1.5 mean control
- Fibrinogen >1.0 g/dL.

Intraoperative anesthetic management:
- Induction:
  - Rapid sequence induction of general anesthesia is preferred techniques
  - Avoid sodium thiopental
  - Propofol should not be used in hypovolemic patients
  - Ketamine (0.5–1.0 mg/kg) and etomidate (0.3 mg/kg) are the best induction agents for bleeding patients
  - Patients with severe hypovolemic shock, intubation may require only a muscle relaxant.
- Maintenance:
  - Nitrous oxide and oxygen with a low concentration of a volatile halogenated agent
  - Concentration of nitrous oxide can be reduced (or omitted) in cases of fetal distress
  - Oxytocin (20 U/L) immediately after delivery
  - Lower uterine segment implantation site does not contract as well as the fundus
  - All uterine segment implantation sites does not contract as well as the fundus
  - Best to eliminate the volatile halogenated agent after delivery
  - Substitute nitrous oxide (70%) and an intravenous opioid.

Abruptio Placenta
- Placental abruption is defined as separation of the placenta from the decidua basalis before delivery of the fetus.
- Incidence is 1 in 100 pregnancies.

Risk factors:
- Hypertension
- Advanced age and parity
- Tobacco use
- Cocaine use
- Trauma
- Premature rupture of membranes
- A history of previous abruption.

Presentation:
- Vaginal bleeding
- Uterine tenderness
- Increased uterine activity.

Complications:
- Hemorrhagic shock
- Acute renal failure (ARF)
- Coagulopathy and disseminated intravascular coagulation (DIC)
- Fetal distress or demise.

Obstetric management:
- Definitive treatment is delivery of the fetus and placenta
- Degree of abruption is minimal fetus shows no signs of distress maternal hemodynamics stable
- Hospitalization fetal heart rate monitoring
- Serial ultrasonography maternal hemodynamic monitoring
- Delivered after fetal lung maturation.

Anesthetic management:
- Preoperative preparation:
  - Airway assessment
  - Assessment of volume status
  - Maternal hemodynamic monitoring
  - Fetal heart rate monitoring
  - Two large bore intravenous catheters
  - Blood for cross matching, hematocrit, and coagulation
  - Maintain supplemental oxygen
  - Left uterine displacement

- For labor and normal delivery:
  - Epidural analgesia can be given only if:
    - Coagulation studies are normal
    - No intravascular volume deficit
  - Observations showed that epidural anesthesia significantly worsened maternal hypotension, uterine blood flow, and fetal. Partial pressures of oxygen (PaO_2) and pH during untreated hemorrhage (20 mL/kg).

Cesarean section:
- General anesthesia is preferred for most of the cases
- Regional anesthesia can be given for a patient with stable hemodynamics, good intravascular volume, minor abruption, and no fetal distress
- Ketamine and etomidate are inducing agents of choice
- Rapid sequence induction is preferred
- Large doses of ketamine may increase uterine tone during early gestation
- So dose of ketamine should be limited to single dose of 1 mg/kg
- Aggressive volume resuscitation with both crystalloids and colloids
  - Blood transfusion
  - Central venous catheter and arterial catheter may be necessary
- High risk for uterine atony and coagulopathy
- Oxytocin 20 U/L infused immediately after the delivery
- Coagulation abnormalities may require FFP
- Prolonged hypotension, coagulopathy, and massive blood volume/product replacement are best monitored in a multidisciplinary intensive care unit.

Uterine Rupture

Rupture of gravid uterus can be disastrous to both mother and fetus. It may be of two types: (1) Uterine scar dehiscence and (2) Complete uterine rupture.

- Uterine scar dehiscence:
  - Fetal distress less common
  - No excessive hemorrhage
  - Rarely require emergency section
- Complete uterine rupture:
  - Fetal distress
  - Massive hemorrhage
  - Requires emergency cesarean section.

Causes:
- Previous uterine surgery
- Trauma
  - Indirect:
    - Blunt (e.g. seat belt injury)
    - Excessive manual fundal pressure
    - Extension of cervical laceration
  - Direct:
    - Manual placental extraction
    - Penetrations wound
    - Intrauterine manipulation
    - Forceps application and rotation
    - Postpartum curettage
    - Version and extraction
    - External version
  - Other causes:
    - Inappropriate use of oxytocin
    - Grand multiparity
    - Uterine anomaly
    - Placenta percreta
    - Tumors (trophoblastic disease and cervical carcinoma)
    - Fetal problems (macrosomia, malposition, and anomaly).

Presentations:
- Vaginal bleeding
- Hypotension
- Cessation of labor
- Fetal distress.

Obstetric management:
- Uterine repair
- Uterine artery ligation
- Hysterectomy definitive treatment.

Anesthetic management:
- Preoperative evaluation, resuscitation, and preparation of operation theater (OT) simultaneously
- General anesthesia is often required
- Regional anesthesia can be given in hemodynamically stable patients who already have an epidural catheter and absence of fetal distress
- Aggressive volume replacement
- Maintenance of urine output
- Invasive hemodynamic monitoring.

Vasa Previa
- Occurs rarely 1 in 2,000 to 3,000 deliveries
- Vasa previa is associated with a velamentous insertion of the cord where fetal vessels traverse the fetal membrane ahead of the fetal presenting part
- Highest fetal mortality rates, 50–75%
- No threat to the mother
- Early diagnosis and treatment are essential to reduce the chance of fetal death
- Requires immediate delivery by cesarean section
- Neonatal resuscitation and neonatal volume replacement
- Choice of anesthetic technique depends on the urgency of cesarean section.

Postpartum Hemorrhage (Flowchart 1)

It is a major cause of maternal morbidity and mortality. Primary postpartum hemorrhage occurs during the first 24 hours after delivery. Secondary postpartum hemorrhage occurs between 24 hours and 6 weeks postpartum.

Causes:
- Uterine atony
- Genital trauma
- Coagulopathy
- Placental abnormalities.

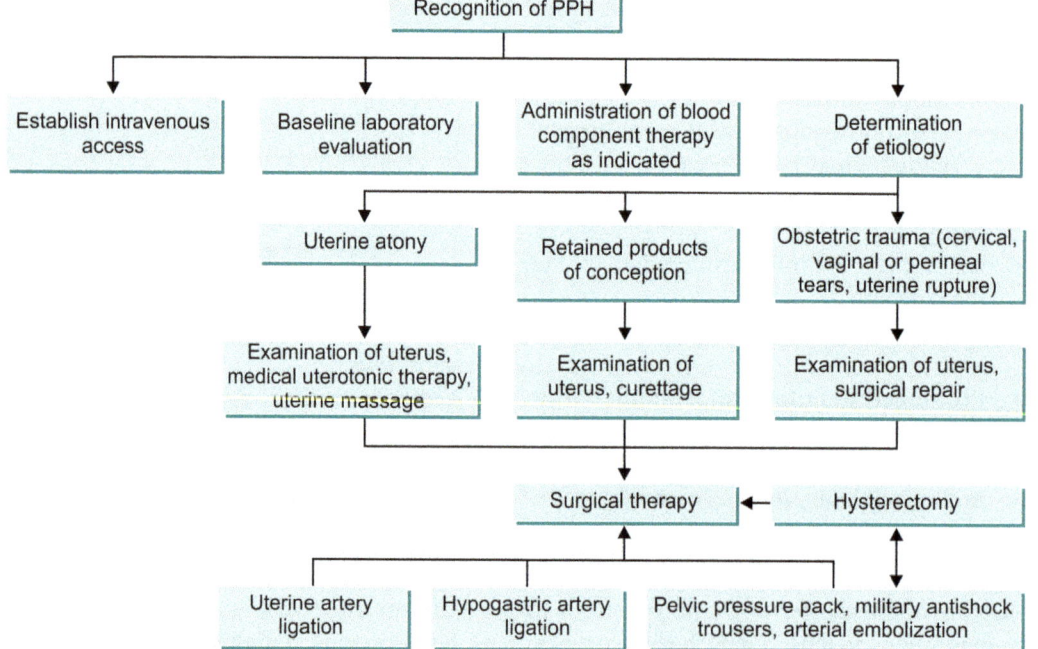

Flowchart 1: Recognition of postpartum hemorrhage (PPH).

Uterine Atony

Risk factors:
- Multiple gestation
- Macrosomia
- Polyhydramnios
- High parity
- Chorioamnionitis
- Precipitous labor
- Augmented labor
- Tocolytic agents
- High concentration of volatile agents
- Prolonged labor.

Drugs:
- **Oxytocin**: It is the first-line drug for the prophylaxis or treatment of uterine atony.
    - Endogenous oxytocin is a 9 amino acid polypeptide produced in posterior pituitary.
    - Exogenous form is a synthetic preparation
    - 20 U of oxytocin to a liter of normal saline (NS) or Ringer's lactate (RL) started as infusion
    - Bolus administration of oxytocin causes peripheral vasodilation and hypotension
    - It increases heart rate, mean arterial pressure (MAP) is decreased, and decreases total peripheral resistance
    - Bolus doses can cause increase in pulmonary artery pressure
    - Cardiovascular changes are short lived (less than 10 minutes).
- **Prostaglandin E2**:
    - Vaginal or rectal suppository 20 mg every 2 hourly
    - Causes bronchodilation
    - Decreased systemic vascular resistance (SVR) and blood pressure
    - Increased heart rate and cardiac output
- **Prostaglandin F2-alpha**:
    - Increases cardiac output
    - Increases systemic and pulmonary artery pressures
    - Increased partial pressures of carbon dioxide ($PaCO_2$) and decreased PaO_2
    - Alterations of ventilation/perfusion ratios
    - Causes bronchospasm
- **15-methyl prostaglandin F2-alpha (carboprost)**:
    - Preferred for treatment of refractory uterine atony
    - 250 mg administered intramuscularly or intramyometrially
    - Causes bronchospasm
    - Disturbed ventilation/perfusion ratios
    - Increased intrapulmonary shunt fraction
    - Hypoxemia
- **Misoprostol**:
    - 800–1,000 µg rectally
    - Prostaglandin E1 analog
    - Effective treatment for postpartum hemorrhage and unresponsive to oxytocin and ergometrine
- **Ergot alkaloids**:
    - 0.2 mg in every 2–4 hours
    - Ergonovine and methylergonovine
    - Restricted to postpartum use
    - Rapidly produce tetanic uterine contraction
    - Act on alpha adrenergic receptors—cause vasoconstriction, hypertension, pulmonary artery pressure, and pulmonary edema

Genital Trauma

- Most common injuries at childbirth are lacerations and hematoma of the perineum, vagina, and cervix
- Pelvic hematomas are of three types:
    1. Vaginal
    2. Vulvar
    3. Retroperitoneal

- Signs and clinical feature:
  - Restlessness
  - Lower abdominal pain
  - A tender mass above the inguinal ligament
  - Vaginal bleeding
  - Abrupt hypotension
  - Ileus
  - Unilateral lung edema
  - Urinary retention
  - Hematuria
- Anesthetic management of genital trauma:
  - For vulval hematomas and small lacerations
    - Local infiltration and a small dose of intravenous opioid
  - For extensive laceration and vaginal hematomas:
    - Pudendal nerve block—technically may not be feasible
    - Neuraxial blockade—may cause hypotension
    - Monitored anesthesia care (MAC)—most preferred. N_2O and O_2 with inhalational agents and low dose ketamine
  - For retroperitoneal hematoma:
    - Laparotomy with general anesthesia
    - Rapid sequence induction
    - Difficult intubation to be anticipated.

Retained Placental Products

Retained placental fragments are a leading cause of both early and delayed postpartum hemorrhage.
- Obstetric management:
  - Manual removal and inspection of the placenta
  - After removal of the placenta, uterine tone should be enhanced with oxytocin.
- Anesthetic management of retained placental products:
  - If epidural catheter is in situ, additional local anesthetic drug can be given
  - Subarachnoid block (SAB) can be given if patient is hemodynamically stable
  - Nitrous oxide analgesia
  - Low-dose ketamine
  - General anesthesia can be given with rapid sequence induction
  - Methods to facilitate uterine relaxation:
    - Halogenated inhalational agents
    - Nitroglycerin.

Placenta Accreta

- Placenta accreta vera is defined as adherence to the myometrium without invasion of or passage through uterine muscle.
- Placenta increta represents invasion of the myometrium.
- Placenta percreta includes invasion of the uterine serosa or other pelvic structures.

Risk factors:
- Previous uterine trauma
- Previous cesarean section
- Low lying placenta.

Diagnosis:
- Antepartum diagnosis rare
- Difficulty in removal of placenta
- Ultrasonography
- Magnetic resonance imaging
- Transvaginal color Doppler.

Obstetric management:
- Uterine curettage followed by oversewing of the bleeding placental bed
- Balloon occlusion
- Embolization techniques
- Postpartum hysterectomy definitive treatment.

Anesthetic management:
- Preoperative diagnosis of placental abnormalities
- Identifying patients with high risk for placenta accreta

- Preparation for hysterectomy
- Availability of blood products.

Uterine Inversion

- Turning inside out of all or part of the uterus
- Occur in 1 in 5,000 to 1 in 10,000 pregnancies.

Risk factors:

- Uterine atony
- Inappropriate fundal pressure
- Umbilical cord traction
- Uterine anomalies
- An abnormally implanted placenta (i.e. placenta accreta).

Obstetric management:

- Early replacement of the uterus is the best treatment. Once the uterus has been replaced.
- Oxytocin (20 U/L) should be infused initially and additional drugs (15-methyl prostaglandin F2) may be needed.

Anesthetic management of uterine inversion:

- Uterine tone precludes immediate replacement
- Uterine relaxation is needed before successful replacement can be performed
- Ideal technique should have:
  - Rapid uterine relaxation
  - No side effects
  - Short duration
  - Restoration of uterine tone after replacement of the uterus.

General anesthesia with inhalational agents more preferred:

- Equipotent doses of all volatile halogenated agents produce a similar degree of uterine relaxation.
- Endotracheal intubation is mandatory
- Others:
  - Terbutaline
  - Magnesium sulfate
  - Organic nitrates.

HYPERTENSIVE DISORDERS IN PREGNANCY

- *Pre-eclampsia*:
  - Blood pressure elevation with proteinuria
  - Occurs after 20 weeks of gestation
  - Proteinuria
  - Urinary excretion of 300 mg or greater of protein in 24 hours
  - Edema no longer diagnostic for poor specifically.
- *Eclampsia*: Seizures
- *HELLP syndrome*: Defined by presence of all three criteria:
  1. Hemolysis:
     - Abnormal peripheral smear
     - Bilirubin 1.2 mg/dL
     - Lactate dehydrogenase 600 IU/L
  2. Elevated liver enzymes (aspartate aminotransferase 2X normal levels)
  3. Thrombocytopenia (platelets <100 × $10^3/\mu L$)

Etiology

Exact cause is unknown. Possible causes are as follows:

- Widespread endothelial dysfunction leading to placental ischemia and multiorgan dysfunction.
- Synthesis of many substances like NO (nitric oxide) and prostaglandin I2 may be decreased in pre-eclampsia.
- Leading to smooth muscle reactivity and platelet adhesion

Complications

- Neurological:
  - Headache
  - Visual disturbance
  - Hyperexcitability
  - Seizures
  - Intracranial hemorrhage
  - Cerebral edema

- Pulmonary:
  - Upper airway edema
  - Pulmonary edema
- Cardiovascular:
  - Decreased intravascular volume
  - Increased arteriolar resistance
  - Hypertension
  - Heart failure
- Hematological:
  - Coagulopathy
  - Thrombocytopenia
  - Platelet dysfunction
  - Prolonged PTT
  - Microangiopathic hemolysis
- Renal:
  - Proteinuria
  - Sodium retention
  - Decreased glomerular filtration
  - Renal failure
- Hepatic:
  - Impaired function
  - Elevated enzymes
  - Hematoma
  - Rupture.

Risk Factors

- Obesity
- Black race
- Chronic hypertension
- Diabetes or insulin resistance
- Collagen vascular disease
- Thrombophilias
- Increasing circulatory testosterone
- Multiple gestation
- Previous pre-eclampsia.

Management

- Definitive treatment of pre-eclampsia is delivery
- Whether or not to deliver the fetus:
  - Gestational age
  - Maternal and fetal condition
  - Severity of pre-eclampsia
- Patients at term—delivered
- Delivery at any gestational age:
  - If maternal end organ dysfunction
  - Nonreassuring tests of fetal well being.

Drug Therapy

- Antihypertensives
  - Oral—methyldopa, labetalol, and nifedipine
  - Intravenous—hydralazine, labetalol infusion, and sodium nitroprusside
- Anticonvulsant
  - Magnesium sulfate

Magnesium Sulfate

- Anticonvulsant of choice in preventing and treating seizures.
- Intravenous bolus 4-6 g and then infusion 1-2 g/hr to keep serum mg in therapeutic range (2-3 mmol/L).

Indicators of $MgSO_4$ toxicity:
- Electrocardiogram (ECG) changes (3-5 mmol/L)
- Loss of deep tendon reflex (5 mmol/L)
- Respiratory depression (6-7.5 mmol/L)
- Cardiac arrest (12 mmol/L)

Anesthetic considerations:
- Preanesthetic assessment
- Fluid balance and hemodynamics
- Hypoalbuminemia
- Increased capillary permeability
- High hydrostatic pressure leads to risk of pulmonary and pharyngolaryngeal edema
- Estimation of cardiac output—if oliguria, pulmonary edema, hypertension resistant to initial therapy
- *Coagulation*: Assessment is essential before regional anesthesia.

Epidural Analgesia

- Early epidural is an ideal form of pain relief in pre-eclampsia patients

- It helps to control the exaggerated hypertensive response to pain and can improve placental blood flow.

Anesthesia for cesarean section:
- Regional versus general:
  - Avoidance of hypertensive response to laryngoscopy (more in pre-eclampsia)
  - Blunting of neuroendocrine response to surgery
  - Prevention of transient neonatal depression associated with general anesthesia.
- Spinal versus epidural:
  - *Advantages*: Quicker and more reliable in onset and less potential trauma in epidural space.
  - *Disadvantages*: Theoretical risk of more abrupt hypotension in a patient:
    - Who may be relatively hypovolemic and with a fetus
    - Who may be compromised by placental insufficiency
    - Alternatively combined spinal and epidural used. Giving small dose of local anesthesia (LA) in spinal anesthesia and option of utilizing the epidural as necessary.

General anesthesia: May be necessary but main concerns are:
- Mucosal edema of upper airway
- Severe hypertensive responses to laryngoscopy and surgery
- Patients on $MgSO_4$ may be very sensitive to effects of nondepolarizing muscle relaxants (NDMRs)
- Difficult intubation cart to be kept ready.

FETAL DISTRESS

Fetal distress is defined as depletion of oxygen and accumulation of carbon dioxide, leading to a state of hypoxia and acidosis during intrauterine life.

Fetal distress causes:
- During labor:
  - Umbilical cord prolapse
  - Umbilical cord compression
  - Variable deceleration
  - Uteroplacental insufficiency (late deceleration)
- At delivery:
  - Shoulder dystocia
  - Major abnormalities of fetal heart rate, in particular prolonged fetal bradycardia, call for immediate delivery, and usually by cesarean section.

Umbilical Cord Accidents (Cord Prolapse)

A cord presentation is defined as the presence of umbilical cord below the fetal presenting part when the membranes are intact. Cord prolapse is the presence of cord below the presenting part when membranes are ruptured.

Most commonly diagnosed by seeing cord at the introitus or feeling it during a vaginal examination. However, an abnormal fetal heart rate pattern may suggest it, as compression of the umbilical vein between the presenting part and the pelvis, reduces or stops the flow of oxygenated blood to the fetus, causing deep variable deceleration, then bradycardia if the situation is not relieved.

Risk factors for cord prolapse:
- Maternal causes:
  - Pelvic tumors (e.g. fibroids in the lower segment)
  - Narrow pelvis
- Fetal causes:
  - Prematurity
  - Malpresentation (e.g. breech, transverse lie, multiple pregnancy, polyhydramnios, placenta previa, and large baby).

Management

Immediate management aims to minimize the pressure of the fetal presenting part on the cord, while plans are made to deliver the baby.

Achieved by moving the woman on to all fours with the head down, applying pressure vaginally the push the presenting part out of the pelvis, or by filling bladder with 500 mL of saline.

With a term baby and a prompt diagnosis in hospital, prognosis is excellent. If prolapse occurs outside hospital, fetus is likely to be dead by the time of admission.

Total cord compression for longer than 10 minutes will cause cerebral damage and if continued for around 20 minutes leads to death.

Shoulder Dystocia

Etiology and Epidemiology

Shoulder dystocia is defined by the RCOG as the need for "additional obstetric maneuvers to release the shoulders after gentle downward traction has failed".

Risk Factors for Shoulder Dystocia

- Maternal
  - Diabetic
  - Short stature
  - Previous shoulder dystocia
  - Obesity
- Fetal
  - Macrosomia
  - Postmaturity
- Intrapartum
  - Long first stage of labor
  - Long second stage of labor
  - Instrumental delivery
  - Induction of labor
  - Use of oxytocin.

Management

- Change maternal position
- Administer supplemental oxygen
- Maintain/improve maternal circulation
- Give a tocolytic for hypertonicity
- Delivery
  - Forceps
  - Cesarean section.

Classification of cesarean section according to urgency:
- *Category 1*: Requiring immediate delivery (threat to maternal and fetal life)
- *Category 2*: Requiring urgent delivery (maternal and fetal compromise that is not immediately life-threatening.
- *Category 3*: Requiring early delivery (no maternal or fetal compromise)
- *Category 4*: Elective delivery (at a time suited to the women and maternity staff).

Sudden Maternal Collapse

- Pulmonary embolism (PE)
- Amniotic fluid embolism.

Pulmonary Embolism

- Thrombosis is consistency the most common cause of maternal death.
- It is important to recognize that although PE is more common in the puerperium, it can occur at any time in the antenatal and postnatal period.

Amniotic Fluid Embolism

- Rare cause
- Caused by amniotic fluid entering the maternal circulation
- Causes acute cardiorespiratory compromise and severe disseminated intravascular coagulation
- Abnormal maternal reaction to amniotic fluid as the primary event.

Diagnosis and Management

- Structured approach
  - A—Airway
  - B—Breathing
  - C—Circulation
- Symptoms:
  - Breathlessness
  - Chest pain
  - Feeling cold
  - Light headedness
  - Restlessness, distress, and panic
  - Pins and needles in fingers
  - Nausea and vomiting.

Assessing the airway (A): The head tilt and chin lift is carried out by placing a hand on the forehead and gently tilting back and two fingers of the other hand under the chin and gently lifting.

Assessing breathing (B) and circulation (C):
- Having opened the airway, the breathing should be assessed for 10 seconds by looking for chest movement and listening and feeling for signs of air movement.
- Although experienced clinicians may also feel the carotid pulse at this stage, the current resuscitation guidelines advise that lack of breathing also indicates a lack of circulation.
- If the airway is open and the patient is breathing, high flow oxygen should be administered via a face mask.
- If there is no circulation or there is some uncertainty, cardiopulmonary resuscitation (CPR) should be commenced immediately.
- This begins immediately with 30 chest compressions followed by two ventilation breaths. Administering chest compressions should be conducted with the patient in the left lateral position.

Reversible causes of cardiac arrest:
- Four H's
- Four T's

Four H's:
- Hyporolemia due to hemorrhage or sepsis
- Hypoxia
- Hyperkalemia and other metabolic disorders
- Hypothermia.

Four T's:
- Thromboembolism
- Toxicity due to drugs, e.g. anesthetic
- Tension pneumothorax
- Tamponade (cardiac).

CONCLUSION

Labor and delivery are one of the most painful experiences a woman is likely to encounter in her lifetime. In order to eliminate/reduce the pain experienced during delivery, we make use of anesthetic techniques. Neuroaxial labor analgesia offers the most complete analgesia and is safe and reliable.

Anesthesia-related maternal morbidity and mortality have decreased steadily in recent years. This may be a result of the more widespread use of neuroaxial analgesia and anesthesia in obstetric patients.

The management of obstetric emergencies is a team work in order to reduce maternal morbidity and maternal mortality. Anesthetist plays a major role in managing obstetric emergencies.

SUGGESTED READING

1. Letsky E, de Swiet M. Thromboembolism in pregnancy and its management. Br J Haematol 1984;57:543-52.
2. Kierkegaard A. Incidence and diagnosis of deep vein thrombosis associated with pregnancy. Acta Obst Gynecol Scand. 1983;62:239-43.
3. Maine D, Rosenfield A, Wallace M, et al. Prevention of maternal deaths in developing countries. New York Centre for Population of Family Health. University of Columbia, 1987.
4. Howell CJ, Clower NWB. The management of major obstetric hemorrhage. Curr Anaesth Crit Care. 1995;6(4):218-23.

5. Berkowitz RL. In: Critical Care of the Obstetric Patient, vol 10. New York: Churchill Livingstone, 1983, pp.288-94.
6. Higgins S. Obstetric hemorrhage. Emerg Med. 2003;15(3):222-31.
7. Li XF, Fortney JA, Kotelchuch M, et al. The postpartum period: the key to maternal mortality. Int J Gynecol Obstet. 1996;54:1-10.
8. Mantel G, Buchmann E, Rees H, et al. Severe acute maternal morbidity : a pilot study of a definition for a "near miss " Br J Obstet Gynecol. 1998;105:985-90.
9. Lewis G, Drife J. Why mothers die 1997-99: the fifth report on the confidential enquiries into maternal deaths in the United Kingdom: Royal College of Obstetrics and Gynecolgy Press, 2001.

CHAPTER 24

Cesarean Delivery

Aishwarya Yerram

■ INTRODUCTION

Cesarean Section

- Cesarean section (CS) is almost certainly one of the oldest operations in surgery with its origins lost in the mists of antiquity and mythology.[1]
- The weak myth that Julius Caesar was born by this route is contradicted by the fact that his mother survived his birth by many years.[1]
- It is likely that the term comes from the Lex caesarea or royal law which proclaimed that women who died before delivering their infant had to have the infant removed through the abdomen before burial 715 BC.[2]

■ INDICATIONS (BOX 1)

- The justification for CS is based on clinical judgment in the interest of the mother, fetus or both in order to avoid the continuation of pregnancy or the onset or the continuation of labor (Box 2).[1]
- The conditions that inform this judgment vary widely depending on the population served and the clinical skills and facilities available.[1]
- Nonetheless, there are four main indications that account for 60-90% of all CS. These include repeat CS (35-40%), dystocia (20-35%), breech (10-15%), and fetal distress (10-15%).[3]

Box 1: Indications for cesarean delivery.[3]

Maternal
- Prior cesarean delivery
- Abnormal placentation
- Maternal request
- Prior classical hysterotomy
- Unknown uterine scar type
- Uterine incision dehiscence
- Prior full-thickness myomectomy
- Genital tract obstructive mass
- Invasive cervical cancer
- Prior trachelectomy
- Permanent cerclage
- Prior pelvic reconstructive surgery
- Pelvic deformity
- Herpes simplex virus (HSV) or Human immunodeficiency virus (HIV) infection
- Cardiac or pulmonary disease
- Cerebral aneurysm or arteriovenous malformation
- Pathology requiring concurrent intra-abdominal surgery
- Perimortem cesarean delivery

Maternal-fetal
- Cephalopelvic disproportion
- Failed operative vaginal delivery
- Placenta previa or placental abruption

Fetal
- Nonreassuring fetal status
- Malpresentation
- Macrosomia
- Congenital anomaly
- Abnormal umbilical cord Doppler study
- Thrombocytopenia
- Prior neonatal birth trauma

Box 2: Classification of urgency of cesarean section.[1,2]

1. *Category I*: Immediate threat to life of woman or fetus, acute fetal distress/fetal bradycardia, cord prolapse, severe placenta abruption, bleeding placenta previa major with maternal hypovolemia, uterine rupture and scar dehiscence, and failed instrumental delivery with fetal distress. These cesareans should occur as quickly as possible and certainly within 30 minutes.[5,6]
2. *Category II*: Maternal or fetal compromise but not immediately life-threatening, malpresentation in labor (e.g. brow presentation and face chin posterior), antepartum hemorrhage without hypervolemia, and failed induction of labor (IOL).[5,6]
3. *Category III*: Needing early delivery but no maternal or fetal compromise, early labor in woman booked for elective lower segment cesarean section (LSCS), macrosomic baby in early labor, and breech in early labor. It is recommended that these women be delivered within 75 minutes.[5,6]
4. *Category IV*: At a time to suit the woman and maternity team, two previous LSCS, breech presentation, multiple pregnancy (first fetus not cephalic), etc.[5,6]

Other Indications[4]

Cesarean Delivery on Maternal Request

Occasionally CS is requested by a pregnant woman, this must be followed by balanced counseling of risks and benefits of CS vis a vis vaginal delivery. The decision thus made by patient should be respected.[4]

▮ PREOPERATIVE CONSIDERATIONS

Consent for Cesarean Section

- Consent should be taken in the language understood by the patient and never implied.[4]
- Patient should be explained that though techniques of anesthesia and surgery, complications like hemorrhage, infection, soft-tissue injuries, and injury to the baby and implications for future pregnancies.[7]
- In case a patient is unable to sign, a left thumb impression is taken. If the patient is not in a position to give a consent and consent should be obtained from relatives. In case of minors <18 years, guardian consent is necessary.[8]
- Patient may opt for refusal of CS being oblivious of benefits to her and her baby's health. She has to be counseled again. Despite this if there is a refusal of consent, it must be documented on paper.[1]

Laboratory Work

- Basic investigations are required—hemoglobin (Hb), blood grouping and Rh typing, human immunodeficiency virus (HIV), hepatitis B virus surface antigen (HBsAg), blood sugar RBS, and urine routine examination. Other investigations like hepatitis C virus (HCV) should be done on availability.[7]
- Cross matching is recommended in cases like Rh negative, anemia, placenta previa, adherent placenta, coagulopathy, sepsis, previous cesarean, and in conditions thought essential by operating surgeon. It is preferable to cross match blood all patients undergoing CS.[7]

▮ PERIOPERATIVE CARE

- *Antibiotic prophylaxis*:
  - *Timing*: American College of Obstetricians and Gynecologists (ACOG) guidelines recommends antimicrobial therapy to all women within 30–60 minutes before making the skin incision to ensure adequate drug tissue levels.[8]
  - *Regimen*: Single dose of cefazolin 2 g intravenous (IV) and add a single dose of azithromycin 500 mg IV to those in

labor or with ruptured membranes. In women with significant penicillin or cephalosporin allergy, a single 600 mg IV dose of clindamycin combined with a weight-based dose of aminoglycoside is an alternative.[8]

In women with more prolonged labor and evidence of chorioamnionitis repeat doses of the same antibiotic can be given for the first 48 hours postoperatively.[1]

- *Advantages*: Reduced the risk of endometritis, wound infection, urinary tract infection, and serious maternal infectious complications were also reduced but did not significantly impact the risk of neonatal sepsis.[9,10]

- If cesarean delivery is scheduled, a sedative may be given at bedtime the night before surgery.
- The guidelines recommend a minimum preoperative fasting time of at least 2 hours from clear liquids, 6 hours from a light meal, and 8 hours from a regular meal.[8]
- Intravenous line to be taken with large bore needle (minimum 16/18 gauge).
- Theater should be kept ready.
- An antacid is given shortly before regional analgesia or induction with general anesthesia.
- Once the woman is supine, a wedge beneath the right hip creates a left lateral tilt to aid venous return and avoid hypotension.
- Fetal heart sounds should be documented in the operating room prior to surgery.
- If hair obscures the operative field it should be removed the day of surgery by clipping. This is associated with fewer surgical site infections compared with shaving (Tanner, 2011).[8]
- An indwelling bladder catheter is placed. Few studies support the nonuse of catheterization in hemodynamically stable women to minimize urinary infections (Li, 2011; Nasr, 2009).
- Thromboembolism is increased with pregnancy and almost doubled in those undergoing cesarean delivery, the ACOG (2011d) recommends initiation of pneumatic compression before cesarean delivery and discontinued once the woman ambulates. Risk factors include bed rest for ≥1 week antepartum, postpartum hemorrhage ≥1,000 mL, previous venous thromboembolism (VTE), thrombophilia, blood transfusion, postpartum infection, and some medical conditions (lupus, heart disease, and sickle cell disease), body mass index (BMI) >30 kg/m^2, multiple gestation, and pre-eclampsia.
- Preparations for surgery in women with medical disorders are discussed in the respective chapters.
- For the newborn, arrangements should be made for suction machine, sterile tubing, laryngoscope, endotracheal tubes, and overhead light/warmer.

TECHNIQUE

Anesthesia[7]

The type of anesthesia should be decided by the anesthesiologist and the obstetrician in conjunction with patient.

- *Spinal*: Spinal anesthesia is reliable, has rapid onset, patient is awake, and there is less risk of aspiration. There is not enough evidence from trials to evaluate use of lateral tilt during CS.[7]
- *Epidural*: Epidural anesthesia has less of hypotension and good postoperative analgesia can be offered.[7]
- *General*: It is mostly used when regional is contraindicated, failure of regional and acute fetal distress and in cases of sepsis, hypotension, thrombocytopenia <75,000, coagulation disorder, and coronary heart disease (CHD). Unusual complications include aspiration and neonatal depression.[6]

- *Local anesthesia*: In an exceptional situation, CS may be performed under local anesthesia.

Skin Incision (Fig. 1)

Transverse Incision

- *Pfannenstiel incision*: It is curved skin incision, two fingers above the symphysis pubis at upper border of pubic hairline. Rectus is cut transversely and separated from the underlying muscles. Muscles are separated from the midline and peritoneum cut transversely.[7]
- *Transverse (Joel-Cohen incision)*: Joel-Cohen incision is a straight skin incision 3 cm above the pubic symphysis. Fascia not separated from muscle and peritoneum opened transversely. Here subsequent tissue layers are opened bluntly, has shorter operating time, and reduced postoperative febrile morbidity.[7]
- *Maylard incision*: Transverse skin incision made 3-8 cm above pubic symphysis. Fascia is incised transversely, muscle is cut transversely and then peritoneum is opened.[1]

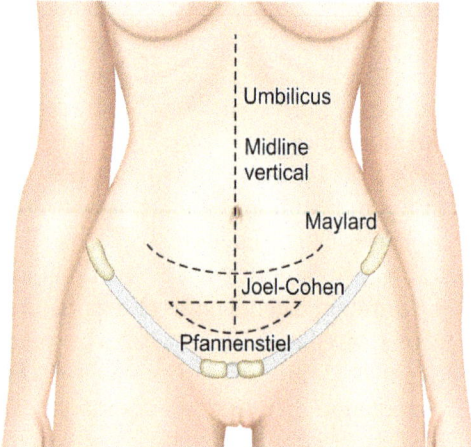

Fig. 1: Types of skin incisions.

Advantages: Less postoperative pain, has cosmetic appeal, low wound dehiscence, and less chances of herniation.

Disadvantages: More bleeding and chance of nerve damage compared to vertical incisions.

Vertical Incision

Traditional (infraumbilical vertical or paramedian): It was used previously extensively.

Advantages: Quick, less blood loss, and nerve damage and extension of incision is easy.

Disadvantages: More postoperative pain, low cosmetic appeal, and more chances of hernia.[8]

Uterine Incision (Figs. 2A to E)

It is an important surgical step and should be planned preoperatively. Type of incision must be mentioned in case notes and all other records.

Lower Segment Transverse (Kerr) Incision

It is most commonly used, 1-2 cm cut, extended transversely with scissors/digitally when lower segment is well formed.

Advantages: Less blood loss, easy repair, can be modified to J or inverted T, and less chance of rupture in future pregnancies.

Disadvantages: Entrapment of preterm head and extension involving uterine arteries.

Lower Segment Vertical (Kronig/DeLee) Incision

It is not commonly used. It may be done in cases of poorly formed lower segment and in preterm patients this incision may be an option.[7]

Advantages: Helpful in malpresentations like transverse lie, can be extended into upper segment in case of necessity, edges are of equal thickness, and easy to approximate.

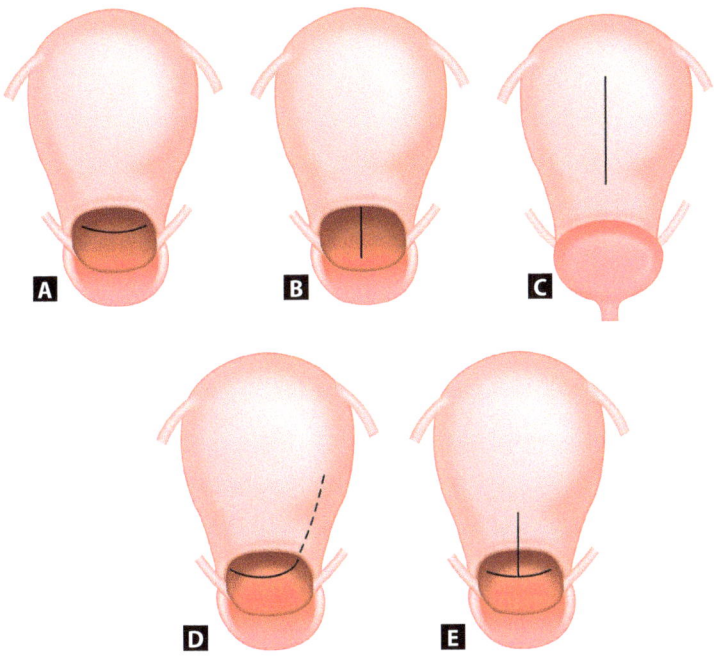

Figs. 2A to E: Types of uterine incisions: (A) Lower segment transverse; (B) Lower segment vertical; (C) Classical; (D and E) "J" and inverted "T" incision.

Disadvantages: Bladder dissection essential, extension into vagina or fundus, and more blood loss than transverse incisions.

Classical Incision[11]

It is a vertical incision over the fundus.

Indications: Extensive adhesions, cervical and lower segment fibroids, placenta previa with or without accrete, carcinoma cervix, postmortem cesarean, and repaired high vesicovaginal fistula.

Disadvantages: Hemorrhage, difficult closure, weak scar, and adhesions.

T-shaped Incisions

If required J-shaped or U-shaped incisions are preferred to T incision.

Indications: These incisions may be required in case of difficult delivery.

Disadvantages: Poor healing, increased postoperative morbidity, and in subsequent pregnancies this will have to be treated as a classical cesarean scar.[12]

Delivery of Baby (Fig. 3)

- Maintaining the flexion of the fetal head during delivery reduces the diameter, prevents extensions, and eases the delivery. One must avoid hasty baby delivery.
- After the delivery of the baby, infant should be rapidly dried and the cord clamped and a specimen kept for cord blood pH analysis. Baby's oral cavity is suctioned and handed over to neonatologist for further care.[1]

Placental Delivery

The placenta should be removed by controlled cord traction once signs of separation

Obstetric Emergencies

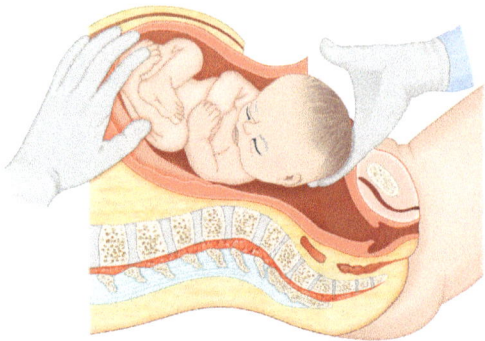

Fig. 3: Manual delivery of the fetal head. Identify the occiput and flex the head through the uterine incision with concomitant fundal pressure by an assistant.

have occurred. Routine manual removal of the placenta is discouraged as it increases blood loss and postoperative sepsis[13] and even occasionally acute uterine inversion. Once the placenta has been delivered the uterine cavity should be checked to ensure there are no retained portions of placenta or membranes.[14]

Measures to Minimize Blood Loss and Prevent Postpartum Hemorrhage

- Oxytocin
  - *Intramuscular*: 10 units are recommended.
  - *Intravenous*: 5–10 units diluted to 5 mL over 1 minute.
  - *Infusion*: 10–20 U in 500 mL (150 mL/hour)
- Ergot-alkaloids-hypertensive side effects
- Misoprostol
- Tranexamic acid.

Closure

Should begin after mops and instruments count is checked and tallied.

Uterus: In Situ versus Exteriorization of Uterus

- Exteriorization of the uterus should not routinely be carried out. This may cause nausea, vomiting, and pain.

- Recommended if there is an extension of the uterine incision or exposure is limited by heavy bleeding.[1]

Uterus: Single- versus Two-layer

- *Two-layer closure*: The first layer should include the cut edges of the muscle only and not the decidua. It should be a running suture, which avoids the bunching and elevation of tissues seen with a continuous locking suture, and facilitates the placement of the second layer which can be either running or locking to undermine the first layer.[15]
- *Single-layer closure*: It is usually with a continuous suture, either running or locked. In general this saves about 7 minutes operating time and results in slightly less blood loss.[15] There are as yet conflicting and inadequate data on the outcome of single- versus double-layer closure upon the integrity of the scar in subsequent labor.[16]
- The most commonly used sutures for uterine closure are No. 0 or No. 1 polyglactin (Vicryl) or chromic catgut.

Peritoneum: Closure versus Nonclosure

- *Nonclosure*: It has been associated with reduces operating time, reduced need for postoperative analgesia, and is associated with quicker return of bowel activity and decreased formation of adhesions.[17]
- *Closure*: However, a recent study has shown that closure of both these peritoneal layers significantly reduces adhesions found at subsequent CS.[18]

Abdomen

- *Rectus muscle*: Gentle approximation with interrupted chromic catgut No.1-0 or polyglactin is done.[17]
- *Rectus sheath*: It is a most important structure for integrity of the abdomen.

Use of delayed or nonabsorbable suture is recommended. Prolene No. 1 is routinely used.[17]
- Vertical incisions should be closed with nonabsorbable suture material in single layer.[17]
- *Subcuticular tissue*: Routine closure is not advocated except when fat is more than 2 cm. Recent data suggests that subcuticular skin closure may reduce the risk of delayed infection.[19]
- *Skin*: Any absorbable or unabsorbable subcuticular suture (Monocryl)/staples/vertical mattress can be used as per need.[19]

COMPLICATIONS OF CESAREAN DELIVERY

Complications of cesarean delivery are given in Table 1.

MISGAV LADACH TECHNIQUE[20-22]

- Developed by Michael Stark at the Misgav Ladach Hospital in Jerusalem[21]
- Joel-Cohen transverse skin incision is used[21]
- The rectus sheath is incised and rectus muscles are pulled apart with the fingers. The parietal peritoneum is then stretched and entered bluntly with the index finger[21]
- The uterus is entered with a scalpel incision then enlarged with the fingers[21]
- Placenta removed manually and the uterus is closed in one layer. Peritoneum is not closed, nor are the rectus muscles[21]
- Shorter operating time, less blood loss, and less postoperative analgesic requirement.[22]

COMPLICATED CESAREAN SECTION

Deeply Engaged Fetal Head[23,24]

In this situation the CS is at full cervical dilatation with the head deeply impacted in the pelvis. The following options are available to deal with this situation:
- With levering movements, push the flat of the lower hand between the uterine incision and the fetal head deep into the vagina.
- An assistant cups the fetal head vaginally in one hand and elevates it to meet the operator's hand.[23]
- *Forceps*: With gentle pressure on the fetal chin rotate the head towards the direct occipitoposterior position and apply the forceps alongside the fetal head with the pelvic curve towards the pubic symphysis.[23]
- *Reverse breech extraction*: The operator reaches up and grasps the fetal feet and pulls them down through the uterine incision, which elevates the fetal trunk and head. Continued traction on the fetal legs, in essence, carries out an internal podalic version and the breech is delivered through the uterine incision first.[25]
- Uterine relaxation as an aid to all the above maneuvers by coordination with the anesthetist.[26]
- Extend the uterine "T" incision.

High Floating Head

- Rupture of membranes followed by suctioning of liquor, allow vertex to

TABLE 1: Complications of cesarean delivery.

Anesthesia related	Surgical complications

- Regional anesthesia:
  – Anaphylaxis
  – Hypotension
  – Postspinal Headache
  – Meningitis
- General anesthesia:
  – Drug reactions
  – Mendelson syndrome
  – Cardiac arrest
  – Pulmonary edema
	- Bleeding
	- Bowel, bladder, and visceral injury
	- Infection
	- Deep vein thrombosis
	- Paralytic ileus
	- Adhesions
	- Incisional hernia
	- Future obstetric complications

descend to incision site, then flexion and delivery.[1]
- Use of vacuum.
- Short forceps is also possible.

Breech Presentation

- Head should be delivered with same care as in vaginal breech delivery. Burn's Marshall technique or Mauriceau-Smellie-Veit method or using forceps.[1]

Transverse Lie

- Internal podalic version followed by breech extraction aided by tocolysis. If the lower segment is inadequately developed, a vertical incision will have to be made, starting low and extending into the upper uterine segment.[1]
- Turn the fetus to a longitudinal lie and find that the lower uterine segment is sufficiently developed to carry out a transverse lower segment incision.[3]

Placenta Previa

There are a number of potential complications of CS specific to placenta previa and placenta accreta.[17]

Obesity

- Cesarean section, which is more commonly indicated in the morbidly obese (BMI >40), presents a major surgical challenge.[27]
- Choice of abdominal incision is Pfannenstiel incision in the healthy skin 3–4 cm above the natural skin crease. In women with a large pannus the umbilicus will be dragged down to the level of the symphysis pubis and a transverse incision made above the umbilicus.[28]
- Other surgical aspects include adequate retraction and full antibiotic and thromboprophylaxis.[28,29]

DOCUMENTATION

After every cesarean delivery a detailed note should be recorded. This should include a summary of events in labor, the indication, and surgical details of the operation. This is necessary for audit purposes and also in a subsequent pregnancy. The perioperative decisions and procedures should also be reviewed with the woman during her postpartum stay in hospital.[1]

POSTOPERATIVE CARE

Monitoring

- Hourly for 6 hours
- 4th hourly for next 24 hours
- Twice daily till discharge
- *Following are monitored*: Temperature, respiration rate, pulse rate, intake/output, cardiorespiratory system, uterine contractility, and vaginal bleeding.

Medications Advised

- *On day 0*:
  - Intravenous fluids
  - Early ambulation should be done and oral fluids should be started early once bowel sounds are heard.[8]
  - *Analgesia*: 8th hourly or as per personnel preference
  - *Antibiotics*: Single dose perioperatively is sufficient as prophylactic measure
  - *Bladder drainage*: Early removal after 12 hours in uncomplicated cases
  - Antiemetics and H2 blockers
  - Breastfeeding is initiated as early possible
- *On postoperative day 1*: Hemoglobin% after 24 hours
- *On postoperative day 3*: Dressing done
- *On postoperative day 7*: Suture removal.

FOLLOW-UP

- *For mother*:
  - Routine follow-up is advised after a week for examining the wound[2]
  - Breastfeeding
  - Hematinics
  - Calcium supplementation
  - Wound care
  - Dietary advice
  - Contraception options
  - Postnatal exercises after 6 weeks.
- *For baby*:
  - Exclusive breastfeeding
  - Immunization.

TRAINING AND AUDIT

Audit is a must to ensure quality and monitoring outcomes. It should include rate of CS, indications of CS, and complications of procedure. Audit should be done for a surgeon as well as entire unit.[2]

CONCLUSION

- Primary cesarean determines future obstetric course of any female and therefore should be avoided whenever possible.
- Patient selection, meticulous asepsis, surgical technique, postoperative care are all factors which are major determinants of the outcome.
- We should respect patient's autonomy but at the same time abide by the principle of "first do no harm".
- The possibility of pelvic floor dysfunction and surgical complications cannot be overlooked and be informed to the patient.

REFERENCES

1. Baskett TF, Calder AA, Arulkumaran S. Munro Kerr's Operative Obstetrics E-Book. Amsterdam, Netherlands: Elsevier Health Sciences; 2014.
2. Fasbender H. Geschichte der geburtshulfe. Jena: Gustav Fisher; 1906. pp. 979-1010.
3. Baskett TF, Arulkumaran S. Intrapartum Care, 2nd edition. London: RCOG Press; 2011. pp. 155-68.
4. Cunningham FG, MacDonald PC, Gant NF. Williams Obstetrics. New York, NY: McGraw-Hill Professional; 2005.
5. National Institute for Clinical Excellence. Clinical guideline: Caesarean section. London: RCOG Press; 2004.
6. Royal College of Obstetricians and Gynaecologists. Classification of urgency of caesarean section—a continuum of risk (Good Practice No. 11). London: RCOG Press; 2010.
7. FOGSI. (2014). Consensus Statement for Cesarean section. [online] Available from: http://www.fogsi.org/wp-content/uploads/2015/11/fogsi_gcpr_ceserean_section.pdf [Last accessed September, 2019].
8. American College of Obstetricians and Gynecologists. ACOG Practice Bulletin No. 120: Use of prophylactic antibiotics in labor and delivery. Obstet Gynecol. 2011;117:1472-83.
9. Smaill FM, Grivell RM. Antibiotic prophylaxis versus no prophylaxis for preventing infection after cesarean section. Cochrane Database Syst Rev. 2014;(10):CD007482.
10. Mackeen AD, Packard RE, Ota E, et al. Timing of intravenous prophylactic antibiotics for preventing postpartum infectious morbidity in women undergoing cesarean delivery. Cochrane Database Syst Rev. 2014;(12): CD009516.
11. Bethune M, Pemezel M. The relationship between gestational age and the incidence of classical caesarean section. Aust NZ J Obstet Gynaecol. 1997;37:153-5.
12. Patterson LS, O'Connell CM, Baskett TF. Maternal and perinatal morbidity associated with classical and inverted 'T' cesarean sections. Obstet Gynecol. 2002;100:633-7.
13. Hema KR, Johanson R. Techniques for performing caesarean section. Best Pract Res Clin Obstet Gynaecol. 2001;15:17-47.
14. Baska A, Kalan A, Ozkan A, et al. The effect of placental removal method and site of uterine repair on postcesarean endometritis and operative blood loss. Acta Obstet Gynecol Scand. 2005;84:266-9.

15. Dodd JM, Anderson ER, Gates S. Surgical techniques for uterine incision and uterine closure at the time of caesarean section. Cochrane Database Syst Rev. 2008;3:CD004732.
16. National Institute for Health and Clinical Excellence: Guidance. Caesarean section. London: RCOG Press; 2004.
17. CAESAR study collaborative group. Caesarean section surgical techniques; a randomised factorial trial (CAESAR). BJOG. 2010;117;1366-76.
18. Lyell DJ, Caughey AB, Hu E, et al. Perinatal closure at primary cesarean delivery and adhesions. Obstet Gynecol. 2005;106:275-80.
19. Clay FS, Walsh CA, Walsh SR. Staples vs subcuticular sutures for skin closure at caesarean delivery: a metaanalysis of randomized controlled trials. Am J Obstet Gynecol. 2011;204:378-83.
20. Holmgren G, Sjoholm L, Stark M. The Misgav Ladach method for cesarean section: method description. Acta Obstet Gynecol Scand. 1999; 78:615-21.
21. Darj E, Nortstrom ML. Misgav Ladach method for cesarean section compared to the Pfannenstiel method. Acta Obstet Gynecol Scand. 1999;78:37-41.
22. Hofmeyr GJ, Mathai M, Shah A, et al. Techniques for caesarean section. Cochrane Database Syst Rev. 2008;(1):CD004662.
23. Allen VM, O'Connell CM, Baskett TF. Maternal and perinatal morbidity of caesarean section at full cervical dilatation compared with caesarean delivery in the first stage of labour. Br J Obstet Gynaecol. 2005;112:986-90.
24. Royal Australian and New Zealand College of Obstetricians and Gynaecologists. Delivery of the fetus at caesarean section. College Statement: C-Obs 3. Melbourne: 7RANZCOG; 2010.
25. Levy R, Chernomoretz T, Appelman Z, et al. Head pushing versus reverse breech extraction in cases of impacted fetal head during caesarean section. Eur J Obstet Gynecol Reprod Biol. 2005;121:24-6.
26. Chopra S, Bagga R, Keepanasseril A, et al. Disengagement of the deeply engaged fetal head during caesarean section in advanced labor: conventional method versus reverse breech extraction. Acta Obstet Gynecol Scand. 2009;88:1163-6.
27. Alanis MC, Goodnight WH, Hill EG, et al. Maternal super-obesity (body mass index > or = 50) and adverse pregnancy outcomes. Acta Obstet Gynecol Scand. 2010;89:924-30.
28. Tixier H, Thouvenot S, Coulange L, et al. Cesarean section in morbid obese women: Supra or subumbilical transverse incision? Acta Obstet Gynecol Scand. 2009;88:1049-52.
29. Kingdom JC, Baud D, Grabowska K, et al. Delivery by caesarean section in super-obese women: beyond Pfannenstiel. J Obstet Gynaecol Can. 2012;34:472-4.

CHAPTER 25

Perimortem Cesarean Delivery

Aishwarya Yerram

■ DEFINITION

Perimortem cesarean delivery (PMCD) or "resuscitative hysterotomy" refers to hysterotomy performed to resuscitate a woman in middle to late pregnancy in the event of cardiac arrest with primary interest of the mother and fetal survival.

■ MATERNAL PHYSIOLOGY

- Cardiac output and plasma volume increase by 30–40% above the nonpregnant state from 6th weeks, which peaks by 30–32 weeks.
- Shock manifests clinically only after loss of 40% blood volume.
- In late pregnancy, compression of the inferior vena cava (IVC) may lead to supine hypotension.
- Decrease in functional residual capacity (−20%) of the lungs due to elevation of the diaphragm (around 4 cm elevation at term).

■ MATERNAL COLLAPSE: CAUSES[1]

The causes of maternal collapse have been described in Table 1.

Management of Maternal Collapse (Flowchart 1)[2,3]

- Focus on resuscitating the mother, not the fetus.

TABLE 1: Maternal collapse—causes.[1]

Reversible causes		Cause in pregnancy
4H	Hypovolemia	Bleeding, septic shock, and neurogenic shock
	Hypoxia	*Cardiac events:* Myocardial infarction, aortic dissection, peripartum cardiomyopathy, and aneurysms-large vessel
	Hyper/hypokalemia and electrolyte disturbances	Same as nonpregnant
	Hypothermia	Same as nonpregnant
	Thromboembolism	Amniotic fluid embolism, pulmonary embolism, air embolism, and myocardial infarction
4T	Toxicity	Anesthesia (local) and other drugs
	Tension pneumothorax	Traumatic causes
	Tamponade	Traumatic causes
Eclampsia and preeclampsia		Includes intracranial hemorrhage

Obstetric Emergencies

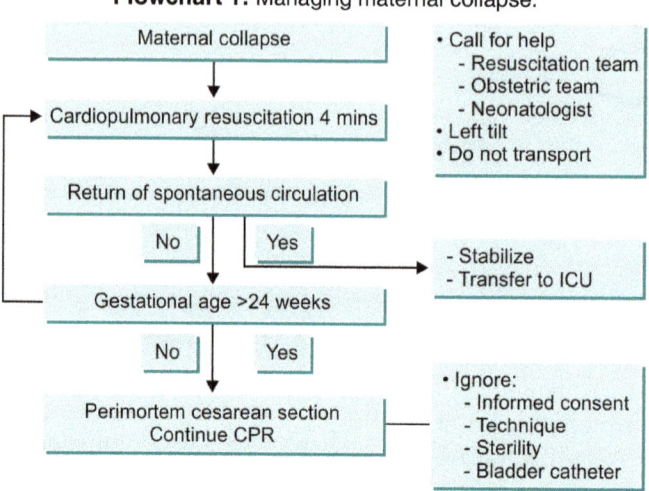

Flowchart 1: Managing maternal collapse.

(CPR: cardiopulmonary resuscitation; ICU: intensive care unit)

- Perform chest compressions on a firm surface with a left lateral tilt of fifteen degrees. This will relieve aortocaval compressions and make compressions to be effective.[4]
    - *Airway*: Use a one size smaller endotracheal tube as there will be physiological narrowing of airways in the third trimester.
        - Intubation medications to be used are the same.
        - Rapid sequence intubation is the preferred method as the chance of aspiration is high in the third trimester.
    - *Breathing*:
        - Supplement 100% O_2
        - Bag and mask ventilation till intubation is achieved.
    - *Circulation*:
        - Compressions to ventilations ratio should be 30:2.
        - If intubated—compressions 100/minute and ventilations at 10/minute
        - Aggressive volume resuscitation with two wide bore cannula regardless of blood pressure
        - *Uterine displacement*: 30° left tilt or manually move the uterus to the left.
    - *Drugs*:
        - Similar drugs in same doses as nonpregnant state.
    - *Delivery*:
        - Consider to deliver if no response after 4 min of cardiopulmonary resuscitation (CPR)
        - Gestational age beyond 20–24 weeks
        - Delivery would assist maternal resuscitation efforts
        - Baby should be out by 5 minutes of collapse.

POTENTIAL BENEFITS[5]

- Perimortem cesarean delivery is resuscitative hysterotomy for the mother—improves maternal and fetal survival chances.
- Aortocaval compression by gravid uterus→ reduces cardiac output by two-thirds.
- *Cardiopulmonary resuscitation→ pregnant mother*: 10% normal cardiac output (*normally*: one-third normal cardiac output).
- Emptying the uterus →↓ compression of inferior vena cava→↑ venous return

(uterine blood flow redistributed to other organs)→↑ 25% cardiac output[6]→↑ functional residual capacity[4]→ diaphragm lowered, respiration improved→↑ oxygenation→ effective CPR[5]→ improves chances of successful maternal resuscitation.

Timing

- Loss of time is crucial. Any delay in decision will lead to increase in the time from cardiac arrest to PMCD.[1]
- Initiate CPR immediately. If response is not seen within 4 minutes of correctly performed CPR, plan for delivery within 5 minutes of collapse, if gestational age beyond 20-24 weeks.[7]
- If gestational age less than 24 weeks, expediting delivery will not have significant effect on maternal outcome.[8]
- Assess gestational age by (1) fundal height two finger breadth or 4cm above umbilicus; (2) ultrasound if available; and (c) medical records for last menstrual period/estimated due date (LMP/EDD).
- *Assess fetal viability*: Not mandatory as (1) delays to time-dependent potential benefit to baby and mother; (2) good neurological outcome in few cases with absent fetal heart tones; (3) ultrasound/Doppler—availability and difficulty to scan during CPR; and (4) fetus may have periods of bradycardia.[9]
- Fetal survival is most successful when performed with 4 minutes of maternal collapse, beyond which resuscitative hysterotomy will still be beneficial for maternal survival. Few case reports have recorded infants with good neurological outcome when delivered after more than 25 minutes of maternal death.[10]

CONTRAINDICATIONS

- Gestational period < 24 weeks
- Successful initial resuscitative efforts.

EQUIPMENT[11]

- *Essential equipment*:
  - Scalpel with No. 10 blade
  - Toothed forceps
  - Bandage
  - scissors
  - Bulb syringe
  - Two umbilical clamps
  - Towels
  - Suction device
  - Packing gauze.
- *Optional equipment*:
  - Antiseptic solution
  - Two medium-sized retractors
  - Foley catheter
  - Needle holder
  - No. 0 or No. 1 delayed-absorbable suture
  - Large needle.

PREPARATION

- *Antibiotic*: Not mandatory. Single dose of any broad-spectrum antibiotic[1]
- *Anesthesia*: Not required
- *Consent*: This is an emergency procedure. Consent is not legally necessary (in case of brain-dead patient on ventilator support, all proceedings have to be undertaken legally).

POSITIONING

- There should be no delay, begin the cesarean at the same place of ongoing resuscitation.[11]
- Should be performed in the supine position with fifteen degree left lateral tilt.
- Preparation of parts and draping the patient are not necessary.

Technique

- *Step 1—Skin incision*:
  - Long vertical incision starting from xiphoid to the pubis
  - Blunt dissection by fingers to separate the layers and enter peritoneum.[12]

- Step 2—displace the bladder, if necessary decompress it by means of needle aspiration.
- *Step 3—incise the uterus*:
  - Lower segment vertical incision. Extend toward fundus as required to access the fetus.[12]
- *Step 4—deliver the infant from vertex position*:
  - Suction mouth and nose with bulb syringe
  - Collect cord blood
  - Clamp cord—assess, clean, and warm infant.
- *Step 5—removing placenta*:
  - Consider direct pressure on aorta,
  - Pack or closure of uterus using one layer closure with delayed-absorbable sutures.
- Step 6—continue full CPR measures during the delivery, if mother responds to resuscitative efforts, closure should be performed in the operating room.[13]

TRAINING AND EDUCATIONAL AIDS

- Advanced Life Support in Obstetrics (ALSO)
- Managing Obstetric Emergencies and Trauma (MOET)
- Advances in Labour and Risk Management (ALARM).

CONCLUSION

- Timing is the key for successful maternal and fetal survival.[12]
- Beyond 24 weeks of gestation, compression of the great vessels by the gravid uterus greatly impact the cardiac output.[4]
- Defibrillation algorithm, drugs and their doses used for resuscitation of the pregnant woman are the same as adults.[13]

REFERENCES

1. Royal College of Obstetricians and Gynaecologists. Maternal Collapse in Pregnancy and the Puerperium. Green-top Guideline No. 56. London: RCOG; 2011.
2. Resuscitation Council (UK). (2010). Resuscitation Guidelines 2010. [online] Available from: http://www.resus.org.uk/pages/guide.htm [Last accessed September, 2019].
3. Soar J, Deakin CD, Nolan JP, et al. European Resuscitation Council Guidelines for Resuscitation 2005. Section 7. Cardiac arrest in special circumstances. Resuscitation. 2005;67(Suppl 1):S135-70.
4. Kinsella SM. Lateral tilt for pregnant women: why 15 degrees? Anaesthesia. 2003;58:835-6.
5. Katz V, Balderston K, DeFreest M. Perimortem cesarean delivery: were our assumptions correct? Am J Obstet Gynecol. 2005;192(6):1916-20.
6. DePace NL, Betesh JS, Kotler MN. 'Postmortem' cesarean section with recovery of both mother and offspring. JAMA. 1982;248(8):971-3.
7. Page-Rodriguez A, Gonzalez-Sanchez JA. Perimortem cesarean section of twin pregnancy: case report and review of the literature. Acad Emerg Med. 1999;6(10):1072-4.
8. Stehr SN, Liebich I, Kamin G, et al. Closing the gap between decision and delivery—amniotic fluid embolism with severe cardiopulmonary and haemostatic complications with a good outcome. Resuscitation. 2007;74(2):377-81.
9. Phelan HA, Roller J, Minei JP. Perimortem cesarean section after utilization of surgeon-performed trauma ultrasound. J Trauma. 2008;64(1):E12-4.
10. Capobianco G, Balata A, Mannazzu MC, et al. Perimortem cesarean delivery 30 minutes after a laboring patient jumped from a fourth-floor window: baby survives and is normal at age 4 years. Am J Obstet Gynecol. 2008;198(1):e15-6.
11. Brown HL. Trauma in pregnancy. Obstet Gynecol. 2009;114(1):147-60.
12. Cunningham FG, MacDonald PC, Gant NF, et al. Williams Obstetrics, 20th edition. Stanford, Conn: Appleton & Lange; 1997.p. 404.
13. American Heart Association. 2010 American Heart Association Guidelines for cardiopulmonary resuscitation and emergency cardiovascular care. Circulation. 2010;122: S829-61.

CHAPTER 26

Postpartum Hemorrhage

Meghana V Nyapathi

INTRODUCTION

According to the WHO South-East Asia region, about one-third of maternal and neonatal deaths occurring all over the world. The highest number of maternal and neonatal deaths is recorded from India.[1] Approximately 6% of women delivering can have postpartum hemorrhage (PPH)[2] which is responsible for 25% of all maternal deaths.[2,3] 66% of the deaths due to PPH are still due to substandard care.[4]

DEFINITION

Postpartum hemorrhage is defined as loss of blood more than 500 mL from the genital tract following the delivery of the fetus (>1,000 mL in cases of cesarean section (Box 1).[3,5]

RISK FACTORS

The risk factors for PPH can be broadly classified as:
1. *Based on etiology*: Factors originating in the antenatal period, intrapartum period and postpartum/postnatal period
2. *Based on pathology*: Classification of PPH based on the four T's—(1) tone, (2) trauma, (3) tissue, and (4) thrombin (Tables 1 and 2).

PREVENTION

Though identification of risk factors, risk modification by timely intervention can prevent PPH to an extent, PPH can also occur in women with no previously identified risk factors. Hence, preparedness for management of PPH is a must for all obstetric units.

Risk modification may include:
- Correction of anemia in the antenatal period
- Proper management of preexisting medical disorders
- Awareness of the site of placentation based on antenatal scans, patient counseling, and preparedness to manage the same
- Unjust use of oxytocics in the first stage of labor to be avoided
- Unnecessary deep episiotomy to be avoided. Episiotomy is associated with 27% of cases of PPH[10] (appropriate management of the first and second stages of labor)
- Anticoagulants to be stopped at least 24 hours before a planned delivery
- Active management of third stage of labor.
- Early identification of PPH and management according to the cause.

Box 1: Classification of postpartum hemorrhage.

Types of postpartum hemorrhage (PPH):
- PPH based on time:
  - *Primary/early/immediate PPH*: From the time of delivery of the baby to 24 hours after delivery
  - *Secondary/late/delayed PPH*: From 24 hours after delivery to 12 weeks postdelivery (Chandrahasan)
- PPH based on blood loss:
  - Minor PPH (500–1.000 mL)
  - Major PPH (>1,000 mL)
    - *Moderate PPH*: Blood loss of 1,000–2,000 mL
    - *Severe PPH*: Blood loss more than 2,000 mL

TABLE 1: Risk factors based on etiology.[6-8]

Antenatal risk factors	Intrapartum factors	Postpartum factors
• *Placental causes:* Placenta previa and abruptio placenta • *Medical causes*: Anemia, bleeding disorders, sepsis, and morbid obesity • *Obstetric*: PIH, HELLP syndrome, grand multipara, elderly gravida • *Uterine:* Myomas in lower segment, overdistended uterus (polyhydramnios and multiple gestation), chorioamnionitis • *Medications*: Anticoagulants and uterine relaxants (MgSO$_4$)	• Labor—induction of labor, prolonged labor, precipitate labor, emergency cesarean section • Episiotomy, trauma to the cervix, uterus, or vagina • Lacerations following operative vaginal deliveries • Amniotic fluid embolism	• Uterine atony • *Placenta:* Abnormal placentation, placenta accreta, retained placenta, and manual removal of the placenta • *Coagulopathy:* Amniotic fluid embolism, sepsis, and bleeding disorders • Uterine inversion • Previous history of severe PPH

TABLE 2: Risk factors based on pathology.[9-12]

Tone (70%)	Trauma (20%)	Tissue (10%)	Thrombin (1%)
Uterine atony due to: • Polyhydramnios • Multiple gestation • Prolonged labor • Precipitate labor • Multiparity • Use of uterine relaxants during labor • Endometritis	• Deep episiotomy • lacerations • Uterine rupture • Uterine inversion	Placenta previa, placenta accreta, retained products of conception, retained blood clots, extension of uterine incision during cesarean delivery	Inherited coagulopathy, clotting disorders, DIC, on anticoagulant therapy, pregnancy induced conditions like PIH, HELLP syndrome, sepsis

■ INVESTIGATIONS

- Complete blood count
- Blood group and type (if not done previously)
- *Coagulation profile*: Prothrombin time (PT), activated partial thromboplastin time (APTT), international normalized ratio (INR), and fibrinogen levels
- Liver function tests (LFT)
- Renal function tests (RFT)
- Serum electrolytes
- ABG and serum calcium
- Thromboelastography (TEG)
- *Thromboelastometry (ROTEM)*: TEG and ROTEM are done on whole blood sample by bedside and give information on the first fibrin strand formation, strength of the clot and fibrinolysis.[13]

■ DIAGNOSIS

- Estimation of blood loss based on blood collection drapes, visual estimation—might underestimate the blood loss by 30–50%
- Soft, boggy uterus suggestive of uterine atony
- Excessive, uncontrolled, or a continuous slow vaginal bleeding
- Swelling and pain in the vulva or vagina could be due to hematoma
- Swelling due to hematoma at the episiotomy site
- Increased pulse rate and low blood pressure
- Signs of dehydration
- Features of hypovolemic shock, if condition not corrected.

MANAGEMENT (FLOWCHART 1)

Management of postpartum hemorrhage is described in Figure 1.

Resuscitative Measures

Should be initiated in all cases where there is more than normal blood loss following delivery:

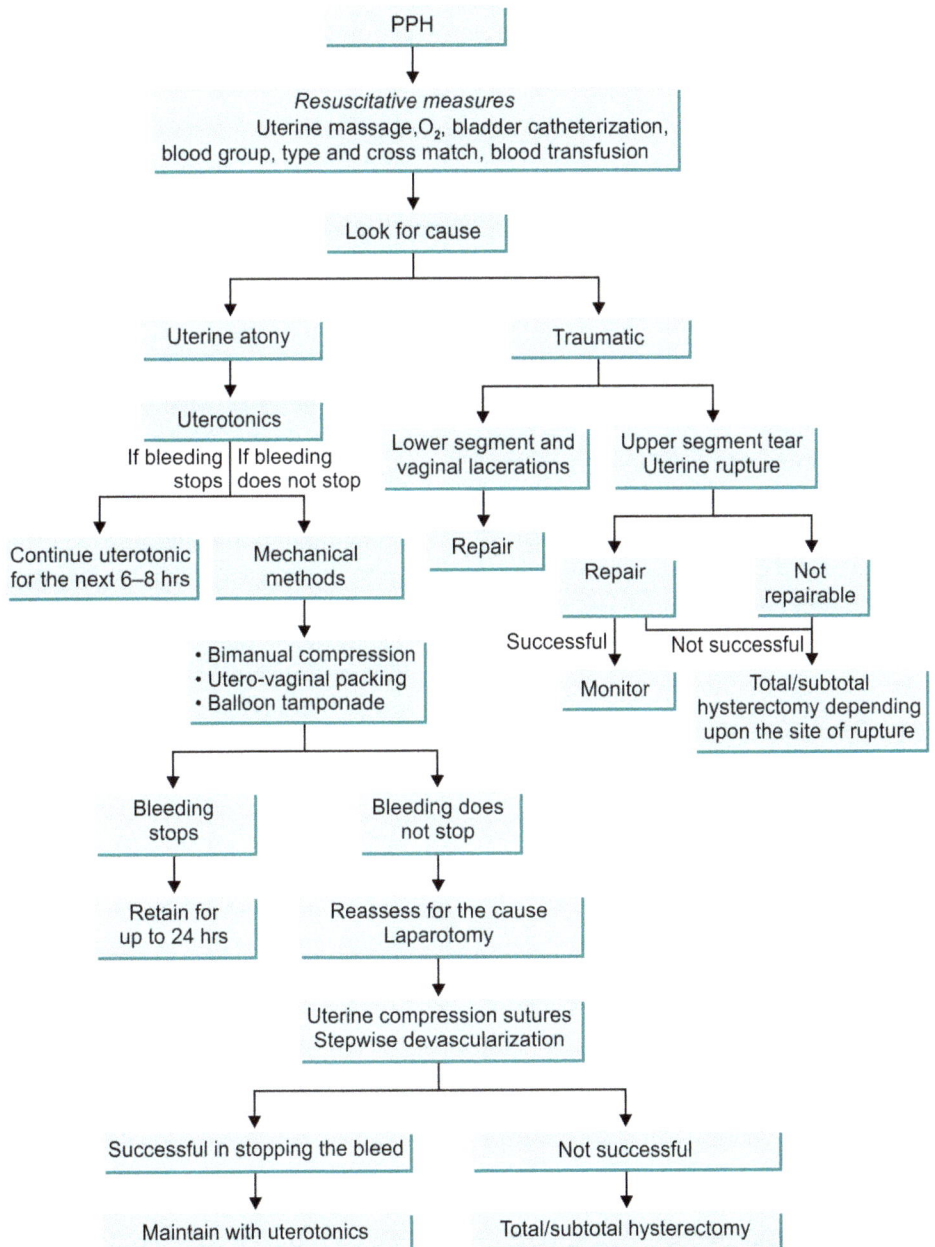

Flowchart 1: Algorithm for PPH management.

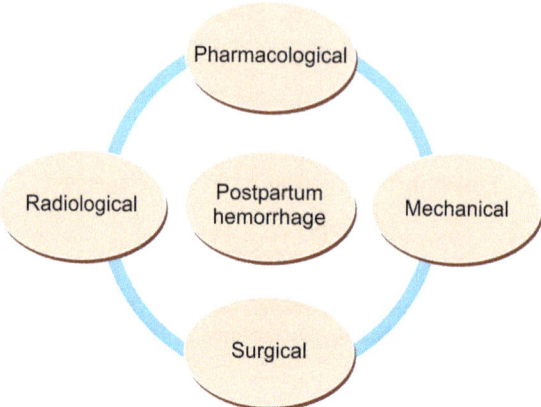

Fig. 1: Management of postpartum hemorrhage.

- Oxygen to be administered
- Foley's catheter to be inserted to measure the urine output
- Continuous monitoring of blood pressure and oxygen saturation
- Administer colloids and crystalloids as required. Fluid overload to be avoided.
- Use of nonpneumatic antishock garment (NASG) is found beneficial.

Pharmacological Methods (Table 3)

Large randomized clinical trials (RCTs) have shown that low-dose intravenous infusions over a period of 1–2 hours are more effective than when given as 10 IU intramuscular. Due to its superior action, oxytocin is considered to be the first line in the PPH prevention and management.[3] Studies have also shown that misoprostol is not as effective as oxytocin in the control of PPH.[17] Routine use of prophylactic oxytocin (RUPO) in a dose of 10 units of oxytocin per 500 mL of normal saline started intravenously after the delivery of the anterior shoulder is a prophylactic measure to reduce blood loss during labor and also decrease the incidence of PPH.[18]

Mechanical Methods

- *Uterine massage*: Manual rubbing of the uterus over the abdominal wall until the uterus hardens or bleeding stops can be routinely done in the immediate postnatal period which can be extended up to 2 hours following vaginal delivery. This is found to be associated with an insignificant reduction of incidence of PPH and a significant reduction in the usage of drugs to contract the uterus.[3]
- *Bimanual uterine compression*: Effective as a temporary measure to stimulate uterine contraction. It can be used following vaginal delivery for PPH management due to uterine atony.
- *Utero-vaginal packing (uterine gauze tamponade)*: Useful in cases of PPH due to uterine atony or persistent bleeding from the placental site in cases of placenta previa or placenta accreta. This tight uterovaginal packing provides a tamponade effect on the open uterine sinuses and thus helps control atonic PPH.[19,20]
- *Intrauterine balloon tamponade*: It can be performed with various devices like Foley's catheter, condom, Bakri balloon,

TABLE 3: Pharmacological management of PPH.

Drug	Group	Dose	Route	Mode of action	Side effects	C/I	ADV/DISADV
Oxytocin	Peptide hormone	10 IU IM or 20–40 IU/LT IV at 250 mL/hr	IM/IV	Through the oxytocin receptor, stimulates the upper uterine segment to contract rhythmically which constricts the spiral arteries and reduces blood flow to the uterus	Antidiuretic effect, hyponatremia	Allergic reaction, genital herpes	Rapid action (within 1–2 mins) temperature to be maintained (2–8°C)
Methergine (methylergonovine)	Semisynthetic ergot alkaloid	0.2 mg can be repeated at 2–4 hrs interval max 1 mg/day	IM	Generalized smooth muscle contraction where in upper and lower uterine segments contract increasing the tone, rate and amplitude of uterine contractions. Sustained and rapid tetanic uterotonic effect	Nausea, vomiting	Preeclampsia and coronary artery diseases	
Prostaglandins	15-methyl PGF2a (carboprost)	0.25 mg repeated every 15 mins for max dose of 2 mg	IM/IV	Enhances uterine contractility and causes vasoconstriction	Nausea, vomiting, diarrhea, headache, flushing	Hypersensitivity, asthma, HTN (relative C/I)	
Misoprostol[14]	Synthetic analog of PGE1	200–1,000 µg (600 µg po) (800 µg sublingual)	Sublingual oral vaginal rectal	Increases uterine tone	Pyrexia, shivering, diarrhea	Hypersensitivity	Long shelf life Stable at room temperature
Tranexamic acid[15]	Antifibrinolytic	1 g/10 mL IV at 10 mL/min over 10 mins 2nd dose after 30 mins	IV	Competitive inhibitor of plasminogen activation by blocking lysine sites. Reduces bleeding by inhibiting breakdown of fibrinogen and blood clots	Headache and diarrhea, fatigue	C/I to antifibrinolytic therapy h/o seizures	Thromboembolism
Carbetocin[16]	Long-acting oxytocin agonist	100 µg	Slow IV	Acts as agonist at peripheral oxytocin receptors mainly at myometrium also functions to thicken the blood	Back pain, chest pain, metallic taste, headache pruritus, hypotension	Allergic reactions, cardiovascular diseases	Room temp stable variant can be stored for up to 36 months at 30°C

Sengstaken–Blakemore catheter, etc. It is effective in the management of atonic PPH though use in cases of traumatic PPH due to extensive vaginal lacerations are also reported.[21,22]

- *Tamponade test*: Described by Condus et al. as a prognostic test for obstetric hemorrhage. When there is no bleeding through the cervix or through the drainage channel of the balloon catheter, the tamponade test is said to be successful upon which it can be retained in place for up to 24 hours. Oxytocin infusion is continued to keep the uterus contracted and antibiotics are administered. The balloon is deflated slowly before removal. This test can be both diagnostic and therapeutic, helps in the identification of cases who require further management. It is found to be effective in controlling hemorrhage in majority of the cases.[22,23]

Surgical Methods

This is employed as the second line in the management of atonic PPH when pharmacological and mechanical methods have proven futile.

- Genital tract lacerations to be identified and repaired accordingly
- *Manual removal of placenta*: It should be performed under anesthesia if the placenta is not expelled from the uterus within 30 mins of delivery of the fetus.[24]
- *Uterine compression sutures*: Pioneered by B-Lynch, these sutures help to achieve hemostasis and also preserve fertility. B-Lynch, Cho, Pereira, Hayman, and Hackethal sutures are some of the compression sutures used in achieving hemostasis.[25] These sutures are effective in achieving hemostasis in approximately 91.7% of cases. The success rates of compression sutures was higher when performed within one hour of delivery in comparison to a delay of more than 2–6 hours or in cases where DIC has already set in (explained in Figs. 2 to 5 and Table 4).[26]
- *Stepwise uterine devascularization*: Done in patients who have not responded to medical or mechanical methods. The steps include:
  - Unilateral uterine artery ligation
  - Bilateral uterine artery ligation
  - Low uterine vessel ligation

B-Lynch suture (brace): To achieve hemostasis in atonic PPH. Salient features of this suture includes:
- Lower uterine segment incision
- Two longitudinal sutures over the surface of the uterus looking like "brace suspenders"
- The whole thickness of both the walls should not be transfixed.

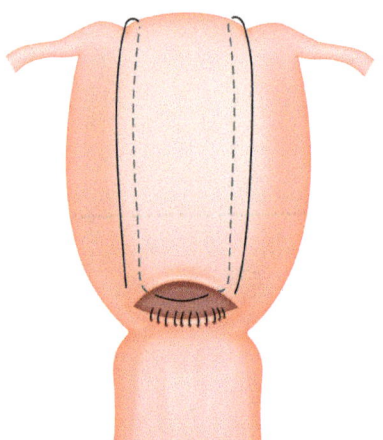

Fig. 2: B-lynch suture.

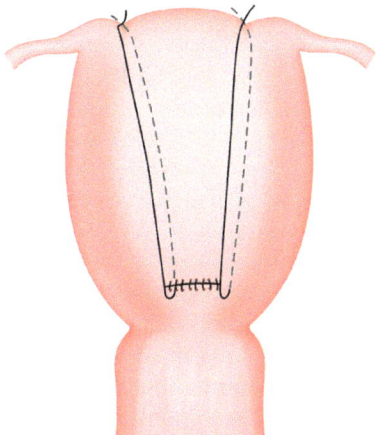

Hayman suture (simple brace): The salient features include:
- The needle transfixes the whole thickness of both anterior and posterior uterine walls at the lower uterine segment level
- The thread is passed over and tied at the fundus to compress it
- Two cervicoisthmic sutures transfixing both the anterior and the posterior cervicoisthmic walls can be done in cases with lower uterine segment bleeding.

Fig. 3: Hayman suture.

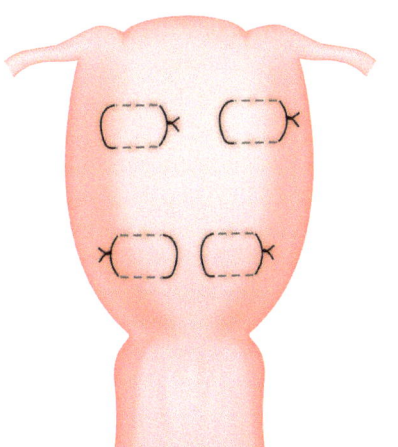

Cho suture (multiple square):
- The suture applied on the uterus from the anterior to the posterior wall and then from the posterior to the anterior wall to approximate the anterior and posterior uterine walls like a square.
- Four to five square sutures may be required to achieve hemostasis in cases of atonic PPH.
- Better hemostasis in lower genital tract bleeding in comparison to other hemostatic sutures.

Fig. 4: Cho suture.

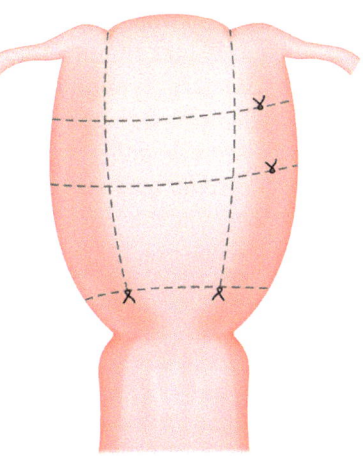

Pereira suture (nonpenetrating multiple transverse and longitudinal):
- Involves wrapping the uterus with many transverse and longitudinal continuous sutures
- Sutures are placed in a circular fashion around the uterus by pricking on the serosa and the subserous myometrium and do not enter the uterine cavity
- The longitudinal sutures are next applied by knotting and fixing the thread at the lowest transverse suture on the dorsal side, going over the fundus and then, knotting on the ventral side
- 2–3 longitudinal and transverse sutures may be required to achieve hemostasis.

Fig. 5: Pereira suture.

TABLE 4: Advantages and disadvantages of compression sutures.

Advantages of compression sutures:	Disadvantages of compression sutures:
<ul><li>Effective in arresting the bleeding</li><li>Helps in preserving future fertility</li><li>Technically less challenging in comparison to arterial ligation and hysterectomy</li></ul>	<ul><li>Need for laparotomy</li><li>Long-term side effects include erosion through the uterine wall, pyometra, uterine necrosis, and Asherman's syndrome</li><li>Not very effective in controlling bleeding from the lower genital tract</li><li>Elective cesarean section might be required for women who have had compression sutures during previous delivery.[27]</li></ul>

- Unilateral ovarian artery ligation
- Bilateral ovarian artery ligation.[28]

Uterine arteries supply about 90% of the uterine blood supply during pregnancy with ovarian and vaginal arteries supplying the remaining 10%. Hence occluding these vessels helps in the control of PPH in cases where medical management has failed.

Uterine artery ligation—After exposing the lower part of the broad ligament, uterine artery is located by feeling the arterial pulsations which are felt near the junction of the uterus and the cervix. The artery is ligated using chromic catgut by passing the needle around the artery and through 2-3 cm of the myometrium. The suture is applied as close to the uterus as possible to prevent ureteric injury.

Ovarian artery ligation—the ligature is placed in the avascular area in the mesovarium around the utero-ovarian arterial anastomosis.[29]

- *Internal iliac artery ligation*: Done in cases of intractable PPH. This is shown to reduce the pelvic blood flow by 49% and pulse pressure by 8%. This reduces the pressures in the arteries to that of venous pressures and can help in achieving hemostasis.[30] After identifying the ureter, peritoneum is dissected and common iliac artery is identified. Internal iliac artery is exposed by blunt dissection, a right angled clamp is applied in close proximity to the artery to prevent internal iliac vein perforation and anterior division of the internal iliac artery is ligated distal to the posterior division after confirming for the presence of femoral artery and dorsalis pedis pulsations. Reported success rates vary from 40% to 100%. Internal artery ligation is more successful in comparison to uterine artery ligation particularly in cases of traumatic PPH like deep forniceal tears, hematomas, uterine rupture, placenta previa.[31]
- Emergency peripartum hysterectomy—subtotal/total (Table 5).

Radiological Methods

- *Uterine artery embolization*: In cases where hemorrhage is not controlled by routine measures and the patient is keen to retain the child-bearing capacity. The procedure involves the introduction of microparticles, polyvinyl alcohol, gel foams, coils, etc. via special catheters to occlude the blood flow to the uterine arteries. This treatment has a success rate of 95% in arresting the hemorrhage and a complication rate of 4.5%.[33] Complications include uterine necrosis, fistula formation, and thromboembolism.[34]
- *Arterial balloon occlusion*: The occlusive balloons are inserted and placed in the internal iliac arteries or in the uterine arteries. These can be inflated in case

TABLE 5: Indications and advantages of subtotal hysterectomy (STH).[32]

Indications	Advantages of STH over TH
• Uterine atony is not managed by other conservative methods • Placenta accreta • Uterine rupture • Vaginal delivery with previous cesarean delivery—15 times higher chance • Rpt cesarean delivery—3.8 times more chance of STH • Grand multiparity >6 • Postpartum thrombin activity <50%	• Lesser operative time • Easier learning curve for the surgeon • Incidence of ureteric injury lesser than TH

there is PPH. Useful in prediagnosed cases of abnormal placentation like placenta accreta, placenta previa, etc.[34]

Transfusion Protocol

- Massive transfusion protocol (MTP) should be initiated when there is uncontrollable hemorrhage or more than 10 units of packed cells may be required.
- Fibrinogen levels of <2 g/L has a good correlation with severe PPH and should be replaced. 30 mL/kg of fresh-frozen plasma (FFP) increases the fibrinogen level by 1 g/L in comparison to 3 mL/kg cryoprecipitate. Also, fibrinogen concentrate of 2 g can be administered intravenously.
- Recombinant activated factor VIIIa 90 µg/kg intravenously can be administered twice in other measures have failed. It requires thromboprophylaxis after the PPH is settled.
- Cell salvage wherever feasible.
- Subsequent thromboprophylaxis may be needed in cases of major PPH or where blood transfusion was required.
- Various studies have shown the ratio of red blood cell (RBC):FFP:Platelets of 6:4:6 to be effective.[35]

■ REFERENCES

1. WHO. Making pregnancy safer: the critical role of the skilled attendant. World health organization. Geneva. 2004.
2. Carroli G, Cuesta C, Abolas E, et al. Epidemiology of postpartum haemorrhage: a systematic review. Best Pract Res Clin Obstet Gynaecol. 2008;22:999-1012.
3. World Health Organization. WHO Recommendations for the prevention and treatment of postpartum haemorrhage. Geneva: WHO; 2012.
4. Cantwell R, Clutton-Brock T, Cooper G, et al. Saving mothers' lives: reviewing maternal deaths to make motherhood safer: 2006-2008. The eighth report of the confidential enquiries into maternal deaths in the United Kingdom. BJOG. 2011;118(Suppl 1):1-203.
5. Chandrahasan E, Krishna A. Diagnosis and management of postpartum haemorrhage. BMJ. 2017;358:j3875.
6. Kumar N. Postpartum haemorrhage; a major killer of woman: review of current scenario. Obstet Gynecol Int J. 2016;4(4):00116.
7. Edhi MM, Aslam HM, Naqvi Z, et al. Postpartum haemorrhage: causes and management. BMC Research Notes. 2013;6:236.
8. Nyflot LT, Sandven I, Stray-pedersen B, et al. Risk factors for severe postpartum haemorrhage: a case-control study. BMC Pregnancy and Childbirth. BMC Series. 2017;17:17.
9. Claroni C, Aversano M, Todde C, et al. Postpartum haemorrhage management: the importance of timing. CME. 2018;12(1):11-5.
10. Carroli G, Mignini L. Episiotomy for vaginal birth. Cochrane Database Syst Rev. 2009;21: CD000081.
11. Buzaglo N, Harlev A, Sergienko R, et al. Risk factors for early postpartum haemorrhage (PPH) in the first vaginal delivery, and obstetrical outcomes of subsequent pregnancy. J Matern Fetal Neonatal Med. 2015;28(8):932-93.

12. ALARM International Program. Fourth edition of the ALARM International Program: Chapter 6. [online] Available from: https://www.glowm.com/pdf/AIP%20Chap1%20SRRH.pdf [Last accessed September, 2019].
13. Pavrd S, Maybury H. How I treat postpartum haemorrhage. Blood. 2015;125:2759-70.
14. Prata N, Weidert K. Efficacy of misoprostol for the treatment of postpartum haemorrhage: current knowledge and implications for health care planning. Int J Womens Health. 2016;8:341-9.
15. Sentilhes L, Lasocki A, Dulcoy-bouthors S, et al. Tranexemeic acid for the prevention and treatment of postpartum haemorrhage. Br J Anaesth. 2015;114(4):576-87.
16. Su LL, Chong YS, Samuel M. Carbetocin for preventing postpartum haemorrhage. Cochrane database Sys Rev. 201215;(2):CDOO5457.
17. Weeks A. The prevention and treatment of postpartum haemorrhage: what do we know, and where do we go next? BJOG. 2015;122:202-12.
18. Kuzume A, Sugumi S, Suga S, et al. The routine use of prophylactic oxytocin in the third stage of labour to reduce maternal blood loss. J Pregnancy. 2017;2017:3274901.
19. Iram Mobusher. Role of uterine packing in control of PPH. PJMHS. 2011;5(3):442-4.
20. Rezk M, Salej S, Shaheen A, et al. Uterine packing versus Foley's catheter for the treatment of postpartum haemorrhage secondary to bleeding tendency in low-resource setting: a four-year observational study. J Matern Fetal Neonatal Med. 2017;30(22):2747-51.
21. Tattersall M, Braithwaite W. Balloon tamponade for vaginal lacerations causing severe postpartum haemorrhage. Br J Obstet Gynecol. 2007;114:647-8.
22. Garg R. Postpartum haemorrhage: Prevention, medical and mechanical methods of management. In: Gandhi A, Malhotra N, Malhotra J, Gupta N, Bora N (Eds). Principles of Critical Care in Obstetrics. New Delhi: Springer; 2016. 153-8.
23. Condous G, Arulkumaran S, Symodns I, et al. The 'Tamponade test' in the management of massive postpartum haemorrhage. Obstet Gynecol. 2003;101:767-72.
24. Urner U, Zimmermann R, Krafft A. Manual removal of the placenta after vaginal delivery: an unsolved problem in obstetrics. J Pregnancy. 2014;2014:274651.
25. Matsubara S, Yano H, Ohkuchi A, et al. Uterine compression sutures for postpartum haemorrhage: an overview. Acta Obstet Gynecol Scand. 2013;92:378-85.
26. Doumouchtsis SK, Papageorghiou AT, Arulkumaran S. Systematic review of conservative management of postpartum haemorrhage: what to do when medical treatment fails. Obstet Gynecol Surv. 2007;62:540-47.
27. Amorim-Costa C, Mota R, Rebelo C, et al. Uterine compression sutures for postpartum haemorrhage: is routine postoperative cavity evaluation needed? Acta Obstet Gynecol Scand. 2011;90:701-6.
28. AbdRabbo SA. Stepwise uterine devascularization: a novel technique for management of uncontrollable postpartum haemorrhage with preservation of uterus. Am J Obstet Gynecol. 1994;171(3):694-700.
29. Atin H, Shyamapada P. Uterine and ovarian arteries ligation: a safe technique to control PPH during caesarean section. J Obstet Gynecol India. 2008;58(4):319-21.
30. Burchell RC. Physiology of internal iliac artery ligation. J Obstet Gynec Brit Cwlth. 1968;75:642-51.
31. Joshi VM, Otiv SR, Majumder R, et al. Internal iliac artery ligation for arresting postpartum haemorrhage. BJOG. 2007;114:356-61.
32. Zhang Y, Yan J, Han Q, et al. Emergency obstetric hysterectomy for life-threatening haemorrhage. Medicine (Baltimore). 2017;96(45):e8443.
33. Ganguli S, Stecker MS, Pune D, et al. Uterine artery embolization in the treatment of postpartum haemorrhage. J Vasc Inter Radiol. 2011;22(2):169-72.
34. El Ayadi AM, Robinson N, Geller S, et al. Advances in the treatment of postpartum haemorrhage. Expert Rev Obstet Gynecol. 2013;8(6):525-37.
35. Dyer RA, Vorster AD, Arcache MJ, et al. New trends in the management of postpartum haemorrhage. Southern African J Anaesth Analg. 2014;20(1):44-7.

CHAPTER 27

Perineal Tears

Nilofer

INTRODUCTION

Lacerations of perineum are the result of overstretching or too rapid stretching of the tissues.

Common in primipara than in multigravida.

1% of all vaginal births.

It is therefore, necessary to inspect the perineum of every parturient woman following a vaginal delivery and suture the tear before transferring her to ward.

ANATOMY

For proper repair of perineal tears, anatomy is very essential.

Perineum is divided into two parts:[1]
1. Anatomical
2. Obstetric

Anatomical

Urogenital Triangle (Anterior Triangle)

- Anteriorly bounded by pubic rami, laterally by ischial tuberosities and posteriorly by superficial transverse perineal muscles.
- It is further divided into compartments by the perineal membrane (Fig. 1).

Superficial Space Colles' Fascia

- Ischiocavernosus muscle
- Bulbocavernosus muscle
- Superficial transverse perineal membrane
- Branches of pudendal vessels and nerve.

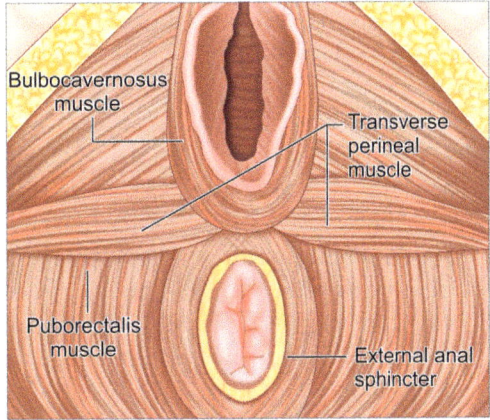

Fig. 1: Anterior and posterior perineal triangle.

Deep Space

- Compressor urethrae
- Urethrovaginal sphincter muscle
- External urethral sphincter
- Internal pudendal artery
- Dorsal nerve and vein of clitoris
- Perineal nerve.

Anal Triangle (Posterior Triangle)

It consists of:
- Ischiorectal fossa bounded anteriorly by posterior border of perineal membrane and posteriorly by sacrotuberous ligament of gluteus maximus.
- Anal canal consists of perineal body anteriorly, laterally by ischiorectal fossa and posteriorly by anococcygeal body.
- Anal sphincter complex.

- Branches of internal pudendal vessels.
- Pudendal nerve.

Obstetric (Perineal Body)

It is the pyramidal shaped area between lower vagina and anal canal. It is the central point where the pelvic floor, perineal muscles, and fascia meet. It measures 4 cm x 4 cm.

It supports perineal organs.

It consists of external anal sphincter (EAS), bulbospongiosus, superficial, and deep transverse perineal muscle.

Anal Sphincters

It is of two types:
1. *External anal sphincter*: It is a striated muscle which is bounded by perineal body anteriorly and coccyx posteriorly. It receives blood supply from inferior rectal artery and nerve supply from inferior anal nerve. Its main function is to relax during defecation.
2. *Internal anal sphincter (IAS)*: It is a smooth muscle. Its main function is to relax prior to defecation. It is innervated by sympathetic S2, S3, and S4 nerve supply.

ETIOLOGY[2,3]

- Asian ethnicity
- *Lack of elasticity of perineal tissue*:
  - Rigidity of the perineum in primipara mainly in elderly.
  - Excessive scarring of the perineum (due to previous surgeries)
  - Friability of the perineum due to edema.
- *Overstretching of the perineum*:
  - Improper management of labor by prolong extension of head.
  - Malpresentations like face to pubis or after coming of head in breech presentation.
  - Forceps delivery.
  - Contracted pelvic outlet.
  - Macrosomic babies.
  - Occipitoposterior delivery.
- Precipitate labor.

Degrees of Perineal Tears (RCOG 2007)[4]

- *First-degree tear*—injury to perineal skin and/or vaginal mucosa (Fig. 2).
- *Second-degree tear*—injury to perineum involving perineal muscles but not involving the anal sphincter (Fig. 3).
- *Third-degree tear*—injury to perineum involving the anal sphincter complex (Fig. 4):
  - Grade 3a tear: Less than 50% of EAS thickness torn.
  - Grade 3b tear: More than 50% of EAS thickness torn.
  - Grade 3c tear: Both EAS and IAS torn
- *Fourth-degree tear*: Injury to perineum involving the anal sphincter complex (EAS and IAS) and anorectal mucosa (Fig. 5).

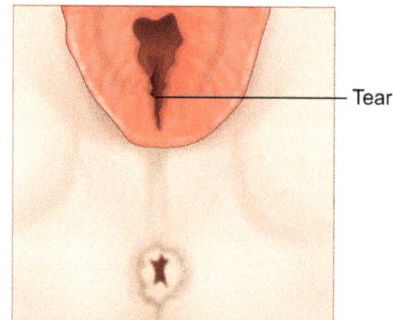

Fig. 2: First-degree perineal tear.

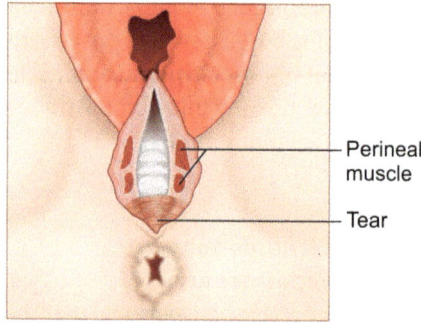

Fig. 3: Second-degree perineal tear.

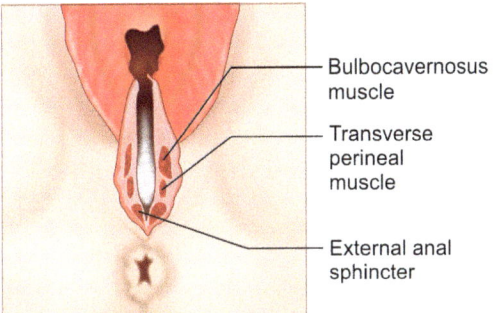

Fig. 4: Third-degree perineal tear.

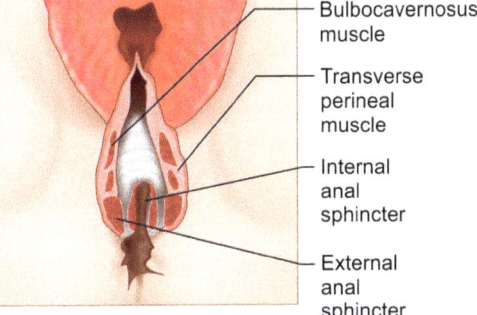

Fig. 5: Fourth-degree perineal tear.

- *Obstetric anal sphincter injuries (OASIS)*—encompass both third and fourth degree perineal tears.

PREDICTION AND PREVENTION[5]

- Mediolateral episiotomy in instrumental deliveries.
- Warm compression during second stage of labor reduces the risk.
- Perineal massage during the last months of pregnancy enables perineal tissue to expand more easily during birth.
- Perineal support during second stage.

MANAGEMENT

First and Second Degree Tear Repair

Recent perineal tears should be repaired immediately or within 24 hours of the delivery. By doing early repair, it reduces the chances of infection and minimizes the blood loss.

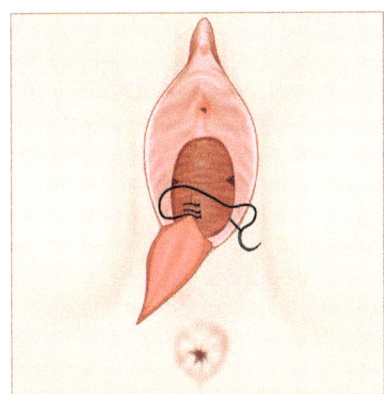

Fig. 6: Closure of vaginal mucosa.

The procedure has to be carried out under aseptic conditions in the operating room with the patient in the lithotomy position.

The preferred suture material is rapidly absorbing polyglactin.

- *First degree*: It is repaired under local anesthesia with proper light exposure. The bleeding tears are identified and ligated. The stitching starts from apex of the vaginal mucosa with continuous locked or interrupted sutures followed by muscle and skin with interrupted sutures.
- *Second degree*: It is also done under local infiltration. The perineal muscle is identified and approximated by interrupted sutures including the torn ends of levator ani followed by vaginal mucosa, muscle, and skin (Figs. 6 to 8).

Obstetrical Anal Sphincter Injuries: Third and Fourth Degree Repairs[6,7]

Repair should be done within 24 hours of delivery or if delayed then repair after 6 weeks. A written consent has to be taken. Repair is done in operation theater under general or spinal anesthesia.

The rectal and anal mucosa is sutured from above downward by interrupted sutures with knots buried inside.

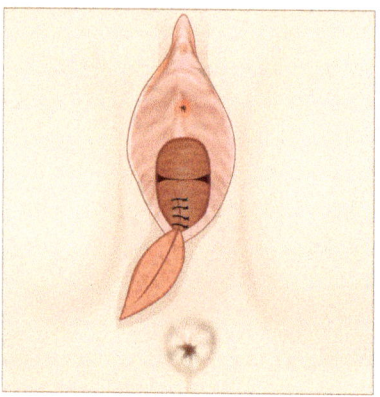

Fig. 7: Closure of vaginal mucosa and perineal muscles.

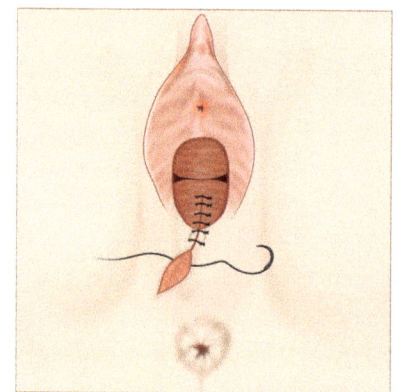

Fig. 8: Approximation of the skin edges.

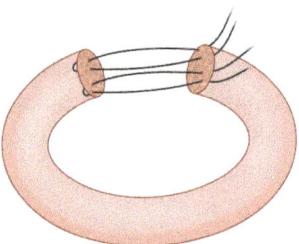

End to end anastomosis

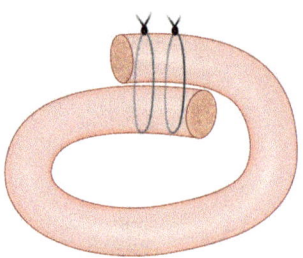

Overlapping anastomosis

Fig. 9: Suturing of external anal sphincter either by end to end or by overlapping method.

The edges of the torn IAS are identified and repair is done by interrupted mattress sutures preferably 3-0.

The torn ends of the external anal sphincter are identified and the edges are held with allis clamp and approximated with interrupted sutures preferably with 2-0 either with overlapping technique or end-to-end technique (Fig. 9). Next levator ani muscles are approximated and sutured followed by vaginal mucosa, perineal muscles, and skin.

After the repair, a rectal examination must be performed to check for any additional injuries that may have been missed and that sutures have not been inadvertently inserted into the anorectal mucosa. If a suture is found, it is safer to remove it so as to minimize the risk of formation of anorectal–vaginal fistula.

Suturing of external anal sphincter either by end to end or by overlapping method (Fig. 9)

POSTOPERATIVE MANAGEMENT[8,9]

- Area should be dry and clean
- Liquid diet for next 24 hours followed by soft diet
- Sitz bath twice daily
- Laxatives
- Antibiotic coverage
- Analgesics
- To avoid intercourse for 2 months.
- Pelvic floor exercises after 3 months of repair.

FOLLOW-UP AND FUTURE DELIVERIES[10]

- Inspection of the perineum.
- Information regarding the symptoms of anal incontinence, if any.

- Counseling regarding the risk of anal incontinence with subsequent deliveries.
- Subsequent deliveries are better by cesarean section for the women who had third or fourth degree perineal tears.
- If there is persistent incontinence of flatus and stools then endoanal ultrasound or transperineal ultrasound or MRI is done to rule out any residual defects.[11]

REFERENCES

1. Cunningham F, Leveno J, Bloom L, et al. Williams Obstetrics. Maternal Anatomy, 23rd edn. New York: Mcgraw Hill Professional; 2009.
2. De leeuw JW, Struijk PC, Vierhout ME, et al. Risk factors for third degree perineal ruptures during delivery. BJOG. 2001;108:383-7.
3. Smith LA, Price N, Simonite V, et al. Incidence of and risk factors for perineal trauma: a prospective observational study. BMC Pregnancy Childbirth. 2013;13:59.
4. Royal College of Obstetricians and Gynaecologists. Guideline no 29, clinical green top guidelines. Classification and terminology. 2015.
5. Royal College of Obstetricians and Gynaecologists. Guideline no 29, clinical green top guidelines. Perineal protection, 2015.
6. Royal College of Obstetricians and Gynaecologists. Guideline no 29, clinical green top guidelines. Management of third and fourth degree perineal tears following vaginal deliveries, June 2015.
7. Aigmueller T, Umek W, Elenskaia K, et al. Guidelines for the management of third and fourth degree perineal tears after vaginal birth from the Austrian urogynecology working group. Int Urogynecol J. 2013;24:553-8.
8. Virkud A. Maternal obstetric injuries. Postoperative care. Modern Obstetrics, 1st edition: 63:364.
9. Royal College of Obstetricians and Gynaecologists. Guideline no 29, clinical green top guidelines. Postoperative management, June 2015.
10. Royal College of Obstetricians and Gynaecologists. Guideline no 29, clinical green top guidelines. Future deliveries. 2015.
11. Sultan AH, Thakar R. Lower genital tract and anal spinchter trauma. Best pract Res Clin Obstet Gynecol. 2002;16:99-115.

CHAPTER 28

Vaginal Birth after Cesarean Section

Sonal Agarwal

INTRODUCTION

Pregnancy with prior cesarean delivery is called postcesarean pregnancy. This is quite prevalent these days in obstetric practice due to liberalization of primary cesarean section with nonrecurrent indications. Management of woman with a prior cesarean delivery is one of the controversial issues in modern obstetrics. It was believed in past that scarred uterus is a contraindication for labor due to fear of uterine rupture. This concept changed with the method of operation from classical vertical uterine incision to transverse uterine incision introduced by Kerr in 1921. Milestone year was 1978 in history of obstetrics when Merrill and Gibbs at San Antonio concluded that vaginal delivery was successful in 83% of cases with prior cesarean deliveries. This was an enlightenment to put a break to cesarean deliveries as cesarean delivery rates were increasing day-by-day. To put a snap to this escalation, the American College of Obstetricians and Gynecologists (ACOG) recommended that woman should be counseled to attempt labor in subsequent pregnancy with one previous low-transverse cesarean delivery in absence of contraindication.[1]

COUNSELING

Counseling is an integral part of any procedure to be undertaken. Couple should be informed properly of all risks, benefits, and consequences regarding any treatment. If there is a history of uterine rupture, then what is required should be properly explained to the couple. Recurrence rate of rupture or dehiscence during labor is 6%, if it is confined to lower segment. It increases to 32%, if upper segment is involved. Such patients should not to go into labor. They should be delivered by repeat C-section at not more than 36 weeks of gestation.[2] As compared to vaginal delivery, cesarean delivery has increased anesthesia risks, hemorrhage, damage to bladder, pelvic infection, scarring, etc. Irrespective of such complications, elective repeat cesarean section is preferred by many women. Reasons for such preference are convenience of scheduling the date and time of delivery and potential fear of a prolonged and painful labor. Abitbol et al. studied 312 women by analyzing their choices after extensive counseling.[3] Of the 312 women, 125 (40%) opted for a repeat cesarean. Extensive counseling thus has a major role in opting for vaginal delivery after cesarean section or not.

HISTORY TAKING FOR CASES WITH PRIOR CESAREAN DELIVERY

- Previous obstetric history should be recorded with more significance on number of deliveries and the method of delivery.
- History of interdelivery interval to be taken.
- Whether that cesarean section was an elective or emergency one.

- What was the stage of labor when it was done.
- History of puerperal infection, wound infection, or resuturing should be taken.

GENERAL AND PHYSICAL EXAMINATION

- Before reaching to a decision, general and systemic examination should be done.
- In abdominal examination, uterine ovoid, hernia sites and details of scar in respect to type, length, and healing should be properly inspected.
- Assessment of fetal lie, presentation, amount of liquor, and fetal weight should be done before deciding for trial of labor.

INFORMED CONSENT

Woman cannot be forced to undergo trial of labor. Risks and benefits of it should be discussed and explained. The American Academy of Pediatrics[4] and the ACOG have recommended that following points should be well addressed:
- Advantages of successful vaginal delivery (short stay, rapid recovery, and less pain)
- Contraindications to trial of labor
- About 1% risk of uterine rupture
- If rupture occurs, there is 10-25% risk of significant adverse fetal complications
- Increased risk of uterine rupture with ≥ 2 prior cesarean delivery
- Risk increases with induction of labor and attempts at cervical ripening
- Perinatal death and permanent neonatal injury are very rare but can occur and this should be explained.

SELECTION CRITERIA FOR TRIAL OF LABOR–VAGINAL BIRTH AFTER CESAREAN (ACOG GUIDELINES)

- Patient consent
- About ≤ 1 prior low transverse cesarean delivery
- Adequate pelvis (assessed clinically)
- Negative history for uterine rupture or scar dehiscence
- Nonrecurrent indication of previous cesarean section
- Senior doctor available for performing emergency cesarean delivery and managing complications
- Blood products available in case of emergency
- Availability of anesthetist
- Labor monitoring equipment is available.

Risks and Benefits of Trial of Labor and Repeat Cesarean Delivery

Levero et al. reported that vaginal birth after cesarean (VBAC) was more riskier than thought of.[5] Scott et al. suggested an alternate viewpoint on mandatory trial of labor based on 12 cases of uterine rupture. There were many other cases of mortality and morbidity reported worldwide and thus these became a concern about safety. Risks and benefits of vaginal birth after cesarean section have been illustrated in Box 1. Uterine rupture and associated complications are there in trial of labor but this should not stop clinicians to attempt VBAC. The absolute risk of uterine rupture is calculated as 7 per 1,000 cases in a study of 18,000 women attempting trial of labor.

Box 1: Risk and benefits of VBAC.

Risks associated with VBAC:
- Failed trial of labor
- Uterine rupture
- Need of emergency cesarean section
- Hemorrhage leading to hysterectomy

Benefits of vaginal birth after cesarean section:
- Maternal morbidity is decreased
- Hospital stay duration is decreased
- Decreased need of blood transfusion
- Decreased risk of abnormal placentation
- Need of successive cesarean delivery is nullified

Suitable Candidates for Trial of Labor

The ACOG practice guidelines say that more cautious approach should be there when VBAC is attempted. Several factors are important for evaluation of women for trial of labor for attempting VBAC.

Factors Affecting Success of Trial of Labor

- Women who have history of vaginal birth have 9–28 times more chances of successful VBAC with success rates of 83–95%.
- History of prior VBAC is the best predictor of success with 87–90% success rates approximately.
- About 50–60% chances with large for gestational age or macrosomic fetus. Elkousy et al. found statistically significant increase in uterine rupture rates amongst women without prior vaginal delivery with fetus >4,000 g.[6] Such cases should not be encouraged.
- Obese and elderly women have lower rates of success.
- Prior lower segment cesarean section (LSCS) due to breech presentation has higher success rates of about 89%.
- On admission, cervical dilatation of more than 4 cm has higher success rates (86%).
- Bishop score >8.
- Spontaneous onset of labor in the present pregnancy has higher success.
- Nonrecurring indications such as breech presentation, fetal distress, and fetal macrosomia.

Absolute Contraindications for Trial of Labor—VBAC[7]

- Prior classic, T-shaped incision
- History of transmural/intrauterine surgery
- Contracted pelvis
- Previous rupture or scar dehiscence
- Nonreassuring fetal status
- Previous two LSCS
- Medical or obstetric complications (preeclampsia, malpresentation, and placenta previa) precluding vaginal delivery
- Patient consent not there
- Unavailability of blood products and anesthetist.

Relative Contraindications

- Women having single layer uterine closure in prior cesarean delivery compared to double layer closure.
- Augmentation of labor [with high-dose oxytocin (>20 mU/min)]
- Interpregnancy interval <24 months.

Prerequisites[8]

- Per speculum and per vaginal examination should be done under aseptic precautions at 36 completed weeks of gestation to look for cervical dilatation and effacement, presentation, flexion, and station of presenting part.
- Status of membranes should be notified.
- Rule out cephalopelvic disproportion.
- Consent for possible cesarean hysterectomy in placenta accreta cases.
- Reserve blood.
- Trial of labor should be done electively in day time in presence of senior doctor and anesthesiologist.
- Crash cesarean operative tray, which has all instruments needed to deliver the baby.
- Practice of fire drills with motive of having shortest time interval should be done.

INDUCTION OF LABOR IN CASES WITH PREVIOUS CESAREAN DELIVERY

Spontaneous labor is preferred than induction of labor. Labor can either be planned as elective case or can be induced due to some indication.

Induction is indicated when it says that benefits to maternal and fetal health are more versus continuing pregnancy.

Advantages of Elective Induction

It helps in proper planning and coordination between staff and hospital. Cervical ripening can be done by many ways for induction of labor.

Disadvantages

Iatrogenic prematurity is there plus very few studies have been done till now.

Always wait for spontaneous labor beyond 40 weeks period of gestation in VBAC candidates. At 41 weeks, induction should be done in women who have favorable cervix, adequate pelvis according to clinical pelvimetry and estimated fetal weight of <4,000 g.

Methods of Induction of Labor

- Oxytocin
- Prostaglandin-E2
- Mifepristone
- Misoprostol.

Oxytocin

Oxytocin can be used for induction and augmentation of labor both, if cervix is favorable. Close monitoring is essential. Standard regimens can be used safely for successful VBAC rates.[9]

Dose of oxytocin:
- Start with 0.4 mu/mL and increase dose of oxytocin every 30 minutes till the patient has adequate contraction that is at least 3 contractions in 10 minutes, each lasting for at least 45 minutes. Maximum dose of 22.8 mu/mL can be used.

- Goetzl et al. observed relation between total oxytocin dose and duration of induction labor and risk of rupture associated with it. Though it was not significant, it directly correlated with rupture rates. The American Academy of Pediatrics and the ACOG (2002) guidelines say that with strict patient monitoring, oxytocin can be used for both induction and augmentation of labor in women undergoing trial of labor. Rate of uterine rupture with different modes of labor[10] is depicted in Table 1.

Prostaglandins-E2 (Dinoprostone)

Only maximum one dose can be used for ripening. Risk of uterine rupture is 1.3% with it and thus there should be a valid reason and compelling indication to use it. Proper counseling[11] and consent should be taken prior to induction (ACOG). Ravasia and colleagues in 2000 made a comparison between rupture rates amongst prostaglandins[12] induced labor and spontaneous labor and found higher uterine rupture rates in the former group (2.9% vs. 0.5%).

Misoprostol

The ACOG contraindicates use of misoprostol because of 5.6% incidence of scar rupture.

Mifepristone

Not much evaluated.

Membrane Stripping

It is done at 38 weeks and repeated, if patient has not delivered yet till next visit. About 1 cm

TABLE 1: Rate of uterine rupture.

Mode of labor	Rate of uterine rupture (%)
Spontaneous	0.4%
Augmented	1%
Induced	2.3%

minimum dilatation of cervix is needed for stripping. It causes increase in phospholipase A2 activity and prostaglandin F2 alpha (PGF2α) levels and causes greater frequency of spontaneous labor and lesser postdated deliveries. Amniotomy with oxytocin augmentation can also be tried, if cervix is ripened and bishop score is > 8.

In cases of unripened cervix, cervical dilatation with Foley's bulb can be attempted.[13]

When to Hospitalize Electively

- *38th week*: To assess cases and formulate line of treatment in cases with previous history of lower segment operation.
- *36th week*: Cases with previous history of classical cesarean section or hysterotomy as risk of rupture more during last 4 weeks of pregnancy.

Monitoring of labor is given in Box 2.

ROLE OF MRI AND DOPPLER IN DIAGNOSING MORBIDLY ADHERENT PLACENTA ACCRETA

Risk of placenta previa accreta in women with history of previous cesarean section is about 30%. Antenatal imaging with magnetic resonance imaging (MRI), color flow Doppler, and power amplitude ultrasonic angiography should be done to make an assessment of deep myometrial, parametrial, and bladder involvement. Doppler ultrasonography gives a sensitivity of 82.4% and specificity of 96.8%. The positive and negative predictive values are 87.5 and 95.3%, respectively.[16]

FACTORS AFFECTING INTEGRITY OF THE SCAR

Scar integrity in classical or hysterotomy scar and lower segment transverse incision is given in Table 2.

Box 2: Monitoring of labor.

- Oral/written consent
- Check for prerequisites
- Intravenous line and blood for cross matching
- Liquid diet only and fluid replacement
- Maternal pulse rate and blood pressure monitoring every half hourly and 2 hourly respectively
- Oxytocin titration and partograph charting
- Electronic fetal heart rate monitoring or intermittent auscultation every half hour in latent labor, every 15 minutes in first stage and after each contraction in second stage of labor[14]
- Vigilant for nonreassuring pattern, severe variable decelerations, prolonged decelerations, or bradycardia
- Epidural analgesia up to 6 cm of dilation but risky as it masks the signs and symptoms of scar dehiscence[15]
- Never use mid-cavity forceps
- Outlet forceps or vacuum can be applied if second stage ≥1 hour
- Digital exploration to be done only in cases with continuous and excessive vaginal bleeding and maternal hypotension in spite of well-contracted uterus
- Surgical correction of scar dehiscence is done only, if significant uncontrollable bleeding is there
- Observation for at least four hours in labor room after delivery.

- Previous operative notes
- *Indication of previous cesarean section:* Placenta previa and prolonged labor are two indications in which scar is weak due to imperfect apposition, thrombosis of placental sinuses, and increased chances of sepsis
- History of lateral extension or tears involving uterine vessels or colporrhexis
- Wedge depression of more than 5 mm may be seen on hysterography in inter-conceptional time
- Complicated twin pregnancy with polyhydramnios
- Placenta previa in the present pregnancy may weaken the scar
- Assessment of uterine scar with ultrasonography.

TABLE 2: Differences between classical and lower segment scar.

	Classical/hysterotomy scar	Lower segment scar
Apposition	Thick muscle layer is difficult to appose. Fibrosis occurs in pockets filled with blood later on. Formation of gutter on inner surface is there	Thin cut margins are better for apposition
State of uterus during healing	Due to contraction and retraction, suture becomes loose leading to imperfect healing	Inert so healing is better
Stretching effect	At right angle to scar	Along the line of scar
Placental implantation in future pregnancy	The placenta is more likely to implant on scar and weakened by trophoblastic penetration or herniation of the amniotic sac through gutter	Unlikely
Scar	Rupture may occur both during pregnancy and labor (4–9%)	Rupture may occur during labor (0.2–1.5%)
Mortality	Maternal death—5% Perinatal death—6 in 8	Maternal death—less Perinatal death—1 in 8

MANAGEMENT OF PREGNANT WOMAN WITH PRIOR CESAREAN SECTION

Management of pregnant woman with prior cesarean section has been given in Flowchart 1.

EFFECTS OF PREVIOUS CESAREAN SECTION ON PREGNANCY AND LABOR

Course of pregnancy is not altered but following complications may occur such as:
- Abortion
- Preterm labor
- Normal pregnancy ailments
- Incidental morbidity and operative interference
- Placenta previa
- Adherent placenta (placenta accreta)
- Postpartum hemorrhage
- Peripartum hysterectomy.

COMPLICATIONS OF AN UNSUCCESSFUL VBAC: TRIAL OF LABOR

- Increased maternal morbidity
- Increased duration of stay in hospital
- Increased risk of hemorrhage
- Need for blood transfusion
- Increased chances of repeat cesarean delivery in future pregnancies
- *Abnormal placentation risk*: Incidence of placenta previa with accreta increases from 3% to 61% from previous one to four cesarean section, respectively
- Increased risk of wound dehiscence and uterine rupture (0.5–1%)
- Increased risk of hysterectomy due to uterine rupture
- Increased risk of infections[17]
- Perinatal complications such as low Apgar score, hypoxic ischemic encephalopathy, admission to neonatal intensive care unit (NICU), still birth, and neonatal death are there.

Complications in Pregnancy with Previous Cesarean Section

Uterine Rupture

Classification of uterine rupture is given in Table 3.

Symptoms of Uterine Rupture

- Pain in incision site or lower abdomen which can range from mild to severe

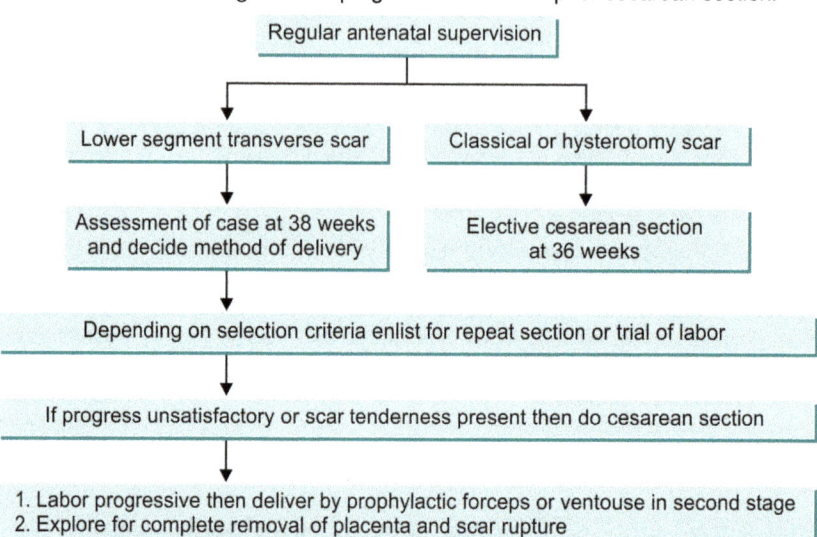

Flowchart 1: Management of pregnant woman with prior cesarean section.

Complete rupture	Incomplete or partial rupture or uterine dehiscence
All layers of uterine wall are separated	Uterine muscle is separated
Breech in visceral peritoneum present	Visceral peritoneum is intact
Extrusion of intrauterine contents in abdominal cavity	Extrusion of intrauterine contents into the broad ligament

TABLE 3: Differences between complete and incomplete uterine rupture.

intensity with tearing sensation. Shoulder pain may be associated
- Decreasing intensity and frequency of uterine contractions
- Dizziness and weakness
- Hematuria.

Signs
- Distension and tenderness on abdomen
- Uterine contour is not appreciable properly
- Fetal parts are palpated superficially and cardiac activity is absent
- Hematuria and bladder tenesmus may be present
- Recession of presenting part per vaginum and sudden cessation of uterine contractions

- Maternal tachycardia
- Tenderness on incision site
- Persistent prolonged or variable decelerations (most specific)
- Meconium stained liquor.

Features of Scar Rupture or Scar Dehiscence[18] during Labor (RCOG 2007)
- Abnormal cardiotocography is the most consistent finding (55–87%)
- Suprapubic pain persisting in between contractions
- Shoulder tip/chest pain or sudden onset of shortness of breath
- Acute onset of scar tenderness
- Abnormal vaginal bleeding or hematuria
- Cessation of adequate uterine contractions

- Loss of presenting part
- Maternal tachycardia/hypotension/shock.

Early diagnosis of scar dehiscence or rupture, if handled as an emergency case will obviously reduce maternal and perinatal morbidity and mortality.

Elicitation of Scar Tenderness

Lower part of uterus between suprapubic region and symphysis pubis should be palpated while patient is engaged in some conversation. Look for wincing on palpation. During labor, it should be elicited during relaxation of uterus and not during contraction.

Risk Factors for Uterine Rupture during Trial of Labor

Risk factors are given in Box 3.
- *Type of incision*: Highest rate of rupture has been reported with incisions extending into fundus that is classical incision. Classical scar can rupture even before onset of labor. Chauhan in 2002 reported one case of complete uterine rupture prior to onset of labor and 15 cases had uterine dehiscence. In women with uterine malformations who have undergone cesarean delivery, the risks for uterine rupture in a subsequent pregnancy are approximately equal to that of classical incision. The ACOG (2004) concluded that women with a prior vertical incision in the lower uterine segment without fundal extension may be candidates for VBAC but there is limited evidence. Whereas prior classical or T-shaped uterine incision is considered as a contraindication to VBAC. Thus, it is very important to make a proper documentation of operative delivery notes for subsequent decision making. Extent of vertical uterine incision in previous delivery should be written in file properly so that no misjudgment occurs by subsequent surgeons.

Box 3: Risk factors for uterine rupture.

Types of uterine incision in previous delivery—estimated percentage of rupture%
- Classical 4–9%
- T-shaped 4–9%
- Low vertical 1–7%
- Low transverse 0.2–1.5%.

Interdelivery interval: 2.3% risk if interval is less than 18 months

Postpartum fever after cesarean: Threefold increased chances of rupture recurrence. Leads to poor wound healing

Uterine anomalies: 8% risk in bicornuate, unicornuate, didelphic, and septate uterus versus 0.6% in women without anomalies

Closure of prior incision: Single layer uterus closure is less prone to rupture

Thickness of previous scar:
- >4.5 mm 0%
- 3.6–4.5 mm 0.6%
- 2.6–3.5 mm 6.6%
- ≤2.5 mm 9.8%

Induction and augmentation of labor

Number of previous cesarean deliveries
- 1–0.7%
- ≥2–1.4%

- *Interdelivery interval*: Risk of uterine rupture increases, if previous scar is not given sufficient time to heal. Studies done with MRI suggest that complete involution of uterus and restoration of anatomy require at least 6 months. Shipp et al. examined interdelivery interval and uterine rupture incidence in 2,409 women and deciphered that duration of 18 months or less was associated with a threefold risk of uterine rupture.[19]
- *Closure of prior incision*: Chapman et al. found no correlation between one or two layer closure and subsequent risk of uterine rupture. According to Mercer and Durnwald, uterine dehiscence has been found to be more common after single-layer closure.[20] Double-layer closure consists of running-lock suture followed by running, nonlocking imbricating suture. In spite of so many evidences, no such

recommendation is there to recommend one particular type of closure.[21]
- *Number of prior cesarean deliveries*: The risk of uterine rupture increases with the number of previous cesarean deliveries. The ACOG recommends VBAC to be attempted only in cases with one prior vaginal delivery amongst women with two prior low-transverse cesarean deliveries.
- *Healing of the uterine wound*: Uterus heals by muscular fiber regeneration and not by development of scar tissue. *Fibroblast proliferation may also be there*. If apposition of margins is perfect, uterine wound is healed by muscles and connective tissues.[22] Factors affecting wound healing are as follows:
    - Imperfect margin apposition
    - Sepsis
    - Hematoma in wound
    - Poor general health condition
    - Excessive stretching of lower segment
    - Decreased vascularity.

MANAGEMENT

Exploratory laparotomy with repair, if feasible and hemostasis can be achieved. Wounds should be approximated properly.[23] If repair is not possible, extension is there into broad ligament vessels, presence of placenta accreta, uncontrollable uterine hemorrhage and patient has completed the family, then hysterectomy should be opted for.[24] In one meta-analysis by Mozurkewich and Hutton in 2000, it was concluded that half women undergoing trial of labor required blood transfusion or hysterectomy undergoing trial of labor as compared to those undergoing elective repeat cesarean delivery. Landon et al. in 2004 observed that risks of blood transfusion and infection were significantly greater for women attempting trial of labor. Failed trial of labor has more chances of major complications as compared to successful VBAC.

PROGNOSIS

Woman is more vulnerable to rupture of uterus late during pregnancy or during labor. Maternal mortality can reach up to 5% with perinatal mortality to 75%. If proper selection of patients for trial of labor and stringent monitoring done then prognosis is quite good and there is equal success rate with planned VBAC and elective repeat cesarean section. Places where meticulous observation and management of complications are not possible then liberal repeat cesarean section offers better prognosis.

Maternal Morbidity and Mortality

Vast majority of maternal deaths is due to hemorrhage, preeclampsia, amniotic fluid embolism, thromboembolism, surgical complications, and uterine rupture. Maternal mortality is high when there is unsuccessful VBAC. There is insignificant difference between a planned VBAC and elective cesarean section.

Perinatal Mortality and Morbidity

Planned vaginal birth after cesarean section carries an additional risk of 2–3/10,000 perinatal birth when compared to elective repeat cesarean section (ERCS). This is similar to risk for women having their first birth. VBAC has 10 in 10,000 risk of antepartum still birth beyond 39 weeks of gestation and 4 in 10,000 risk of perinatal death. Incidence of intrapartum hypoxic ischemic encephalopathy is more in planned VBAC as compared to ERCS. Whereas, VBAC reduces risk of transient tachypnea of newborn and respiratory distress syndrome.[25]

Sterilization

Couples should be counseled about risks of further pregnancies after ≥2 cesarean section.[26] To further stop such complications, sterilization option should be given and emphasized upon before attempting third time cesarean delivery.

Different Situations

Role of External Cephalic Version in Scarred Uterus

Some studies suggest that this will not likely affect uterine rupture rates but more studies are required pertaining to it.

Role of VBAC in Twins

Safety of VBAC has no differences between singleton gestation and twins but these findings are not yet confirmed with larger sample sizes.

Role of VBAC with Preterm Birth

Planned preterm VBAC has similar success rates to term VBAC but with a lower risk of uterine rupture.

CONCLUSION

Maximum cases of previous CS done for nonrecurrent indications can be delivered safely by the vaginal route with least chances of any major complication to both mother and neonate. The utmost pre-requisite is that such deliveries should be conducted in well-equipped institution having facilities for emergency ceserean section.

REFERENCES

1. American College of Obstetricians and Gynaecologist. ACOG Practice Bulletin No 54: Vaginal birth after previous Cesarean delivery. Obstet Gynecol. 2004;104:203-12.
2. Wagner M. Choosing caesarean section. Lancet. 2000;356:1677-80.
3. Abitbol MM, Castillo I, Taylor UB, et al. Vaginal birth after cesarean section: the patient's point of view. Am Fam Physician. 1993;47:129-34.
4. American Academy of Pediatrics, the American College of Obstetricians and Gynecologists. Guidelines for Perinatal Care, 5th edition. Elk Grove, Ill: American Academy of Pediatrics; 2002.
5. Hibbard JH, Gilbert S, Landon MB, et al. Increased success of trail of labor after previous vaginal birth after cesarean. Obstet Gynecol. 2006;108:125-33.
6. Elkousy MA, Sameul M, Steven E, et al. The effect of weight on vaginal birth after cesarean delivery success rate. Am J Obstet Gynecol. 2003;188:824-30.
7. Maudin JG, Newman RB. Prior cesarean: a contraindication to labor indication? Clin Obstet Gynecol. 2006;49(3):684-97.
8. American College of Obstetricians and Gynecologists. Committee Opinion No. 271: Induction of labor for vaginal birth after cesarean delivery. Obstet Gynecol. 2002;99: 679-80.
9. Goelze L, Shipp TD, Zelop CM, et al. Oxytocin dose and risk of uterine rupture in trail of labor after cesarean section. Obstet Gynecol. 2001;97:381-84.
10. Zelop CM, Shipp TD, Repke JJ, et al. Uterine rupture during or augmented labor in gravid women with one cesarean delivery. Am J Obstet Gynecol. 1999;18:882-6.
11. Benjamin P. VBAC: Contemporary issues. Clin Obstet Gynecol. 2001;44(3):553-629.
12. Flamm BL, Anton D, Goings JR, et al. Prostaglandin E2 for cervical ripening: a multicenter study of patients with previous cesarean delivery. Am J Perinatol.1997;14: 157-60.
13. Bujold E, Blackwell SC, Gaudier F, et al. Cervical ripening with transcervical Foley catheter and the risk of uterine rupture. Obstet Gynecol. 2004;103:18-23.
14. Thacker SB, Stroup D, Chang M. Continuous electronic heart rate monitoring for fetal assessment during labor. Cochrane Database Syst Rev. 2001;2:CD000063.
15. Yost NP, Bloom SL, Sibley MK, et al. A hospital-sponsored quality improvement study of pain management after cesarean delivery. Am J Obstet Gynecol. 2004;190:1341-6.
16. Chou MM, Ho ES, Lee YH. Prenatal diagnosis of placenta praevia accret by transabdominal color Doppler Ultrasound. Ultrasound Obstet. Gynecol. 2000;15:28-35.
17. Vermillion ST, Lamoutte C, Soper DE, et al. Wound infection after cesarean: Effect of subcutaneous tissue thickness. Obstet Gynecol. 2000;95:923-6.

18. Royal College of Obstetricians and Gynecologists: Clinical green top guidelines No. 45 Feb 2007. (2007). Birth after previous cesarean birth. [online] Available from: http://www.jsog.org/GuideLines/Birth_after_previous_caesarean_birth.pdf [Last accessed, September, 2019].
19. Shipp T, Zelop CM, Repke JT, et al. Inter delivery interval and risk of symptomatic uterine rupture. Obstet Gynecol. 2001;97(2):175-7.
20. Durmold C, Mercer B. Uterine rupture, perioperative and perinatal morbidity after single layer closure at cesarean delivery. Am J Obstet Gynecol. 2003;189:925-29.
21. Bujold E, Bujold C, Hamilton EF, et al. The impact of a single-layer or double-layer closure on uterine rupture. Am J Obstet Gynecol. 2002;186:1326-30.
22. Tulandi T, Al-Jaroudi D. Nonclosure of peritoneum: A reappraisal. Am J Obstet Gynecol. 2003;189:609-12.
23. Chelmow D, Rodriguez EJ, Sabatini MM. Suture closure of subcutaneous fat and wound disruption after cesarean delivery: A meta-analysis. Obstet Gynecol. 2004;103:974-80.
24. Learman LA, Summitt RL, Varner RE, et al. A randomized comparison of total or supracervical hysterectomy: surgical complications and clinical outcomes. Obstet Gynecol. 2003;102:453-62.
25. Landon MB, Hauth JC, Leveno KJ, et al. Maternal and perinatal outcomes associated with a trial of labor after prior cesarean delivery. N Engl J Med. 2004;351:2581-9.
26. American College of Obstetricians and Gynecologists. Practice Bulletin No. 54: Vaginal birth after previous cesarean delivery. Obstet Gynecol. 2004;104(1):203-12.

CHAPTER 29

Drug Therapy in Pregnancy

Vignata N

INTRODUCTION

Drug usage in pregnancy requires special consideration because both mother and child are affected. The efficacy and the outcome of drug therapy in pregnancy are enumerated from the evidences available.[1] Drug use in pregnancy has a very important concern because of the teratogenicity effect and also the physiologic changes that occur in pregnant mother. About 44-99% of the pregnant women use one or the other medication.[2] Majority of the drugs given in the antenatal period are for pregnancy-related complications and minor infections, and also in some cases for chronic diseases.[2] Hence, fetus is accidentally exposed to drugs in the early embryonic period. While prescribing drugs, a risk benefit assessment should be made.

Events in the past like thalidomide crisis in 1960s and adverse effects caused by the usage of diethylstilbestrol in 1971 led to initiate strict rules regarding the usage of drugs in pregnancy, drug labeling, and checking the reliability and effectiveness of any medicine before it is made available commercially.[3,4]

PHARMACOKINETICS OF PREGNANCY

The physiological changes which take place in pregnancy modify the actions of the drug significantly (Fig. 1). The effectiveness of a drug depends on the following:

- The uptake, distribution, metabolism, and excretion by the mother
- The passage and metabolism through the yolk sac and the placenta
- The distribution, metabolism, and excretion by the embryo or fetus
- Reabsorption and swallowing of substances by the unborn from the amniotic fluid.[5]

The capacity of the drug distribution and clearance is high in pregnancy, resulting in decreased plasma concentration of the drugs.[6]

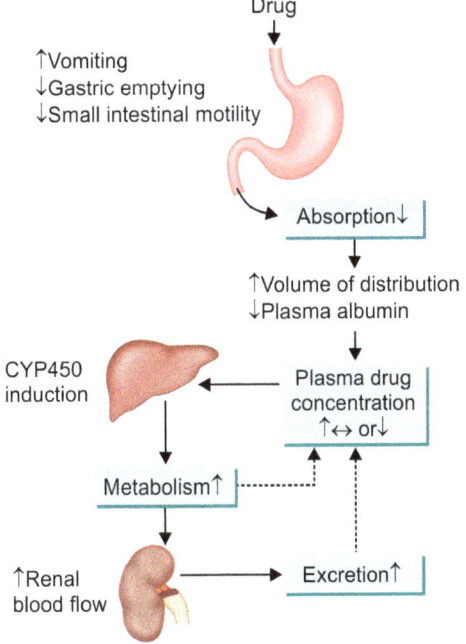

Fig. 1: Pharmacokinetic changes in pregnancy.

In Pregnancy

- Drug absorption is reduced because of the increased progesterone levels which, in turn reduces the gastric emptying and intestinal motility.
- Increased total body weight and fat distribution leads to large volume of distribution.
- Increased renal elimination of drugs due to increased glomerular filtration rate.
- Increased blood flow to the liver, causes more amount of drug available to metabolize.

■ DRUGS: PLACENTAL TRANSFER

Drugs cross from the mother to unborn fetus by diffusion across placenta.[7] Only free unbound drug crosses the placenta. Transfer of drugs rises in 7th–9th month gestation due to large surface area, increased blood flow and decreased thickness of placenta.[8]

Consequence of the drug usage on the fetus depends on:
- Stage of development of fetus
- Dosage of the drug
- Amount of the drug which is actively available.

Guidelines for Prescribing Drugs in Pregnancy

- Do not use drug unless it is absolutely necessary
- Rule out the likelihood of pregnancy in every female between 15 years and 45 years of age.
- Risk benefit ratio should be calculated
- Use lower doses of drugs if necessary for short-term.

■ CATEGORIZATION OF DRUGS

United States Food and Drug Administration (USFDA) has classified all the drugs into five categories (Table 1).

- Categories A and B medications usually are considered safe in humans.
- Category C drugs have not been definitively shown to be unsafe to human fetus, but reasons exist to be cautious while prescribing them.
- Category D drugs are those with evidence of human fetal risk based on previous human studies, but the benefits of treatment prevail over the risks.

TABLE 1: Food and Drug Administration (FDA) categorization of drugs.[9]

Category	Description
A	Adequate, well-controlled studies in pregnant women have not shown an increased risk of fetal abnormalities
B	• Animal studies have revealed no evidence of harm to fetus, there are no adequate and well-controlled studies in pregnant women (or) • Animal studies have shown an adverse effect, but adequate and well-controlled studies in pregnant women have failed to demonstrate a risk to fetus
C	• Animal studies have shown an adverse effect and there are no adequate and well-controlled studies in pregnant women (or) • No animal studies have been conducted and there are no adequate and well-controlled studies in pregnant women
D	Studies, adequate and well-controlled or observational, in animals or pregnant women have demonstrated a risk to fetus; however, benefits of therapy may outweigh the potential risk
X	Studies, adequate and well-controlled or observational, in animals or pregnant women have demonstrated positive evidence of fetal abnormalities. The use of product is contraindicated in women who are or may become pregnant

Drug Therapy in Pregnancy

COMMONLY USED DRUGS AND CATEGORIES

Nausea and Vomiting (Table 2)

- It occurs in about 60–70% of pregnant women.
- First, nonpharmacologic options should be given like avoiding spicy, fatty or fried foods, and supplements containing iron.
- Women who are unable to maintain adequate hydration should be admitted to the hospital for intravenous (IV) fluids and electrolyte replacement.

Hypertension (Table 3)

- The main aim of treating hypertension in pregnant women is to prevent the grave adverse effects and to give birth to a healthy neonate.[11]
- There is no clear evidence that preeclampsia can either be prevented or delayed by treating the antenatal women suffering with mild or moderate hypertension.
- Gestational hypertension, preeclampsia, and chronic hypertension can be effectively treated with antihypertensive drugs.
- In pregnant women, these drugs move through the placenta and reach the fetal circulation in higher concentrations. The possible complications caused by these drugs had not been appropriately evaluated.
- Methyldopa is a very effective antihypertensive in pregnant women as it has distinctive safety for the fetus and has been accepted considerably till date.
- Hydralazine is the most commonly used antihypertensive in cases of severe toxemia. But the adverse effect of this drug is it may cause hypotension and severe uteroplacental insufficiency leading to fetal distress.
- The National Heart, Lung, and Blood Institute (NHLBI) guidelines stated alpha-methyldopa as a first-line drug for hypertension in pregnant women. Other options available are oral labetalol, beta-blockers, and calcium antagonists.[12]

TABLE 2: Drugs used in treatment of nausea and vomiting in pregnancy.[10]

Drug	Pregnancy risk category
Metoclopramide	B
Ondansetron	B
Cyclizine	B
Prochlorperazine	C
Promethazine	C
Chlorpromazine	C

TABLE 3: Drugs for treatment of hypertension.[13]

Drug	Example	Pregnancy risk category
Centrally acting agonist	Aldomet	C
Alpha-blockers	• Labetalol • Metoprolol • Atenolol	C C C
Calcium antagonists	• Verapamil • Diltiazem	C C
Angiotensin-converting enzyme (ACE) inhibitors	Captopril	D
Angiotensin II receptor blockers	• Analapril • Lisinopril • Losartan • Valsartan	D D D D
Diuretics	• Bumetanide • Furosemide • Hydrochlorothiazide • Indapamide • Spironolactone • Triamterene	D C C B B D
Direct vasodilators	• Hydralazine • Minoxidil	C C

- Angiotensin-converting enzyme (ACE) inhibitors are contraindicated in pregnancy, as they may cause lethal renal failure at birth.

Epilepsy (Table 4)

Management of epilepsy in pregnant women still remains as a challenge. The main aim of treating epilepsy in pregnancy is such that the patient would be free from seizures in the antenatal and immediate postpartum period. Care should also be taken in a way that the drugs given for management of epilepsy would not harm the unborn fetus.[14]

During pregnancy, the plasma concentrations of antiepileptic drugs (AEDs) reduce. Less is known regarding the potency and safety profile of the usage of newer AEDs during pregnancy.

Use of phenytoin and other AEDs had caused severe teratogenic effects.[15,16] Higher numbers of birth defects had been noted in fetus exposed to AEDs in utero. Exposure of pregnant women to newer AEDs had not increased the risk of neural tube defects.[17]

The fetal hydantoin syndrome, which occurs due to exposure to AEDs, is identified by abnormal facies, hypoplasia of digits and nails, growth and mental retardation, along with other congenital anomalies. It has been associated with the occurrence of neural crest tumors.[18]

In antenatal women taking AEDs, folate deficiency is noted.[19,20] Usage of single drug is recommended in most cases. The drug is chosen based on its efficacy to provide optimal seizure control with fewer side effects.

No drug has been proven to be completely safe in pregnancy.

Monitoring of the plasma drug levels is done regularly in view of higher requirements in pregnant women.

It is advised that any patient on AEDs should continue the same drugs after conception. However, if pregnancy is to be planned better avoid valproate or switch to some other drugs. Carbamazepine, lamotrigine, and levetiracetam are much safer. Phenobarbitone is the drug of choice, in case where antiepileptics are to be initiated.

Antibiotics (Table 5)

The physiologic changes in pregnancy may affect plasma levels of antibiotics. Only limited studies are available about the plasma antimicrobial levels, except for the ones about amoxicillin.[21] Infections in pregnancy should be treated on a more conservative manner, like 5 days treatment for urinary tract infection (UTI) as compared to 3 day treatment in general population.

Gestational Diabetes (Table 6)

In pregnant women with gestational diabetes, insulin—most preferred drug, if they do not respond to diet control.[22]

There had been development of newer antidiabetic drugs, in the recent times, keeping in consideration of rise in the incidence of type 2 diabetes. However, usage of these drugs in pregnancy has been limited in view of teratogenicity.[23]

Routine use of glyburide and other new antidiabetic drugs in pregnancy can be approved only after further research.

TABLE 4: Drugs for treatment of epilepsy.

Drug	Pregnancy risk category
Topiramate	C
Lamotrigine	C
Levetiracetam	C
Phenobarbital	D
Phenytoin	D
Carbamazepine	D
Valproic acid	D

TABLE 5: Antibiotic drugs.

Drug	Example	Pregnancy risk category
Aminoglycoside	Amikacin, gentamicin, neomycin	D
Cephalosporins	• First-generation—cephalexin, cefazolin • Second-generation—cefuroxime, cefoxitin • Third-generation—cefotaxime, ceftazidime, ceftriaxone	B B B
Linezolid		C
Clindamycin		B
Chloramphenicol		C
Macrolides	Azithromycin, erythromycin	B B
Metronidazole		B
Nitrofurantoin		B
Penicillins	• First-generation—penicillin G, benzathine penicillin • Second-generation—oxacillin, dicloxacillin • Third-generation—ampicillin, amoxicillin • Fourth generation—ticarcillin, piperacillin-tazobactam	B B B B
Tetracycline		D
Sulfonamides		C
Vancomycin		C
Doxycycline		D
Quinolones	• First-generation—nalidixic acid • Second-generation—ciprofloxacin, norfloxacin, ofloxacin • Third-generation—levofloxacin • Fourth-generation—moxifloxacin, gatifloxacin	C C C C

TABLE 6: Drugs for treatment of gestational diabetes.

Drug	Pregnancy risk category
Insulin	B
Metformin	C
Glipizide	C
Glyburide	C
Sulfonylurea	Limited data available

TABLE 7: Anticoagulant drugs.

Drug	Pregnancy risk category
Heparin	B
Low-molecular-weight heparin	B
Warfarin	C

Anticoagulants (Table 7)

Heparin is the most commonly used anticoagulant, as only negligible amount crosses through placenta, and hence, it has almost nil effect on the unborn fetus. Few disadvantages with this drug are parenteral administration and the difficulty in monitoring.

Low-molecular-weight heparin (LMWH) usage had been increased as compared to unfractionated heparin in view of its properties like it does not bind to plasma protein immediately, has high expected dose response, and half-life.[24] LMWH monitoring done by measurement of antifactor Xa activity, which is at lower level in pregnant women.[25] Current evidence states in order to prevent postpartum hemorrhage, LMWH should be stopped at least 12 hours prior to delivery. Fondaparinux is administered as a substitute to unfractionated heparin in cases suffering from heparin-induced thrombocytopenia.[26]

Warfarin diffuses through the placenta and has an immense effect on the fetal prothrombin time. Its usage in first trimester in women with prosthetic heart valves has increased chances of birth defects. Exposure to warfarin in first trimester leads to "fetal warfarin embryopathy" that includes chondrodysplasia punctata, midface hypoplasia, short proximal limbs, short phalanges, scoliosis, increased risk of low intelligence quotient (IQ), and mental retardation.[27]

Exposure during the second half of pregnancy is associated with central nervous system (CNS) abnormalities like agenesis of corpus callosum, Dandy–Walker malformation, optic atrophy, and midline cerebellar atrophy.[27]

The risk of outstanding abnormalities is low (6.4%).[27] High incidence of miscarriages and intrauterine fetal death are noted with usage of warfarin in pregnancy.[28] Warfarin should only be used in cases where it is not possible to use heparin or dicumarol.[29]

Cardiac Medications (Table 8)

Antiarrhythmic drugs are given in cases of refractory arrhythmias, where the benefits may outweigh the risks to the fetus.

Antidepressants

About 7-23% of pregnant women suffer from depression. Usually, selective serotonin reuptake inhibitors (SSRIs) are only used in such cases. The benefits of treating depression usually outweigh the risks during pregnancy.

TABLE 8: Cardiac medications.

Drug	Pregnancy risk category
Lidocaine	B
Adenosine	C
Digoxin	C
Ibutilide	C
Amiodarone	D
Procainamide	C
Flecainide	C
Quinidine	C

Thyroid Medications

Medications for thyroid disorders in pregnancy are given in Table 9.

Antituberculous Drugs (Table 10)

In developing countries, tuberculosis is more vigorous during pregnancy with human immunodeficiency virus (HIV) coinfection resulting in greater mortality.[30]

Antituberculosis compounds during pregnancy have been reviewed regarding their teratogenicity.[31] The first-line drugs are safer in pregnancy, i.e. isoniazid, ethambutol, and rifampin. Ethionamide and streptomycin have increased teratogenic effects and hence are contraindicated in pregnancy.[32]

Other Respiratory Medications (Table 11)

For the treatment of upper respiratory infections, allergies, and asthma.

Migraine (Table 12)

- Acetaminophen is the preferred drug for pregnant women with migraine headaches, up to maximum of 1,000 mg per dose.
- Selective serotonin receptor agonists (e.g. sumatriptan, naratriptan, zolmitriptan, and rizatriptan are not recommended during pregnancy).

TABLE 9: Thyroid medications.

Drug	Pregnancy risk category
Levothyroxine	B
Propylthiouracil	D
Methimazole	X

TABLE 10: Antituberculous drugs.

Drug	Pregnancy risk category
Isoniazid	C
Rifampin	C
Ethambutol	C

TABLE 11: Respiratory medications.

Drug	Example	Pregnancy risk category
Anticholinergic	Ipratropium	B
Beta adrenergic	• Albuterol	C
	• Epinephrine	C
	• Terbutaline	B
Corticosteroids	• Methylprednisolone	C
	• Prednisolone	C
	• Prednisone	C
Antihistamines	• Chlorpheniramine	C
	• Diphenhydramine	B
	• Hydroxyzine	C
	• Meclizine	B
	• Cetirizine	B
	• Fexofenadine	C
	• Loratadine	B
Decongestants	Pseudoephedrine	C

TABLE 12: Drugs for treatment of migraine.

Drug	Pregnancy risk category
Acetaminophen	B
Ibuprofen	B
Zolmitriptan	C
Sumatriptan	C
Naratriptan	C
Prochlorperazine	C
Ergotamine tartrate	D
Dihydroergotamine	X

TABLE 13: Gastrointestinal medications.

Drug	Example	Pregnancy risk category
Antacids	Ranitidine	B
	Cimetidine	B
	Famotidine	B
Proton pump inhibitors	Pantoprazole	B
	Omeprazole	C
	Esomeprazole	B
	Lansoprazole	B

TABLE 14: Antifungal agents.

Drug	Pregnancy risk category
Clotrimazole	C
Nystatin	C
Ketoconazole	C
Fluconazole	D
Terbinafine	B

TABLE 15: Antiviral agents.

Drug	Example	Pregnancy risk category
Antiherpetic	Valacyclovir	B
	Acyclovir	B
	Famciclovir	B
Anti-influenza	Amantadine	C
	Oseltamivir	C

- Nonsteroidal anti-inflammatory drugs (NSAIDs), ergotamine, and dihydroergotamine not to be used in pregnancy.

Gastrointestinal Medications

Medications in relation to gastrointestinal system are given in Table 13.

Antifungal Agents

Antifungal agents are given in Table 14.

Antiviral Agents

Antiviral agents are given in Table 15.

CONCLUSION

- The physiology of pregnancy makes treating the chronic and acute disorders a challenge
- Treatment must always be focused on benefit versus risk
- Therefore, it is very important to counsel the patients and giving them accurate information about the benefits and risks associated with the drug usage.

REFERENCES

1. Rubin PC, Craig GF, Gavin K, et al. Prospective survey of use of therapeutic drugs, alcohol, and cigarettes during pregnancy. BMJ. 1986;292:813.
2. Bakker MK, Jentink J, Vroom F, et al. Drug prescription patterns before, during and after pregnancy for chronic, occasional and pregnancy-related drugs in the Netherlands. BJOG. 2006;113:559-68.
3. Melton MW. Take two Aspirin or not? Risk of medication use during pregnancy. Mother Baby J. 1999;4:25-32.
4. Ward RW. Difficulties in the study of adverse fetal and neonatal effects of drug therapy during pregnancy. Semin Perinatol. 2001;25:191-5.
5. Loebstein R, Lalkin A, Koren G. Pharmacokinetic changes during pregnancy and their clinical relevance. Clin Pharmacokinet. 1997;33:328-43.
6. Dawes M, Chowienczyk PJ. Drugs in pregnancy. Pharmacokinetics in pregnancy. Best Pract Res Clin Obstet Gynaecol. 2001;15:819-26.
7. Sorensan MK, Phillips BB, Mutnick AH. Drug use in specific patient populations: pediatric, pregnant, geriatric. In: Shargel L, Mutnick A (Eds). Comprehensive Pharmacy Review, 5th edition. Philadelphia: Lippincott Williams & Wilkins; 2004. pp. 673-82.
8. Yankowitz J, Niebyl JR (Eds). Drug Therapy in Pregnancy, 3rd edition. Philadelphia: Lippincott Williams & Wilkins; 2001.
9. Pangle BL. Drugs in Pregnancy and Lactation. In: Herfindal ET, Gourley DR (Eds). Textbook of Therapeutics, Drug and Disease Management, 8th edition. Philadelphia: Lippincott Williams & Wilkins; 2006. pp. 434-48.
10. Nelson-Piercy C. Treatment of nausea and vomiting in pregnancy. When should it be treated and what can be safely taken? Drug Saf. 1998;19(2):155-64.
11. Coppage KH, Sibai BM. Treatment of hypertensive complications in pregnancy. Curr Pharm Des. 2005;11(6):749-57.
12. The Seventh Report of the Joint National Committee on Prevention, Detection, Evaluation, and Treatment of High Blood Pressure. US: National Heart, Lung and Blood Institute; 2004.
13. The sixth report of the joint national committee on prevention, detection, evaluation, and treatment of high blood pressure. Arch Intern Med. 1997;157:2413-46.
14. Meador KJ, Pennell PB, Harden CL, et al. Pregnancy registries in epilepsy: a consensus statement on health outcomes. Neurology. 2008;71(14):1109-17.
15. Hanson JW, Smith DW. The fetal hydantoin syndrome. J Pediatr. 1975;87:285-90.
16. Feldman GL, Weaver DD, Lourien EW. The fetal trimethadione syndrome: Report of an additional family and further delineation of this syndrome. Am J Dis Child. 1977;131:1389-92.
17. Yerby MS. The use of anticonvulsants during pregnancy. Semin Perinatol. 2001;25:153-8.
18. Allen RW, Ogden B, Bentley FL, et al. Fetal hydantoin syndrome, neuroblastoma and hemorrhagic disease in a neonate. JAMA. 1980;244:1464-5.
19. Dansky LV, Andermann E, Rosenblatt D, et al. Anticonvulsant, folate levels, and pregnancy outcome: a prospective study. Ann Neurol. 1987;21:176-82.
20. Mosley BS, Cleves MA, Siega-Riz AM, et al. Neural tube defects and maternal folate intake among pregnancies conceived after folic acid fortification in the United States. Am J Epidemiol. 2009;169(1):9-17.
21. Nahum GG, Uhl K, Kennedy DL. Antibiotic use in pregnancy and lactation: what is and is not known about teratogenic and toxic risks. Obstet Gynecol. 2006;107(5):1120-38.
22. Metzger BE, Buchanan TA, Coustan DR, et al. Summary and recommendations of the Fifth International Workshop-Conference on Gestational Diabetes Mellitus. Diabetes Care. 2007;30 Suppl 2:S251-60.

23. Klieger C, Pollex E, Koren G. Treating the mother—protecting the unborn: the safety of hypoglycemic drugs in pregnancy. J Matern Fetal Neonatal Med. 2008;21(3):191-6.
24. Hirsch J, Warkentin TE, Raschke R, et al. Heparin and low-molecular-weight heparin: mechanisms of action, pharmacokinetics and safety. Chest. 1988;114:489S-510S.
25. Casele HL, Laifer SA, Woelkers DA, et al. Changes in the pharmacokinetics of the low-molecular-weight heparin enoxaparin sodium during pregnancy. Am J Obstet Gynecol. 1999;181:1113-7.
26. Deruelle P, Coulon C. The use of low-molecular-weight heparins in pregnancy—how safe are they? Curr Opin Obstet Gynecol. 2007;19(6):573-7.
27. Chan WS, Anand S, Ginsberg JS. Anticoagulation of pregnant women with mechanical heart valves: a systematic review of the literature. Arch Intern Med. 2000;160:191-6.
28. Hall JG, Pauli RM, Wilson K. Maternal and fetal sequelae of anticoagulation during pregnancy. Am J Med. 1980;68:122-40.
29. Chang MK, Harvey D, de Swiet M. Follow-up study of children whose mothers were treated with warfarin during pregnancy. Br J Obstet Gynaecol. 1984;91:1070-3.
30. Keskin N, Yilmaz S. Pregnancy and tuberculosis: to assess tuberculosis cases in pregnancy in a developing region retrospectively and two case reports. Arch Gynecol Obstet. 2008;278(5):451-5.
31. Holdiness MR. Teratology of the antituberculosis drugs: a review. Early Hum Dev. 1987;15:61-74.
32. Holdiness MR. Neurological manifestations and toxicities of the antituberculosis drugs: a review. Med Toxicol. 1987;2:33-51.

CHAPTER 30

Peripartum Cardiomyopathy

Shalini MA

Peripartum cardiomyopathy (PPCM) is a rare cardiac condition associated with idiopathic dilated cardiomyopathy (DCM).

DEFINITION

It is defined by *the onset of heart failure in the last month of pregnancy or the first 5 months of postpartum, with no other identifiable cause for heart failure and no history of cardiac disease prior to the last month of pregnancy.* Incidence of PPCM differs by locality and affects <0.1% of all pregnancies globally and it has 5–32% risk of morbidity and mortality.[1]

Echocardiography parameters require at least one of the following features to be present.
- Ejection fraction < 45%
- M-mode fractional shortening < 30%
- Left ventricular (LV) end-diastolic dimensions > 2.7 cm/m² body surface area.[1]

Although PPCM has the appearance of DCM, it can be differentiated from other DCM, due to its *rapid development*. It affects an apparently healthy women, severity varying from severe cardiac failure up to heart transplantation. Around 80% of symptomatic patients recover, although <30% achieve complete recovery (normalization of LV function and chamber size).[2]

EPIDEMIOLOGY

Peripartum cardiomyopathy showed regional variability in the population; higher rates in black population reaching 1:100 births at Nigeria and very low rates with the Japanese population (1:20,000 births).[1] Recent studies such as Silwa et al. stated that PPCM condition was seen equally amongst the Black and Caucasians.[3] Women with lower socioeconomic status were more likely to be affected by PPCM (outside of Europe).[1]

RISK FACTORS

- Multiparity[4]
- Maternal age >30 years[4]
- Twin pregnancies[4]
- History of hypertension, preeclampsia, and eclampsia[4]
- Human immunodeficiency virus (HIV) considered as potential risk factor and mostly diagnosed in cases outside of Europe.[1]

ETIOLOGY AND PATHO-PHYSIOLOGY

Genetic Factors

Peripartum cardiomyopathy has tendency of familial occurrence, even though it is nonfamilial and nongenetic form of cardiomyopathy, suggesting a genetic propensity. Initially, it may manifests as a familial DCM. An overlap in the clinical spectrum was observed as many genetic variants are common between PPCM and DCM.

Geographic or ethnic variations may be associated with the incidence of PPCM.[5]

Angiogenesis Imbalance

Physiologically in late gestation, the placenta secretes vascular endothelial growth factor inhibitors (antiangiogenic factor). Excess antiangiogenic signaling causes systemic or cardiac specific antiangiogenic environment in PPCM. This hypothesis suggests that PPCM is a vascular disease, which contributes to the development of PPCM in late gestation, and why multiple gestations and preeclampsia are commonly seen with PPCM.[5]

Myocardial Inflammation

Evidence for and against a role of inflammation in PPCM is questionable.[4] On one hand, endomyocardial biopsy samples in PPCM patients showed high rate of active myocarditis, ranging from 29% to 100%.[4,5] Some articles even showed that interstitial inflammation with viral genome in 31% of PPCM patients.[5] On the other hand, the rates of myocarditis is not universally high among PPCM cases.

C-reactive protein (CRP), interferon γ, tumor necrosis factor-α (TNF-α), Fas/apoptosis antigen 1, and interleukin-6 were obtained in high concentration in PPCM. During pregnancy, inflammatory cytokines may create hostile cardiac adaptations leading to cardiac fibrosis. Till to date, etiology of myocardial inflammation is unknown in PPCM.[5]

Oxidative Stress and the Prolactin Theory

The level of oxidative stress in PPCM is exaggerated to normal pregnancy. The oxidative stress in pregnancy is due to insulin resistance and metabolic shift towards fatty acids.[5]

Full length prolactin has proangiogenic effect via reactive oxygen species scavenging, while the 16-KDa cleaved has antiangiogenic and proapoptotic properties; resulting in destruction of cardiac and vascular tissue.

Fetal Chimerism

During pregnancy, fetal cells which enter into the maternal circulation are destroyed by the maternal immune system. In certain occasions, when the maternal immune system is weak, chimeric cells with paternal haplotype enter and settle in the heart of the pregnant women.[1] When the immune system normalizes in postpartum, these chimeric cells residing in maternal heart trigger a response leading to high titers of antibody directed against cardiac myosin heavy chain (not found in idiopathic DCM or in healthy population). This explains the higher incidence in multiple gestation and recurrence, but the relation between the antibodies and PPCM still remains unclear.[4]

CLINICAL PRESENTATION

Even though we consider multiparity and increasing maternal age as the risk factors for PPCM, up to one-third of cases are younger in age group and primigravida.[6]

Clinical features mimic DCM with systolic heart failure:
- Fatigue
- Exertional dyspnea
- Paroxysmal nocturnal dyspnea
- Orthopnea
- Engorged neck vein
- Pulmonary crackles
- Hepatic congestion
- Third heart sound
- Leg edema.[5]

Early symptoms mimic the physiological changes in normal pregnancy. Mostly, the symptoms occur in first 4 months after delivery and <10% of cases present in antepartum. The severity varies from New York Heart Association (NYHA) functional class I to IV.[6]

Peripartum cardiomyopathy has rapid progression (within days) to a slow course over months. Morbid complications include cardiogenic failure, refractory heart failure, severe ventricular arrhythmia, thromboembolism, multiorgan failure, and even death. Individuals with severe LV dysfunction are more prone to systemic embolism and LV thrombosis.[5]

DIAGNOSIS (BOX 1)

Diagnosis requires a high degree of suspicion and often delayed, as the symptoms of PPCM are similar to physiological changes during late trimester.[4] PPCM should be suspected in a case of heart failure or in those with delayed recovery to a prepregnant state (Flowchart 1).[5]

Detailed history to be obtained to know the familial pattern of the condition.[5] Chest X-ray may show pulmonary congestion, pleural effusion, and cardiomegaly. Although, electrocardiogram is not specific, several findings such as QT interval prolongation, non-specific ST-T wave abnormality, QRS widening, atrial fibrillation, and LV hypertrophy urges cardiac analysis.[5]

Recent studies suggest some biomarkers, which might be specific for PPCM; the 16-KDa prolactin, MicroRNA-146a and soluble fms-like tyrosine kinase-1 of diagnostic value in clinical practice, requires verification.[5]

Endomyocardial biopsy is warranted in some cases to exclude the inflammatory pathology of acute heart failure.[5]

Brain-type Natriuretic Peptide or N-terminal Pro-brain Natriuretic Peptide

Brain-type natriuretic peptide (BNP) or N-terminal pro-BNP (NT-proBNP) is useful in screening potential PPCM patients, as it has high sensitivity and high specificity. In spite of the hemodynamic stress during pregnancy, blood concentration of BNP or NT-proBNP does not increase during pregnancy. High values of BNP or NT-proBNP during or before pregnancy predict adverse maternal outcomes in pregnancy.[5]

Normal BNP or NT-proBNP levels (<100 pg/mL)—high negative predictive value for adverse maternal complications, where as BNP or NT-proBNP >300 pg/mL predicts complications during peripartum period with DCM.[5]

Box 1: Diagnostic testing for peripartum cardiomyopathy.
- Blood tests:
  - Complete blood picture
  - Blood urea nitrogen, serum creatinine, and serum electrolytes
  - Cardiac enzymes including troponin
  - BNP or N-terminal BNP
  - Liver function test
  - Thyroid stimulating hormone
- Chest radiograph
- Electrocardiogram
- Transthoracic echocardiogram
- Cardiac magnetic resonance imaging (if needed)

(BNP: brain-type natriuretic peptide)

Flowchart 1: Suspected peripartum cardiomyopathy.[5]

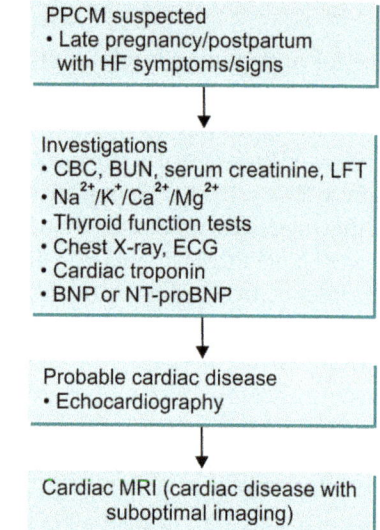

(BNP: brain-type natriuretic peptide; BUN: blood urea nitrogen; CBC: complete blood count; ECG: electrocardiogram; HF: heart failure; MRI; magnetic resonance imaging; NT-proBNP: N-terminal brain type natriuretic peptide; LFT: liver function test)

Brain-type natriuretic peptide or NT-proBNP levels rise in certain cardiac conditions during pregnancy:[5]
- Preeclampsia/eclampsia
- Congenital heart disease with structural defects
- Various forms of cardiomyopathy.

Echocardiography

The echocardiography criteria for PPCM were strict; ejection fraction <45%, M-mode fractional shortening <30%, and LV end-diastolic dimensions >2.7 cm/m² body surface area. The latest guidelines quotes that LV dilatation is not mandatory for diagnosis of PPCM. However, echocardiography is a useful investigation for excluding the differential diagnosis.
- Significant diastolic dysfunction with preserved systolic functions suggests hypertensive heart diseases such as preeclampsia.
- Marked right ventricular dysfunction suggests pulmonary embolism.
- Regional wall motion abnormality of the LV suggests myocarditis or acute coronary syndrome.[5]

Cardiac Magnetic Resonance Imaging

Cardiac magnetic resonance imaging (MRI) complements echocardiography, especially in patients with suboptimal echocardiography imaging. MRI demarcates the global and segmental LV contraction and differentiates the ischemic heart disease and acute myocarditis.[5]

Late gadolinium enhancement (LGE) levels provide prognostic information in ischemic and nonischemic cardiac conditions, but the clinical significance of LGE in PPCM is not established. Extensive LGE in PPCM may show myocarditis like-transitory feature, which is not necessarily an adverse predictor for the long-term LV recovery.[5]

In antepartum period, the administration of gadolinium, benefits versus risks must be carefully weighed, as it crosses the placenta.[5]

Endomyocardial Biopsy

Endomyocardial biopsy is not routinely recommended in the current guidelines. It can be considered when the clinical course deteriorates during standard medical treatment, in the diagnosis of acute myocarditis or other forms of cardiomyopathy.[5]

Box 2 describes the criteria for diagnosis of PPCM.

DIFFERENTIAL DIAGNOSIS

Peripartum cardiomyopathy is a diagnosis of exclusion. Box 3 enlisted the conditions that are considered.

Box 2: Current diagnostic criteria for peripartum cardiomyopathy.[4]

- Development of heart failure in last month of pregnancy or 5 months postpartum
- Absence of pre-existing heart disease
- Independent cause
- Echocardiographic findings (a, together with b or c, and all of these)
  a. Ejection fraction <45%
  b. M-mode fractional shortening <30%
  c. Left ventricular end-diastolic dimensions >2.7 cm/m² body surface area.

Box 3: Differential diagnosis of peripartum cardiomyopathy.[5]

- Pre-existing valvular heart disease, particularly valvular stenosis
- Pre-existing congenital heart disease
- Familial dilated cardiomyopathy
- Pre-existing other forms of cardiomyopathy
- Acute pulmonary embolism
- Pre-eclampsia and eclampsia (hypertensive heart disease)
- Thyrotoxicosis
- Acute myocarditis
- Maternal sepsis
- Acute coronary spasm, dissection, thrombosis, and myocardial infarction

Pre-existing or Familial Dilated Cardiomyopathy

Time frame of the clinical disease is an important factor to differentiate DCM and PPCM. In majority of the cases of DCM, heart failure develops in second trimester as the hemodynamic stress peaks rapidly, whereas PPCM develops in last month of pregnancy. Women who develops DCM in third trimester, current approaches are difficult to differentiate from PPCM.[5]

Acute Myocarditis

Rapidly progressing acute heart failure mimics PPCM. Endomyocardial biopsy is low yielding and an invasive procedure, therefore cardiac MRI is an alternative modality to diagnose acute myocarditis.[5]

Pre-eclampsia with Heart Failure

Critical diastolic dysfunction and heart failure can be due to severe hypertension including preeclampsia in pregnant women. These adverse maternal complications occur due to pregnancy-related blood volume overload which leads to cardiac decompensation in these hypertensive patients. Echocardiography differentiates this condition from PPCM. Elevated left atrial filling pressure with preserved LV ejection fraction indicates preeclampsia.[5]

■ MANAGEMENT

Management of PPCM involves:
- Heart failure therapy
- Arrhythmia management
- Anticoagulation
- Mechanical circulatory support and transplantation
- Targeted therapy.

Heart Failure Therapy

Lack of evidence-based clinical data in heart failure around pregnancy poses a challenge to the physicians. Well-coordinated multidisciplinary approach involving; cardiovascular medicine, obstetrics, immunology, pathology, and other specialities for managing a case of PPCM with complication.[4]

- *First aim*: Improve the symptoms through conventional pharmacologic therapies and nonpharmacologic therapies, if required.
- *Second aim*: Cure through the administration of targeted therapies.

Currently, European Society of Cardiology (ESC) guidelines for heart failure in pregnancy is used for the treatment of PPCM[7] (Table 1). Oxygen, angiotensin-blocking agents, and diuretics are used for acute management of PPCM.[4]

In late pregnancy; beta blockers, thiazide diuretic, or furosemide treatment may be required in some patients of PPCM. Diuretic therapy to be used with caution as it may impair the perfusion of placenta, which may cause potential harm to the fetus.[7]

After delivery, standard therapy for heart failure is recommended in PPCM (Table 2). Inotropes should be considered in patients with severe hypotension and/or signs of cardiogenic shock. Inotropes (e.g. dobutamine) are to be used cautiously, as the data on its use is not available and catecholamines may aggravate myocardial damage. PPCM patients with severely depressed ejection fraction, early treatment with beta blockers in very low dosages also has protective effect. Beta blockers usage is limited in cases of persistent sinus tachycardia, where ivabradine can be used.[7]

Risk of sudden death is increased in PPCM patients and seems to benefit from implantable cardioverter-defibrillator (ICD) and cardiac resynchronization therapy (CRT). Wearable cardioverter/defibrillator (3–6 months) would be an alternative option versus ICD or CRT defibrillator (CRT-D) implantation as a primary prophylaxis in patients with least marked improvement in systolic LV function.[7]

TABLE 1: Medications for peripartum cardiomyopathy.[5]

Category	Drug	Dosage	Comment
ACEI (neurohormonal blockade)	Captopril	6.25 mg TID up to 25–30 mg TID	Contraindicated during pregnancy
	Enalapril	1.25 mg BID up to 10 mg BID	Contraindicated during pregnancy
	Ramipril	2 mg BID up to 5 mg BID	Lack of data during pregnancy
ARB (neurohormonal blockade)	Candesartan	2 mg OD up to 32 mg OD	Contraindicated during pregnancy and lactation
	Valsartan	40 mg TID up to 160 mg TID	Contraindicated during pregnancy and lactation
MRA	Spironolactone	12.5 mg OD up to 50 mg OD	Contraindicated during pregnancy and lactation
β-blockers (long-term management of systolic dysfunction)	Extended release metoprolol	0.125 mg OD up to 0.25 mg OD	Risk of bradycardia or respiratory distress in new born
	Carvedilol	3.125 mg BID up to 25 mg BID	Same as metaprolol
Vasodilators (nitroprusside; causes potential cyanide toxicity—not recommended)	Hydralazine	10 mg TID up to 40 mg TID	
	Nitroglycerin	10–20 µg/min IV Adjust the dose according to BP	Risk of hypotension
Diuretics (reduces preload—treats pulmonary congestion or peripheral edema)	Hydrochlorothiazide	12.5–50 mg OD	Risk of uteroplacental circulatory insufficiency
	Furosemide	20–80 mg OD-BID (oral/IV)	Risk of uteroplacental circulatory insufficiency
Inotropics (only in severe low output cases)	Digoxin	0.125–0.25 mg OD	Risk of drug toxicity
	Dobutamine	2.5–10 µg/kg/min	
	Milrinone	0.125–0.5 µg/kg/min	
Prolactin inhibition	Bromocriptine	2.5 mg BID for 2 weeks, then 2.5 mg OD for 2 weeks	Risk of thrombosis

(AECI: angiotensin-converting enzyme inhibitor; ARB: angiotensin receptor blocker; BID: twice a day; BP: blood pressure; IV: intravenous; MRA: mineralocorticoid receptor antagonist; OD: once a day; TID: three times a day)

TABLE 2: Proposed strategy for heart failure drug therapy in peripartum cardiomyopathy patients after delivery before and after complete recovery of left-ventricular structure and function.[7]

Drug	Safety during lactation[a]	Absence of complete recovery	Complete and sustained recovery of left-ventricular structure and function (echocardiographic follow-up every 6 months)
β-blocker	In rare cases, bradycardia of the newborn reported. Best drug during lactation—metoprolol	It is essential for every patient.	6 months: Continue all drugs for at 6 months after full recovery to avoid relapse. 6–12 months: Continue β-blocker and ACE inhibitor/ARB for at least 6 months after stopping MRA >12 months: Continue β-blocker for at least 6 months after stopping ACE inhibitor/ARB. >18 months: Discontinue β-blockade, ensure echocardiographic follow-up
ACE inhibitors	Enalapril and captopril—less transfer into breast milk	It is essential for every patient	Reduce dosage and then discontinue ACE inhibitor/ARB
ARB	Should be avoided as there is very limited data available	Recommended for patients who cannot tolerate	
MRA	Should be avoided as there is very limited data available	Recommended for all patients with LVEF <40%. Eplerenone may be considered due to less hormonal side effects	Discontinue only if complete and sustained recovery of left-ventricular structure and function
Ivabradine	Should be avoided as there is no data available	• Heart rate >75/min, when β-blocker uptitration is not possible. • When β-blocker uptitration is possible and/heart rate is <60/minute	• Continue when heart rate is >75/min despite β-blocker uptitration • Discontinue only if complete and sustained recovery of left ventricular structure and function
Diuretics	Thiazides—well tolerated. Furosemide and torasemide should be avoided as there is very limited data available. They may decrease milk production	• Only when edema/congestion is present • Even before full recovery of left ventricular function, early tapering of dose according to symptoms	Continue only symptoms (edema/congestion) are present without diuretic therapy as part of an antihypertensive drug therapy

[a]According to the ESC guidelines, the manufacturer's instructions are mainly based on the fact that drugs are not tested sufficiently during pregnancy and breastfeeding. For this and for legal reasons, drugs are frequently considered prohibited during pregnancy and lactation.
(ACE: angiotensin-converting enzyme; ARB: angiotensin receptor blocker; ESC: European Society of Cardiology; LVEF: left ventricular ejection fraction; MRA: mineralocorticoid receptor antagonist)

Arrhythmia Management

Most common arrhythmia in PPCM is atrial fibrillation. Quinidine and procainamide are considered as first-line of antiarrhythmic management and relatively safer in puerperium. Digoxin can also be used in the first-line therapy. Permanent pacemakers and ICDs may be required in cases of refractory atrial fibrillation.[4]

Anticoagulation

Pregnancy and heart failure are both considered as independent risk factors for venous thromboembolism. Anticoagulation is recommended when left ventricular ejection fraction (LVEF) <30% in heart failures. In antepartum, low-molecular-weight heparin (LMWH) is recommended; whereas in postpartum, heparin/LMWH/warfarin can be used. Warfarin is to be avoided during pregnancy due to its teratogenicity.[4]

The optimal approach is to follow-up the patients and gradually taper the dosage over a period of 6–12 months, when there is evidence of recovery (clinical and echocardiographic findings).

Mechanical Circulatory Support and Transplantation

Mechanical circulatory support and even heart transplantation may be required in severe cases of PPCM. In the awaiting period before heart transplantation, intra-aortic balloon pumps and LV assist devices (LVADs) have been used as a bridge. Prolonged circulatory support has dramatically decreased the percentage of PPCM patients requiring heart transplant, from 33% to 4–7%.[4] Few studies compared the outcome of heart transplantation in PPCM versus idiopathic DCM. These studies show that, PPCM has high chance of organ rejection due to increased prevalence of autoimmune mechanisms. Some studies showed that heart transplant at a younger age and closer to onset of the disease improves prognosis.[4]

Targeted Therapy

- *Immunosuppressive drugs*: This therapy is not universally successful and empirically not recommended as myocarditis is not seen in all cases. But it remains as an option, when active myocarditis has been confirmed by endomyocardial biopsy.[4]
- *Intravenous immunoglobulin*: This therapy has a promising approach in improvement of cardiac function. In few retrospective studies of women with PPCM with LVEF <40%, the improvement was greater in group treated with intravenous immunoglobulin than in control group (26% vs. 13%, P = 0.042). However, these results has not been replicated.[4]
- *Pentoxifylline*: A nonrandomized study was conducted in patients with PPCM, 29 were administered with pentoxifylline 400 mg three times daily versus 30 control patients receiving standard care. The pentoxifylline treated group had showed clear survival benefit over control group at 6 months (1 death vs. 8 deaths). The survival benefit of pentoxifylline has been attributed to TNF-α, CRP, and Fas/apoptosis-1 reducing actions.[4]
- *Bromocriptine*: In a pilot study of PPCM, bromocriptine showed better survival benefit compared to control group receiving standard care (1 vs. 4 death, greater LVEF recovery from 27% at baseline to 58% vs. 36% at 6 months). In this study, the prolactin inhibitor bromocriptine, 2.5 mg twice daily for 2 weeks and then 2.5 mg twice daily for 4 weeks was used along with standard care.[4]

DELIVERY

Delivery should be managed by the multidisciplinary team in a high-risk care setting. Based on the maternal hemodynamic stability, obstetric indications including fetal conditions, the timing, and the mode of delivery is chosen.[5]

Spontaneous vaginal delivery is preferred when the women is hemodynamically stable. The advantages of vaginal delivery are as follows:
- Avoids abdominal surgery
- Less blood loss
- Low risk of thromboembolism
- Early recovery
- Regional anesthesia does not cause LV depression.

Hemodynamic changes are significant during antenatal period and 24 hours after delivery, so close monitoring is required. Heparin to be stopped when patient goes in to spontaneous labor or 24 hours before the planned caesarean section.

Epidural anesthesia is preferred as a pain management to minimize the hemodynamic stress for vaginal delivery. Cut short the second stage of labor using assisted delivery by ventouse or forceps. In third stage of labor, autotransfusion of the blood from contracted uterus increases the preload leading to pulmonary congestion. To prevent the pulmonary congestion, intravenous furosemide may be needed.

A planned cesarean-section is preferred in critically ill women or hemodynamic unstable women. It requires intensive care monitoring, which includes inotropes, mechanical ventilation or continuous invasive monitoring. General anesthesia is often needed.[5]

OUTCOMES

Peripartum cardiomyopathy mortality rates have decreased to as low as 3% within 6 months postpartum due to current improvised management of heart failure. Recovery of LV function is markedly higher in PPCM compared to other cardiomyopathies. Around 50% of the cases recover ejection fraction within 6 months to 5 years. In spite of the improvised management, 4% of patients require heart transplant.[1]

SUBSEQUENT PREGNANCIES

About 50% of the patients who recover to normal or near normal ejection fraction after developing PPCM, have significantly lower mortality rates and better chance of improved cardiac function. Other women who continue to have diminished ejection fraction has 25% mortality rate and further decline in cardiac function. Bromocriptine therapy immediately after delivery has significantly improved LV function and 0% mortality.[1] In subsequent pregnancy, team involving cardiology, high-risk obstetrics, and perinatology is required to provide best management strategy. Dobutamine stress echo is a better predictor of woman's ability to withstand the subsequent pregnancy.[1]

PREVENTION

Heart healthy lifestyle, a well-balanced diet, regular exercise, and refraining from alcohol consumption and smoking are recommended. Bromocriptine helps in reducing mortality and prevents further reduction in ejection fraction for a subsequent pregnancy.[1]

CONCLUSION

Over the past few years, mortality rates in women with peripartum cardiomyopathy have decreased, which could be accounted for the recent advances in medical therapy. Risk of sudden deaths have been significantly reduced due to vigorous use of implantable defibrillators. Left ventricular function normalizes in >50% of individuals with PPCM with pharmacologic therapy, but there is almost always risk of PPCM recurrence in subsequent pregnancies.

REFERENCES

1. Gupta D, Wenger NK. Peripartum cardiomyopathy: Status 2018. Clin Cardiol. 2018;41:217-9.
2. Hilfiker-Kleiner D, Schieffer E, Peter Meyer G, et al. Postpartum cardiomyopathy. Dtsch Arztebl Int. 2008;105(44):751-6.
3. Silwa K, Mebazaa A, Hilfiker-Kleiner D, et al. Clinical characteristics of patients from worldwide registry on peripartum cardiomyopathy (PPCM): EURObservational Research Programme in conjunction with Heart Failure Association of the European Society of Cardiology Study Group on PPCM. Eur J Heart Fail. 2017;19:1131-41.
4. Bhattacharyya A, Basra SS, Sen P, et al. Peripartum cardiomyopathy: a review. Tex Heart Inst J. 2012;39(1):8-16.
5. Mi-Jeong K, Mi-Seung S. Practical management of peripartum cardiomyopathy. Korean J Intern Med. 2017;32:393-403.
6. Silwa K, Fett J, Elkayam U. Peripartum cardiomyopathy. Lancet. 2006;368:687-93.
7. Hilfiker-Kleiner D, Haghikia A, Nonhoff J, et al. Peripartum cardiomyopathy: current management and future perspectives. Eur Heart J. 2015;36:1090-7.

CHAPTER 31

Uterine Inversion

Priyadharsini S

INTRODUCTION

Uterine inversion is one of the most dreaded complications during third stage of labor, though very rare. It requires rapid diagnosis and immediate clinical action. Incidence varies from 1 case in 2,000 to 1 case in every 20,000 deliveries, 1 in 8,537 (India).[1]

DEFINITION

Uterine inversion is defined as the passage of uterine fundus through the cervix, turning inside out of uterus, either partially or completely.

ETIOLOGY

Uterine inversion may be spontaneous or induced. It occurs mainly due to mismanagement of third stage of labor, pulling the cord before separation.[2]

Risk factors include:
- Atonic uterus
- Fundal implantation of placenta
- Placenta accreta
- Excessive fundal pressure
- Cord traction, while uterus is relaxed.

CLASSIFICATION

Based on Extent of Inversion (Fig. 1)

- *First degree*: Dimpling of fundus (above internal os)
- *Second degree*: Fundus comes out through the internal os to enter the vagina
- *Third degree*: Fundus protrudes through the vaginal introitus (outside vulva) and complete inversion.

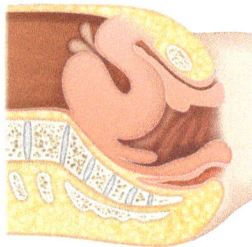
1st degree
Inverted fundus
up to cervix

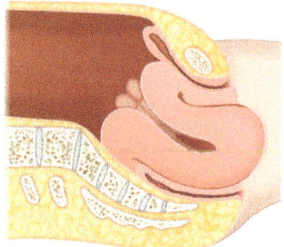
2nd degree
Body of uterus
protrudes through
cervix into vagina

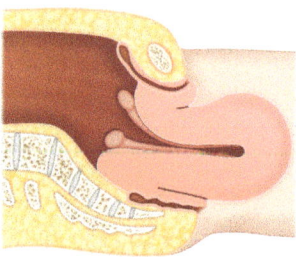
3rd degree
Prolapse of
inverted uterus
outside vulva

Fig. 1: Degrees of inversion.

According to Time of Diagnosis

- *Acute*: Occurs within first 24 hours of delivery, before contraction of cervical ring
- *Subacute*: Occurs after 24 hours but before 4 weeks of delivery, after contraction of cervical ring
- *Chronic*: Occurs after 4 weeks postpartum.

DIAGNOSIS (FIG. 2)

- In case of unexplained postpartum collapse, always suspect inversion
- Neurogenic shock and hemorrhage, shock out of proportion to bleeding (neurogenic shock is due to stretching of infundibulopelvic ligament, pressure on ovaries and peritoneal irritation)
- *Per abdominal examination*: Not able to feel the fundus of uterus (dimpling of fundus)
- *Per vaginal examination*: Soft globular swelling in the vagina or cervical canal.

MANAGEMENT (FLOWCHART 1)

- Call for help
- Resuscitation and replacement of uterus are the mainstay of treatment. Both should go hand in hand.

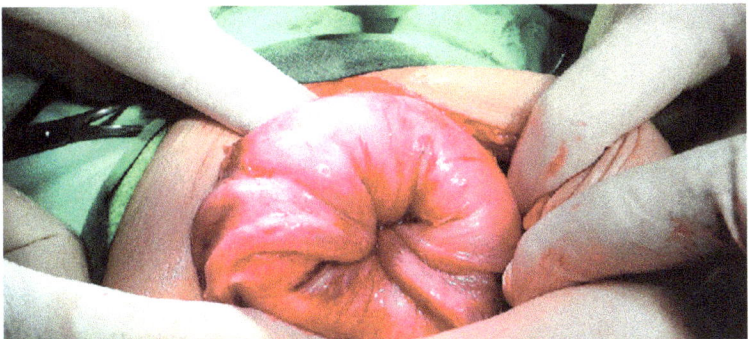

Fig. 2: Uterine inversion.

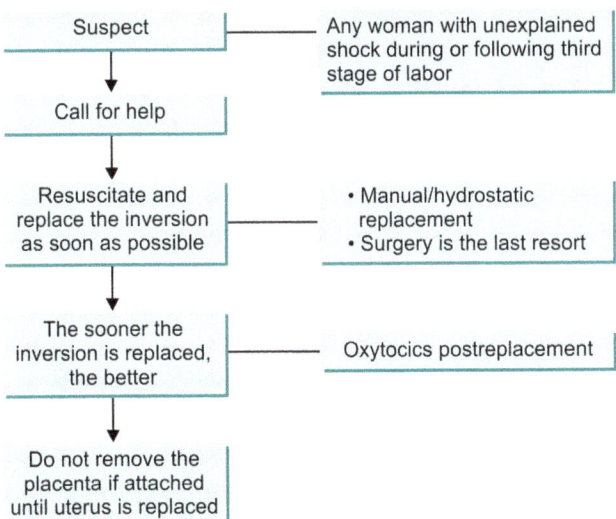

Flowchart 1: Management of inversion of uterus.

- Treat vasovagal shock [i.e. airway, breathing and circulation (ABC) and intravenous (IV) access]
- No attempts should be made to remove placenta before correction.

Manual Replacement (Fig. 3)

- If diagnosed immediately, inversion can be corrected even without anesthesia. If not, general anesthesia is required for manual replacement.
- After completely relaxing the uterus, the part that comes out first, i.e. the fundus should be pushed in the last *(Johnson maneuver)*.
    - After replacement, the placenta is removed and oxytocics given to promote contraction.
    - Oxytocics should not be given before repositioning.
    - Tocolytics can be used to relax uterus while repositioning (nitroglycerine, terbutaline, ritodrine, and magnesium sulfate).[3]

Hydrostatic Method of O'Sullivan

Under general anesthesia, warm sterile saline is passed into the vagina with labia kept manually closed to prevent backflow. The vagina balloons with fluid and the inversion corrects on its own.

New Technique (Ogueh and Ayida)

- A modified form of the O'Sullivan technique (Fig. 4).
- Attach the IV tubing to silicone cup used in vacuum extraction.
- Place the cup in the vagina, an excellent seal is created.

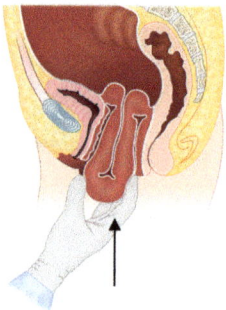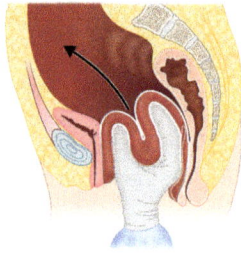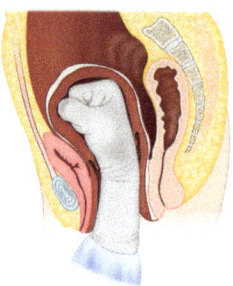

Fig. 3: Manual replacement.

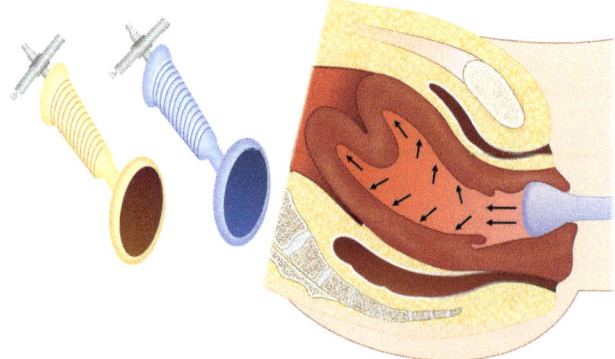

Fig. 4: Modified O'Sullivan method.

Surgical Method

Laparotomy[4]

- Final option of management, if other measures fail.
- *Huntington's repair*:[5] Traction is given on round ligaments with Allis forceps[6] to pull the fundus of uterus. If this method fails, Haultan's repair is alternative method.
- *Haultan's repair*:[7] Vertical incision is made in posterior cervix to relieve the cervical constriction ring.
- *Newer methods*: Laparoscopic reduction,[8] use of obstetric ventouse at laparotomy.[9]

PREVENTION

Preventive measures for uterine inversion have been specified in Table 1.

CHRONIC PUERPERAL INVERSION

After 4 weeks of delivery, recurrent episodes of bleeding and signs of infection suggest chronic inversion.

Differential Diagnosis

- *Uterine prolapse*: Velvety surface, ring of cervical canal above the mass, and absence of external os at its lower end points to chronic inversion.
- *Fibroid polyp*: Fundus will be palpable in normal position on bimanual examination in case of fibroid polyp. Ultrasound will help in diagnosis.

Treatment

- Treat infection with broad-spectrum antibiotics.
- Surgical repositioning after 2–3 months by abdominal route (Haultain) or vaginal route (*Spinnell*[10]—dissection of bladder from inverted uterus, a midline split made in cervix and carefully separated from bladder, uterus is turned outside in by pressure).

CONCLUSION

- Uterine inversion is one of the most dreaded complications in obstetrics.
- Though very rare, it is a life-threatening complication which should be diagnosed and tackled immediately.

REFERENCES

1. Van Vugt PJ, Baudoin P, Blom VM, et al. Inveriso uteri puerperalis. Acta Obstet Gynaecol Scand. 1981;60:353-62.
2. Horsager R, Roberts S, Rogers V, et al. Williams Textbook of Obstetrics and Gynecology, 24th edition. New York: McGraw-Hill; 2014. pp. 787-8.
3. Hong RW, Greenfield ML, Polley LS. Nitroglycerin for uterine inversion in the absence of placental fragments. Anesth Anal. 2006;103:511-2.
4. Kochenour N. Diagnosis and management of uterine inversion. In: Gilstrap LG III, Cunningham FG, Van Dorsten JP (Eds). Operative Obstetrics. New York: McGraw-Hill; 2002. p. 241.
5. Huntington JL, Irving FC, Kellogg FS. Abdominal reposition in acute inversion of the puerperal uterus. Am J Obstet Gynecol. 1928;15:34-40.
6. Robson S, Adair S, Bland P. A new surgical technique for dealing with uterine inversion. Aust NZ J Obstet Gynecol. 2005;45:250-1.

TABLE 1: Preventive measures for uterine inversion.

Do's	Dont's
• Active management of third stage of labor • Wait for signs of placenta separation • Controlled cord traction only after the placenta has separated	• Do not pull placenta when uterus is relaxed • No fundal pressure • Avoid excessive traction

7. Haultain FWN. The treatment of chronic uterine inversion by abdominal route. Br Med J. 1901;2:974-80.
8. Rajagopalan V, Sujatha Y. Acute postpartum uterine inversion with haemorrhagic shock with laparoscopic reduction: a new method of management. BJOG. 2006;113:1100-2.
9. Antonelli E, Irion O, Tolck P, et al. Subacute uterine inversion: description of a novel replacement technique using the obstetric ventouse. BJOG. 2006;113:846-7.
10. Shivanagappa M, Bhandiwad A, Mahesh M. A Case of Acute on Chronic Uterine Inversion with Fibroid Polyp. J Clin Diagn Res. 2013; 7(11):2587-8.

32. Peripartum Collapse

Smitha Avula

INTRODUCTION

Maternal collapse is defined as an acute event involving the cardiorespiratory systems and/or brain, resulting in a reduced or absent conscious level (and potentially death), at any stage in pregnancy and up to 6 weeks after delivery.[1]

INCIDENCE

The breakthrough in maternal mortality statistics was when the literature review in 1996 revealed more than 60% deaths were in postnatal period, 45% within a day, 65% within a week, and 80% within 2 weeks.

Hence World Health Organization (WHO) recommends at least three postnatal visits following delivery: first within 48–72 hours, second between 7 days and 14 days, and third at 6 weeks.

RISK REDUCTION

American College of Obstetricians and Gynecologists (ACOG) (2018) recommended a comprehensive postpartum visit take place within the first 6 weeks after birth. ACOG now recommends that postpartum care should be an ongoing process, rather than a single encounter and that all women have contact with their obstetrician-gynecologist or other obstetric care providers within the first 3 weeks of postpartum. Reemphasizing on the fourth trimester up to 12 weeks postpartum.[2]

Also it provides a window for long-term follow-up in women with chronic pre-existing condition, as numbers go as high as 1 in 10.

STRATEGIES TO IMPROVE OUTCOMES AFTER MATERNAL COLLAPSE

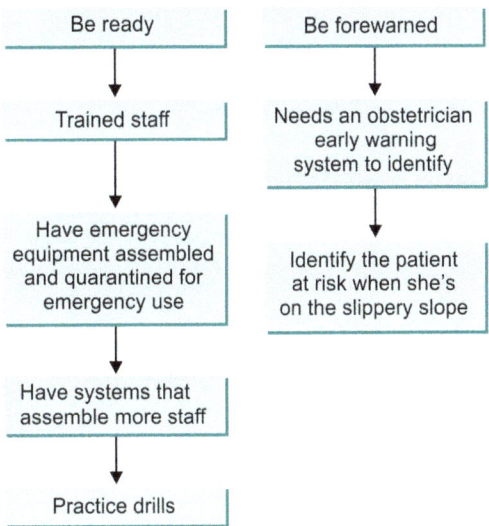

RISK FACTORS UNIQUE TO PREGNANCY

- There is a significant reduction in cardiac output to 10% in pregnant woman with cardiopulmonary resuscitation (CPR) versus a 30% in nonpregnant women
- Reduced oxygen carrying capacity due to hemodilution

- Increased heart rate and cardiac output increase CPR demand
- Increased uterine blood flow (10% of CO) causes rapid obstetric hemorrhage
- Due to decreased systemic vascular resistance there is sequestration of blood in peripheries
- Respiratory changes predispose to hypoxia and acidosis
- Gastrointestinal (GI) changes of relaxed lower esophageal sphincter and decreased gastric motility predispose to aspiration due to sphincter relaxation.

ETIOLOGY

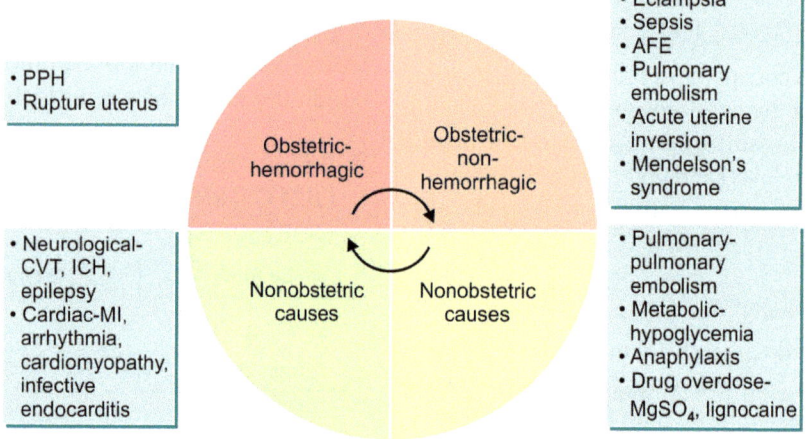

(AFE: amniotic fluid embolism; CVT: cerebral venous thrombosis; ICH: intracerebral hemorrhage; MI: myocardial infarction; PPH: postpartum hemorrhage)

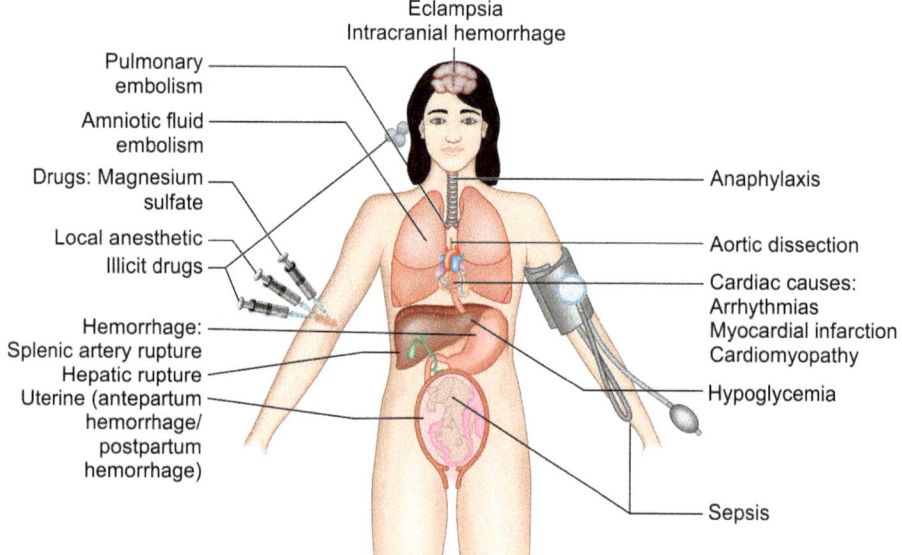

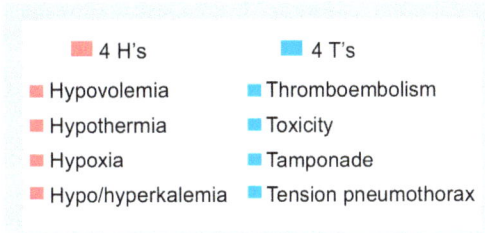

WHAT TO DO IN A MATERNAL COLLAPSE?[3]

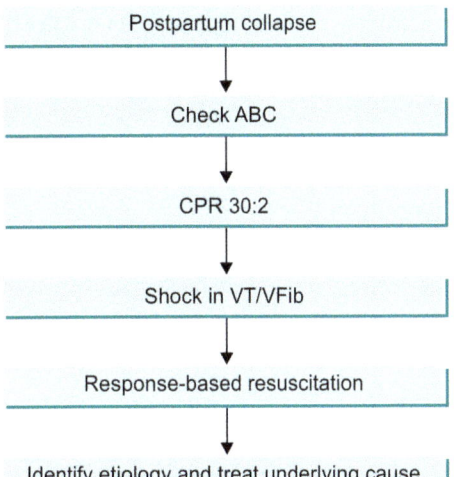

(ABC: airway, breathing, and circulation; CPR: cardiopulmonary resuscitation; VFib: ventricular fibrillation; VT: ventricular tachycardia)

POINTS TO REMEMBER

- *Hypovolemia:*
  - Bleeding may be concealed as in placental abruption
  - Placenta previa
  - *Consider sepsis*: A leading cause of death masked by the physiological changes in pregnancy
- *Hypoxia:*
  - Pulmonary embolism
- Hypothermia, hypo/hyperkalemia, and electrolyte disturbances
- *Pregnancy specific causes:*
  - Intracranial hemorrhage and eclampsia
- Thromboembolism and amniotic fluid embolism
- Toxicity and trauma
- Tension pneumothorax and tamponade

BASIC LIFE SUPPORT: DO'S AND DON'TS

- Rapid notification to the maternal cardiac arrest response team
  (Class 1 Level C)
- High level of CPR with uterine displacement and a firm backboard
- Rapid automated defibrillation wherever indicated appropriate by rhythm analysis
  (Class 1 Level C)
- Appropriate basic life support (BLS) protocols
- A member of first responder team to perform bag-mask ventilation with 100% O2 at 15 L/min
  (Class 2b Level C)
- A minimum of four staff members should respond for BLS resuscitation of a pregnant woman.[4]

PERIMORTEM CESAREAN TO RESUSCITATIVE HYSTEROTOMY

Shift in mindset from the fetocentric 4-minute rule for perimortem cesarean section to initiating preparations at the time of arrest thereby shifting priorities to the mother. There was a dramatic 67% chance of return of spontaneous circulation (ROSC) with 75% neonatal survival and 50% chances of improvement in maternal hemodynamics.[5]

CONCLUSION

- Peripartum collapse can have fatal consequences on the unborn child when occuring antenatally.
- More importantly, the care of the pregnant woman does not end with delivery. The woman in the postpartum period is particularly vulnerable and appropriate interventions can avert more than two-thirds of these fatalities, making healthy mother and healthy baby a reality.

REFERENCES

1. RCOG. (2011). Maternal collapse in pregnancy and puerperium (Green-top Guideline No. 56). [online] Available from: https://www.rcog.org.uk/en/guidelines-research-services/guidelines/gtg56/ [Last accessed September, 2019].
2. ACOG. (2018). Optimizing Postpartum Care. [online] Available from: https://www.acog.org/Clinical-Guidance-and-Publications/Committee-Opinions/Committee-on-Obstetric-Practice/Optimizing-Postpartum-Care?IsMobileSet=false [Last accessed September, 2019].
3. Sharma C, Kewal M. Postpartum collapse. A Practical Guide to Third Trimester of Pregnancy and Puerperium. New Delhi: Jaypee Brothers Medical Publishers (P) Ltd.; 2016.
4. Jeejeebhoy FM, Zelop CM, Lipman S, et al. Cardiac Arrest in Pregnancy: A Scientific Statement From the American Heart Association. Circulation. 2015;132:1747-73.
5. Rose CH, Faksh A, Traynor KD, et al. Challenging the 4- to 5-minute rule: from perimortem cesarean to resuscitative hysterotomy. Am J Obstet Gynecol. 2015;213(5):653-6, 653.e1.

CHAPTER 33

Acute Abdomen in Pregnancy

Smitha Avula

INTRODUCTION

Incidence of acute abdomen in pregnancy varies from 1:500 pregnancies to 1:635 pregnancies[1-3] and increasing assisted reproductive technology (ART) pregnancies have added to the brunt of the burden by increasing the incidence of ectopic/heterotopic pregnancies, torsion ovary, and ovarian hyperstimulation syndrome (OHSS). Pregnancy in itself poses a diagnostic dilemma with regards to establishing a single causative entity for pain abdomen. What adds to the complexity of the situation is that the clinical picture of nausea, vomiting can coexist even in a normal pregnancy. The altered physiology of pregnancy makes it worse for the clinician to diagnose based on clinical/laboratory findings. Conventional radiological investigations are limited by the risk of exposure of the fetus to ionizing radiation. However, prompt diagnosis and treatment are quintessential considering the well being of both patients—the mother and the fetus.

PREGNANCY: ALTERED MILIEU

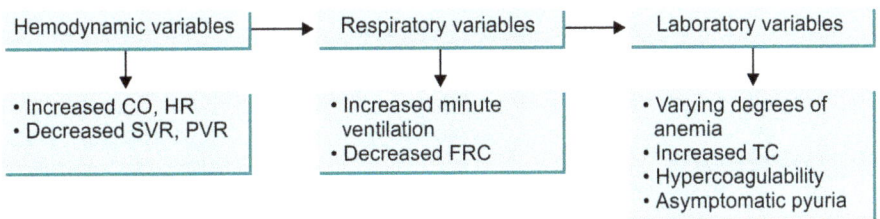

(BP: blood pressure; CO: carbon monoxide; FRC: functional residual capacity; HR: heart rate; PVR: pulmonary vascular resistance; SVR: systemic vascular resistance; TC: total cholesterol)

Obstetric Emergencies

DIFFERENTIAL DIAGNOSIS OF ACUTE ABDOMEN

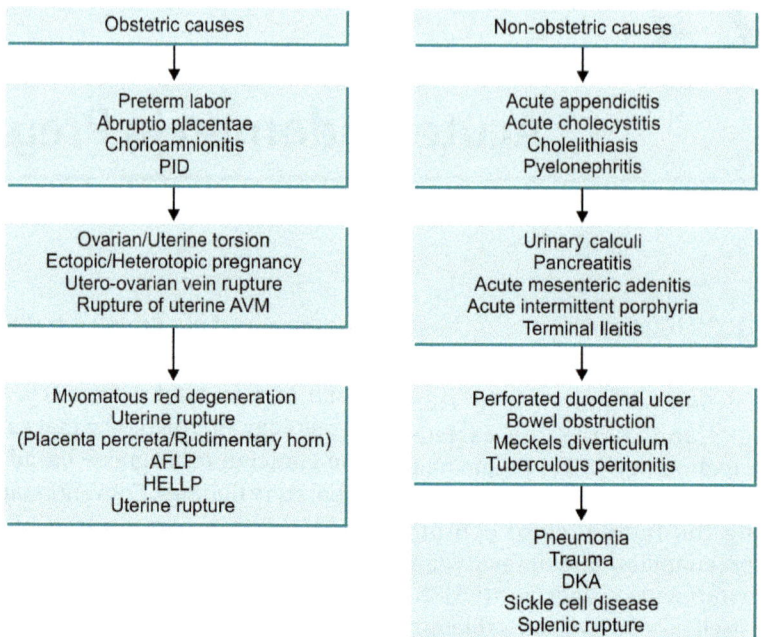

(AFLP: acute fatty liver of pregnancy; AVM: arteriovenous malformation; DKA: diabetic ketoacidosis; PID: pelvic inflammatory disease)

ETIOLOGY BASED ON ONSET, NATURE, AND LOCALIZATION OF PAIN

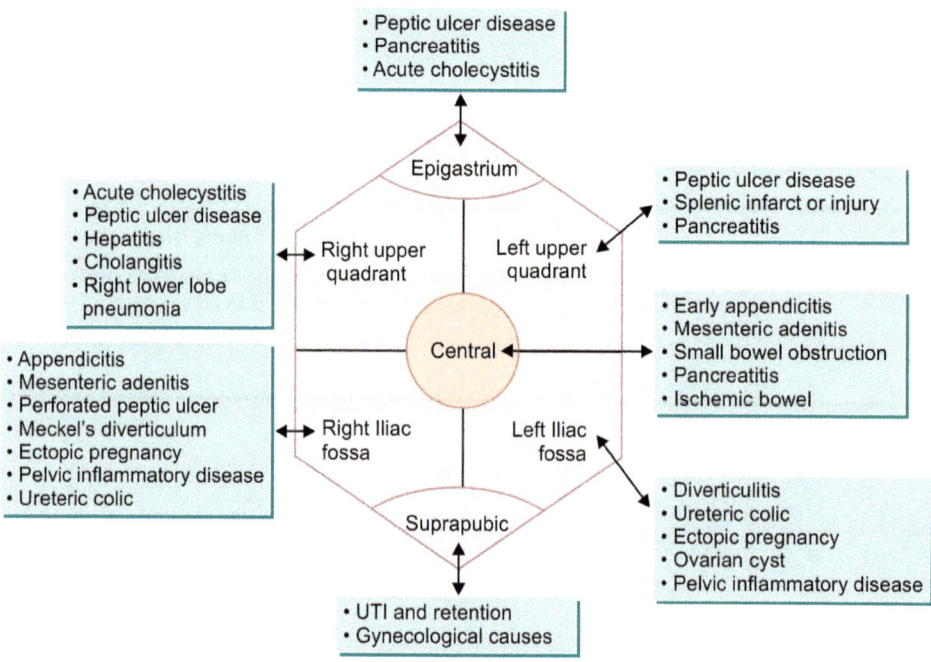

(UTI: urinary tract infection)

Acute Abdomen in Pregnancy

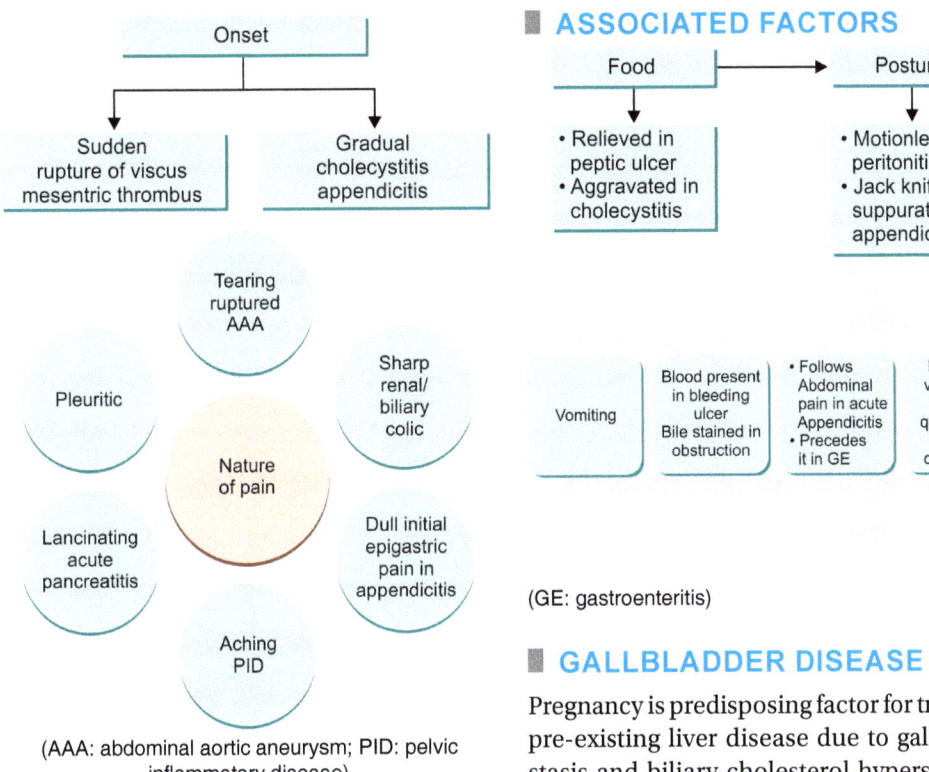

(AAA: abdominal aortic aneurysm; PID: pelvic inflammatory disease)

The longer the duration the more likely a surgical condition.

(GE: gastroenteritis)

GALLBLADDER DISEASE

Pregnancy is predisposing factor for triggering pre-existing liver disease due to gallbladder stasis and biliary cholesterol hypersecretion and is the second most common emergency in pregnancy.[4,5]

In acute cholecystitis, sonographic evidence of cholelithiasis with positive Murphy's sign has a high predictive value (92%).[6]

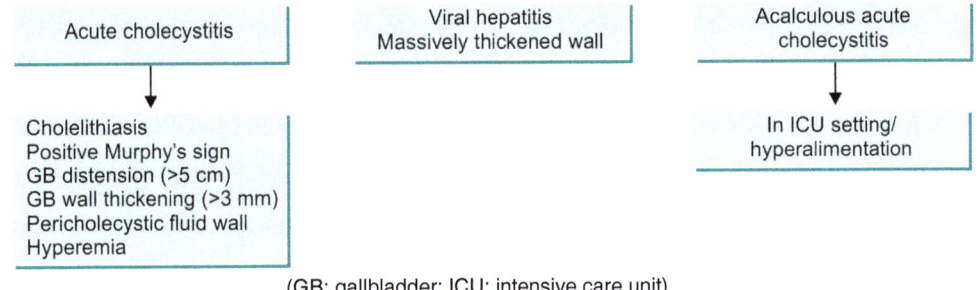

(GB: gallbladder; ICU: intensive care unit)

Management of acute cholecystitis is generally surgical in midtrimester of pregnancy and is conservative in the first and third trimester. Laparoscopic approach is the preferred modality due to its less invasive nature. Both conservative and surgical management have comparable results though in the former 25% patients fail to respond to therapy.[7-9]

PREGNANCY AND THE BOWEL

Acute Appendicitis

Acute appendicitis is the most common cause of acute abdomen in pregnancy. It complicates 1:1,500 pregnancies,[10] delay in diagnosis leads to higher incidence of perforation and higher fetal loss rates (30%)[11] more so in the third trimester.

Other bowel disorders in pregnancy are:

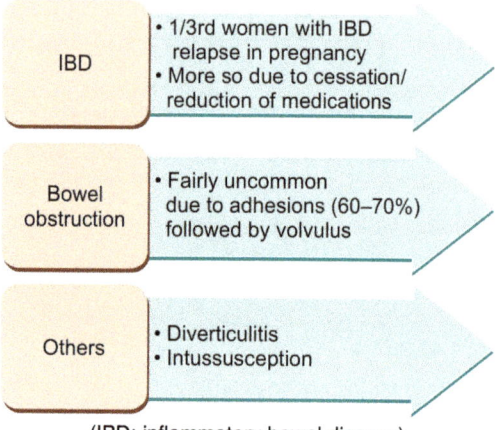

(IBD: inflammatory bowel disease)

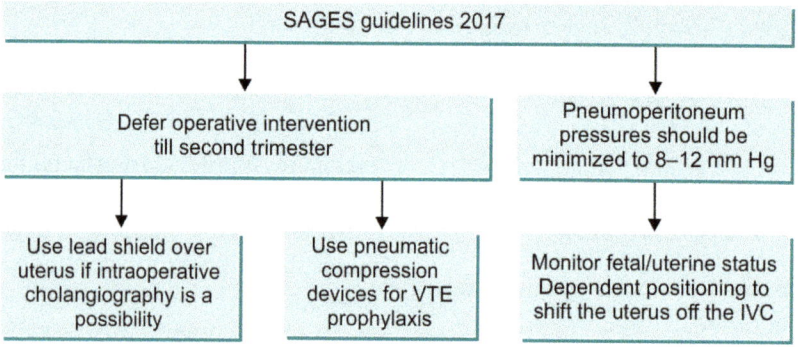

(IVC: inferior vena cava; SAGES: Society of American Gastrointestinal Endoscopic Surgeons; VTE: venous thromboembolism)

Diagnosis is with the help of sonography. In acute appendicitis, it is the presence of tender, nonperistaltic tubular structure with 6 mm diameter with obvious clinical presentation of pain abdomen, vomiting, and fever. Leukocytosis is evident in most cases.

If sonography is inconclusive in establishing diagnosis, MRI may be required to avoid delays in diagnosis.[12,13]

PREGNANCY AND THE KIDNEY

Pregnancy predisposes to hydronephrosis due to pressure of the gravid uterus and smooth muscle relaxation due to progesterone effect, hence considered physiological. It can occur in 70–90% of women more so in third trimester.

Acute pain in the lower abdomen with hematuria and flank pain is pathognomonic of urinary calculi and occurs in 1:1,500 pregnancies.[14] Diagnosis is a challenge in itself and is wrongly diagnosed in a third of cases.[15,16] In absence of evidence of calculi, indirect evidence of renal pathology and in terms of renal enlargement, perinephric fluid and focal hyperechogenicity could indicate pyelonephritis. The significance of pyelonephritis is it predisposes to preterm labor and warrants appropriate antibiotic therapy.

TRAUMA IN PREGNANCY

A leading nonobstetric cause of maternal death, occurring in 5% of pregnancies,[17] can have fatal implications due to abruption. Initiating trauma protocols for management with maternal/fetal surveillance under admission for a 24-hour period is recommended. Prompt delivery where fetal compromise is evident as in an abruption.

Abdominal CT has second place over conventional ultrasound in detecting abdominal injury and is highly specific,[18] though most specific only in first trimester.

After the initial screen patients can be further triaged into those requiring further evaluation. Splenic, bowel, and liver injuries are commonly encountered other than placental abruption.

MINIMIZING RADIATION EXPOSURE TO FETUS

Effects on fetus depend on the dose of exposure, cumulative exposure, and gestational age at exposure. It is recommended not to exceed the cumulative exposure of 50–100 mGy in pregnancy.

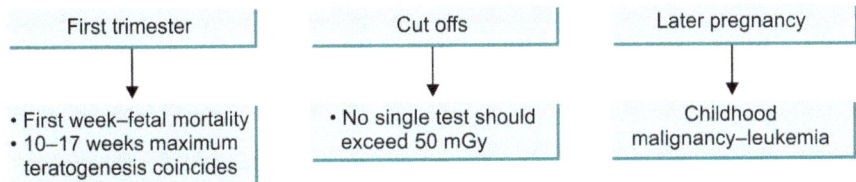

TAKE HOME MESSAGES

- Acute abdomen can be masked by exaggerated physiological states in pregnancy, which should not lead to delay in establishing diagnosis.
- Diagnostic modalities are limited by risk of radiation exposure to the fetus; however, when ultrasonography (USG) is inconclusive more appropriate X-ray or CT scan should be considered without minimizing the lag time which can worsen the morbidity/mortality rates in both mother and the fetus.
- Treatment modalities can vary from less invasive ones in first and third trimesters to more aggressive surgical interventions in the midtrimester and should be individualized for every patient considering the gestational age of pregnancy.
- Laparoscopy is a safe and effective tool when performed by a skilled and experienced surgeon.

Acting in the golden hour is the dictum...
Lost, yesterday, somewhere between sunrise and sunset, two golden hours, each set with sixty diamond minutes. No reward is offered for they are gone forever...
—Horace Mann

CONCLUSION

Acute abdomen in pregnancy can be intriguing to the clinician and distressing to the pregnant woman. Prompt diagnosis with appropriate investigations can lead to accurate diagnosis. Clinical judgment and systematic evaluation form the crux of diagnosis backed by array of laboratory and radiological investigations in management of confounding and complex scenarios encountered in pregnancy.

REFERENCES

1. Kammerer WS. Nonobstetric surgery during pregnancy. Med Clin North Am. 1979;63(6):1157-64.
2. Kort B, Katz VL, Watson WJ. The effect of nonobstetric operation during pregnancy. Surg gynecol obstet. 1993;177(4):371-6.
3. Augustin G, Majerovic M. Non-obstetrical acute abdomen during pregnancy. Eur J Obstet Gynecol Reprod Biol. 2007;131(1):4-12.
4. Ko CW. Risk factors for gallstone-related hospitalization during pregnancy and the postpartum. Am J Gastroenterol. 2006;101(10):2263-8.
5. Ko C. Biliary sludge and acute pancreatitis during pregnancy. Nat Clin Pract Gastroenterology Hepatol. 2006;3(1):53-7.
6. Ralls PW, Colletti PM, Lapin SA, et al. Real-time sonography in suspected acute cholecystitis: prospective evaluation of primary and secondary signs. Radiology. 1985;155(3):767-71.
7. Date RS, Kaushal M, Ramesh A. A review of the management of gallstone disease and its complications in pregnancy. Am J Surg. 2008;196(4):599-608.
8. Hanan IM. Inflammatory bowel disease in the pregnant woman. Compr Ther. 1998;24(9):409-14.
9. Graham G, Baxi L, Tharakan T. Laparoscopic cholecystectomy during pregnancy: a case series and review of the literature. Obstet Gynecol Surv. 1998;53(9):566-74.
10. Sharp HT. The acute abdomen during pregnancy. Clin Obstet Gynecol. 2002;45(2): 405-13.
11. Mazze RI, Källén B. Appendectomy during pregnancy: a Swedish registry study of 778 cases. Obstet Gynecol. 1991;77(6):835-40.
12. Pedrosa I, Lafornara M, Pandharipande PV, et al. Pregnant patients suspected of having acute appendicitis: effect of MR imaging on negative laparotomy rate and appendiceal perforation rate. Radiology. 2009;250(3):749-57.
13. Pedrosa I, Levine D, Eyvazzadeh AD, et al. MR imaging evaluation of acute appendicitis in pregnancy. Radiology. 2006;238:891-9.
14. Bailey LE, Finley RK Jr, Miller SF, et al. Acute appendicitis during pregnancy. Am Surg. 1986;52:218-21.
15. McAleer SJ, Loughlin KR. Nephrolithiasis and pregnancy. Curr Opin Urol. 2004;14(2):123-7.
16. Stothers L, Lee LM. Renal colic in pregnancy. J Urol. 1992;148:1383-7.
17. Goldman SM, Wagner LK. Radiologic ABCs of maternal and fetal survival after trauma: when minutes may count. Radiographics. 1999;19:1349-57.
18. Richards JR, Ormsby EL, Romo MV, et al. Blunt abdominal injury in the pregnant patient: detection with US. Radiology. 2004;233:463-70.

CHAPTER 34

Umbilical Cord Prolapse

Taswin Kaur Reddy

INTRODUCTION

Pregnancy and childbirth is always expected to be a safe and satisfying adventure for the laboring woman and her family as well as her healthcare providers. Little does anyone hope for a mishap; especially an unforeseen one. However, the reality is far from the contrary. According to the World Health Organization; it is estimated that 830 women die daily from preventable causes related to pregnancy and child birth.[1] Almost all of them occur in developing countries. As an obstetrician, it is of utmost importance to assure that child birth is a safe experience and ensure that both the lives—the mother and the fetus are safeguarded.[2] Unfortunately, there are unforeseen startling incidences that catch the healthcare providers out of the hook needing a vigilant lookout and action. Umbilical cord prolapsed is an infrequent sporadic obstetric emergency situation requiring swift identification and intervention to reduce fetal morbidity and mortality.[3]

INCIDENCE AND EPIDEMIOLOGY

The reported risk of umbilical cord prolapsed is between 0.1% and 0.62%.[4-6] Umbilical cord prolapse occurs more frequently in fetus having abnormal presentations; especially a transverse lie or a breech presentation.[7,8] However, over the last century; the incidence of umbilical cord prolapse has been decreasing with almost 94% fetal survival rate.[9,10] This has been attributed to meticulous monitoring and expeditious management—more widespread availability of cesarean section and advanced neonatal resuscitation techniques. According to a study by Murphy et al.; 77% of cases were singleton pregnancies; in twin pregnancies, the first twin was less affected (9%) compared to the second twin (14%).[3]

DEFINITION AND TYPES (FLOWCHART 1 AND TABLE 1)

Cord prolapse is defined as the descent of the umbilical cord into the lower uterine segment where it may lie adjacent to the presenting part or below the presenting part without an intact fetal membrane.

Other types of cord accidents:
- *True knot*: It is an intertwining segment of umbilical cord which is commonly formed by the fetus slipping through the

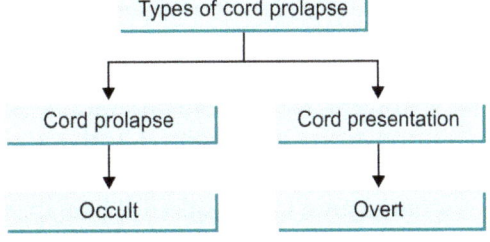

Flowchart 1: Types of cord prolapse.

TABLE 1: Different types of cord prolapse.

	Occult cord prolapse	Overt cord prolapse	Cord (funic) presentation
Definition	Prolapse of the umbilical cord through the cervix alongside the presenting part	Prolapse of the umbilical cord past the presenting part into the vagina or vulva	Prolapse of the umbilical cord below the level of the presenting part before the rupture of the amniotic membranes
Membrane status	Amniotic membranes have ruptured	Occurs after the amniotic membranes have ruptured	Intact amniotic membranes
Cord position	Beside the presenting part	Below the presenting part	Below the presenting part
Vaginal examination	Cannot be palpated on vaginal examination Palpable only by passing the examining finger into the cervical canal	Can be palpable on vaginal examination	Can be palpated through the membranes Presence of one or more loops of umbilical cord between the fetal presenting part and the fetal membrane overlying the cervical os
Other features	May lead to variable decelerations on the cardio topography (CTG) or unexplained fetal distress		Harbinger of cord prolapse

loop of the cord; usually does not cause circulation obstruction.
- *Nuchal cord*: The umbilical cord is wrapped around the fetus in utero or when the baby is being born. It is usually possible to slip the loops gently over the head of the baby during delivery. Occurs in more than 25% of deliveries; especially in those with longer cord length.

■ RISK FACTORS

Multiple risk factors have been enlisted to be associated with umbilical cord abnormalities (Box 1).[8] Numerous studies have attempted to identify and rank these risk factors. However, due to the uncommon occurrence of umbilical cord prolapse, there is no consensus at present attempting to assign a relative risk for each of the available assumed associated risk factor. The attributed factors causing umbilical cord prolapse can be broadly classified into spontaneous and iatrogenic causes.

Spontaneous umbilical cord prolapse can otherwise occur in uncomplicated

Box 1: Risk factors associated with umbilical cord prolapse.[8,11-13]

Spontaneous
- Malpresentation—transverse lie and breech[14]
- Polyhydramnios—associated with an unstable lie
- Multiple pregnancy—especially during delivery for the aftercoming twin[15]
- Grand multipara—due to laxity of the muscles and uterine dystonia
- Cord abnormalities—long umbilical cord
- Preterm delivery
- Low birth weight (<2,500 g)—includes intrauterine growth restriction and prematurity
- Fetal anomalies
- Spontaneous rupture of membranes—prior to the engagement of the presenting part [premature rupture of membrane (PROM) and preterm PROM (PPROM)]

Iatrogenic[16]
- Artificial rupture of membranes with a high presenting part[12]
- Fetal invasive procedures—placement of intrauterine pressure catheter/fetal scalp electrode
- External cephalic version in a patient with ruptured amniotic membranes
- Amnioinfusion
- Induction of labor using a large balloon catheter.

pregnancies, which usually occurs due to a fetal or maternal underlying cause that prevents the engagement of the fetal head into the maternal pelvis or due to cord abnormalities, hence allowing space for the escape of the umbilical cord. Fetal malpresentation is the most widely accepted risk factor.

Iatrogenic umbilical cord prolapse can usually be prevented by a meticulous approach and wholesome assessment of the laboring woman. The most common iatrogenic cause described is by virtue of an amniotomy prior to engagement of the presenting part.

PATHOPHYSIOLOGY[17,18]

The failure of the fetal presenting part to engage into the maternal pelvis causes the umbilical cord to slip downwards and to plunge through the cervix after the membranes are ruptured. The intrauterine pressure (amniotic sac) is higher than the external environment. Consequently, with the aid of gravity, when the membranes rupture, the amniotic fluid gushes out.[19] Owing to the slit available between the maternal pelvis and fetus; the loosely dangling mobile cord finds its way downwards along with the amniotic fluid. The sudden lower temperature of the vagina causes vasospasm of the umbilical vessels, which leads to a decreased fetal preload.

Situation is worse when the labor contraction begins; causing the umbilical cord to be compressed between the presenting part and the maternal bony pelvis, uterus and cervix which culminate with the uterine artery compression. The compression of the artery is reflected as fetal heart decelerations. Normally, as much as 50% of the fetal circulation passes through the umbilical arteries.[20] Therefore, compression of these vessels makes a humongous difference in the fetal cardiovascular status and the unaccustomed fetal heart has to work double to overcome the resistance by the increased vascular pressure.

To increase the pulse pressure, the heart rate is decreased which is reflected by the fetal heart rate (FHR) tracing. There is a sudden severe reduction in FHR, especially after the rupture of the amniotic membranes. This causal nexus of reduced blood flow to the circulation produces fetal hypoxia resulting in adverse fetal outcomes and morbidity. The FHR abnormalities are an indirect indicator of the poor perfusion of the placenta—fetus plexus which if left untreated dwindles to a mishap.

DIAGNOSIS

Umbilical cord prolapse is suspected when there is sudden FHR deceleration with prolonged bradycardia or moderate to severe variable decelerations; after the rupture of fetal membranes.

The diagnosis of cord prolapse can be confirmed on examination with an umbilical cord loop extruding out of the introitus or the cord is visualized in the vagina on per speculum examination. A soft pulsatile mass is felt on palpation during internal examination.

Umbilical cord prolapse can only be definitely diagnosed if the cord is palpable. Hence, overt cord prolapse is easier to diagnose than occult cord prolapse. Majority cases of occult cord prolapse go undiagnosed and the pregnancy is terminated by an emergency cesarean section in view of fetal bradycardia or repeated variable decelerations of the fetal heart tracing. During internal examination, if the cord or soft pulsating mass is felt through the fetal membranes; an assumption of cord presentation is made. Thus, it is of utmost importance to perform an internal examination prior to artificial rupture of membranes to exclude a cord presentation and to avoid cord prolapse. The umbilical cord pulsations may be absent in cases of cord prolapse with intrauterine fetal demise.

The soft umbilical cord may sometimes be confused with abnormal presentations—fetal limb or face presentation and severe caput succedaneum; by amateur obstetricians. Since umbilical cord prolapse is a rather rare phenomenon in this century; other causes of FHR decelerations including maternal hypotension, after receiving spinal anesthesia, rupture of vasa previa, placental abruption, and uterine rupture should be ruled out simultaneously; and these conditions also require an urgent delivery.

MANAGEMENT[8]

Umbilical cord prolapse is one of the acute obstetric emergencies encountered in a laboring woman with ruptured amniotic membranes. Cord prolapse can lead to fetal compromise, which results in long-term morbidity and even fetal mortality.[4] The yardstick of a successful cord prolapse management is based on speed; as the perinatal outcome is largely dictated by the diagnosis to delivery interval.[21] Therefore, patients diagnosed with an umbilical cord prolapse with a live fetus in general undergo a cesarean section; unless she is in second stage of labor, delivery is imminent and shall be achieved quicker than a cesarean section.

Three main components of management are:
1. Prevent or relieve cord compression and vasospasm
2. Fetal assessment
3. Prompt delivery of the fetus, if alive.

Initial Management of Umbilical Cord Prolapse in Hospital Setting

Initial management of umbilical cord prolapse in hospital setting has been described in Flowchart 2.

Manual Elevation

This procedure is done by inserting a gloved hand or two fingers into the vagina where the presenting part is gently pushed upwards.

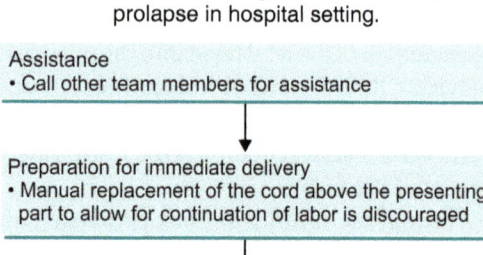

Flowchart 2: Initial management of umbilical cord prolapse in hospital setting.

Assistance
• Call other team members for assistance

↓

Preparation for immediate delivery
• Manual replacement of the cord above the presenting part to allow for continuation of labor is discouraged

↓

Prevent vasospasm
• Colder temperature outside the vagina and excessive handling of the cord can exaggerate the vasospasm
• If the cord is outside the introitus, gently replace it into the vagina
• Cover the hanging umbilical cord with sterile surgical packs soaked in warm saline (unproven benefit)

↓

Prevent cord compression (primary prevention until delivery)
• Options available:
 • Manually
 • Filling the urinary bladder
 • Adjusting the maternal position-knee-chest position, left lateral tilt or head down tilt

↓

Tocolysis
• While preparing for lower segment cesarean section (LSCS) or when delivery is expected to be slightly delayed

Utmost care is taken to prevent excessive pressure on the umbilical cord. A variation of this maneuver is to remove the hand from the vagina once the presenting part is above the pelvic brim and apply continuous suprapubic pressure upwards. However, excessive displacement may encourage more room for umbilical cord prolapse.

Bladder Filling

This maneuver was introduced by Vago in 1970 where the patient's anatomy is altered to alleviate the compression on the umbilical cord. The patient is placed in Trendelenburg position and by inserting the Foley catheter into the bladder, the urinary bladder is

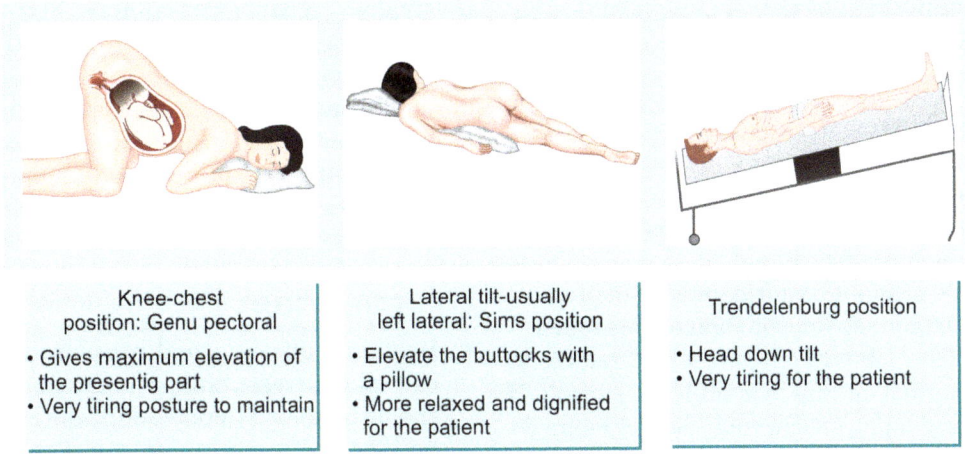

Fig. 1: Maternal positions.

distended. After infusing around 500–750 mL of saline, the catheter is clamped. In addition, the procedure is said to physiologically inhibit contractions. The contractions that may be present are not strong enough for the presenting part to effectively cause cord compression.

Adjusting the Maternal Position

The principle of altering maternal positions is to allow gravity aid in decompressing the pressure on the umbilical cord (Fig. 1).

The cornerstone of a successful cord prolapse management is delivery of a nonmorbid baby and this can be ensured by prompt delivery of the fetus with continuous FHR monitoring. The delivery should be planned as soon as possible after diagnosis to forestall hypoxia and acidosis to the fetus (Flowchart 3).[22]

Management in a Community Setting

There is an increased risk in perinatal mortality in cases of umbilical cord prolapse occurring outside the hospital setting; even compared with an unmonitored fetus that

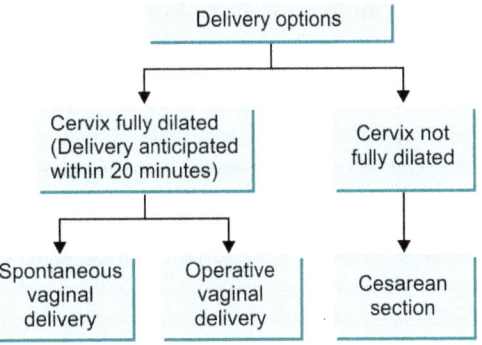

Flowchart 3: Delivery options.

had a cord prolapse while being in the hospital. While awaiting a hospital transfer to the nearest healthcare facility, the patient is advised to assume the knee-chest position or a steep Trendelenburg position. However, during an emergency ambulance transfer; the left lateral position should be used as the knee-chest position is potentially unsafe. If a midwife is available with the patient, she can be instructed to elevate the presenting part by manual or by bladder filling method to relieve the compression on the umbilical cord. Strict instructions for minimal handling of the prolapsed umbilical cord which is outside the introitus should be ensured.

Management of Occult Umbilical Cord Prolapse

When occult cord prolapse is suspected, the line of suggested management is as follows:
- Immediate vaginal examination to rule out cord prolapse
- Left lateral position to avoid compression on the umbilical cord
- Discontinue oxytocin infusion (if present)
- Oxygen supplementation to the mother
- Allow labor to progress if FHR returns to normal and there is no further insult. If any doubt, patient counseled for cesarean section
- Continuous FHR monitoring.
- Amnioinfusion—if required
- If cord compression pattern continues on fetal heart tracing, to avoid perinatal morbidity and mortality; an urgent cesarean section is performed.

CONSEQUENCES OF UMBILICAL CORD PROLAPSE

Different consequences of umbilical cord prolapse have been described in Figure 2.

OUTCOME

Overall, the perinatal outcome of umbilical cord prolapse is good and the fetal survival rate has increased over the past years owing to the higher index of suspicion and quicker timely delivery and safer cesarean section deliveries. Umbilical cord prolapse occurring in a hospital setting has lesser perinatal morbidity and mortality rates compared to those further away. On the whole, fetuses delivered within 30 minutes of diagnosis generally do well without any long-term sequelae.

PREVENTION

- Women with abnormal presentations such as transverse, oblique or unstable lie should be offered elective admission to the hospital at 37 weeks of gestation or sooner if there are signs of labor or suspicion of ruptured membrane.
- Women with noncephalic presentations and preterm rupture of membranes should be offered admission.
- Artificial rupture of membranes should be avoided whenever possible if the presenting part is unengaged or is mobile. If it is essential to rupture the membranes prior to engagement of the presenting part; facilities for immediate cesarean section should be available.
- Speculum or a digital vaginal examination should be performed to confirm the diagnosis whenever cord prolapse is suspected; regardless of the period of gestation.
- Artificial rupture of membranes should be avoided if on vaginal examination the umbilical cord is felt below the presenting part in labor (cord presentation). A cesarean section should be performed.
- Inpatient care will minimize delay in diagnosis to delivery of a patient with cord prolapse.

CONCLUSION

Umbilical cord prolapse is an acute, frightening, and life-threatening obstetric emergency

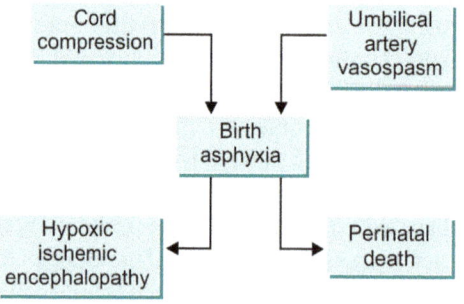

Fig. 2: Consequences of umbilical cord prolapse.

Flowchart 4: Management of umbilical cord prolapse.

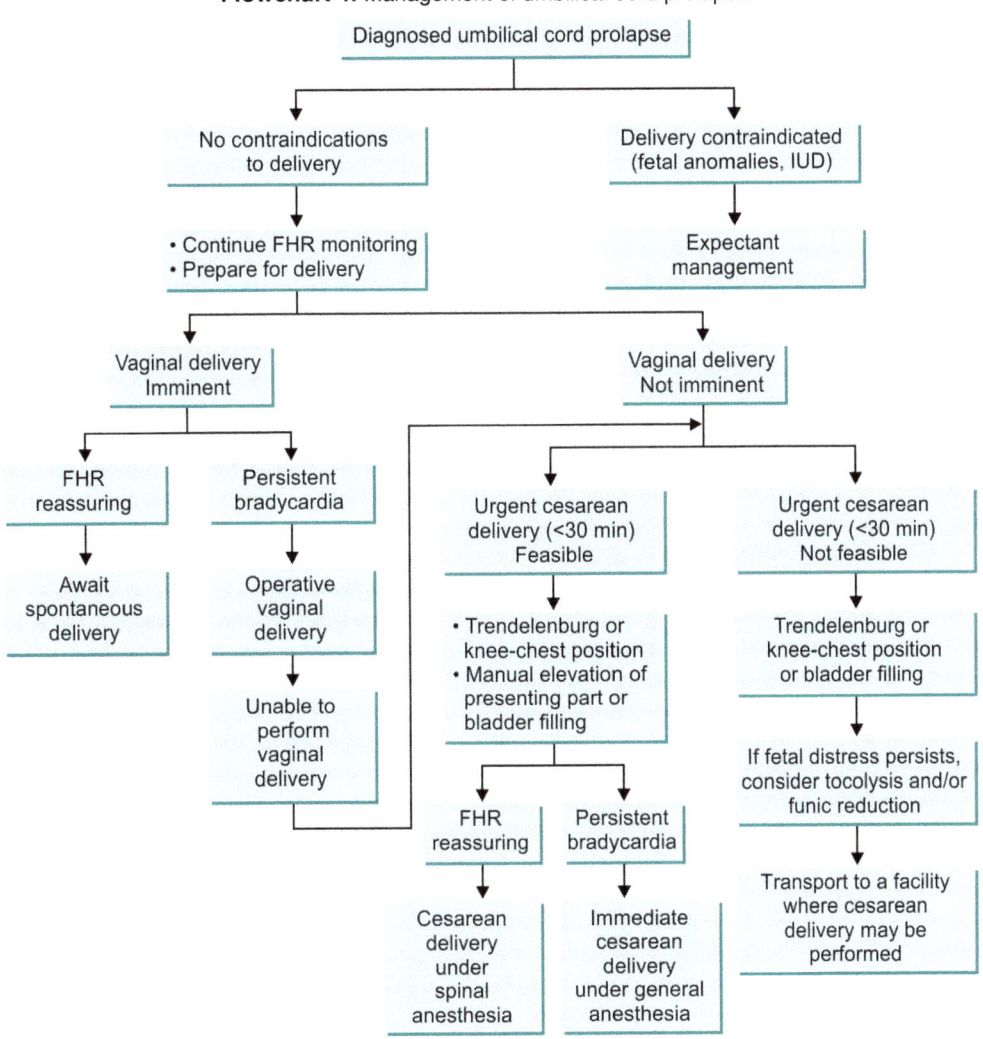

(FHR: fetal heart rate; IUD: intrauterine device)

requiring a timely management that occurs in labor. Rapid identification and an immediate dash are required to save the life of the neonate. Therefore, although uncommon, the clinician should be knowledgeable in its recognition and management as it leaves no minutes for a mishap.

Algorithm for the management of umbilical cord prolapse has been shown in Flowchart 4.[23]

REFERENCES

1. World Health Organization. (2018). Maternal mortality. [online] Available from: https://www.who.int/News-Room/Fact-Sheets/Detail/Maternal-Mortality [last accessed September, 2019].
2. Steer PJ. Saving Mothers' Lives. Reviewing maternal deaths to make motherhood safer: 2006-2008. Br J Obstet Gynaecol. 2011;118(11):1404.

3. Murphy DJ, Mackenzie IZ. The mortality and morbidity associated with umbilical cord prolapse. Br J Obstet Gynaecol. 1995; 102(10):826-30.
4. Hehir MP, Hartigan L, Mahony R. Perinatal death associated with umbilical cord prolapse. J Perinat Med. 2017;45(5):565-70.
5. Kahana B, Sheiner E, Levy A, et al. Umbilical cord prolapse and perinatal outcomes. Int J Gynecol Obstet. 2003;84(2):127-32.
6. Qureshi N, Taylor D, Tomlinson A. Umbilical cord prolapse. Int J Gynecol Obstet. 2004; 86(1):29-30.
7. Savage E, Kohl, S, Wynn R. Prolapse of the umbilical cord. Obstet Gynecol. 1970;36(4): 502-9.
8. RCOG. (2014). Umbilical Cord Prolapse (Green-top Guideline No. 50) [online] Available from: https://www.rcog.org.uk/En/Guidelines-Research-Services/Guidelines/Gtg50/[Last accessed September, 2019].
9. Silver RM. Umbilical cord prolapse—progress! Br J Obstet Gynaecol. 2014;121(13):1709.
10. Gibbons C, O'Herlihy C, Murphy J. Umbilical cord prolapse—changing patterns and improved outcomes: A retrospective cohort study. Br J Obstet Gynaecol. 2014;121(13):1705-8.
11. Dilbaz B, Ozturkoglu E, Dilbaz S, et al. Risk factors and perinatal outcomes associated with umbilical cord prolapse. Arch Gynecol Obstet. 2006;274(2):104-7.
12. Huang C, Landy H, Kawakita T. Risk factors for umbilical cord prolapse at the time of artificial rupture of membranes. AJP Rep. 2018; 08(02):e89-e94.
13. Behbehani S, Patenaude V, Abenhaim H. Maternal risk factors and outcomes of umbilical cord prolapse: A population-based study. J Obstet Gynaecol Can. 2016;38(1):23-8.
14. Hasegawa J, Ikeda T, Sekizawa A, et al. Obstetric risk factors for umbilical cord prolapse: a nationwide population-based study in Japan. Arch Gynecol Obstet. 2015;294(3):467-72.
15. Hembram M, Sagili H. Risk factors, maternal and neonatal outcome in umbilical cord prolapse in south Indian population. J SAFOG. 2017;9(4):323-6.
16. Roberts W, Martin R, Roach H, et al. Are obstetric interventions such as cervical ripening, induction of labor, amnioinfusion, or amniotomy associated with umbilical cord prolapse? Am J Obstet Gynecol. 1997;176(6): 1181-5.
17. Clark DO, Copeland W, Ullery JC. Prolapse of the umbilical cord. A study of 117 cases. Am J Obstet Gynecol. 1968;101(1):84-90.
18. Mcdaniels HR, Umezaki H, Harer WB, et al. Is umbilical cord prolapse secondary to fetal acidemia? Prenat Neonatal Med. 2001;6(2): 129-32.
19. Fisk NM, Tannirandorn Y, Nicolini U, et al. Amniotic pressure in disorders of amniotic fluid volume. Obstet Gynecol. 1990;76(2):210-4.
20. Fineman JR, Clyman R. Fetal Cardiovascular Physiology. In: Creasy RK, Resnick R, Iams JD (Eds). Creasy and Resnick's Maternal-Fetal Medicine: Principles and Practice, 6th edition. Philadelphia: Saunders Elsevier; 2009.pp. 161–2.
21. Copson S, Calvert K, Raman P, et al. The Effect of a multidisciplinary obstetric emergency team training program, the in time course, on diagnosis to delivery interval following umbilical cord prolapse. Obstetric Anesthesia Digest. 2018;38(2):83-5.
22. Pereira S, Chandraharan E. Umbilical cord prolapse. In: Jha S, Ferriman E (Eds). Medicolegal Issues in Obstetrics and Gynaecology. Berlin, German: Springer; 2018.
23. Holbrook BD, Phelan ST. Umbilical Cord Prolapse. Obstet Gynecol Clin North Am. 2013; 40(1):1-14.

CHAPTER 35

Epilepsy in Pregnancy

Surbhi Gupta

INTRODUCTION

Epilepsy is defined as a group of brain diseases; heterogeneous in nature with the common feature of seizure. Epilepsy as a neurological condition has an incidence of 0.5–1% in pregnancy.[1] One-third of women with epilepsy (WWE) are in their reproductive age group. The number of infants born to WWE per year in the United Kingdom approximates to about 2,500.[2] There is almost ten times increased risk of death in pregnant WWE than those without epilepsy.[1] Epilepsy has been shown to account for 5% of the maternal deaths in the United Kingdom in 2011–2013 triennium.[3]

The risk of major congenital malformations is also increased with the use of antiepileptic drugs (AEDs).[4-10] This can result in stoppage or decrease in the dose of the AEDs because of anxiety among women; thus, leading to increased risk of seizures.

PATHOPHYSIOLOGY

A seizure is defined as a paroxysmal disorder of the central nervous system characterized by an abnormal neuronal discharge with or without loss of consciousness.

The various causes of convulsive disorders include head trauma, alcohol and other drug-induced withdrawals, cerebral infections, brain tumors, biochemical abnormalities and arteriovenous malformations. Idiopathic epilepsy is a diagnosis of exclusion. The cardinal feature of epilepsy encompassing different syndromes is predisposition to unprovoked seizures.

CLASSIFICATION OF SEIZURE DISORDERS

Classification of epilepsy syndrome is essential for choosing appropriate AED, for determining prognosis and for identifying and preventing factors responsible for seizure determination. It will also help in identifying provoking factors and for formulating the plan of management.

The various seizure disorders in pregnancy are shown in Table 1.

The strongest risk factor for sudden unexpected death in epilepsy (SUDEP) is uncontrolled tonic-clonic seizures. SUDEP is the main cause of death in epilepsy.[12] SUDEP is defined as a sudden, unexpected, witnessed or unwitnessed, nontraumatic and nondrowning death in patients with epilepsy, with or without evidence for a seizure and excluding documented status epilepticus, in which postmortem examination does not reveal a toxicologic or anatomic cause for death.[13]

DIAGNOSIS OF EPILEPSY

Neurologist should be consulted for making definitive diagnosis of epilepsy and epileptiform seizures. This condition in pregnancy should be assessed on the basis

TABLE 1: Types of seizure disorders.[11]

S. no.	Common types of seizures	Clinical features	Effect on mother and baby
1.	Tonic-clonic seizures (Previously grand mal seizures)	Dramatic events with stiffening, bilateral jerking and a postseizure state of confusion and sleepiness	• Sudden loss of consciousness with an uncontrolled fall without prior warning • Associated with variable period of fetal hypoxia • Associated with highest risk of SUDEP
2.	Absence seizures	Generalized seizures consisting of brief spells associated with unresponsiveness; followed by rapid recovery	• Brief loss of awareness with modest physiological effects • Increased the risk of tonic-clonic seizures with worsening absence seizures
3.	Juvenile myoclonic epilepsy	• Myoclonic jerks are a key feature and often precede tonic-clonic convulsion • Jerks present as sudden and unpredictable movements and represent a generalized seizure	• Provoked with sleep deprivation and in the period soon after waking or when tired • May lead to falls or to dropping of objects, including the baby
4.	Focal seizures (Previously "complex partial" if seizures impair consciousness and "simple partial" if consciousness impaired)	• Variable symptoms depending on regions and networks of brain affected • Consciousness may be impaired • Primary focal seizures can undergo generalization • An aura is a primary focal seizure	• Impairment of consciousness increases risk of injuries like fractures, dental or head injury, electrocution or burns compared to retained consciousness (epileptic aura only) • Can be associated with variable period of hypoxia and risk of SUDEP

of duration and severity, the type of seizures, their frequency and any aggravating factors. The impact of these seizures on mother in her daily routine activities should also be assessed. The drug history of effective and ineffective medications and adverse effects, if any, should be considered.

Women with seizure-free period of at least 10 years with last 5 years off AEDs should be considered epilepsy free. Also, women who had epilepsy in childhood but have reached adulthood without any episodes of seizure and without any treatment are also considered to be epilepsy free.[14] These women are categorized as low risk in absence of other risk factors.

Any seizure in pregnancy not because of epilepsy should be treated as eclampsia unless proved otherwise.[15]

Other differential diagnosis includes:
- Cardiac causes like cardiac arrhythmia, aortic stenosis, carotid sinus sensitivity, vasovagal syncope
- Metabolic causes like hypoglycemia, hyponatremia, Addisonian crisis
- Other intracranial conditions like cerebral venous sinus thrombosis, posterior reversible encephalopathy syndrome, space-occupying lesions, reversible cerebral vasoconstriction syndrome
- Neuropsychiatric conditions including nonepileptic attack disorder.

The diagnostic considerations also include past history of epilepsy or other risk factors for developing pre-eclampsia.

Magnetic resonance imaging (MRI) and computerized tomography (CT) scans can be performed in women with episodes of seizures. Single exposure to these presents minimal risk to fetus.[16-18]

PRECONCEPTIONAL COUNSELING AND MANAGEMENT

Women having epilepsy should be counseled in detail about the effect of pregnancy on epilepsy and both short-term and long-term effects on the health of their offspring. WWE should be counseled in detail regarding prenatal screening, risks of stopping AEDs on their own and the effects of epilepsy and the drugs for its treatment on the pregnancy, fetus, breastfeeding and contraception.[11] Drowning is a known risk factor for both maternal and fetal death and thus, advice should be given regarding bathing in shallow water and with assistance for both themselves and the babies.[19]

Consultation with a neurologist or a clinician with expertise in epilepsy management should be done regarding the type and dose of AEDs, based on their efficacy and risk to the fetus.

Embryofetal Malformations

Women with epilepsy should also be counseled regarding the congenital malformations in the fetus with the use of AEDs. The incidence of major congenital malformations is same as in WWE not exposed to AEDs.[20] The risk of major congenital malformations is dependent on the type, number and dose of AEDs. The risk of major congenital malformations is least with lamotrigine and carbamazepine monotherapy at low doses.[10] A meta-analysis of 31 studies found lamotrigine and levetiracetam to carry the lowest risk of malformations.[21] The most common major congenital malformations with the use of AEDs are neural tube defects (NTDs), congenital heart diseases, urinary tract and skeletal abnormalities and cleft palate (Table 2). The risk is reduced with monotherapy as compared to polytherapy. There is insufficient evidence regarding congenital malformations associated with AEDs like gabapentin, oxcarbazepine, pregabalin, topiramate, zonisamide or eslicarbazepine.

A systematic review and meta-analysis of 59 studies suggested that the risk of congenital malformations was highest with sodium valproate or AED polytherapy.[8] The risk of major congenital malformations is high in WWE with a previous child having major congenital malformation. The association of congenital malformations with type of epilepsy or first trimester tonic-clonic seizures was not significant.

Effect of Antiepileptic Drugs on Neurodevelopmental Outcome

In utero exposures of AEDs have also shown to affect neurodevelopmental outcomes in the offspring. This is seen most commonly with sodium valproate. Carbamazepine and lamotrigine exposure in utero is not associated with adverse neurodevelopmental outcome. There is insufficient evidence for other drugs. As per 2014 Cochrane review, the developmental quotient of children exposed to the AEDs like carbamazepine, lamotrigine and phenytoin when compared to infants of mothers without epilepsy or those with epilepsy not taking AEDs was not significantly different.[23] The exposure of sodium valproate in the antenatal period resulted in a significantly lower developmental quotient.[23] There is negative effect of high doses of sodium valproate on the verbal ability, intelligence

TABLE 2: Teratogenic effects of common antiepileptic drugs.[22]

Drug	Associated congenital malformations	Affected	Embryofetal risks
Valproate	• Neural tube defects • Cardiac anomalies • Facial cleft • Hypospadias • Developmental delay	10% with monotherapy; higher with polytherapy	Yes
Phenytoin	Fetal hydantoin syndrome—craniofacial anomalies, fingernail hypoplasia, growth deficiency, developmental delay, cardiac anomalies, facial clefts	5–11%	Yes
Carbamazepine	• Fetal hydantoin syndrome • Spina bifida	1–2%	Yes
Phenobarbital	• Facial clefts • Cardiac anomalies • Urinary tract malformations	10–20%	Suggested
Lamotrigine	Increased risk for facial clefts (Registry data)	Up to 1% (4- to 10-fold higher than expected)	Suggested
Topiramate	Facial clefts	2–3% (15- to 20-fold higher than expected)	Suggested
Levetiracetam	Theoretical risk—skeletal abnormalities, impaired growth in animals	Preliminary observation	Suggested

quotient (IQ), nonverbal ability, memory and executive function.[24] There is increased risk of childhood autism with antenatal exposure of sodium valproate.[25,26]

Reducing the Risk of Congenital Malformations

Women with epilepsy should be prescribed 5 mg/day of folic acid 1 month prior to conception till the end of first trimester to minimize the risk of major congenital malformations. The risk of AED-related cognitive defects is also reduced with its intake. The minimum effective dose of the appropriate AED should be prescribed. The exposure to sodium valproate should be kept at a minimum. AED polytherapy should be avoided after consultation with an epilepsy specialist and after analyzing potential risks and benefits. AED monotherapy is preferred.

Effect of Pregnancy on Seizures

Women should also be counseled regarding the effect of pregnancy on seizures. About two-thirds (67%) of women will not have seizure deterioration or seizure in pregnancy. The most important factor for assessment of risk of seizure deterioration is the seizure-free period. If the seizure-free duration is at least 9 months to 1 year prior to pregnancy, 74–92% women will not have any seizures during pregnancy.[27-29] As compared to focal epilepsies, where there is 60% incidence of seizure-free episodes, idiopathic generalized epilepsies are more likely to have seizure-free period (74%).[30]

There is insufficient evidence to assess the risk of status epilepticus in WWE. Status epilepticus is defined as 30 minutes of continual seizure activity or a cluster of seizures without recovery. Currently, no tests are available to predict seizure deterioration in pregnancy.[11]

ANTEPARTUM MANAGEMENT

Pregnant WWE should have regular antenatal care which should happen in a multidisciplinary setting. It should involve obstetrician, neurologist or a physician with expertise in epilepsy, nurses trained to manage epilepsy patients and other specialists like neuropsychiatrist if required. Women on AEDs with an unplanned pregnancy should consult the neurologist on an urgent basis. They should be managed on an individualized basis. It may require change in the type or dose of AED. There should not be abrupt discontinuation or change of AEDs. Continuation of high-risk drugs like sodium valproate might be required depending on the associated risks and benefits. The following points should be kept in mind during the antenatal period in WWE.

Screening for Fetal Abnormalities

All WWE should undergo a detailed anomaly scan between 18^{+0} weeks and 20^{+6} weeks of gestation to identify major cardiac defects, NTDs or other structural abnormalities. The detection rate of NTDs is increased to 94–100% with combined use of ultrasonography with biochemical screening for maternal serum alpha-protein.[31]

Monitoring of Antiepileptic Drugs

There is decrease in the levels of most AEDs in pregnancy due to changes in pharmacokinetics of absorption, metabolism, hemodilution and excretion.[32-34] But routine monitoring of serum AED levels is not recommended in pregnancy.[11] The levels of lamotrigine fall by up to 70% in pregnancy.[35]

The monitoring of AEDs can be done in two ways; either regular therapeutic drug monitoring or monitoring based on clinical features to adjust the AED dose.[36,37] There is insufficient evidence to recommend either of the two methods for monitoring on a routine basis. So clinical judgment has to be taken on the basis of suspicion of nonadherence, toxicity and intractable seizures.

Adverse Effects of Antiepileptic Drugs on Mother

Certain epilepsies and AEDs have the potential to cause depression with features like low mood, inability to plan and organize thoughts, poor concentration, tiredness, irritability or anger.[38] Women should be advised for self-monitoring of these symptoms to improve quality of life.

Antiepileptic drugs also affect maternal cognition; especially with high doses or polytherapy. So early referral to neuropsychiatrist or perinatal mental health team should be done in these cases.

Obstetric Complications in Women with Epilepsy

There is increased risk of spontaneous miscarriage, antepartum hemorrhage, hypertensive disorders, fetal growth restriction, cesarean section and postpartum hemorrhage in WWE as compared to women without epilepsy.[39]

Women on AEDs have higher risk of undergoing induction of labor and cesarean delivery, fetal growth restriction and postpartum hemorrhage than those not on any AEDs.[39] The risk of cesarean delivery is also increased in women on polytherapy as compared to those on monotherapy.

Also, children of epileptic mothers have a 10% risk of developing a seizure disorder.

Antenatal Monitoring in Women with Epilepsy

Women with epilepsy should be regularly assessed in the antenatal period for risk factors for seizures such as sleep deprivation and stress, adherence to AEDs and seizure type and frequency. Precipitants of seizures such as fasting, sleep deprivation and stress should be identified and appropriately managed.[40] Women having active seizures should be advised not to remain alone or unobserved because unwitnessed seizures carry the highest risk of SUDEP; with nocturnal seizures being an independent risk factor.

Fetal monitoring should be done by serial growth scans beginning from 28 weeks of gestation for detection of growth restriction. There is no role for routine antepartum fetal surveillance with tocography in women on AEDs.[11]

Role of Vitamin K in Women on Antiepileptic Drugs

Enzyme-inducing drugs like carbamazepine, phenytoin, phenobarbital, primidone, oxcarbazepine, topiramate and eslicarbazepine competitively inhibit the precursors of clotting factors and affect fetal microsomal enzymes that degrade vitamin K, thus increasing the chances of hemorrhagic disease of the newborn (HDN). Hence, it is recommended to administer 1 mg of intramuscular vitamin K to all babies born to WWE on AEDs to prevent HDN. But, there is insufficient evidence to recommend routine use of vitamin K to mothers to prevent HDN or postpartum hemorrhage.[11]

Optimal Timing and Mode of Delivery in Women with Epilepsy

Most of the WWE will have a normal labor and delivery without any complications. Epilepsy per se is not an indication for induction of labor and cesarean section.

The mode of delivery and its appropriate time in WWE is not defined. Recurrent and prolonged seizures, with high risk of status epilepticus, are indications for elective cesarean section.[11]

Role of Steroids in Women with Epilepsy

Women at risk of preterm labor should be administered the routine dose of corticosteroids to prevent respiratory distress in the newborn. Enzyme-inducing AEDs may increase the metabolism of corticosteroids with reduced therapeutic effectiveness but no studies have assessed the effectiveness of higher or frequent doses of corticosteroids.[41] Hence, routine doubling of dose of steroids is not recommended.

INTRAPARTUM MANAGEMENT

Management of Seizures in Labor

The risk of seizures in labor is low. The frequency of tonic-clonic seizures in labor is about 1–2% and within 24 hours occurs in a further 1–2%.[42] Seizures in labor can lead to maternal hypoxia; thereby causing fetal hypoxia and acidosis due to uterine hypertonus.[43,44] Risk factors for seizures in labor are sleep deprivation, nonintake of AEDs, pain, tiredness, stress and dehydration. AED intake should not be stopped during labor. If oral administration is not possible, then parenteral administration should be done (phenytoin, phenobarbital, sodium valproate and levetiracetam). Adequate hydration and analgesia must be maintained to minimize the risk of seizures.

There should be written guidelines for management of seizures in labor.

There should be one-to-one monitoring during labor with appropriate facilities available for resuscitation of mother and neonate.

Benzodiazepines (like clobazam) are the drugs of choice for management of seizures in labor. Prophylactic clobazam should be given in cases of recent episode of seizures, or a past history of intrapartum seizures.

Continuous fetal monitoring should be done in women at high risk of seizure in labor and following an intrapartum seizure.

Any seizure lasting for more than 5 minutes represents a high risk for progression to status epilepticus and is a life-threatening medical emergency affecting 1% of pregnancies in WWE.[45] They should be managed as status epilepticus. Left lateral tilt along with maintenance of airway and oxygenation should be done.

Benzodiazepines are the drug of choice in status epilepticus:
- Lorazepam should be administered intravenously at a dose of 0.1 mg/kg (initially bolus dose of 4 mg). Diazepam at a dose of 5–10 mg can be administered intravenously as an alternative.
- If intravenous access is not there, diazepam 10–20 mg per rectally is administered every 15 minutes or midazolam 10 mg is given as a buccal preparation.
- If seizures are still not controlled, phenytoin or fosphenytoin should be administered as a loading dose of 10–15 mg/kg intravenously; with the usual dosage of about 1,000 mg for an adult.[36]

Tocolytic agents should be administered in case of persistent uterine hypertonus. In case of persistent fetal bradycardia, emergency cesarean section should be done. The neonatal team should be informed because of high risk of neonatal withdrawal syndrome with the use of benzodiazepines and AEDs.[46]

Analgesia in Labor in Women with Epilepsy

Importance should be given to pain relief in labor in WWE. The various suitable and safe methods of analgesia are transcutaneous electrical nerve stimulation (TENS), nitrous oxide and oxygen (Entonox) and regional analgesia (epidural, spinal, combined spinal epidural). Epidural analgesia can be administered early to minimize the factors which can provoke seizures in labor like sleep deprivation, overbreathing, pain and emotional stress.

In case of requirement for general anesthesia, avoid anesthetic agents like pethidine, ketamine and sevoflurane. Pethidine is metabolized to norpethidine which is a known epileptogenic agent. Ketamine also lowers seizure threshold and sevoflurane has epileptogenic potential.[47-49]

Effects of Induction of Labor

Epilepsy per se is not an indication for induction of labor. The use of induction agents is not contraindicated in women on AEDs. Also, there is no evidence regarding effect of any AED on induction agents. Care should be taken regarding provoking factors for seizures like stress, insomnia and dehydration in cases of prolonged induction.[11]

POSTPARTUM MANAGEMENT

Risk of Seizures in Postpartum Period

There is a high risk for exacerbation of seizure frequency in the immediate postpartum period which is higher than that during the antenatal period. This is because of increased stress, sleep deprivation, anxiety and missed medication. It should be ensured that WWE continue to take AEDs postnatally. There should be adequate support during the postnatal period to minimize seizure provoking factors.

Postpartum Antiepileptic Drug Dose Modification

The physiological changes of pregnancy like increased renal and hepatic clearance and hemodilution are reversed in the postnatal period.[50,51] This can put the women at high risk for drug toxicity. Thus, a review for the dose of AED should be made within 10 days of delivery with the neurologist and gradually tapered to avoid toxicity.

Effect of Antiepileptic Drug on the Newborn

The rates of transfer of AEDs to the neonate through placenta and breast milk are different for different drugs. The newborns should be monitored for adverse effects like lethargy, difficulty in breathing, excessive sedation and withdrawal symptoms. Monitoring for signs of toxicity by measuring serum AED levels should be done in premature babies.[11,52]

Drugs such as phenobarbital, carbamazepine, phenytoin, lamotrigine, oxcarbazepine have free transfer across placenta with umbilical cord to maternal serum AED concentration (U/S) close to one. Fetal accumulation is slightly higher for levetiracetam, sodium valproate and gabapentin.

The magnitude of AED transfer to the baby through breast milk required to affect neonatal outcome is not known. WWE on AEDs are encouraged to breastfeed and they are not associated with adverse cognitive outcomes at 3 years of age.[53]

■ CONTRACEPTION

Advice regarding effective contraception should be given to all WWE to prevent unplanned pregnancies. Copper intrauterine devices (Cu-IUDs), levonorgestrel-releasing intrauterine system (LNG-IUS) and medroxyprogesterone acetate injections are the methods of choice for contraception as they are not affected by enzyme-inducing AEDs.

Drugs with enzyme inducing properties like carbamazepine, phenytoin, phenobarbital, primidone, oxcarbazepine, topiramate and eslicarbazepine increase the risk of failure of hormonal contraceptives. The expected failure is three times higher in women on AEDs as compared to general population.[54-56] The contraceptive efficacy for women on enzyme-inducing AEDs wishing for hormonal contraception can be improved by administering increasing doses of estrogen component (50 μg to maximum 70 μg), reducing the pill-free interval from 7 days to 4 days and by tricycling (taking three packs back to back).[57] They should also be advised regarding additional use of barrier contraceptives.

The efficacy of other methods like transdermal patches, vaginal ring and progestogen-only implants is also reduced with enzyme-inducing AEDs.

Copper-IUD is the only method of choice for emergency contraception in women on enzyme-inducing AEDs.[11]

All methods of contraception can be offered to women on nonenzyme-inducing AEDs like sodium valproate, levetiracetam, gabapentin, tiagabine and pregabalin.[11]

Oral hormonal contraceptives can also alter the efficacy of some AEDs. Lamotrigine is not an enzyme inducer but oral contraceptives have shown to decrease its level by 25–70%; with a drop of more than 20% in the first 3 days after taking contraceptive pills. This is more in cases of lamotrigine monotherapy and estrogen-containing contraceptives. The fall in lamotrigine levels can lead to seizure deterioration.[58,59]

■ CONCLUSION

The clinical management of WWE on AEDs during pregnancy is a challenge for both obstetrician and neurologist. The main goal of treatment focuses on adequate seizure control with minimal exposure of AEDs in utero in order to minimize the risks of structural and neurodevelopmental teratogenic effects. There is no seizure deterioration in two-thirds of the women during pregnancy but the altered physiological changes and pharmacokinetics during pregnancy can result in increased seizure deterioration. The management of epilepsy during pregnancy should involve a multidisciplinary approach with careful adjustment of the doses of AEDs during the antenatal and the postpartum period. Patients should be appropriately counseled about risk of major congenital malformations, neurodevelopmental outcomes, obstetrical risks, perinatal complications and breastfeeding. It is important to monitor WWE during pregnancy, and despite multiple complexities in the care of WWE, majority of the WWE have healthy pregnancies. They should also be appropriately educated about the need for contraception so as to avoid unplanned pregnancies.

REFERENCES

1. Edey S, Moran N, Nashef L. SUDEP and epilepsy-related mortality in pregnancy. Epilepsia. 2014;55:e72-4.
2. UK Epilepsy and Pregnancy Register. [online] Available from: http://www.epilepsyandpregnancy.co.uk/ [Last accessed September, 2019].
3. Knight M, Tuffnell D, Kenyon S, Shakespeare J, Gray R, Kurinczuk JJ (Eds). Saving Lives, Improving Mothers' Care: Surveillance of the Maternal Deaths in the UK 2011-2013 and Lessons Learned to Inform Maternity Care from the UK and Ireland Confidential Enquiries into Maternal Deaths and Morbidity 2009-2013. Oxford: National Perinatal Epidemiology Unit, University of Oxford; 2015.
4. Artama M, Auvinen A, Raudaskoski T, et al. Antiepileptic drug use of women with epilepsy and congenital malformations in offspring. Neurology. 2005;64:1874-8.
5. Hernández-Díaz S, Smith CR, Shen A, et al. Comparative safety of antiepileptic drugs during pregnancy. Neurology. 2012;78:1692-9.
6. Hernández-Díaz S, Werler MM, Walker AM, et al. Folic acid antagonists during pregnancy and the risk of birth defects. N Engl J Med. 2000;343:1608-14.
7. Mawhinney E, Craig J, Morrow J, et al. Levetiracetam in pregnancy: results from the UK and Ireland epilepsy and pregnancy registers. Neurology. 2013;80:400-5.
8. Meador K, Reynolds MW, Crean S, et al. Pregnancy outcomes in women with epilepsy: a systematic review and meta-analysis of published pregnancy registries and cohorts. Epilepsy Res. 2008;81:1-13.
9. Morrow J, Russell A, Guthrie E, et al. Malformation risks of antiepileptic drugs in pregnancy: a prospective study from the UK Epilepsy and Pregnancy Register. J Neurol Neurosurg Psychiatry. 2006;77:193-8.
10. Tomson T, Battino D, Bonizzoni E, et al. Dose-dependent risk of malformations with antiepileptic drugs: an analysis of data from the EURAP epilepsy and pregnancy registry. Lancet Neurol. 2011;10:609-17.
11. Royal College of Obstetricians and Gynaecologists. Epilepsy in pregnancy. Green-top Guideline No. 68. RCOG; 2016.
12. Shorvon S, Tomson T. Sudden unexpected death in epilepsy. Lancet. 2011;378:2028-38.
13. Nashef L. Sudden unexpected death in epilepsy: terminology and definitions. Epilepsia. 1997;38(11 Suppl):S6-8.
14. Fisher RS, Acevedo C, Arzimanoglou A, et al. ILAE official report: a practical clinical definition of epilepsy. Epilepsia. 2014;55:475-82.
15. Altman D, Carroli G, Duley L, et al. Do women with pre-eclampsia, and their babies, benefit from magnesium sulphate? The Magpie Trial: a randomised placebo-controlled trial. Lancet. 2002;359:1877-90.
16. Gaillard WD, Cross JH, Duncan JS, et al. Epilepsy imaging study guideline criteria: commentary on diagnostic testing study guidelines and practice parameters. Epilepsia. 2011;52:1750-6.
17. Dineen R, Banks A, Lenthall R. Imaging of acute neurological conditions in pregnancy and the puerperium. Clin Radiol. 2005;60:1156-70.
18. ACOG Committee on Obstetric Practice. ACOG committee opinion. Number 299, September 2004 (replaces no. 158, September 1995). Guidelines for diagnostic imaging during pregnancy. Obstet Gynecol. 2004;104:647-51.
19. Knight M, Kenyon S, Brocklehurst P, Neilson J, Shakespeare J, Kurinczuk JJ (Eds). Saving

Lives, Improving Mothers' Care: Lessons Learned to Inform Future Maternity Care from the UK and Ireland Confidential Enquiries into Maternal Deaths and Morbidity 2009-12. Oxford: National Perinatal Epidemiology Unit, University of Oxford; 2014.
20. Fairgrieve SD, Jackson M, Jonas P, et al. Population based, prospective study of the care of women with epilepsy in pregnancy. BMJ. 2000;321:674-5.
21. Weston J, Bromley R, Jackson CF, et al. Monotherapy treatment of epilepsy in pregnancy: congenital malformation outcomes in the child. Cochrane Database Syst Rev. 2016;11:CD010224.
22. Leveno KJ, Spong CY, Dashe JS, Casey BM, Hoffman BL, Cunningham FG, Bloom SL. Williams Obstetrics, 25th edition. New York: McGraw-Hill; 2018.
23. Bromley R, Weston J, Adab N, et al. Treatment for epilepsy in pregnancy: neurodevelopmental outcomes in the child. Cochrane Database Syst Rev. 2014;(10):CD010236.
24. Meador KJ, Baker GA, Browning N, et al. Fetal antiepileptic drug exposure and cognitive outcomes at age 6 years (NEAD study): a prospective observational study. Lancet Neurol. 2013;12:244-52.
25. Bromley RL, Mawer GE, Briggs M, et al. The prevalence of neurodevelopmental disorders in children prenatally exposed to antiepileptic drugs. J Neurol Neurosurg Psychiatry. 2013;84:637-43.
26. Christensen J, Grønborg TK, Sørensen MJ, et al. Prenatal valproate exposure and risk of autism spectrum disorders and childhood autism. JAMA. 2013;309:1696-703.
27. Vajda FJ, Hitchcock A, Graham J, et al. Seizure control in antiepileptic drug-treated pregnancy. Epilepsia. 2008;49:172-6.
28. Gjerde IO, Strandjord RE, Ulstein M. The course of epilepsy during pregnancy: a study of 78 cases. Acta Neurol Scand. 1988;78:198-205.
29. Tomson T, Lindbom U, Ekqvist B, et al. Epilepsy and pregnancy: a prospective study of seizure control in relation to free and total plasma concentrations of carbamazepine and phenytoin. Epilepsia. 1994;35:122-30.
30. Battino D, Tomson T, Bonizzoni E, et al. Seizure control and treatment changes in pregnancy: observations from the EURAP epilepsy pregnancy registry. Epilepsia. 2013;54:1621-7.
31. Nadel AS, Green JK, Holmes LB, et al. Absence of need for amniocentesis in patients with elevated levels of maternal serum alpha-fetoprotein and normal ultrasonographic examinations. N Engl J Med. 1990;323:557-61.
32. Adab N. Therapeutic monitoring of antiepileptic drugs during pregnancy and in the postpartum period: is it useful? CNS Drugs. 2006;20:791-800.
33. Pennell PB. Antiepileptic drug pharmacokinetics during pregnancy and lactation. Neurology. 2003;61 Suppl 2:S35-42.
34. Pennell PB, Hovinga CA. Antiepileptic drug therapy in pregnancy I: gestation-induced effects on AED pharmacokinetics. Int Rev Neurobiol. 2008;83:227-40.
35. Miškov S, Gjergja-Juraški R, Cvitanovi´c-Šojat L, et al. Prospective surveillance of Croatian pregnant women on lamotrigine monotherapy—aspects of pre-pregnancy counseling and drug monitoring. Acta Clin Croat. 2009;48:271-81.
36. National Institute for Health and Care Excellence. The epilepsies: the diagnosis and management of the epilepsies in adults and children in primary and secondary care. NICE clinical guideline 137. Manchester: NICE; 2012.
37. Scottish Intercollegiate Guidelines Network. Diagnosis and management of epilepsy in adults: a national clinical guideline. SIGN publication no. 143. Edinburgh: SIGN; 2015.
38. Jackson MJ, Turkington D. Depression and anxiety in epilepsy. J Neurol Neurosurg Psychiatry. 2005;76 Suppl 1:i45-7.
39. Viale L, Allotey J, Cheong-See F, et al. Epilepsy in pregnancy and reproductive outcomes: a systematic review and meta-analysis. Lancet. 2015;386:1845-52.
40. Malow BA. Sleep and epilepsy. Neurol Clin. 2005;23:1127-47.
41. Patsalos PN, Fröscher W, Pisani F, et al. The importance of drug interactions in epilepsy therapy. Epilepsia. 2002;43:365-85.
42. Bardy A. Epilepsy and pregnancy: a prospective study of 154 pregnancies in epileptic women (thesis). Helsinki, Finland, University of Helsinki; 1982.
43. Teramo K, Hiilesmaa V, Bardy A, et al. Fetal heart rate during a maternal grand mal epileptic seizure. J Perinat Med. 1979;7:3-6.

44. Nei M, Daly S, Liporace J. A maternal complex partial seizure in labor can affect fetal heart rate. Neurology. 1998;51:904-6.
45. EURAP Study Group. Seizure control and treatment in pregnancy: observations from the EURAP epilepsy pregnancy registry. Neurology. 2006;66:354-60.
46. McElhatton PR. The effects of benzodiazepine use during pregnancy and lactation. Reprod Toxicol. 1994;8:461-75.
47. Kuczkowski KM. Seizures on emergence from sevoflurane anaesthesia for caesarean section in a healthy parturient. Anaesthesia. 2002;57:1234-5.
48. Hsieh SW, Lan KM, Luk HN, et al. Postoperative seizures after sevoflurane anesthesia in a neonate. Acta Anaesthesiol Scand. 2004;48:663.
49. Kuczkowski KM. Sevoflurane and seizures: déjà vu. Acta Anaesthesiol Scand. 2004;48:1216.
50. Tran TA, Leppik IE, Blesi K, et al. Lamotrigine clearance during pregnancy. Neurology. 2002;59:251-5.
51. de Haan GJ, Edelbroek P, Segers J, et al. Gestation-induced changes in lamotrigine pharmacokinetics: a monotherapy study. Neurology. 2004;63:571-3.
52. Davanzo R, Dal Bo S, Bua J, et al. Antiepileptic drugs and breastfeeding. Ital J Pediatr. 2013;39:50.
53. Meador KJ, Baker GA, Browning N, et al. Effects of breastfeeding in children of women taking antiepileptic drugs. Neurology. 2010;75:1954-60.
54. Zupanc ML. Antiepileptic drugs and hormonal contraceptives in adolescent women with epilepsy. Neurology. 2006;66(6 Suppl 3):S37-45.
55. Beghi E, Cornaggia C; RESt-1 Group. Morbidity and accidents in patients with epilepsy: results of a European cohort study. Epilepsia. 2002;43:1076-83.
56. Coulam CB, Annegers JF. Do anticonvulsants reduce the efficacy of oral contraceptives? Epilepsia. 1979;20:519-25.
57. Faculty of Sexual and Reproductive Healthcare. Faculty of Sexual and Reproductive Healthcare Clinical Guidance: Combined Hormonal Contraception. London: FSRH; 2011.
58. Stodieck SR, Schwenkhagen AM. Lamotrigine plasma levels and combined monophasic oral contraceptives or a contraceptive vaginal ring: a prospective evaluation in 30 women. Epilepsia. 2004;45(Suppl 7):187.
59. Wegner I, Edelbroek PM, Bulk S, et al. Lamotrigine kinetics within the menstrual cycle, after menopause, and with oral contraceptives. Neurology. 2009;73:1388-93.

CHAPTER 36

Diabetic Ketoacidosis in Pregnancy

Sunil Gupta

INTRODUCTION

Diabetic ketoacidosis (DKA) is one of the most serious acute complications of diabetes and is characterized by uncontrolled hyperglycemia, anion gap metabolic acidosis and ketosis.[1] The incidence of diabetes in pregnancy ranges from 6% to 7% with 90% of cases constituted by women affected by gestational diabetes mellitus (GDM). Many studies have reported incidence of DKA between 0.5% and 10% of all diabetic pregnancies.[2-4] Earlier it was considered to happen exclusively in typical of type 1 diabetes mellitus (DM), but now it is reported to occur in type 2 DM and GDM patients also. DKA in pregnancy is a rare but an urgent complication, which can compromise both fetus and mother. Historically, most of the studies have reported the risk of fetal demise after DKA in pregnancy as high as 25–60%.[5,6] A recently published retrospective cohort study from Boston[7] included pregnancies between 1996 and 2015 with at least one DKA event in women with type 1 diabetes. Amongst 77 DKA events in 64 pregnancies, 62 were included in the study. Complications like fetal demise, preterm birth, and neonatal intensive care unit (NICU) admissions found in 15.6%, 46.3%, and 59% of pregnancies, respectively. Pregnant mothers suffered from DKA between 5 weeks and 38 weeks of gestation. Approximately 60% of fetal demise occurred at the time of or within 1 week of the DKA event while 40% fetal demise occurred between 1 week and 11 weeks. Maternal intensive care unit (ICU) admission ($P = 0.024$) and higher serum osmolality ($P = 0.045$) due to DKA were associated with increased risk of fetal demise. The risk of fetal demise after DKA during pregnancy has decreased over time but remains substantially higher than the baseline risk (2–3%) in women with type 1 diabetes.[8,9]

PATHOGENESIS

Diabetic ketoacidosis is the result of an absolute or relative deficiency of insulin, which causes a state of starvation of cells accompanied by an increased secretion of the counter-regulatory hormones. All these conditions result in hyperglycemia which results from increased hepatic gluconeogenesis and decreased utilization of glucose in muscle. There is an increased lipolysis resulting in large quantities of free fatty acids being mobilized from fat storage into the circulation. Hepatocyte mitochondria become more permeable to fatty acids resulting in increased fatty acid oxidation with the formation of large quantities of acetyl coenzyme A (acetyl-CoA), which is then converted by the liver into ketone bodies [beta-hydroxybutyrate (β-OHB) and acetoacetate]. Acetoacetate undergoes decarboxylation and conversion into acetone. The abundant ketone bodies, and particularly β-OHB and lactic acid are the main contributors to the metabolic acidosis.[10]

Metabolic characteristics of DKA trigger a chain of events that will self-perpetuate in a vicious circle. Hyperglycemia gives rise to an osmotic gradient which results in an excessive diuresis, which leads to severe dehydration and hypovolemia. This further aggravates the hyperglycemia and acidosis due to the activation of other stress hormones and osmotic diuresis causes low sodium levels. In the condition of acidosis, hydrogen ions move into the intracellular space from the extracellular compartment resulting in a shift of potassium in the opposite direction which determines a depletion of intracellular potassium.

DIABETIC KETOACIDOSIS IN PREGNANCY

Pregnancy is characterized by insulin resistance, accelerated starvation and respiratory alkalosis, especially in the second and third trimesters. Sensitivity to insulin decreases in pregnancy, reaching its nadir in the third trimester and rapidly returning to prepregnancy levels after delivery. Specific mechanisms underlying the gradual onset of insulin resistance, often with a concomitant increase in insulin secretion, have not been fully elucidated. Endocrine changes characteristic of pregnancy, such as increased levels of estrogen, progesterone, human placental lactogen (hPL), cortisol and tumor necrosis factor-alpha (TNF-α) have contribution to it. The gradual decline in insulin sensitivity is considered to be a physiological mechanism which helps in helping fetus to provide glucose. There is a gradual increase of the secretion of insulin to maintain normal glucose tolerance.

High levels of human chorionic gonadotropin in early pregnancy are often associated with nausea and vomiting, which may give rise to a state of starvation, dehydration and acidosis, with the subsequent activation of stress-related hormones. Progesterone also reduces gastrointestinal motility and increases carbohydrate absorption, thus raising plasma glucose levels. Greater alveolar ventilation in pregnant women gives rise to a state of respiratory alkalosis that is overcome by means of an increased renal excretion of bicarbonate, which leads to a lower buffering capacity. These changes can trigger the onset of ketoacidosis at lower glycemic levels than those seen in diabetic women who are not pregnant.[11] In pregnant women with type 2 diabetes, the pregnancy-related drop in insulin sensitivity overlaps the patient's pre-existing insulin resistance, meaning that these patients need insulin therapy early in their pregnancy to avoid ketoacidosis.

EUGLYCEMIC KETOACIDOSIS

Euglycemic ketoacidosis was defined as severe ketoacidosis with serum bicarbonate levels of 10 mEq/L or less, in the absence of pronounced hyperglycemia. Euglycemic ketoacidosis has been reported in women with both pregestational diabetes (type 1 and type 2), and gestational diabetes. True euglycemic ketoacidosis is rare, with only 0.8–1.1% of all episodes meeting the above-mentioned plasma bicarbonate concentration criterion.[12] Pregnancy predisposes the mother to accelerated starvation characterized by the switch from use of hepatic glycogen to lipolysis during fasting and associated with development of hypoglycemia, raised plasma levels of free fatty acids and increased plasma and urinary ketones, even after an overnight fast. It is hypothesized to be associated with increased excretion of glucose from the kidney due to the increased renal blood flow by 60% and raised glomerular filtration rate during pregnancy.

RISK FACTORS OF DIABETIC KETOACIDOSIS

The risk factors for DKA in pregnancy are extreme lack of food, protracted vomiting, infections, insulin pump failure, undiagnosed DM, poor metabolic control of diabetes and/or poor therapy compliance, use of β-sympathomimetic drugs for tocolysis, steroid therapy for fetal lung maturation, diabetic neuropathic gastroparesis. Most common precipitating event is emesis from any cause, accounting for 42% of DKA. The second most common precipitating event is use of β-sympathomimetic agents (which increase blood glucose values, free fatty acids and ketones stimulating gluconeogenesis, glycogenolysis and lipolysis) and when combined with emesis, these events accounted for 57% of episodes of DKA. Schneider et al.[13] evaluated pregnant women with diabetes treated with insulin therapy presented with DKA. In these patients, 27% of cases were due to intercurrent infections and 18% were due to missing doses of insulin therapy.

CLINICAL SIGNS AND SYMPTOMS

The symptoms of diabetic DKA in pregnancy are no different from those seen in women who are not pregnant, except that they tend to develop more rapidly in pregnancy. Patients usually present with a generalized malaise, nausea, vomiting, polyuria, polydipsia, weakness, tachypnea and signs of dehydration. Abdominal pain due to a reduced peripheral perfusion may be severe mimicking an intra-abdominal process and accompanied by uterine contractions. If infection is the precipitating factor, patients may have fever or, paradoxically, hypothermia due to the vasodilatory effects of the hydrogen ions in excess when severe ketoacidosis develops. In the advanced stages of the disease, patients may have Kussmaul respirations and a breath with a classic fruity smell. Lethargy and signs of central nervous system involvement such as disorientation, obtundation and coma due to cerebral edema can be present.

INVESTIGATIONS

Investigations must include serum glucose levels, serum electrolytes, osmolarity, blood urea nitrogen, creatinine, arterial blood gas and serum bicarbonate levels, anion gap, serum ketones, a complete blood cell count, liver function tests, and urine analysis. Hyperglycemia (plasma glucose levels > 300 mg/dL,) an increased anion gap, an arterial pH < 7.3, ketosis (positivity for serum and urine ketosis) and decreased serum bicarbonate levels are characteristic of DKA. However, as previously documented, pregnant women with DKA are more likely to present with lower blood glucose levels, even in normoglycemia, making the diagnosis more challenging.

The predominant ketone produced in DKA is β-OHB and neither acetone nor β-OHB reacts as strongly as acetoacetate with nitroprusside which is used to test for the presence of ketosis in urine. Moreover, as ketones may be detected in blood before urine, blood testing allows for more rapid diagnosis of ketosis and when DKA is treated with insulin infusion, β-OHB is rapidly converted into acetoacetate so the ketone body levels in urine increase—even though the patient's ketoacidosis is regressing. So the blood β-OHB testing is to preferred to urine acetoacetate testing.[14] Patients may have normal or high potassium levels, but it is important to consider that their total body potassium is generally low, and they are dehydrated and hypokalemic. Creatinine levels and blood urea nitrogen may be high as a result of renal damage.

MANAGEMENT OF DIABETIC KETOACIDOSIS

Diabetic ketoacidosis during pregnancy is an obstetric and medical emergency that warrants intensive treatment at a specialized care unit. The principles of DKA management in pregnancy are same as for patients who are not pregnant. Treatment for DKA includes fluid replacement, insulin therapy, correcting acidosis and abnormal electrolytes and treating the underlying disease associated with intensive monitoring of maternal and fetal conditions.

Fluids Therapy

Use isotonic saline solution for a total replacement in the first 12 hours with 4–6 L (1 L in the first hour; 500–1,000 mL/h for 2–4 hours; 250 mL/h up to 80% fluid replacement). In cases of hypernatremia, use 0.45% saline solution. Use glucose infusion, starting with a 5% dextrose, when glucose levels drop <250 mg/dL (14 mmol/L).

Electrolytes

Potassium: If normal or low, begin with 15–20 mEq/h; if high, wait until it drops to within normal range, then 20–30 mEq/L. Bicarbonate infusion of 44 mEq only if pH < 7.

Insulin Therapy

An initial bolus of 10–15 U of regular insulin (0.2–0.4 U/kg). Intravenous infusion with 2–10 U/h may be used.

PREVENTION OF DIABETIC KETOACIDOSIS

Women with pregestational diabetes should be educated about the risk of DKA before conception as well as during pregnancy. In particular, they should be instructed about the importance of compliance with diet, exercise, measurements and recordings of glucose values and therapy (especially insulin dose and device as insulin pumps). In addition, they need to be educated about precipitating factors, signs and symptoms of DKA. Moreover, all women should know that if glucose levels are >200 mg/dL, it is necessary to check blood β-OHB and, if positive, they have to contact their physician.

CONCLUSION

Diabetic ketoacidosis is a rare but serious complication of diabetes in pregnancy and whereas it has a devastating effect in pregnancy, its real impact on fetal outcomes has not yet well-evaluated. Further studies need to be conducted to clarify this point. It must be emphasized that women affected by diabetes in pregnancy have to be educated to recognize signs and symptoms of DKA and to check blood β-OHB in presence of risk factors of DKA in order to improve maternal and fetal outcomes. It is also important to bear in mind the euglycemic ketoacidosis, even in nondiabetic pregnant women, because early diagnosis and prompt treatment of this condition could reduce the adverse fetal and maternal outcomes.

REFERENCES

1. Kitabchi AE, Umpierrez GE, Murphy MB, et al. Hyperglycemic crises in adult patients with diabetes: a consensus statement from the American Diabetes Association. Diabetes Care. 2006;29:2739-48.
2. Montoro MN, Myers VP, Mestman JH, et al. Outcome of pregnancy in diabetic ketoacidosis. Am J Perinatol. 1993;10:17-20.
3. Kilvert JA, Nicholson HO, Wrigth AD. Ketoacidosis in diabetic pregnancy. Obstet Gynecol. 2003;102:278-81.
4. Parker JA, Conway DL. Diabetic ketoacidosis in pregnancy. Obstet Gynecol Clin North Am. 2007;34:533-43.
5. Shimizu I, Makino H, Imagawa A, et al. Clinical and immunogenetic characteristics

of fulminant type 1 diabetes associated with pregnancy. J Clin Endocrinol Metab. 2006;91: 471-6.
6. Lufkin EG, Nelson RL, Hill LM, et al. An analysis of diabetic pregnancies at Mayo Clinic, 1950-79. Diabetes Care. 1984;7:539-47.
7. Morrison FJ, Movassaghian M, Seely EW, et al. Fetal outcomes after diabetic ketoacidosis during pregnancy. Diabetes Care. 2017;40:e77-9.
8. Goldenberg RL, Culhane JF, Iams JD, et al. Epidemiology and causes of preterm birth. Lancet. 2008;371:75-84.
9. Cordero L, Treuer SH, Landon MB, et al. Management of infants of diabetic mothers. Arch Pediatr Adolesc Med. 1998;152:249-54.
10. Laffel L. Ketone bodies: a review of physiology, pathophysiology and application of monitoring to diabetes. Diabetes Metab Res Rev. 1999;15: 412-26.
11. Montelongo A, Lasuncion MA, Pallardo LF, et al. Longitudinal study of plasma lipoproteins and hormones during pregnancy in normal and diabetic women. Diabetes. 1992;41:1651-9.
12. Chauhan SP, Perry KG, McLaughlin BN, et al. Diabetic ketoacidosis complicating pregnancy. J Perinatol. 1996;16:173-5.
13. Schneider M, Umpierrez G, Ramsey R, et al. Pregnancy complicated by diabetic ketoacidosis: maternal and fetal outcomes. Diabetes Care. 2003;26:958-9.
14. National Institute for Health and Care Excellence. NICE guideline. Diabetes in pregnancy: management from preconception to the postnatal period. Published on 25 February 2015. [online] Available from: https://www.nice.org.uk/guidance/ng3 [Last accessed September, 2019].

CHAPTER 37

Laparoscopy in Pregnancy

Arathi Sreedhara

■ DEFINITION

It is a minimal access surgical procedure allowing endoscopic access to peritoneal cavity after gas insufflation for safe manipulation of instruments and performing surgery.[1-5]

■ TYPES

1. Intraperitoneal
2. Extraperitoneal
3. Gasless laparoscopy
4. Hand-assisted laparoscopy.

■ INDICATIONS

Obstetrics
- Excision of rudimentary horn
- Heterotopic pregnancy
- Ectopic pregnancy

Gynecology
- Adnexal mass
- Ovarian tumors
- Torsion

Other nongynecological conditions
- Abdominal surgeries like appendicitis, cholecystitis, and hernia surgery.[6-9]

■ CONTRAINDICATIONS

Advantages

Maternal: Laparoscopy is associated with:
- Shorter operative time
- Shorter length of hospital stay, and
- Fewer intraoperative complications compared.

Open surgery is associated with a threefold increased risk of postoperative obstetric complications:
- Including preterm delivery
- Preterm labor without preterm delivery
- Miscarriage.[10,11]

Fetal: There are no significant differences between laparotomy and laparoscopy with respect to congenital malformations, gestational duration, birth weight, intrauterine growth restriction, stillbirth, or neonatal deaths.

Note
1. There is no evidence to suggest fetal acidosis could develop from carboperitoneum.
2. The fetus possibly be injured directly if uterus is perforated by a trocar or Veress needle. This is avoided by introducing tracer under vision/placing Veress needle at Palmer's point.
3. No evidence to suggest rise in intra-abdominal pressure with carbon dioxide decreases uteroplacental blood flow and causes fetal hypoxia.

For mother
- Pneumoperitoneum can alter arterial oxygenation, and acid-base balance as a result of CO_2 absorption. Use capnometer in anesthesia machine reduces this risk.
- Pressure on uteroplacental vessels can decrease uterine blood flow, reduce residual lung volume and functional residual capacity.

- Carboperitoneum can cause decreased cardiac index and increased mean arterial pressure and systemic vascular resistance.[12]

PREOPERATIVE INSTRUCTIONS

- Technical
- Patient
- Surgeon.

COMPLICATIONS

- Intraoperative
- Delayed postoperative.

INDICATIONS

Advantages of Laparoscopy

- Small abdominal incision
- Early postoperative recovery
- Early mobilization
- Decreased risk of thromboembolism
- Shorter hospitalization time and early return to work
- Fewer incisional hernias
- Decreased manipulation of the bowel during surgery, thus reducing adhesions
- Decreased postoperative pain and less narcotic use, thus reducing chances of fetal depression.

Safety

- No significant difference between in laparoscopic surgery versus open surgery.
  - Intrauterine growth restriction
  - Congenital malformations
  - Stillbirths or nconatal deaths
  - No adverse long-term effects.

Timing

- There is no absolute maximum gestational age for performing laparoscopy; the operation can be performed in any trimester.[13,14]
- Optimal time to operate is the early second trimester.
- Laparoscopy during the last trimester can be difficult because of gravid uterus interfering with adequate visualization.

Indications for Thromboprophylaxis

- When duration of laparoscopic procedure is long, prolonged pneumoperitoneum contributes to the venous stasis and possibly thrombosis, these patients should receive pneumatic compression devices on the lower limbs.[15]
- There is no recommendation on routine use of unfractionated or low-molecular-weight heparin.[16]

Prophylactic Tocolysis

- Use of prophylactic tocolysis or glucocorticoids is not indicated routinely.
- May be indicated in the event of threatened preterm delivery presenting with premature contractions.
- If *monopolar cautery* is used, a grounding pad will reduce flow of electric current through the amniotic fluid.

PREMEDICATION

- Nil by mouth for 6 hours
- No enema
- Antibiotics
- Written informed consent for laparoscopy/conversion to laparotomy by the operating surgeon
- Anxiolytics/Antiemetic/H_2 receptor antagonist/Analgesic
- Deep vein thrombosis (DVT) prophylaxis.

PATIENT POSITION

- Supine or low lithotomy position for the first port. Patient position can be changed later for secondary ports.

- Hands should be extended position or by the side of patient well protected to prevent cautery burns/dislocation.

BASIC GUIDELINES FOR LAPAROSCOPY

1. Primary port can be Hasson's/Veress or direct technique aided by elevating the abdominal wall.[17]
2. Laparoscopic ports in pregnancy—when uterus is <18 weeks, the initial trocar placement is in through umbilicus or supraumbilical, in pregnancies with uterine size >18 weeks, the initial trocar is placed at Palmer's point. All secondary ports are inserted and removed under direct visualization.[18-19]
3. Suggest positioning the secondary port at least 6 cm above the uterine fundus. This placement provides an adequate distance between the tip of the laparoscope and the uterus to allow better visibility and instrument manipulation.
4. Pneumoperitoneum—intra-abdominal pressure usually is maintained 12 mm Hg and not exceeding 15 mm Hg. Recommended end-tidal CO_2 at 32–34 mm Hg, to minimize respiratory acidosis.
5. All specimens should be preferably removed in an Endobag to avoid spillage and port site events like infection, especially infected material and suspected malignant specimen.

Fetal Assessment

- Fetal heart rate should be confirmed and documented before and after the procedure, and is usually done with hand held Doppler device.
- Intraoperative fetal monitoring is necessary, transabdominal fetal monitoring can be performed through the left abdominal wall.

Postoperative Care

- A cardiotocography (CTG) (nonstress test) is performed in the recovery room.
- Opioids analgesics and antiemetics are kept to minimum.
- Nonsteroidal anti-inflammatory drug (NSAID) is avoided, especially after 32 weeks of gestation.

Complications and Risks

- The risk of spontaneous abortion is high in first trimester of pregnancy.
- Anesthesia-related complication is directly proportional to duration of the surgery.

Intraoperative Events

Pneumoperitoneum

1. Cardiac:
   - Arrhythmia
   - Hypo/hypertension
2. Pulmonary:
   - Gas embolism
   - Hypercarbia
3. Extravasation:
   - Subcutaneous emphysema
   - Pneumothorax
   - Pneumomediastinum

CONCLUSION

- Laparoscopic may be performed safely and effectively in pregnant women.
- The procedure has been performed as late as 34 weeks of gestation, but the optimal time is the early second trimester.
- We suggest use of pneumatic compression devices for low-risk pregnant women undergoing short laparoscopic procedures for surgical problems, and low molecular weight heparin for procedures >45 minutes.
- There is no evidence that open procedures are safer than blind procedures.

Modification of port sides is necessary when the uterus is significantly enlarged.
- We suggest intra-abdominal pressure be maintained between 8 to 12 mm Hg and not exceed 14 mm Hg.
- We suggest keeping the end-tidal carbon dioxide at 32 to 34 mm Hg, as respiratory acidosis is unlikely at this level.

REFERENCES

1. Soriano D, Yefet Y, Seidman DS, et al. Laparoscopy versus laparotomy in the management of adnexal masses during pregnancy. Fertil Steril. 1999;71:955.
2. Reedy MB, Källén B, Kuehl TJ. Laparoscopy during pregnancy: a study of five fetal outcome parameters with use of the Swedish Health Registry. Am J Obstet Gynecol. 1997;177:673.
3. Nasioudis D, Tsilimigras D, Economopoulos KP. Laparoscopic cholecystectomy during pregnancy: a systematic review of 590 patients. Int J Surg. 2016;27:165.
4. Cox TC, Huntington CR, Blair LJ, et al. Laparoscopic appendectomy and cholecystectomy versus open: a study in 1999 pregnant patients. Surg Endosc. 2016;30:593.
5. Pearl JP, Price RR, Tonkin AE, et al. SAGES guidelines for the use of laparoscopy during pregnancy. Surg Endosc. 2017;31:3767.
6. Lee D, Abraham N. Laparoscopic radical nephrectomy during pregnancy: case report and review of the literature. J Endourol. 2008;22:517.
7. Felbinger TW, Posner M, Eltzschig HK, Kodali BS. Laparoscopic splenectomy in a pregnant patient with immune thrombocytopenic purpura. Int J Obstet Anesth. 2007;16:281.
8. Alouini S, Rida K, Mathevet P. Cervical cancer complicating pregnancy: implications of laparoscopic lymphadenectomy. Gynecol Oncol. 2008;108:472.
9. Wai PY, Ruby JA, Davis KA, et al. Laparoscopic ventral hernia repair during pregnancy. Hernia. 2009;13:559.
10. Affleck DG, Handrahan DL, Egger MJ, Price RR. The laparoscopic management of appendicitis and cholelithiasis during pregnancy. Am J Surg. 1999;178:523.
11. Sachs A, Guglielminotti J, Miller R, et al. Risk factors and risk stratification for adverse obstetrical outcomes after appendectomy or cholecystectomy during pregnancy. JAMA Surg. 2017;152:436-41.
12. Steinbrook RA, Bhavani-Shankar K. Hemodynamics during laparoscopic surgery in pregnancy. Anesth Analg. 2001;93:1570.
13. Andreoli M, Servakov M, Meyers P, Mann WJ Jr. Laparoscopic surgery during pregnancy. J Am Assoc Gynecol Laparosc. 1999;6:229.
14. Stepp K, Falcone T. Laparoscopy in the second trimester of pregnancy. Obstet Gynecol Clin North Am. 2004;31:485.
15. Levy T, Dicker D, Shalev J, et al. Laparoscopic unwinding of hyperstimulated ischaemic ovaries during the second trimester of pregnancy. Hum Reprod. 1995;10:1478.
16. Guyatt GH, Akl EA, Crowther M, et al. Executive summary: antithrombotic Therapy and Prevention of Thrombosis, 9th edition: American College of Chest Physicians Evidence-Based Clinical Practice Guidelines. Chest. 2012;141:7S.
17. Yuen PM, Ng PS, Leung PL, Rogers MS. Outcome in laparoscopic management of persistent adnexal mass during the second trimester of pregnancy. Surg Endosc. 2004;18:1354.
18. O'Rourke N, Kodali BS. Laparoscopic surgery during pregnancy. Curr Opin Anaesthesiol. 2006;19:254.
19. Kodali BS, Chandrasekhar S, Bulich LN, et al. Airway changes during labor and delivery. Anesthesiology. 2008;108:357.

CHAPTER 38

Pregnancy as a Result of Rape

Rahul Wani

INTRODUCTION

Rape is a forceful violent act which has far seeking implications on the survivor which include physical, psychological, social, and emotional effects. Pregnancy as a result of rape aggravates this trauma and suffering to unsurmountable levels.

Rape and forced continuation of pregnancy by confining the woman has been known to be used as a tactic to demoralize the enemy psychologically during war in olden days.

The offence of rape has a deep impact on the overall wellbeing of the victim and is a serious condition to be dealt with sensitivity by health workers.

Physically the patient may suffer from injuries and bleeding from the genital tract, pelvic infection (pelvic inflammatory disease), pain, sometimes pregnancy and in rare cases perforation of genital organs.

These patients may also suffer psychologically and are likely to experience various forms of psychological distress. Psychological distress could be severe with tendency for suicide. Mental health outcomes depend on the circumstances the victim faces and the psychological support such victims get. Instead of supportive and caring attitude, if the caregivers blame the victim, do not allow the patient to express herself, and suppress the emotions of the patient, such patients are likely to have poor outcomes.

Role of Medical Professionals

The medical fraternity has a crucial role in the treatment as well as in securing justice for those who have been sexually assaulted. Law in India has specific provisions which medical professionals need to follow. These provisions are in line with recommendations of bodies like the World Health Organization.

Insensitive Response of Society

Most often these crimes are not reported due to the stigma attached with such crimes. Victims who overcome the fear and stigma to come forward and report such incidences often face hurdles at the police stations and hospitals. Police as usual try to discourage them from filing complaints to avoid increasing their work load. Hospitals resist treating such cases with the fear of medicolegal implications. Such attitude of police officials and the healthcare workers lead to further traumatization of the victim.

INCIDENCE

Reported incidences of the number of pregnancies due to rape vary widely. One report from United States suggested that pregnancies as a result of rape occurs between 25,000 and 32,000 times each year.[1]

A study of 44 cases in the United States, which dealt with pregnancies as a result of rape, showed that pregnancy occurred in 5%

of the victims of reproductive age group aged between 12 years and 45 years. Similar study in 1987 among college students aged between 18 years and 24 years in the United States also estimated a pregnancy rate of around 5% in rape victims. A 2005 study placed the rape-related pregnancy rate at around 3–5%.

A study from Ethiopia estimated a pregnancy rate of 17% among rape-related adolescent victims, while reports from Mexico reported a rate of pregnancy as a result of rape as 15–18%.

Incidence in India

National Crime Records Bureau (NCRB) in 2012 reported 24,923 cases of rape and 45,351 cases of molestation in India.[2]

Though there are no direct figures in India as to the number of pregnancies as a result of rape, in one of the studies in Mumbai, 5 out of 95 survivors who reported to the hospital between the age group of 13 years and 18 years reported with a pregnancy as a result of rape.

Indirectly from this report, incidence of pregnancy as a result of rape could be estimated at around 5%.

RAPE-RELATED PREGNANCIES

Obstetric Consequences

There are many adverse outcomes associated with rape-related pregnancies which could affect both the mother and the child such as lower birth weight and failure to thrive for the child and complications both during and after pregnancy for the mother. These patients are more prone to developing pregnancy induced hypertension, intrauterine growth restriction (IUGR) while postdelivery they tend to have lactational failure and postpartum depression. Victims of intimate partner rape reported fewer live births.

Health Consequences

The health consequences as a result of rape include physical and psychological effects.[3]

Physical Consequences

Physical injuries: Genital and nongenital.
Genital injuries are commonly seen on the external perineal surface, which include injuries to posterior fourchette, the labia minora, the hymen, and the fossa navicularis. The types of injuries vary from lacerations, tears, bruises, abrasions, inflammatory redness, and swelling.

Nongenital physical injuries depend upon the nature of assault and the force used. These injuries could vary from bruises, contusions, and lacerations to ligature marks to ankles, wrists, and neck if the assault included tying up the patient with rope. Hand prints, finger marks, belt marks, and bite marks if the victim was beaten to physically overpower the victim. Anal or rectal trauma may be seen in unnatural means of intercourse.

These victims may end up with mortality because of murder by the preparators to avoid detection of crime, honor killings by the community due to the stigma attached to such crimes or suicide by the victim due to grave mental and physical trauma.

Victim could land up with unwanted pregnancy as a result of such assault and seek unsafe abortion.

Such victims are at risk of sexually transmitted infections (STIs) like gonorrheal, chlamydial, human papillomavirus (HPV), and hepatitis B including human immunodeficiency virus/acquired immunodeficiency syndrome (HIV/AIDS).

These patients could land up with chronic consequences like sexual dysfunction, infertility, pelvic pain, PID, and urinary tract infections.

Psychological Consequences

Psychological consequences may vary depending on the victims personality and the support system such victim has. Some of the common psychological effects include rape trauma syndrome (RTS), post-traumatic stress disorder (PTSD), depression, withdrawal from society, anxiety, overdependence, and misuse of drugs leading to addictions and suicidal tendencies.

Chronic consequences include:
- Headaches
- Chronic tiredness
- Sleep disorders due to nightmares and flashbacks
- Anorexia
- Dysmenorrhea
- Sexual dysfunction.

Rape Trauma Syndrome

One of the common psychological effects of sexual violence is RTS.

Definition: "The stress response pattern of a person who has experienced sexual violence". Rape trauma syndrome has physical, neuropsychological, psychological, and/or behavioral symptoms and usually manifests in two distinct phases: (1) the immediate phase and (2) the long-term phase.

The immediate phase is characterized as a phase when the victim is disorganized. The onset is along with the incident and lasts for about 2–3 weeks. This phase manifests with physical and emotional symptoms.

Emotional symptoms may be either overt or suppressed, for example frequent crying spells; smiling or laughing without any obvious reason or the victim may present herself as very calm and controlled suppressing all her internal emotions.

Emotions may manifest as feeling hurt, shaken with nervousness or anxiety. Some may show intense feelings of sorrow and grief; others may suppress their feelings and overtly appear as though everything is fine. The immediate response arises due to fear of bodily trauma disfigurement or death. After recovery from the immediate trauma they begin to experience abrupt change of moods; lower self esteem; disrespected, disappointed with self; guilt; feeling of inadequacy; self-blame; despairing; anger; and revenge and vulnerable to another assault.

The long-term phase is termed as period of restructuring or reorganizing, usually starts from 2–3 weeks from the incidence. During this phase the person starts to restructure and reorganize her lifestyle, which may depend on her ability or inability to adapt to the prevailing circumstances. The way the person responds during this stage, depends on various factors like age; circumstances in her own life and the incidence; her own personality; and support systems she has.

Survivor may bring in changes in her life such as change of residence and contact number. Few may choose to take a break from daily routine and embark on traveling. Some of them may face difficulties in coping up with work or at home or school. Panic reactions in crowds or when alone may set in which could be related to the circumstances of the incidence. Sexual aversion leading to change in sexual life can occur. This may even lead to break in relationship with existing intimate partner.

Some of the sexual problems that women often encounter postassault include sexual dysfunction due to flashbacks of the rape during sex like vaginismus and inability to experience orgasm. Victims who have a pre-existing psychological disorder (pathology) or who have suffered of sexual violence in the past are likely to have worsening of their trauma and may complicate their recovery.

Post-traumatic Stress Disorders

One of the common psychological disorders faced by victims of sexual assault is PTSD.

PTSD often occurs in victims who experienced extreme overpowering physical violence, often with a threat of dangerous weapon like a gun or a knife, were raped by unknown persons, and in cases where physical injuries were inflicted. PTSD may manifest with symptoms of intrusions and avoidance.

Intrusions involve re-experiencing the traumatic incidence and include flashes of memories of the incidence; frightening and unpleasant dreams; and frequent unpleasant involuntary thoughts that stay in the mind.

Avoidance symptoms include lack of physical or emotional feelings; withdrawal from socialization; reasoning out the incident; lack of attention in routine activities; increased substance use or abuse like drugs and alcohol; indulging in dangerous behaviors; and keeping away from places, work or people that remind them of the assault. Some other features of PTSD include disconnect, hypervigilance, ill temper, and emotional dysregulation.

EXAMINATION AND REPORTING

Patients could report directly to the clinic or could be brought by the police for examination. Role of the medical practitioner is not limited to collecting evidence for medicolegal purposes, but comprehensive medical management of the patient.

Examination should be conducted without delay. Consent needs to be taken for examination, collection of evidence, and information to police. Even if patient denies examination, treatment has to be offered. Patient may deny passing on the information to police. Even when the patient refuses consent for information to police the medical practitioner is bound by law to inform, with a clear note of patient's refusal to such information.

Time of starting examination and time when examination was completed needs to be noted for medicolegal purposes. Following examination, a complete report needs to be sent to the police officer in charge of the investigation.

TREATMENT GUIDELINES AND PSYCHOSOCIAL SUPPORT[4]

Immediate Management

Physical Injuries

Patients received in the casualty need to be screened those with serious injuries requiring immediate attention should be referred for emergency treatment. While those with simple injuries like minor bruises, cuts, and abrasions wounds can be managed by the examining doctor himself. All wounds should be cleaned and treated as necessary.

The patients should be treated with prophylactic antibiotics to prevent secondary infection of the wounds. Tetanus toxoid injection should be administered. Analgesics and anxiolytics may also be required depending on case to case basis.

Sexually Transmitted Infections

Victims of sexual violence are prone to contact STI as a result of the assault. Infections sexually transmitted could be bacterial or viral. The common bacterial infections which these victims are prone to contract are:
- Chlamydial
- Gonorrheal
- Syphilis
- Trichomonal.

While frequently contracted, viral infections could be HPV, herpes simplex virus type 2 (HSV-2), HIV, and the hepatitis B virus.

If patients have clinical signs suggestive of sexually transmitted disease (STD), swabs for diagnosis should be collected and empirical management of STI should be started; however if there are no clinical signs and symptoms suggestive of STI, treatment can be withheld till the results from the laboratory are obtained.

The recommended treatment for STI in nonpregnant patient is azithromycin 1 g stat or doxycycline 100 mg bd for 7 days with metronidazole 400 mg for 7 days along with a antacid.

While in pregnant women, amoxicillin/ azithromycin with metronidazole is preferred. Metronidazole is contraindicated in the first trimester of pregnancy.

Hepatitis B

Hepatitis B immunoglobulin (HBIG) in not required unless the assailant is suffering from acute hepatitis B. The administration of HBIG or the hepatitis vaccine is not contraindicated in pregnant women.

If immunoglobulin needs to be administered then collect blood for hepatitis B virus surface antigen (HBsAg) test and then administer 0.06 mL/kg HBIG immediately (preferably within 72 hours after sexual act if the victim has not been immunized earlier.

If the victim has been immunized, there is no need to revaccinate or administration of immunoglobulins.

Postexposure Prophylaxis for Human Immunodeficiency Virus

A victim of sexual assault is at risk of contracting HIV. It would be difficult to ascertain the status of the assailant unless he is known person. Postexposure prophylaxis (PEP) should be started immediately preferably not later than 72 hours of the incidence and should be continued for 28 days. Strict compliance is necessary to get maximum benefit. Antiemetics can be administered to counter the side effects of the medication. Complete blood count (CBC) and liver function test (LFT) should be done prior to commencement of the treatment to record baseline values, which can be compared latter. If preliminary HIV test is negative repeat testing should be done at 6, 12, and 24 weeks.

The patient needs to be counseled well about the efficacy of PEP, length of treatment, side effects, and strict compliance.

Emergency Contraception

Pregnancy Prophylaxis

Victims of rape are also at risk of pregnancy. Emergency contraception needs to be offered to these patients. Emergency contraception is effective if given within 72 hours, while CuT can be used as an emergency contraceptive method for up to 5 days postexposure.

Emergency contraceptive pills (ECPs) act by preventing or delaying ovulation, by blocking fertilization, or by interfering with implantation. There are no known contraindications for the use of ECP. Commonly marketed ECPs are I-pill and unwanted 72 containing 1.5 mg of levonorgestrel. ECPs have a failure rate of around 1–2%. Hence if the victim misses her period, pregnancy should be checked for.

Follow-up

Follow-ups are important so as to repeat investigations after window periods and to assess any psychological effects post-trauma of sexual assault.

Patient Reporting with Pregnancy after Rape

More often than not such victims report late due to the social stigma attached to such incidences and hence pregnancies get detected late in second trimester limiting the choices available to the girl. In case if the patient is pregnant she needs to be counseled about choices available to her.

The options available to the patient are either continuing with the pregnancy or termination of pregnancy.

If the patient decides to continue with the pregnancy she also has the option to either keep the child under her care or to give it in adoption.

Medical professionals should be aware of laws which are applicable in such issues so as to counsel the victim appropriately and help them take an informed choice. Even in countries where abortion is legally not provided for, provisions are made for termination of pregnancies arising out of rape. After due consideration of all her choices, if the victim choses to terminate the pregnancy, she should be referred to center approved to carry out medical termination of pregnancies.

Decisions about emergency contraception and termination of pregnancy are best left to the patient. It is her choice and no decisions can be forced onto her. The role of the medical professional is to provide appropriate information and to encourage the victim to make her own choices which she feels is appropriate to her.

Counseling and Social Support

Sexual violence victims behave differently to the incident, some victims may be psychologically affected for short time while others may have a prolonged course. There could be recurrence of psychological disturbances after recovery. The course of recovery depends on individual personality as well as support systems the victim has. Victim may require counseling sessions depending on the severity of affection. Counseling sessions could be in the form of individual, family or group sessions.

Group sessions are helpful as it helps in getting free of isolation, victims can share their experiences which helps them reduce the burden of guilt and overcome their low self-esteem. However in cases with pre-existing psychological disorders, group therapy may not work well and in such cases individual treatment would be better.

Referrals

Victims may require various forms of support services and services of rape crisis centers, shelters or safe houses, HIV/AIDS counseling centers, agencies providing legal aid, and various forms of other support groups may be required. They should be provided with verbal and written information or referrals of such services.

■ HURDLES FACED BY THE SURVIVOR

Very often these patients report to hospitals, but hospitals are not willing to treat these patients for the fear of medicolegal implications.

If the victim is a child she may not be aware of she being sexually exploited and pregnancy may be detected beyond legal limits of termination and approaching the courts are only option left to her. Even after detecting pregnancy the girl and family members may not muster courage to report and may seek illegal abortion.

Due to these reasons, rape survivors, especially children, are denied abortion services. There have been two such reported incidences; one was a 10-year-old girl with 28 weeks pregnancy and other was a 13-year-old girl with 26 weeks pregnancy. Both these cases had reported to hospitals, but were denied termination due to pregnancies being beyond the legal gestational age of termination.[5] These cases approached the Supreme Court appealing for permission for termination of pregnancies. Supreme Court allowed termination of pregnancy of 26 weeks while termination of pregnancy to 28 weeks was denied.

There have been several such cases seeking permission to terminate pregnancies that are as a result of rape. Reasons for reaching late to seek medical assistance could be varied. Child may not realize that she is being sexually exploited. She may not be aware that such acts lead to pregnancy. The child might have been threatened with dire consequences to her life and her near ones. Pregnancy is detected only when the child starts having symptoms of morning sickness or abdominal pain or a swelling in the abdomen is noticed.

Role of the Medical Boards

Through the various cases reaching the courts, courts have directed formation of committee of medical experts (medical boards) to opine on the safety of termination of such pregnancies. More often than not the medical boards have based their opinion on the legal limits of termination and interpretation of law rather than assessing the physical, mental, and emotional trauma the survivor is going through.

Limit of gestational age for termination of pregnancy as per the Medical Termination of Pregnancy (MTP) Act is set at 20 weeks of gestation. However, there is a provision under Section 5 of Act, which allows termination irrespective of the gestational age if continuation of pregnancy is threat to the life of the mother.

The question here is can we consider the mental and psychological trauma of pregnancy as a result of rape so grave as to endanger the life of the victim to apply Section 5 and terminate such pregnancies irrespective of the gestational age, especially because such patients have a tendency for suicide.

LEGAL ASPECTS

The MTP Act is an enabling act which provides for termination of pregnancies under certain specified conditions.[6]

Indication for Termination of Pregnancy

Pregnancy as a result of rape is one such valid condition. Hinderance being the limit of gestational age.

Consent for Termination

If the victim is a major, only her consent is required. If the victim is minor, then consent of guardian is required. However, MTP Act does not do away with the consent of the minor, especially in the age group between 12 years and 18 years. Consent for termination of pregnancy if the guardian gives consent cannot be presumed, the view of the minor child has to be taken into consideration.

In a landmark judgment, a two-judge bench of the Madras High Court recognized the right of the minor girl to bear a child under the fundamental right of Article 21, Right to life and personal liberty. Indian constitution does not make any distinction between minor and major in as far as fundamental rights are concerned.

Information to Police

The Protection of Children from Sexual Offences (POCSO) casts a duty upon any person to intimate to the police, knowledge or suspicion of sexual assault on the child.[7]

Child under the act is any child less than 18 years of age irrespective of whether the child is married or had a consensual relationship. In short what these provisions imply is, if we come across any child less than 18 years of age with pregnancy it is our legal duty to inform police.

In case of adult patients Section 357C of criminal procedure code lays down that as soon as we come across patients with sexual assault such patients have to be examined without delay, first aid, and treatment has to be provided free of cost and immediate information to police has to be provided.[8]

What is important here is treatment and information to police is mandatory. Collection of evidence is not mandatory.

Treatment of Victims

Section 357C of criminal procedure code mandates that all hospitals whether public or private have to provide first aid or medical treatment free of cost to victims of sexual assault.

Punishment

Failure to treat a patient of sexual assault or failure to provide information to police is a criminal offence and invites punishment.

Under the Indian Penal code Section 166B, failure to treat a patient of sexual assault invites punishment of imprisonment for a period up to 1 year or fine or both.[9]

Section 21 of POCSO provides that failure to report commission of sexual assault on minor could invite punishment of imprisonment up to 6 months or fine or both.

CONCLUSION

Pregnancy as a result of rape throws various challenges to the clinician. Focus has to be on holistic management providing medical, psychological, emotional, and legal support.[10] Having a positive attitude towards such victims and providing quick and supportive care would go a long way in reducing the trauma and psychological distress faced by these victims.

In India, though there has been steady increase in such crimes and it has been a burning issue since long, the necessary and important aspect of provision of psychosocial support and crisis intervention services has remained neglected.

Provision of abortion services to such victim is an important integral part of this immediate treatment. Longer the pregnancy continues longer is the suffering and trauma of the incidence making early recovery from the incidence difficult for the survivor. Denying abortion services and asking such victims to continue with the pregnancy and suggesting giving the child up for adoption is worsening the trauma of the survivor. A serious thought needs to given by the medical fraternity, judiciary, and legislators to consider rape-related pregnancies as grave as to endanger life of the victim and legalizing termination for such indication irrespective of gestational age.

REFERENCES

1. Edmond T, Slator M. Prevention and response to rape-related pregnancy: issues in Missouri. Brown School, Washington University in St. Louis, No. 3: Center for Violence and Injury Prevention; 2013.
2. CEHAT. (2012). Establishing a Comprehensive Health Sector Response to Sexual Assault. [online] Available from: http://www.cehat.org/go/uploads/Publications/R87%20Establishing%20a%20Comprehensive%20Health%20Sector%20Response%20to%20Sexual%20Assault.pdf [Last accessed September, 2019].
3. Munro ML, Foster Rietz M, Seng JS. Comprehensive care and pregnancy: the unmet care needs of pregnant women with a history of rape. Issues Ment Health Nurs. 2012;33(12):882-96.
4. World Health Organization. (2003). Guidelines for medico-legal care for victims of sexual violence. [online] Available from: https://www.who.int/violence_injury_prevention/publications/violence/med_leg_guidelines/en/ [Last accessed September, 2019].
5. Padma D, Sangeeta R. (2017). Rape Survivors' Right to Abortion: Are Doctors Listening? [online] Available from: https://thewire.in/175257/rape-survivors-right-to-abortion/ [Last accessed September, 2019].
6. MTP Act, 1972.
7. Protection of Children from Sexual Offences Act, 2012.
8. Criminal Procedure Code, 1973.
9. Indian Penal Code, 1852.
10. Coleman GD. Pregnancy after rape. Int J Womens Health Wellness. 2015;1(1):1-4.

CHAPTER 39

Obstetric Emergencies: Medicolegal Issues and Implications

*SV Joga Rao**

INTRODUCTION

Obstetric emergencies are health issues that arise most frequently in pregnant women and their babies. These health issues pose a high risk to the health and life of the mother as well as to the baby. An obstetric emergency may arise at any time during the subsistence of the gestation period[1] and at any time during parturition.[2] The associated risks with obstetric emergencies are premature birth, miscarriage, or increased peril to the women's life and health. Owing to this, hospital care under the supervision of a specialist is advised to the pregnant woman in the event of an obstetric emergency.

There are many kinds of obstetric emergencies, and there exists a plethora of cases pertaining to the subject. The following are types of obstetric emergencies and some cases relating to the same.

PLACENTAL ABRUPTION

Placental abruption is a condition that transpires when the placenta partially or completely detaches from the inner wall of the uterus prior to delivery. This condition more often than not diminishes or stops flow of oxygen and nutrients to the fetus. It results in heavy loss of blood in the mother.

Placental abruption has the increased chance of occurring in the last trimester of pregnancy, especially in the last few weeks prior to the birth. Placental abruption is characterized by vaginal bleeding and/or abdominal/back pain, and uterine tenderness/contractions.[3]

In certain cases, placental abruption is witnessed to be a slow and gradual development, which is marked by light vaginal bleeding. Sometimes the bleeding is merely intermittent.

Treatment

Once the placenta gets detached from the uterine wall, reattachment is not an option for the same and is not possible. Treatment options for placental abruption are circumstantial:

- *The baby is not close to full term*: In the scenario where abruption seems mild, the fetus's heart rate is normal and it is too soon delivery—generally before 34 weeks of pregnancy—one might be hospitalized for close monitoring. Later in the event that the bleeding stops and the fetus's condition is stable, rest at home may be prescribed. In some cases, medication may be administered to help

---

*Advocate and Healthcare Consultant, Legalexcel, Bengaluru and Visiting Professor, NLSIU, Bengaluru
Author sincerely appreciates the research contribution of Ms Kritika and Ms Manogna, Interns at Legalexcel. Similarly he conveys his sincere thanks to Ms Sanidhya, Associate, Legalexcel for her research and content contribution.

the baby's lungs mature, in case early delivery becomes necessary.
- *The baby is close to full term*: Generally, after 34 weeks of pregnancy, if the placental abruption seems minimal, a closely monitored vaginal delivery might be possible. If the abruption progresses or endangers the health of the mother or the child, an immediate delivery—usually by cesarean section is undertaken. In the instance of severe bleeding, one might need a blood transfusion.[4]

Case Study I[5]

Facts:
- The complainant, suffered from a lot of pain during her pregnancy and consulted the doctor at the maternity and surgical nursing home.
- The doctor after examination, informed her that the bleeding was due to separation of fetus from placenta. And, without giving any emergency treatment, the doctor referred her to another doctor at another hospital
- The doctor without examining her, informed her about the need of an immediate operation and, accordingly, the doctor performed cesarean operation [lower segment cesarean section (LSCS)], took out the dead fetus
- The complainant alleged that, the consent was taken afterwards. Even though the bleeding did not stop, hence the doctor proceeded for hysterectomy operation without her and her husband's consent
- Hence, alleging that, both the doctors acted negligently, it and deficiency in service to remove the uterus, the complainant filed a complaint before State Commission and prayed for compensation of ₹5,30,000 from both the doctors.

Issue: Was the doctor negligent in her duties?

Analysis: The Complainants argued that the doctors were negligent on several counts:
  i. No proper consent was taken.
  ii. Unnecessary hysterectomy was performed.

The Doctors contended that:
  i. Consent was taken via a form
  ii. Since the case was an emergency, and the uterus was flabby (atonic uterus), the hysterectomy was a life-saving treatment.

The Judges relied upon:
  i. "Obstetric Hemorrhages", the Anesthetic and Obstetric Management of High-Risk Pregnancy by Sanjay Datta, Springer edition. A Textbook of Postpartum Hemorrhage: A Comprehensive Guide to Evaluation, Management and Surgical Intervention edited by Christopher B-Lynch. According to these sources, the Abruptio Placentae is an emergency condition, which, when left untreated, puts both the mother and baby in jeopardy.
  ii. The consent form and deemed that valid consent was given.
  iii. *Kusum Sharma v. Batra Hospital* (2010) 3 SCC 480 which laid down many principles pertaining to medical negligence including—"*(xi) The medical professionals are entitled to get protection so long as they perform their duties with reasonable skill and competence and in the interest of the patients. The interest and welfare of the patients have to be paramount for the medical professionals.*"

Conclusion

Relying upon the Bolam test and several judgments of the Hon'ble Supreme Court, the NCDRC did not find any negligence in the actions of OP-2 who took a proper decision to save the life of the patient.

PLACENTA PREVIA

Placenta previa is a condition that arises when a fetus's placenta gets attached to the lower part of the uterus, resulting in partial or total covering of the mother's cervix—the outlet for the uterus. The consequence of which is that it can cause severe bleeding during pregnancy and delivery.

Bright red vaginal bleeding sans pain during the second half of pregnancy is the major symptom of placenta previa. In certain cases, contractions have also been observed as a symptom.

In numerous cases, women diagnosed with placenta previa early in their pregnancies, it has been found that the condition got resolved by itself. With the growth of uterus, there is a good possibility that the distance between the cervix and placenta may increase. But more the placenta covers the cervix and the later in the pregnancy that it remains over the cervix, the less likely it is to resolve.[6]

Treatment unavailable can only be managed. No medical or surgical treatment exists to cure this condition, one only seeks to manage the bleeding caused by it. If placenta previa does not resolve during pregnancy, the goal is to help one get as close to one's due date as possible. Almost all women with unresolved placenta previa require a cesarean delivery.[7]

Case Study II[8]

Facts: The complainant's late wife was admitted for her delivery at a Nursing Home under care of a doctor on 29/10/2006. She had delivered a female child on the same day and was discharged on 07/11/2006. At the time of delivery of the complainant's late wife, it was a case of Adherent Placenta and the complainant was duly warned about it with advice at the time of discharge to ensure removal of piece of placenta attached to the part of Uterus within next 40 days.

On 24/11/2006 the complainant's wife complained of bleeding and therefore, she was readmitted around 09.30 pm on that day at the same Nursing Home. While the complainant had gone to fetch blood as per the Doctor's instructions, it shocked him to return to the fact that the Doctor had already initiated the operation without blood as required and therefore, he inferred that such act on the part of doctor led to the deterioration of his late wife's condition.

The Doctor then suddenly asked for the patient to be shifted to another Hospital for further treatment. However, she died there due to excessive bleeding. Postmortem of the complainant's late wife was also carried out.

It is alleged by the complainant that had the placenta tissue attached to the lower uterus segment been removed she would not have died, and that the Doctor's actions could constitute a deficiency in service.

Issue: Were the Nursing Home and Doctors negligent the duties?

Analysis:
- It was revealed from the evidence and material placed on record that doctor could not remove the piece of placenta as it was not possible unless the entire uterus was removed and since the complainant had two daughters, did not consent for the removal of the uterus at the time of delivery.
- As far as case of adherent placenta is concerned, when the fertilized zygote gets attached to the lower uterine segment, it later on gives rise to placenta previa, which is natural in its formation and doctors play no role in its occurrence. Adherent placenta occurred when chorionic villus gets anchored to the myometrium. Depending on its penetration into the myometrium one gets placenta accreta (serious medical condition that occurs when the placenta grows too deeply into the uterine wall), increta (when all or a part of the placenta attaches abnormally to the muscular layer of the uterine wall—known

as the myometrium) or percreta (condition wherein the placenta grows through the uterine wall). Whenever the deciduas of the uterus which is thin, there are chances of developing an adherent placenta. The incidence of adherent placenta is high in placenta previa, or on previous LSCS scar. Therefore, adherent placenta previa is natural in its formation and doctors play no role in its occurrence. Therefore, it could be further inferred that there is no medical negligence shown either by OP-1 and 2 on the date of delivery.

- When the complainant's wife was brought back to the hospital because of excessive bleeding, the primary line of treatment identified was to carry out blood transfusion and arrest further bleeding. The Nursing Home and the Doctor [OPs] proved that while the Complainant had gone to bring blood, only a conservative procedure of packing had been carried out to arrest the bleeding. Under the circumstances, precious time would have been lost and the patient could bleed to death. Arrest of bleeding had to be undertaken with or without blood.

Conclusion

There is no contra evidence to disbelieve this fact. Under the circumstances, it could be seen that the normal medical protocol was duly followed by the Nursing Home and the Doctor.

Considering the condition of the complainant's wife and the availability of required facilities to meet her critical condition, she was further advised to shift to another Hospital. She was accordingly shifted, but there is no record available as to her condition on arrival at the Hospital. The only fact which further emerged as an undisputed fact is that she ultimately died at the Hospital.

Her postmortem was carried out, but there was no final opinion as to her cause of death on record. It is alleged by the opponents that it was not a case of unnatural death as recorded in the record. Since the Complainant did not contradict said statement of the Nursing home and the Doctor and since no other better material is on record to hold otherwise, we find no reason to disbelieve said statement.

Thus, in light of no concrete evidence against the Nursing Home's and Doctors' evidence and considering all the circumstances, the court dismissed the consumer complaint and did not hold the Doctors and the Nursing Hoem liable.[9]

PRE-ECLAMPSIA AND ECLAMPSIA

Pre-eclampsia is the condition where pregnant women suffer from high blood pressure, which as a consequence of the pregnancy. This causes water retention which results in severe swelling and bloating. It can lead to kidney and liver failure. This condition usually sets in post 20 weeks of pregnancy in women whose blood pressure had been normal prior. Eclampsia is the onset of seizures or coma in a pregnant woman with pre-eclampsia. These seizures are not a result of pre-existing brain condition.[10]

Treatment:
- Usually hospitalization and sometimes antihypertensive treatment
- Delivery, depending on factors such as gestational age and severity of pre-eclampsia
- Magnesium sulfate for prevention or treatment of seizures.[11]

Case Study III[12]

Facts: The Complainant/Patient was admitted with labor pains on completion of full-term pregnancy in a Nursing Home on 25.05.1993 and that on the following day she underwent a cesarean section, from which she never fully recovered consciousness and finally passed away in a vegetative state in 2004.

Issue: Were the doctors, who performed the cesarean, negligent in their duties?

Analysis:

Complainants/patient's arguments:
i. Patient did not suffer from pre-eclampsia or eclampsia, and was only rendered comatose from the administration of the wrong treatment and negligence of the Doctors and the Nursing Home.
ii. Care provided to the patient throughout was inadequate, deficient, and negligent history was no recorded properly, no laboratory tests were taken and delay in conducting cesarean.

Arguments of the Nursing Home and Doctors:
i. All the necessary tests were conducted and indicated that the patient, by virtue of the symptoms of high blood pressure, protein in the urine, and swelling of the feet, suffered from pre-eclampsia.
ii. Due to the administration of medication and her serious condition, monitoring was required and dictated as per protocol, and only when fetal distress was observed the next morning, was the cesarean conducted.
iii. All the doctors involved were qualified and performed their duties diligently and thoroughly.
iv. The sudden discharge by the Complainants the day after the cesarean, adversely affected the patient.
v. *Expert evidence*: In addition to the medical literature provided by both parties, the opinion of two medical experts was taken on record because as the State Commission felt that the decision of the case necessitated the imperative need of obtaining experts' opinions before the issues were decided.
vi. The parties counsels were requested to give names of two experts, one of whom should be dealing with Neurology and another with Obstetrics and Gynecology. From amongst the names, Professor and Head of Department of Neurosurgery and a Professor of Obstetrics and Gynecology from a College were requested to guide the Commission with reference to the facts available on the record.
vii. Apart from filing their affidavits based on the records of the case, Commission permitted cross examination of the two experts by the Counsel for all parties and the State Commission framed the following three questions, which it felt were pertinent to enable it to reach a decision in the matter.

Q1: What was the time of arrival of the Complainant into the Nursing Home and what happened till she left the said Nursing Home?

Finding: The extract of the views of the two experts do not leave any manner of doubt that at the time of admission, sufficient steps had not been taken for controlling the blood pressure as per the claim that it was on the higher side. It was further observed that her condition had only worsened 12-14 hours after admission. Such a condition obviously was preventable by administering adequate medicines and attempting to have the child delivered through cesarean section earlier than the delivery which had taken place the next day. Only one conclusion was possible at the time of admission, i.e. the patient was not having any immediate signs of pre-eclampsia much less eclampsia. If the doctors noted that she was having immediate presence of pre-eclamptic signs, steps could have been at once taken to prevent the eclampsia from overpowering the patient. Both these actions are absent. It was observed that nothing prevented them from taking suitable steps to save the child as well as the mother.

The statement of the Professor of Obstetrics and Gynecology is very clear that it should have been better for the doctors in the Nursing Home to administer specific antihypertensive drugs. It is also her clear statement that what may have been excessive dose of scoline after the operation.

The Professor and Head of the Department of Neursurgery was also candid in his statement that hypoxic ischemic brain damage was the result of the state of affairs of the Complainant. On looking at the data available and the documents, i.e. alleged bed head ticket and the anesthetist's report, it was said to be obvious that there was no pathological confirmation of any of the allegations of the Nursing Home and the Doctors about the meconium coming out of the child in the womb or that there was actual presence of albumin in excessive quantity so as to invite eclampsia to overtake the patient. The attempt to argue that pathological report was removed by the complainant or her relatives is mentioned only to be rejected. If they were to carry away only the pathologist's report, they could very well have taken out the bed head ticket also.

The two learned experts belonged to the same medical fraternity as the Doctors.

Q2: Whether the documents produced by the parties are correct and reliable?
Finding: It was observed there were several omissions and commissions in the documents produced, but since the complainant's case was proved and certainly neither disproved nor rendered unproved by either the Nursing Home's or the Doctors' documents, no finding about their being otherwise or being not genuine is called for.

Q3: Whether the case of the Complainant if believed will earn compensation as originally claimed or as claimed through the amendment?

Finding: On considering the lapse in time from when the complaint was filed and the judgment delivered, the expenses incurred during this time, the attachment of liability on the Nursing Home and the Doctors, it was observed that the Nursing Home and the Doctors were liable to pay ₹ 3 lakhs each in cash or by bank draft to the Complainant, through her mother.

NCDRC observations:
i. *Medical treatment and care at the time of admission till surgery:*
   a. The patient did suffer from pre-eclampsia.
   b. The Nursing Home and the Doctors were negligent in not recording previous case history, tests, etc. —this is a minimum requirement.
   c. Applied the principle laid down in *Achutrao Haribhau Khodwa and Others v State of Maharashtra and Ors.* [(1996) 2 SCC 634]—merely because a doctor chooses one course of action in preference to the other one available, he would not be liable if the course of action chosen by him was acceptable to the medical profession.
   d. Medicines prescribed in the pre-operative period were correctly administered.
ii. *Medical treatment and care at the time of surgery:* No clear case of medical negligence or deficiency is made out, and the patient clearly suffered from eclampsia and its repercussions during the surgery. It was also observed that despite the contention that the patient did not have a high blood pressure and therefore could not have suffered from pre-eclampsia and eclampsia, the Commission relied on *"Textbook of Obstetric"* by Dr DC Dutta, which clarified that eclamptic convulsions can

occur even with moderate rise of blood pressure.
iii. *Medical treatment and care postsurgery*:
   a. No conclusive evidence to point out deficiency and medical negligence, even after consultation with experts.

Conclusion

Based on a catena of judgments by the Hon'ble Supreme Court, the NCDRC could only find the two of the three Doctors negligent for their failure to record the case history of the Complainant/Patient at the time of her admission and thereafter to get conducted the required laboratory tests, which are essential in a high risk first pregnancy case detected with pregnancy-induced hypertension (PIH) and pre-eclampsia. However, did not find the other Doctor guilty of either negligence or deficiency in service in the treatment and care of the patient during surgery, including anesthesia.

Case Study IV[13]

Facts: The Appellant's spouse, (hereinafter "patient"), went to Vijayawada to her parent's home, where she was under the medical care of Respondents No. 1 and 2.

On 2.8.2000, she underwent cesarean operation and delivered healthy twin babies. In the evening of 03.08.2000, fluids were coming out of the stitches and there was blockage of urine. After consulting the doctors over it, it was decided that her condition necessitated a reoperation for it was observed that her kidneys had been affected by increased pressure of the twin pregnancy.

On 04.08.2000, Respondents No. 1 and 2 had operated upon the patient to investigate the presence of any disease or injury (exploratory laparotomy). After which she was sent for dialysis, as was directed by the nephrologist. Thereafter, she was put on ventilator owing to the condition of her lungs which also had got affected. After every 2 days the patient was sent for dialysis. However, the health of the patient only became worse and she passed away on 07.08.2000.

A postmortem report concluded the cause of the death to be septicemia resulting from postoperative complications. The Appellant alleged that the doctors were negligent.

Issue: Were the doctors negligent and could their actions amount to deficiency in service?

Analysis

Appellant's arguments:
i. Because of the negligence during the surgery which caused a wound in the urinary bladder, the patient suffered from septicemia and subsequent death. This is confirmed by the postmortem report.
ii. No specific explanation was given by the Doctors as to why this problem occurred within 24 hours of the surgery apart from the patient being a high-risk case, which itself had not been recorded anywhere in the case sheet.

Arguments of the Doctors:
i. No medical evidence that the surgery conducted by the Doctors had caused septicemia.
ii. Patient died 4 days after the surgery, and even during this time she was attended by many doctors, including a nephrologist.
iii. When the urinary output of the patient stopped and some fluid started leaking from the site, a urologist was immediately called and an abdominal scanning and blood test revealed kidney damage because of a high serum creatinine. The urinary bladder was opened and sutured on the same day to control the fluid leakage and the exploration did not reveal any urological problem.
iv. The patient had pregnancy-induced complications, i.e. eclampsia and kidney failure which were not the result of the

surgery but a pre-existing condition which caused her death.

Relevant SCDRC observation: The standard care that was due to the patient should have been provided by the Doctors. Especially, in the light of the complications that arose post the surgery conducted for the purposes of delivery. Furthermore, the Doctors have conceded that cause of blockage of urine was not found. The Hon'ble Supreme Court had laid down, in the case of Savita Garg v. National Heart Institute, that it is the duty of the treating doctor and hospital to explain the line of treatment to the patient. Also, the burden of proof is shifted onto the hospital and doctors to prove that their acts were not negligent and conform very much to standard medical practices. The documentation of the case by the Doctors was faulty, for it did not reflect the patient to be a high-risk patient. The cause for the fluid leak or the urinary blockage had not been identified. Also, it was said that the bladder showed no injury but the postmortem said the contrary. Owing to all these reasons the Doctors are held to be negligent.

NCDRC's observations:
i. The postmortem report proves an injury, of the nature of an incision, to the bladder measuring 1.5 cm. It was because of this injury that urine leaked. Such an injury could have been inflicted only during the cesarean operation. This establishes a nexus between the operation conducted by the doctors and the subsequent ill health and death of the patient.
ii. If the patient was to be considered a high-risk patient because of eclampsia, records of the same should be kept as case history. No such condition was notes in the case history of the patient in this case.
iii. Relied upon the principle of what constitutes medical negligence as has been established by the Hon'ble Supreme Court in the case of *Jacob Mathew v State of Punjab and Anr (2005) 6 SCC 1*. It is to be seen that whether the impugned Doctor has done or failed to do something in a given context, no doctor would do; and whether the negligence was in the lines of res ipsa loquitur, i.e. its manifest nature was such that no doctor in ordinary sense could have done such an act.

Conclusion

Both the Doctors are jointly and severally guilty of medical negligence in the instant case with a compensation of ₹50,000/- each and a total of ₹150,000/-.

■ PREMATURE RUPTURE OF MEMBRANES

Premature rupture of membranes (PROM) is the condition where the amniotic sac ruptures before the onset of labor. Preterm PROM (PPROM) is the term used when the pregnancy is less than 37 weeks.

The rupture of amniotic sac puts mother and the unborn child at a higher risk of infection and increases the chance of the premature birth or early delivery.[14,15]

Treatment: Delivery—in case of risk of infection to the fetus, or the fetus is in distress, or gestational age ≥34 weeks.

Otherwise, pelvic rest, close monitoring, antibiotics, and sometimes corticosteroids.

A PROM management requires balancing risk of infection when delivery is delayed with risks due to fetal immaturity when delivery is immediate.[16]

Case Study V[17]

Facts: The patient was brought to the Nursing Home in the morning on 29-12-2003, with the leaking of fluid throughout the night and a chance of infection and danger to the child. Accordingly, the Treating Doctor gave medication and suggested for an immediate cesarean operation, but the patient's husband and father-in-law did not consent to the operation. After consent was obtained later, the operation was conducted.

After operation, the condition of the patient was satisfactory. The Doctor had to go to Nagpur due to a family emergency, and in her absence, her husband, an Assistant Surgeon and a Gynecologist looked after the patient every day.

On 01-01-2004, the Gynecologist examined the patient, in consultation with the Assitant Surgeon, called the Physician. Her blood pressure dropped and after treatment, while the BP did normalize, there was no urine output; therefore, on return of the Treating Doctor, the patient was referred to another Hospital for the dialysis as it was not available in the city.

The Treating Doctor submitted that due to delay in LSCS operation, there were more chances of infection which could result in septicemia, disseminated intravascular clotting (DIC), and amniotic fluid embolism (AFE). At the other Hospital, on admission the patient was in serious condition, developed septicemia with DIC, acute renal failure (ARF), and acute respiratory distress syndrome (ARDS). Despite the best treatment, the patient died on 14-01-2004 at the Hospital that she was referred to.

Analysis: The NCDRC relied on "Bacteriological study of premature rupture of membranes" by R Kondal/Rao and Nandan Singh— *"The fetal membranes provide protection against infection. The amniotic fluid has antibacterial activity due to zinc protein complex. Bacterial colonization of the amniotic cavity is known to occur after rupture of the fetal membranes through direct ascent for endogenous vaginal flora".* Therefore, to counter the risk and to control the infection, the Treating Doctor gave broad-spectrum antibiotics pre- and postoperatively but despite the precautions, patient developed infection further septicemia and shock and further renal complications and DIC.

Conclusion

Relying upon the *Jacob Mathews* Case, and other Supreme Court judgments pertaining to medical negligence, the NCDRC was of the view that the death was not due to any negligence, on the part of the Treating Doctor.

■ SHOULDER DYSTOCIA

The main mechanism behind the occurrence of shoulder dystocia is the retention of the anterior shoulder behind the pubic symphysis, while the posterior shoulder is usually located in the maternal pelvis. In rare situations, both shoulders are retained above the pelvic brim.[18,19]

Treatment is with physical maneuvers to reposition the fetus, operative vaginal delivery, or cesarean delivery.[20]

Case Study VI[21]

Facts: The complainants conceived a child 10 years after marriage and for the purpose of delivery they got themselves registered with the Hospital. The Complainant No. 2 was admitted in the hospital on 4.6.2007, with the clear condition of the PIH requiring qualitative caution and appropriate procedure while handling the delivery case. The Complainant No. 2 delivered reportedly a healthy male baby in the evening of 5.6.2007 through full time normal vaginal delivery apparently with no complications as per obstetric report.

However, soon after an abnormality in the left arm of the baby was discovered and that abnormality was attributed to "shoulder dystocia". It is alleged that the abnormality in the functioning of the left arm termed as stricken with Erb palsy was due to crude and violent pulling of the newborn baby during the latter's delivery irreversibly damaging the neuromotor functioning of the left arm. The baby was subjected to violence through pulling which caused the destruction of the nerve roots through an exercise of unprofessional and intransigent use of violence and the consequent pseudomeningocele.

Since no complications were noted during delivery, the apparent dysfunction of the left arm was deemed to be attributable to some defect in the bone. Therefore, an X-ray test was advised to the baby and accordingly the Complainant No. 1 was referred to the physiotherapy department. No further scans were taken.

On visiting other doctors for advice in the matter, the damage done to the newborn was confirmed. The Complainants, based on the confirmations, accuse the Hospital of medical negligence and state that their actions amount to deficiency in service.

Issue: Were the Hospital in the instant matter, negligent?

Principle: Res ipsa loquitur.

Analysis:

Arguments by the Hospital:
i. No negligence or failure in duties by the doctors.
ii. The baby was diagnosed with "shoulder dystocia" which is the result of natural complication that can happen in any childbirth despite total and absolute precaution having been taken. It happens in a very small number of cases but this is something which cannot be predicted. One comes to know of such an abnormal event only in the process of delivery when head of the baby is out of the womb but remaining part remains to be taken out. Thus, it is not the result of any negligence or deficiency.
iii. No expert was called upon to prove such negligence.

Complainant's arguments:
i. The Hospitals were not well aware of the seriousness of the situation when they termed the delivery as normal. It is a case where it was incumbent on the part of the doctor to observe precaution which was not done leading to this avoidable untoward situation.
ii. Principle of res ipsa loquitor was relied upon.

Commission's Observations:
i. Relying upon the Supreme Court case of V Kishan Rao v Nikhil Super Specialty Hospital (2010), in cases of res ipsa loquitor, the commission need not rely upon expert evidence, and may apply their own mind to the facts and circumstances of the case. Thereby, allowing for efficient adjudication and speedy justice.
ii. Relying on a catena of Supreme Court decisions pertaining to medical negligence, including Dr V Srinath & Anr. v Gaurav Lamba (2011)—which held that "wrongful surgery causing permanent disability amounts to negligence", the SCDRC was of the opinion that no due care was exercised.

Conclusion

Considering the standard of care established by the Hon'ble Supreme Court, the SCDRC was of the view that the matter was one of *res ipsa loquitor*, and that the doctors were negligent in the instant matter. A compensation of ₹ 30 Lakhs was awarded to the complainants.

Case Study VII[22]

Facts: On 16.08.2002, complainant No. 3 was taken for an emergency surgery where she delivered the baby. After the delivery the Gynecologist informed the mother that owing to the baby's excessive weight and since the shoulder did not expel normally, forceps had been used for the delivery. This procedure of delivery had resulted in paralysis of the upper right limb of the baby. It was also observed that the baby's head had been squashed on both sides. Owing to bleeding under skin the baby's neck and shoulders had turned blue.

The parents of the baby sought medical aid and service from various eminent medical professionals who then told them that five nerves of the baby had got damaged during the time of delivery. Despite all the medical treatment and corrective surgeries sought, the condition of the child had not been alleviated.

The parents alleged that this occurred because of the medical negligence and deficiency in service on the part of the doctors and hospital.

Issue: Were the the Maternity and Medical Center and the Doctors negligent in the instant matter?

Analysis:

Arguments by the Medical Center and the Doctors:
   i. All required prenatal tests were conducted and as per medical literature on the subject both in India and in the developed world (USA, etc.) only a baby that weighs more than 4.5 kg can be termed as macrosomic.
   ii. Doctors took the correct decision to opt for a normal delivery since there were no clinical or other medical conditions to indicate the necessity of a cesarean.
   iii. Relying upon Williams Obstetrics (21st edition), most of the cases of shoulder dystocia cannot be predicted or prevented because there are no accurate methods and it can occur in both normal weight and also large weight babies.
   iv. When shoulder dystocia was noticed, the standard protocol/procedure to deal with such cases was undertaken. Relying upon medical literature, it was argued that the use of forceps in this situation was ideal, vis-à-vis the use of vacuum delivery since forceps operation can quickly expedite delivery in case of fetal distress whereas vacuum will be unsuitable as it takes a longer time.
   v. Appropriate medical care was given to Complainant-1 postdelivery, and despite there being no need for a neurosurgeon to be consulted, the doctors recommended one by way of caution.
   vi. A team of medical experts from Maulana Azad Medical College were sought to give their opinion by the State Commission with regard to progress of pregnancy of the Complainant 3. They had opined after perusing the ultrasound records that there was normal progress of pregnancy with no evidence of macrosomia. *(expert opinion—evidence)*

Complainant's arguments:
   i. Crucial antenatal investigations, for example, pelvic assessments, gestational diabetes test, correlation of ultrasounds, etc. were not conducted. Therefore, it is submitted that the antenatal checks and care was incomplete.
   ii. Vacuum should have been employed for the delivery—it would have been ideal. For extensive, medical literature has given us enough proof that wrongful delivery by forceps can also cause shoulder dystocia, it was evident that the forceps were used with unnecessary and excessive force for there exists no other plausible explanation to demonstrate the extensive brachial plexus injury, breaking all the five nerves of the upper right limb and damage to the face and head.

iii. The indifference and callous attitude of the Medical Center and the Doctors were evident by the lack of due care given postdelivery. Also, a neurosurgeon was brought in only after insistence on the third day.

NCDRC's observations:
i. Antenatal investigations are a crucial component of medical care during pregnancy for it is through these that one is able to identify, assess, and consequently reduce the risks to both the mother and the fetus. In the instant matter, antenatal care which was provided with was inadequate.
ii. As per the Supreme Court judgment of Achutrao Haribhau Khodwa v State of Maharashtra [(1996) 2 SCC 634], when a doctor chooses one treatment option, when faced with many, he is not to be held liable for negligence if the line of treatment chosen by him is in conformity with the standard medical protocols and practices. Therefore, the Anesthesiologist cannot be held negligent for exercising his discretion in his professional choice.
iii. But, the method by which the procedure was conducted can be tested according to the reasonable standard established in the Bolam case, and thus, by not using the single most effective procedure, i.e. McRoberts maneuver, it can be said that shoulder dystocia was not adequately handled.
iv. The Medical Center and the Doctors were not found to be negligent in the postdelivery ministrations.

Conclusion

In failing to give appropriate antenatal care and by not using the McRoberts maneuver, the NCDRC held the Medical Center and Doctors negligent of their medical duties.

Case Study VIII[23]

Facts: Appellants 2 and 3 (the parents of Appellant 1), under the care of the Doctors, were told that the development of the fetus was normal. On 7.3.2001, the mother was admitted to Hospital due to unbearable labor pains and also profuse bleeding. After a physical examination and insertion of a pill in her vagina, she was kept in the labor room with instructions that delivery is likely to take place in the morning. No investigations were carried out during this period nor anybody attended to her.

Only the next morning, following severe bleeding and the appearance of the head of the baby, was the mother taken for delivery which was conducted by the use of forceps. No primary medical check was done on the infant and in fact appellant's mother-in-law observed that the baby was dropped by the nurse to whom she was handed over following delivery. When the infant was brought before the appellants for the first time, they noted that there were marks of injury on the side of his head and they were informed that these were minor and were caused because of use of forceps.

After examination by other doctors, damage to the brain and sensory nerves was confirmed and was observed to have been caused at the time of birth. Appellant 1 subsequently developed brachial palsy and is now permanently disabled. The Appellants allege gross negligence by the Respondents.

Issue: Were the Respondents in the instant matter negligent in their conduct and duties?

Principle: Res ipsa loquitur.

Analysis:

Appellants' arguments:
i. Negligence is evident and this is a case of res ipsa loquitor.

ii. Delay in conducting the delivery, and leaving the patient in pain and allowing the excessive bleeding, was highly negligent conduct.
iii. The delivery was not handled with due care as there was excessive unnecessary use of force with the forceps and by the fact that the nurse dropped the baby after he was born.
iv. Inadequate postdelivery care was given to the mother and child, which only exacerbated the condition of the latter.

Arguments by the Doctors and the Maternity Home:
 i. Due care, treatment and precautions were taken during the pregnancy and at the time of delivery.
 ii. Ultrasonography was done regularly to determine the growth and status of the fetus. During delivery, the shoulder dystocia was unexpected, and only after trying an episiotomy, was a delivery by forceps resorted to. And unfortunately, despite all precautions, in 20% of all cases of shoulder dystocia, brachial palsy does occur.
 iii. No injury was caused by the nurse dropping the baby.
 iv. When the case was in the State Commission forum the expert opinion by Gynecologist was relied upon as evidence which said that the treatment given by the opposite doctor was within the acceptable norms.

NCDRC's observations:
 i. On perusing the medical literature, there is an inherent risk of brachial palsy in cases of shoulder dystocia. No evidence of negligence in this connection.
 ii. Injury caused by dropping the baby does not inspire confidence as there exists no further proof of such an incident happening.
 iii. Adequate prenatal care and postdelivery care was given, including administration of medication, etc.

Conclusion

The SCDRC was unable to conclude that there was any medical negligence by the Maternity Home and the Doctors in the instant matter, and therefore dismissed the appeal.

■ RUPTURE OF THE UTERUS

Uterine rupture is defined as a defect in the uterine wall associated with fetal distress or maternal hemorrhage sufficient to require cesarean delivery or postpartum laparotomy.

Uterine rupture is a condition usually associated with the acute and dramatic collapse of the mother's health condition. The mother may go into shock, symptoms of the same can be seen by pallor, rapid pulse, shallow breathing, and a fall in blood pressure. This condition is characterized by severe pain and bleeding as well.[24]

Treatment of uterine rupture is immediate laparotomy with cesarean delivery and, if necessary, hysterectomy.[25]

Case Study IX[26]
Facts: On 20.11.1995, the deceased patient had developed labor pains and was admitted to Nursing Home.

During the delivery, the patient suffered from rupture of the uterus through previous surgical scar which caused profuse blood loss. The baby was delivered at 3.30 pm but the bleeding did not stop despite measures taken. Thereafter, an attempt at blood transfusion was made but the patient suffered from renal failure thereafter.

The Complainants allege negligence on the part of doctors, and claim that no due care was given to the patient and thus, there was a deficiency in service.

Issue: Were the Nursing Home and the Doctors negligent in the instant matter?

Analysis:

Complainant's arguments:
  i. Inadequate prenatal tests and investigations were conducted.
  ii. Emergency cesarean should have been conducted instead of vaginal delivery.
  iii. Syntocinon drip was administered at a higher rate which resulted in uterine contractions and rupture of the uterus.
  iv. While attempting blood transfusion, due to nonavailability of "A" Negative blood, "A" Positive blood was transfused to the patient without consulting any specialist, which further caused renal failure.

Arguments by the Nursing Home and the Doctors:
  i. Prior to the delivery, necessary tests and periodical checkups were advised, but the patient did not turn up.
  ii. On arrival to the hospital, she was sent to the labor room directly and was administered medication immediately. The dosage of syntocinon given was lesser than the usual dose.
  iii. The patient was constantly monitored, and so was the fetal heart rate.
  iv. No negligence during delivery, no need for LSCS was seen.
  v. The mother unexpectedly began to bleed, and despite being given the appropriate medication, the bleeding did not stop. There was a fall in pulse and blood pressure, the uterus of patient became flabby. The patient was found to be "A" Negative. Due to nonavailability of "A" Negative blood, she was transfused "A" Positive blood initially and thereafter, the patient was given six units of "A" Negative blood along with dopamine drip to revive her condition but instead of that, the patient did not recover.

NCDRC's observations:
  i. As per Book of Obstetrics by DC Dutta," *Previous history of Cesarean Section does not appreciably alter the course of pregnancy and labor. However, the following complications are likely to increase (1) Abortion, (2) Premature labor, (3) Normal pregnancy ailments, (4) Operative interference and incidental morbidity, and (5) Retained placenta and postpartum hemorrhage (PPH)".* Thus, previous history need not be taken and choosing the different treatment was not medical negligence.
  ii. As per the Supreme Court judgment of *Achutrao Haribhau Khodwa v State of Maharashtra* [(1996) 2 SCC 634], merely because the doctor chooses one course of action in preference to the other one available, he would not be liable if the course of action chosen by him was acceptable to the medical profession.
  iii. Syntocinon was administered in a controlled manner.
  iv. The medical record did not show that there was uterine rupture as alleged by the Complainant. The death of patient was due to PPH and DIC.

Conclusion

The doctors have acted in accordance with accepted standards of medical practice and therefore cannot be said to have been negligent of their duties.

Case Study X[27]

Facts: On 10.6.1999, a patient was admitted to the hospital for her delivery. By the midnight of 11/12-6-1999 it was observed that the heart rate of the unborn child was decreasing rapidly. Owing to which the doctors conducted cesarean. A female baby was born but it took 5 minutes to get her to cry. She was then kept on a ventilator in neonatal ICU.

Even with the assertions of the Doctors that the reports of the baby were normal, the health of the baby further worsened. Later when the baby stabilized, she was discharged. But the child could suckle and at 2.5 months she underwent a few tests which revealed that she suffered from atrophy of the brain.

Expert opinion posited that the atrophy of the brain was a result of birth asphyxia. It meant that the child could remain mentally retarded for her life.

Thus, the doctors were alleged to be negligent by the parents of the child.

Issue: Were the Doctors and the Hospitals negligent in their duties?

Principle: Res ipsa loquitur.

Analysis:

Complainant's arguments:
i. The cesarean was supposed to have been conducted within 12–18 hours after rupture of membrane. The delay was for 27 hours.
ii. The dose of Syntocinon was excessive and it was the trigger for the fetal distress, and subsequently resulted in cerebral anoxia-palsy.
iii. The patient was in a condition that required immediate care from the Doctors, the same was not meted out to her. This had an adverse impact on the child because of the seizures.
iv. The Doctors and the Hospitals have meddled, suppressed, and fabricated relevant and crucial medical records.
v. Due care was not observed by the doctor during delivery which resulted in the asphyxiation of the baby.
vi. *Evidence* relied upon was *medical textbooks and other medical literature*.

Arguments by the Doctors and the Hospitals:
i. No unusual amount of Syntocinon was administered.
ii. Prior check and monitoring were routinely conducted and the patient was advised accordingly. However, the advice was ignored.
iii. There was no delay in taking the decision for the need for a C-section, however, due to the noncooperation of the patient, the doctors waited. Thereafter, due to nonprogress and cervical dystocia, the C-section was performed.
iv. Both, the baby and the patient were given due care postdelivery and were monitored appropriately.
v. As *evidence expert opinion* of three doctors were sought, but since they belonged to the hospital impugned in the case it was not taken into consideration.

NCDRC's observations:
i. The Doctors should not have waited more than 24 hours after the administration of Syntocinon, and thus, there was a delay in the performing of the cesarean.
ii. Inappropriate dosage of Syntocinon was administered which made it possible, as per the extensive literature relied upon, for the baby to suffer from adverse effects.
iii. No proper consent was obtained.
iv. Residents and nurses failed to appreciate the signs of distress on the fetal heart monitor.

Conclusion

The corporate hospitals and specialists are expected to provide medical services at a higher level, i.e. with more care and expertise, than other hospitals/general practitioners. For they pose themselves to have better skills and infrastructure. This is also reflected in the fees they charge.

The Hospital and its nursing staff failed in their duty of care of rendering medical services with the reasonable skill and diligence prevailing in the medical profession to the delivery of the child.

Thus, the Doctors and Hospital in this case were held to be negligent and their actions were said to amount to deficiency of service. Appropriate compensation of ₹ 1 Crore was awarded.

AMNIOTIC FLUID EMBOLISM

Where fluid moves from the amniotic sac and ends up in the mother's blood. This is a very rare complication and can happen during pregnancy, but usually occurs during strong contractions in labor and causes serious complications including death of the mother. The onset of AFE is unforeseen and fast. It is characterized by sudden shortness of breath, pulmonary edema, sudden low blood pressure, cardiovascular collapse, blood clotting issues, uterine bleeding, cesarean incision or intravenous (IV) sites, chills, rapid/disturbed heart rate, seizures, fetal distress, loss of consciousness, and an altered mental status.[28][29]

Treatment: Amniotic fluid embolism necessitates a quick response aimed at addressing lack of oxygen and decreasing blood pressure. Emergency treatments include but are not limited to the following:
- Catheter placement—it allows intravenous administration of nutrients and medicines
- Oxygen mask—for ease of breathing and to counter lack of oxygen intake
- Medications—to help with the heart function and for its support. Also, for the purpose of countering the effects of the fluid entering the heart or lungs
- Blood transfusion—in the event of severe loss of blood, one may require blood transfusion.[30]

Case Study XI[31]

Facts: The wife of the Complainant (since deceased and hereafter referred to as "the patient") was under the care of the Gynecologist at the Hospital, and on 29.8.2000, she was admitted into Hospital, wherein the Gynecologist assured her of normal delivery and shifted her to the labor room.

Thereafter, on 30.8.2000, the Gynecologist informed the patient about decision to conduct delivery by C-section (LSCS) to save the child and the mother. The patient gave birth to the baby at 2:*45 am, and the baby was handed over to* the Complainant. However, the patient was under a coma, which, according to the Hospital and the Doctors was due to a cardiac arrest caused by a Monocef injection being administered without a pre-sensitivity test. The patient's condition only deteriorated further, despite the Complainant seeking treatment from different hospitals. The patient passed away in 2004. The Complainant alleges that the patient's death was due to the negligent conduct of the Hospital and the Doctors and since no due care was given.

Issue: Were the Hospital and the Doctors negligent in their duties and could their actions amount to deficiency in service?

Analysis:

Complainant's arguments:
i. The Doctors did not perform timely resuscitation in its hospital, which resulted in permanent damage to the brain.
ii. The Hospital did not give any discharge slip or medical records, while shifting the patient to the other hospital. Thus, it was negligence committed by Hospital and the Doctors; the patient remained in coma, throughout for about 4 years and died, on 21.8.2004.
iii. No due care was given to the patient during the delivery, and the anesthesia was wrongly administered.

Arguments by the Hospital and the Doctors:
i. Due care was given to the patient prior to the delivery, and the decision to conduct LSCS was taken so as to save the life of the

fetus, and was in the best interest of both the mother and the fetus.
ii. Procedure was only performed after informed consent was obtained.
iii. The patient was operated under spinal anesthesia because the patient was not fasting and has taken a glass of water also.
iv. After delivery of baby, injection "Monocef" was administered to the patient with presensitivity test. Therefore, the doctor may not be held responsible for the anaphylactic reaction.
v. There was no delay in resuscitation soon after cardiac arrest. Even the discharge ticket issued by the other hospital did not indicate that the cardiac arrest was due to Monocef injection allergy.
vi. Expert opinion was sought from the Medical Board of AIIMS and the same was relied upon which was in favor of the Doctor.

NCDRC's observations:
i. The surgical notes clearly mention about the actual events that took place in the OT. The patient was properly resuscitated after the cardiac arrest. Thereafter, the patient was shifted to the other hospital, the admission and treatment records shows that the patient was admitted in the other hospital, in emergency, patient was intubated.
ii. Relying on Goodman and Gilman's *"The Pharmacological Basis of Therapeutics"* it was observed that "there are no skin tests that can reliably predict, whether a patient will manifest an allergic reaction to the cephalosporins".
iii. Regarding whether the patient suffered an anaphylactic reaction due to an AFE, it was noted that the cause may be due to anaphylaxis or by AFE. Since, as per medical literature, the injection Monocef rarely causes anaphylaxis, whereas, the signs of AFE are also similar to anaphylaxis. Such occurrence is not intentional or in anybody's hands, hence the Hospital and the Doctors could not be held liable.
iv. With respect to whether the Doctor handled the cardiac arrest (emergency) by cardiac resuscitation properly, the clinical notes clearly indicate that the patient was intubated and oxygen saturation was maintained. Proper emergency medicines like atropine, steroids, etc. were given to save the life of patient. Thus, resuscitation was done by the Doctor, as per standards of practice. Thereafter, patient was timely referred to the other hospital for further treatment. Therefore, we do not find any lapse in treatment of cardiac arrest.

Conclusion

Based on the plethora of Supreme Court judgments on the standard of care, and the facts and arguments advance, the NCDRC were not of the view that the doctors acted negligently.

However, in the instant case, the Hospital did not provide medical records to the Complainant within time, even before the Commission the Hospital produced the medical records at a belated stage. It was seen with suspicion, and deemed to be unethical conduct. Therefore, punitive costs of ₹10 lakhs were imposed on the Hospital to pay the Complainant.

Case Study XII[32]

Facts: The deceased Patient, wife and mother of the Complainants, was admitted in the Nursing Home run by the Doctor and was administered Cerviprime gel to induce labor pains. She was assured that her labor would be normal.

After the labor pains started, she was taken to the labor room where she gave birth via normal vaginal delivery. After the delivery, she was shifted to a room. Soon after, the family of the patient started noticing blood on her garments, and requested the staff to call the the Doctors to come and examine her. However, the staff could not get in touch with the Doctors as she was not in the Nursing Home. By the time the Doctor returned, which was approximately 2 hours later, the patient was unconscious and pale. She was taken to the operation theatre, but was declared dead within a short time.

The doctors stated that the cause of death was due to AFE, whereas the attendants were of the belief that she died of excessive bleeding, i.e. PPH.

The Complainants allege that the Doctor was negligent of her duties and that her actions and inaction can amount to deficiency in service.

Issue: Was the Doctor negligent of her duties?

Analysis:

Complainant's arguments:
  i. The doctor was absolutely callous and negligent of her duties.
  ii. Her absence during delivery and at the critical time of postdelivery makes a clear case of negligence.
  iii. No conclusive evidence by the doctor.
  iv. No proper cause of death was opined, as no proper postmortem was carried out.

Doctor's arguments:
  i. Due care was taken of the patient before, during and after delivery by the Doctors and the staff of the Nursing Home.
  ii. She was present in the Nursing Home for the delivery and during post-delivery.
  iii. The cause of death is AFE.

NCDRC's observations:
  i. There exists no conclusive proof as to the presence of the Doctor in the Nursing Home at the time of delivery and postdelivery.
  ii. Relying on medical literature, the Commission was of the view that the cause of death was most likely to be PPH rather than AFE, as the latter has ambiguous symptoms, is rare and causes instantaneous death. Only a postmortem could have determined an absolute answer.

Conclusion

Based on a catena of Supreme Court judgments which laid down the principles of medical negligence, the Commission found that the Doctor was negligent, and thereby, deficient in her service towards the deceased.

REFERENCES

1. The period during which a fertilized egg cell develops into a baby that is ready to be delivered; Oxford Medical Dictionary, 6th edition. PP. 314.
2. Childbirth; Oxford Medical Dictionary, 6th edition. PP. 314.
3. https://www.mayoclinic.org/diseases-conditions/placental-abruption/symptoms-causes/syc [Last accessed on 30-09-2019].
4. https://www.mayoclinic.org/diseases-conditions/placental-abruption/diagnosis-treatment/drc. [Last accessed on 30-09-2019].
5. Kirti B Nayak v Sonalben S Vyas (NCDRC 2014).
6. https://www.mayoclinic.org/diseases-conditions/placenta-revia/symptoms-causes/syc [Last accessed on 20-09-2019].
7. https://www.mayoclinic.org/diseases-conditions/placenta-previa/ diagnosis-treatment/drc [Last accessed on 30-09-2019].
8. Shree Nursing Home v Chandrashekar Singh (Mah SCDRC 2013).
9. https://www.betterhealth.vic.gov.au/health/HealthyLiving/pregnancy-obstetric-emergencies [Last accessed on 30-09-2019].
10. https://medlineplus.gov/ency article/000899.htm [Last accessed on 30-09-2019].
11. https://www.msdmanuals.com/professional/gynecology-and-obstetrics/abnormalities-of-pregnancy/preeclampsia- and-eclampsia [Last accessed on 30-09-2019].
12. KK Kakkar v Neetu Singh (NCDRC 2014).

13. Dr Atluri Ravindranath and Anr v Jangamgunta Balasubramanium and Ors. (NCDRC 2012).
14. https://www.betterhealth.vic.gov.au/health/HealthyLiving/pregnancy-obstetric-emergencies [Last accessed on 30-09-2019].
15. https://www.urmc.rochesteredu/encyclopedia/content.aspx? Content Type D = 90 & Content ID = P02496 [Last accessed on 30-09-2019].
16. https://www.msdmanuals.com/professional/gynecology-and-obstetrics/abnormalities-and-complications-of-abor-and-delivery/prematurerupture-of-membranes-prom [Last accessed on 30-09-2019].
17. Ajay Khandel and Ors. v Prakash Nursing Home and Ors. (NCDRC 2017).
18. Ayres-de-Campos D. Obstetric Emergencies: APractical Guide, 1st edition. Berlin, Germany: Springer; 2017.
19. https://www.betterhealth.vic.gov.au/health/HealthyLiving/pregnancy-obstetric-emergencies [Last accessed on 30-09-2019].
20. https://www.msdmanuals.com/professional/gynecology-and-obstetrics/abnormalities-and-complications-of-labor-and-delivery/fetal-dystocia [Last accessed on 30-09-2019].
21. Ritesh Kumar Garg and Ors. v Max Hospital (Del. SCDRC 2018).
22. Singhal Maternity and Medical Center v Master Nishant Verma (NCDRC 2014).
23. Harsh Amit Kumar Sheth (Minor) and Ors. v Sheth Hospital and Maternity Home and Ors. (NCDRC 2012).
24. Source: West Z. Complications in anesthesia. Accupuncture in Pregnancy and Childbirth, 2nd Edition. London, United Kingdom: Churchill Livingstone; 2007. (pg. 151-2).
25. https://www.msdmanuals.com/professional/gynecology-and-obstetrics/abnormalities-and-complications-of-labor-and-delivery/uterinerupture [Last accessed on 30-09-2019].
26. Katra Satyanarayana and Ors. v Lakshmi Nursing Home and Ors. (NCDRC 2017).
27. Indu Sharma v Indraprastha Apollo Hospital and Ors. (NCDRC 2017).
28. https://www.betterhealth.vic.gov.au/health/HealthyLiving/pregnancy-obstetric-emergencies [Last accessed on 30-09-2019].
29. https://www.mayoclinic.org/diseases-conditions/amniotic-fluid-embolism/symptoms-causes/syc [Last accessed on 30-09-2019].
30. https://www.mayoclinic.org/diseases-conditions/amniotic-fluid-embolism/diagnosis-treatment/drc [Last accessed on 30-09-2019].
31. Vivek Jaimini and Ors. v Metro Hospital and Ors. (NCDRC 2016).
32. Sabita v Shreepad and Ors. (NCDRC 2015).

40
Puerperal Sepsis

Sudeepti Mummadi

INTRODUCTION

- Puerperal sepsis (childbed fever) was a major cause of maternal death in Europe in the 19th century. In 1843, Oliver Wendell Holmes made the unpopular suggestion that it was carried on the hands of doctors, and 4 years later Ignaz Semmelweis in Vienna showed how it could be prevented if doctors and midwives washed their hands before attending a woman in labor and practiced aseptic techniques.
- "Sepsis", as defined as the presence of infection along with features of systemic inflammation. These features are characterized by criteria which define systemic inflammatory response syndrome (SIRS).
- Many physiological changes associated with pregnancy, such as tachycardia and hypotension, are similar like in sepsis.
- *"Sepsis-induced hypotension"* is defined as a systolic blood pressure (SBP) <90 mm Hg or mean arterial pressure (MAP) <70 mm Hg or a SBP decrease >40 mm Hg or more than two standard deviations below normal for age in the absence of other causes of hypotension.
- *"Septic shock"* is defined as sepsis-induced hypotension persisting despite adequate fluid resuscitation.

ESSENTIALS OF DIAGNOSIS[1]

- History of recent delivery.
- Systemic signs of infection.
- Abdominal pain and vaginal discharge.
- Peritoneal signs.
- Boggy, tender uterus, and purulent lochia.

CRITERIA FOR SYSTEMIC MANIFESTATION OF INFECTION[2]

Criteria for systemic manifestation of infection have been given in Table 1.

ETIOLOGY AND PRESENTATION

Infectious complications in pregnancy may be divided into the following:[3]

Pregnancy-related Infection

Sepsis in early pregnancy may be associated with a miscarriage or follow a termination of pregnancy. In the second or third trimester, premature rupture of membrane (PROM) is associated with a risk of chorioamnionitis. Perineal infections, endometritis, wound infections, and mastitis should be considered in the postnatal period.

Nonpregnancy-related Infection

A few predisposing factors, including human immunodeficiency virus (HIV), comorbid illness (e.g. cystic fibrosis), or steroids and immunosuppressants may predispose to infection.

Nosocomial Infection

Prolonged hospital stay, intravenous (IV) lines or catheters, and overcrowding may predispose to hospital-acquired infections.

TABLE 1: Criteria for systemic manifestation of infection.

Variable	Infection (documented/suspected) and some of the following:
General	• Fever (>38.3°C) or hypothermia (temperature <36°C) • Heart rate >90 beats/min • Tachypnea • Altered mental status • Significant edema or positive fluid balance (>20 mL/kg over 24 hours) • Hyperglycemia in the absence of diabetes
Inflammatory	• WBC count >12,000/mL • WBC <4,000/mL • Normal WBC count with greater than 10% immature forms • Plasma C-reactive protein >2 SD above the normal value • Plasma procalcitonin >2 SD above the normal value
Hemodynamic	Arterial hypotension (SBP <90 mm Hg, MAP <70 mm Hg, or an SBP decrease >40 mm Hg in adults or more than 2 SD below normal for age)
Organ dysfunction	• Arterial hypoxemia (PaO_2/FiO_2 <300) • Acute oliguria (urine output <0.5 mL/kg/hr for at least 2 hours despite adequate fluid resuscitation) • Creatinine rise >0.5 mg/dL or 44.2 µmol/L • Coagulation abnormalities (INR >1.5 or aPTT >60 s) • Ileus • Platelet count <100,000/mL • Plasma total bilirubin >4 mg/dL or 70 mmol/L
Tissue hypoperfusion	• Hyperlactemia >1 mmol/L • Decreased capillary refill or mottling

(aPTT: activated partial thromboplastin time; FiO_2: fraction of inspired oxygen; INR: international normalized ratio; MAP: mean arterial pressure; PaO_2: partial pressure of oxygen; SBP: systolic blood pressure; SD: standard deviation; WBC: white blood cell)

In severe cases of puerperal pyrexia, group A beta-hemolytic *Streptococcus* [*Streptococcus pyogenes* and group A *Streptococcus* (GAS)] should be suspected. Streptococcal throat infections are relatively common in the community. Cautions against hand to genital tract transmission should be taken, including hand washing before and after using the lavatory and changing sanitary towels. This is particularly important when the mother has had a recent contact with someone with a sore throat or upper respiratory tract infection. GAS causes a wide spectrum of illness ranging from bacteremia without a focus of infection, to endometritis, and peritonitis. "Invasive GAS" is associated with necrotizing fasciitis and toxic shock syndrome.[3]

The single most important risk factor for postpartum infection is cesarean section. Retained products of conception may also result in endometritis. Patients often present with uterine tenderness, abdominal pain, purulent foul-smelling lochia, and features of systemic infection. Cervical and high vaginal swabs must be obtained for culture. The rate of endometritis is approximately threefold higher in nonelective cesarean sections compared to elective sections. The use of prophylactic antibiotics prior to section is associated with a significant reduction in the rates of wound infection and endometritis.[4]

Ascending bacterial colonization of the genital tract may result in uterine contractions and can result in preterm prelabor rupture of membranes. This may result in chorioamnionitis, which typically presents with abdominal tenderness and fever following preterm premature rupture of membrane (PPROM). The use of prophylactic antibiotics is associated with prolongation of pregnancy, fewer neonatal infections, and a reduction in rates of chorioamnionitis.[5] It is recommended that a 10-day course of erythromycin is administered following PPROM. If GAS is isolated, penicillin should be administered or administer clindamycin to women who are allergic to penicillin.[6]

The principal risk factors for endometritis are cesarean delivery, young age, low socioeconomic status, extended duration of labor and ruptured membranes, and multiple vaginal examinations. In addition, pre-existing infection or colonization of the lower genital tract [gonorrhea, group B *Streptococcus* (GBS), and bacterial vaginosis] also predisposes to ascending infection. Other risk factors for maternal sepsis include maternal anemia, obesity, poor nutrition, induced labor, and prolonged labor (>12 hours).[3]

MICROBIOLOGY

Endometritis is a polymicrobial infection caused by organisms which are part of the normal vaginal flora. They gain access to the upper genital tract, peritoneal cavity, and occasionally the bloodstream because of vaginal examinations during labor and manipulations during surgery.

The most common organisms are GBS, anaerobic Gram-positive cocci, aerobic Gram-negative bacilli—mainly *Escherichia coli*, *Klebsiella pneumoniae*, and *Proteus* species— and anaerobic Gram-negative bacilli, mainly *Bacteroides* and *Prevotella* species. *Chlamydia trachomatis* is not a usual cause of early-onset puerperal endometritis but has been implicated in late-onset infection. The genital mycoplasmas may be pathogens in some patients, and are usually are present in association with more highly virulent bacteria.

Group A *Streptococcus* infection is a rare, life-threatening cause of puerperal fever due to *Streptococcus pyogenes*. GAS infections are invasive and toxin production allows the organism to spread across tissue planes and cause necrosis while evading containment and abscess formation by the maternal immune system.

Bacteria commonly responsible for female genital infections are given in Box 1.[7]

Box 1: Bacteria commonly responsible for female genital infections.

Aerobes
Gram-positive cocci: Group A, B, and D streptococci, Enterococcus, Staphylococcus aureus, Staphylococcus epidermidis
Gram-negative bacteria: Escherichia coli, Klebsiella, Proteus
Gram-variable: Gardnerella vaginalis
Others
Mycoplasma and Chlamydia, Neisseria gonorrhoeae
Anaerobes
Cocci: Peptostreptococcus and Peptococcus species
Others: Clostridium, Bacteroides, Fusobacterium, Mobiluncus

CLINICAL FINDINGS

Fever, diarrhea, vomiting, abdominal pain, generalized maculopapular rash (staphylococcal or streptococcal sepsis), offensive vaginal discharge, and visible evidence of infection in cesarean wounds are the common symptoms of puerperal sepsis.[8]

Symptoms of puerperal sepsis in the early postpartum period are fever, peritoneal pain, and vaginal discharge. Examination reveals abdominal tenderness, exquisite uterine tenderness, and purulent lochia with leukocytes and bacteria on Gram stain.

DIAGNOSIS

Differential diagnoses of puerperal fever are endometritis, atelectasis, pneumonia, viral syndrome, pyelonephritis, and appendicitis. Differentiation among these disorders usually can be made on the basis of physical examination and laboratory investigations such as white blood cell count, urinalysis and culture, and in selected patients, chest radiograph. Blood cultures are not done routinely because of their expense and their lack of impact on clinical decision making. However, blood cultures are indicated in patients who have a poor initial response to therapy and in those who seem seriously ill, are immunocompromised, or are at increased risk for bacterial endocarditis. Also, blood cultures could be considered in women with exceedingly high temperature spikes that may mean virulent infection with group A streptococci.[9]

Presentation of GAS is atypical and may involve extremes of temperature, unusual and vague pain, and pain in extremities. Endometrial biopsy may be a useful rapid diagnostic tool.

MANAGEMENT

The management of the patient is divided into the resuscitation phase, antimicrobial treatment (including obtaining blood cultures and source control), and subsequent supportive treatment.

Overview

Urgent and repeated blood cultures should be taken in systematically ill women. Swabs should be taken from the genital tract to identify the offending organism. Ultrasound may help in identifying retained products, which may be a source of infection. Treatment should be started promptly without awaiting results of cultures. In view of polymicrobial nature of infections, broad spectrum IV antibiotics should be commenced.

If retained products are present, evacuation should be performed after antibiotics have been given for 24 hours. Earlier intervention in presence of active sepsis may trigger septicemia and should be avoided.

If there is lack of improvement, causes of refractory pelvic infection should be looked for. These include parametrial cellulitis, abscesses, infected hematomas, and septic thrombophlebitis.

Septic shock should be treated aggressively in an intensive care facility, as these patients will require accurate fluid replacement, respiratory and circulatory support and possible hemodialysis in addition to antibiotics.

Resuscitation

Tissue hypoxia can develop due to low blood flow. Fluid resuscitation should be initiated promptly in patients with hemodynamic instability or if there is elevated lactate, to achieve an adequate oxygen delivery. Controversy exists as to the best type of fluid [colloid vs. crystalloid, type of colloid (e.g. albumin vs. gelatin vs. starch), balanced vs. unbalanced solutions, the optimal filling target, etc.]. Excessive amount of starch-based solutions should be avoided as this has been associated with increased rates of acute kidney injury.[10]

Antimicrobial Therapy and Source Control (Table 2)

Patients who have moderately severe infections, especially after vaginal delivery, can be treated with short IV courses of single agents such as the extended-spectrum cephalosporins, penicillins or carbapenem antibiotics like imipenem-cilastatin and meropenem.

Once antibiotics are begun, approximately 90% of patients get better within 48-72 hours. When the patient has been afebrile and asymptomatic for 24 hours, parenteral antibiotics are to be discontinued and the patient should be discharged. An extended course of oral antibiotics is not necessary after discharge. However, oral antibiotics may be needed in the following cases. First, patients who have had a vaginal delivery and who defervesce within 24 hours are candidates for early discharge. In these individuals, a short course of an oral antibiotic such as amoxicillin-clavulanate (875 mg every 12 hours) may be substituted for continued parenteral therapy. Second, patients who have had staphylococcal bacteremia may require a more extended period of administration of parenteral and oral antibiotics with specific antistaphylococcal activity.

Patients who fail to respond to the antibiotic therapy mentioned earlier usually have one of two problems. The first is a resistant organism (Table 3).

The next major cause of treatment failure is a wound infection, in the form of incisional abscess or a cellulitis with no actual purulent collection. Abscesses should be opened completely to provide drainage and a specific antistaphylococcal antibiotic should be added to the treatment regimen.

If extensive cellulitis at the margin of the incision is present, an antibiotic with specific coverage against staphylococci should be added, but the wound should not be opened. vancomycin (1 g IV every 12 hours) is a good antistaphylococcal antibiotic, particularly against methicillin-resistant *Staphylococcus aureus (MRSA)*.[11] Other possible antistaphylococcal agent is linezolid (600 mg IV every 12 hours). Antibiotics may be discontinued once the patient has been afebrile and asymptomatic for a minimum of 24 hours.

When changes in antibiotic therapy do not result in clinical improvement and no evidence of wound infection is present, several unusual disorders should be considered.

TABLE 2: Combination antibiotic regimens for treatment of puerperal endometritis.

Antibiotics	Intravenous dose
Regimen 1	
Clindamycin plus	900 mg every 8 hours
Gentamicin	7 mg/kg every 24 hours
Regimen 2	
Clindamycin plus	900 mg every 8 hours
Aztreonam	1–2 g every 8 hours
Regimen 3	
Metronidazole plus	500 mg every 12 hours
Penicillin	5 million U every 6 hours
Ampicillin plus	2 g every 6 hours
Gentamicin	7 mg/kg ideal body weight every 24 hours

▍ DIFFERENTIAL DIAGNOSIS OF PERSISTENT PUERPERAL FEVER[12]

Differential diagnosis of persistent puerperal fever has been given in Table 4.

▍ EFFECTS

The long-term morbidity associated with maternal sepsis includes chronic pelvic inflammatory disease, chronic pelvic pain,

TABLE 3: Treatment of resistant microorganisms in patients with puerperal endometritis.

Initial antibiotics	Principal weakness in coverage	Modification of therapy
Extended-spectrum cephalosporins	Some aerobic and anaerobic Gram-negative bacilli, enterococci	Change treatment to clindamycin or metronidazole plus penicillin or ampicillin plus gentamicin
Extended-spectrum penicillins	Some aerobic and anaerobic Gram-negative bacilli	Same as above
Clindamycin plus gentamicin or aztreonam	Enterococci, some anaerobic Gram-negative bacilli	Add ampicillin or penicillin Consider substitution of metronidazole for clindamycin

TABLE 4: Differential diagnosis of persistent puerperal fever.

Condition	Diagnostic tests	Treatment
Resistant microorganism	Blood culture	Combination antibiotics
Wound infection	• Physical examination • Needle aspiration • Ultrasound	Incision and drainage if abscess is present; add antibiotic to cover staphylococci
Pelvic abscess	• Physical examination • Ultrasound • Computed tomography • Magnetic resonance imaging	Drainage; combination antibiotics
Septic pelvic vein thrombophlebitis	• Ultrasound • Computed tomography • Magnetic resonance imaging	Heparin anticoagulation; combination antibiotics
Drug fever	• Temperature graph • White blood cell for eosinophilia	Discontinue antibiotics
Mastitis	Physical examination	Add antibiotic to cover staphylococci

bilateral tubal occlusion and impaired fertility, and also impacts neonatal morbidity.

PREVENTION

Prophylactic antibiotics are valuable in reducing the frequency of postcesarean delivery endometritis, especially in women having surgery after a prolonged period of labor and ruptured membranes.

Historically, IV prophylactic antibiotics for cesarean delivery were delayed until cord clamping based on several prior studies,[13] which showed that the delay decreased the probability that neonates would require evaluations for sepsis without compromising effectiveness. However, a recent Cochrane review of the timing of IV prophylactic antibiotics for cesarean delivery showed that preoperative administration significantly decreases the incidence of composite maternal postpartum infectious morbidity, as compared with administration after cord clamping, with no differences in adverse neonatal outcomes reported.[14] Women undergoing cesarean delivery should receive antibiotic prophylaxis preoperatively to reduce maternal infectious morbidities.[15]

Cochrane database[16] evaluated 15 randomized trials (n = 4,694 patients) to compare different methods of removing the placenta. A consistent finding in these trials was a decreased rate of endometritis in women where placenta was removed by gentle traction on the umbilical cord than for manual extraction.

It is recommended that low- and high-risk patients having cesarean delivery receive antibiotics 30–60 minutes before the start of surgery. American College of Obstetricians and Gynecologists (ACOG) recommends use of cefazolin, 1 g if body mass index (BMI) is less than 30 m²/kg (or <80 kg) and 2 g if BMI is greater than 30 m²/kg (or >80 kg), given as a rapid IV infusion.[17]

The WHO guidelines on "the five cleans" needed during delivery have led to the introduction of clean birth kits that contain soap, plastic sheeting, gloves, sterile gauze, a razor, and cord ties for use at home births.[18]

CONCLUSION

Most women of childbearing age are healthy. However, in a small proportion of childbearing age, severe complications can occur. Due to physiological changes in pregnancy, early sepsis can be easily missed. A high index of suspicion should be held particularly in the presence of risk factors. Early resuscitation and antibiotics form the cornerstone of management.

REFERENCES

1. Marshall B, Marshall K. Obstetric and gynecologic emergencies and sexual assault. In: Stone KC, Humphries RL (Eds). Current Diagnosis and Treatment: Emergency Medicine, 8th edition. New York, NY: McGraw-Hill; 2017.
2. Dellinger R, Levy MM, Rhodes A, et al. Surviving Sepsis Campaign: international guidelines for management of severe sepsis and septic shock, 2012. Intensive Care Med. 2013;39(2):165-228.
3. Arulkumaran N, Singer M. Puerperal sepsis. Best Pract Res Clin Obstet Gynaecol. 2013;27(6):893-902.
4. Smaill FM, Gyte GM. Antibiotic prophylaxis versus no prophylaxis for preventing infection after cesarean section. Cochrane Database Syst Rev. 2010;20(1):CD007482.
5. Kenyon S, Boulvain M, Neilson JP. Antibiotics for preterm rupture of membranes. Cochrane Database Syst Rev. 2003;(2):CD001058.
6. RCOG. (2010): Preterm Prelabour Rupture of Membranes (Green-top Guideline No. 44). [online] Available from https://www.rcog.org.uk/en/guidelines-research-services/guidelines/gtg44/ [Last accessed September, 2019].
7. Cunningham FG, MacDonald PC, Gant NF. Puerperal complications. Williams Obstetrics, 25th edition. New York, NY: McGraw-Hill Professional; 2018.
8. Wilkinson H. Saving mothers' lives. Reviewing maternal deaths to make motherhood safer: 2006-2008. BJOG. 2011;118(11):1402-3.
9. Gabbe SG, Niebyl JR, Simpson JL, et al. Maternal and perinatal infection in pregnancy: Bacterial. Obstetrics: Normal and Problem Pregnancies. Amsterdam, Netherlands: Elsevier Health Sciences; 2017.
10. Zarychanski R, Abou-Setta AM, Turgeon AF, et al. Association of hydroxyethyl starch administration with mortality and acute kidney injury in critically ill patients requiring volume resuscitation: a systematic review and meta-analysis. JAMA. 2013;309(7):678-88.
11. Duff P. Antibiotic selection in obstetrics: making cost-effective choices. Clin Obstet Gynecol. 2002;45(1):59-72.
12. Duff P. Pathophysiology and management of postcesarean endomyometritis. Obstet Gynecol. 1986;67(2):269-76.
13. Dinsmoor MJ, Gilbert S, Landon MB, et al. Perioperative antibiotic prophylaxis for non-laboring cesarean delivery. Obstet Gynecol. 2009;114(4):752-6.
14. Mackeen AD, Packard RE, Ota E, et al. Timing of intravenous prophylactic antibiotics for preventing postpartum infectious morbidity in women undergoing cesarean delivery. Cochrane Database Syst Rev. 2014;(12): CD009516.
15. Costantine MM, Rahman M, Ghulmiyah L, et al. Timing of perioperative antibiotics for cesarean delivery: a metaanalysis. Am J Obstet Gynecol. 2008;199(3):301.e1-6.
16. Anorlu RI, Maholwana B, Hofmeyr GJ. Methods of delivering the placenta at cesarean section. Cochran Database Syst Rev. 2008;(3):CD004737.
17. American College of Obstetricians and Gynecologists. ACOG Practice Bulletin No. 120: Use of prophylactic antibiotics in labor and delivery. Obstet Gynecol. 2011;117(6):1472-83.
18. World Health Organization (WHO). Essential newborn care. Report of a technical working group (Trieste, 25–29 April 1994). Geneva: WHO, Division of Reproductive Health (Technical Support); 1996.

CHAPTER 41

Obstructed Labor

Rajitha Yarlagadda

INTRODUCTION

Normal labor depends on three components adequate power (uterine contractions and maternal pushing efforts), passage (good pelvis), and passenger (normal size baby). Obstructed labor is due to the disproportion of the fetal presenting part and maternal pelvis, i.e. when vertex is in the occipitoanterior position or relative disproportion due to deflexion and malpresentation.[1] In the 21st century obstructed labor is a life-threatening complication that increases significantly maternal and perinatal morbidity.

World Health Organization (WHO) defined obstructed labor as the failure of the descent of presenting part of the fetus to progress into the birth canal due to mechanical obstruction despite good uterine contractions.[2] It is the fourth leading cause of MMR in India and 8% of maternal mortality is the result of obstructed labor in developing countries.[3]

Even though timely identification of risk factor for obstructed labor at the antenatal period, i.e. big baby, short stature, and nulliparity has not shown sufficient positive predictive value to serve as screening tool.[4,5] Timely clinical diagnosis, resuscitation, and correction of obstruction by an assisted vaginal delivery that is vacuum extraction or cesarean delivery prevents complications of obstructed labor. So identifying the risk factors of obstructed labor in pregnant women in antenatal period and taking effective measures for the prevention, diagnosis, and management of the obstructed labor is very essential in the postmillennium developmental era.

INCIDENCE

In India, obstructed labor accounts to 160/1,000 perinatal mortality.[6]

Incidence of obstructed labor in referral hospital is between 0.56–1.89% in India.[7]

RISK FACTORS

- *Age*: 20–30 years
- Primigravida (64.3%)
- Unbooked case
- Inadequate antenatal care
- Low socioeconomic status
- Delivery by untrained person in rural areas
- Extremes of age in reproductive period, pregnancy in adolescence causes problem as bones of pelvis may not yet have achieved its full dimensions
- Childhood rickets, adolescent and adulthood osteomalacia results in poor or distorted pelvis[8]
- Short stature maternal height is an indirect sign of a woman's general health and nutritional status from her childhood along the genetic factors. They are various cut- off values in different studies as being associated or predicting an increased risk of obstructed labor, less than 140 cm in India.[9]

ETIOLOGY

The causes of obstructed labor have been given in Table 1.

PATHOPHYSIOLOGY OF OBSTRUCTED LABOR

Normal physiology of labor consists of series of uterine contractions, on contraction calcium binds to calmodulin on entering into the myometrium and activates enzyme myosin light chain kinase (MLCK) which in turn phosphorylates myosin thus stimulating interaction with actin and subsequent cross-bridge cycling and contraction.

By increasing the glycogen store and fatty acid droplets, myometrium prepares for labor biochemically. Adenosine triphosphate (ATP) is needed for cross-bridge cycle and acidification is produced as the result of ATP hydrolysis.

In labor, uterine blood vessels are compressed by the powerful uterine contractions lead to transient hypoxic condition. Thus myometrium responds by producing ATP anaerobically, i.e. more pyruvate is formed into lactic acid due to increased LDH activity, instead of entering the Krebs cycle for oxidative metabolism. In obstructed labor, the initial labor pattern of uterine activity will be same as long as metabolic demands are met, in case of restricted intake of food and water during labor, the metabolic stores, i.e. glycogen during labor gradually decreases and finds difficulty to maintain ATP levels. Hence continuous production of lactic acid coupled with decreased ability to extrude protons will lead myometrial acidification. The hypothesis for decreased contractility in primigravid women in obstructed labor is because of myometrium acidification.

This acidification is due to myometrium energy depletion, anaerobic metabolism, and systemic ketoses.

In multigravida, an unknown mechanism drives the myometrium to become tolerant to the effects of acidification and continue to contract in the presence of myometrial energy depletion and hypoxia leads to myometrial edema and necrosis leading to uterine rupture.[10]

Bandl's ring is an hour glass constriction ring of the uterus. Incidence is 1 in 5,000 live births and is associated with obstructed labor in second stage.

TABLE 1: Etiology of obstructed labor.

Maternal factors	Fetal factors

• Bony pelvis:
  – Childhood malnutrition
  – Rickets and osteomalacia
  – Poliomyelitis causes bony deformities, i.e. structure of hip
  – Contracted pelvis
  – Pelvic fractures damaging normal pelvic anatomy 8–12 weeks of fracture healing is required before considering for vaginal delivery
  – Nutritional deficiencies such as Ca, Vit-D, folic acid, zinc, and iron in association with various biological factors.[8]
• Soft tissue:
  – Cervical fibroids
  – Broad ligament fibroid
  – Ovarian tumors
  – Rectal tumors
  – Vagina—septum, stenosis, or tumors
	• Malpositions:
	  – Asynclitism
	  – Occipitoposterior position
	  – Persistent-occipito transverse position
	  – Deep transverse arrest
	• Malpresentation (27%):
	  – Brow presentation
	  – Face presentation
	  – Shoulder presentation
	  – Breech presentation
	  – Compound presentation
	  – Transverse lie.
	• Malformation:
	  – Hydrocephalus
	  – Abdominal tumors (e.g. Wilm's tumor)
	  – Cystic hygroma
	  – Conjoined twins
	  – Locked twins.

In obstructed labor, the uterus overcomes the obstruction by powerful uterine contractions with very little relaxation. Thus pushing the fetus down into the lower uterine segment, resulting in the formation of a pathological retraction ring of Bandl's ring between the markedly thickened and retracted upper contractile segment of the uterus and the abnormally thinned and stretched out lower uterine segment.

CLINICAL FEATURES

Signs and Symptoms

- History of prolong duration of labor pain of more than 18 hours
- Hot and dry skin with loss of tissue turgor
- Decreased urine output
- Tachycardia, tachypnea, and pyrexia
- Acetone smell in breath and urine due to ketoacidosis
- Distention of bowel and atony due to hypokalemia
- Purulent vaginal discharge
- Signs of septic shock.

Abdominal Examination

- Compression of bladder between posterior surface of pubic symphysis and presenting part resulting difficulty in emptying the bladder. Bladder forms a palpable tender swelling above pubic symphysis. Blood-stained urine is due to prolonged compression traumatizing the bladder is a feature of obstructed labor, but does not necessarily imply the rupture of uterus
- Uterus is hard and tender, with frequent uterine contractions with no relaxation in between (tetanic contractions)
- Rising retraction ring is seen and felt as an oblique groove across the abdomen
- Fetal parts cannot be felt easily
- Fetal heart rate (FHR) is absent or shows fetal distress due to interference with the uteroplacental blood flow.

Per Vaginal Examination

- *Vaginal findings*: Offensive vaginal discharge, edema of the lower vagina, and vulva. In case of rupture uterus, patient presents with vaginal bleeding.
- *Cervical finding*: Cervix is fully or partially dilated, edematous loose hanging cervix in shoulder or malpresentation.
- Membranes are ruptured.
- The caput succedaneum makes identification of the presentation and position very difficult. More importance should be given to the abdominal findings when deciding the level or station of the head, a large caput on the apex of a severely-molded head may reach the outlet when the greatest diameter is still above the brim.

PREVENTION

General

- Assessing the high-risk patients
- Good nutrition during the childhood, adolescence, and pregnancy.[11] Antenatal period supplementation of macro and micronutrient to the mother can influence childhood and adolescent growth, hence it takes few generations to eliminate obstructed labor.
- Delaying early marriage
- Training of primary healthcare workers and traditional birth attendant.

Intrapartum

- Use of partograph is the best diagnostic tool to early detect prolonged labor—early referral to health center if cervical dilatation is approaching the action line
- Skilled birth attendance
- Efficient referral system in case of emergency
- Identify causes of obstructed labor and preventing it
- Diagnosing obstructed labor and appropriate management.

COMPLICATIONS

Maternal Complications

- Increase in operative delivery—(cesarean section, forceps, and vacuum deliveries)
- Postpartum hemorrhage (PPH)—atonic/traumatic
- Annular detachment of cervix
- *Rupture uterus*: Worldwide obstructed labor is the leading cause of uterine rupture. It is very commonly seen in multipara and very rarely in primigravida. There are several impending/early signs and symptoms of rupture uterus, which help in prevention of rupture uterus:
    - Persistent lower uterine segment pain and tenderness between contractions
    - Vaginal bleeding
    - Swelling and crepitus of lower uterine segment
    - Tachycardia and hypotension
    - Hematuria
    - *Fetal heart rate abnormalities*: Tachycardia, variable, and late deceleration.
    - Late signs:
        - Sudden onset of tearing abdominal pain
        - Cessation of uterine contractions
        - Recession of the presenting part
        - Absent fetal heart
        - Signs of intra-abdominal hemorrhage with hypovolemic shock are the signs of complete rupture uterine.
        - Avascular rupture of previous lower uterine segment scar site is presented with minimal bleeding and labor continued uneventfully is diagnosed in the postpartum period.
- *Infection*:
    - Sepsis, peritonitis, and wound infection
    - Puerperal sepsis—due to:
        - Prolonged rupture of membranes
        - Repeated vaginal examinations
        - Instrumental delivery.
- *Injury to genital treat*: It occurred during destructive surgeries
- *Fistula*: Most common complication, accounts for 20% of all cases of fistula formation. In developing regions, the incidence of rectovaginal and vesicovaginal fistula is 0.01–0.08% of births,[12] it is due to avascular pressure necrosis from part of soft tissues of the pelvic floor and bladder base and urethra between the presenting part and pelvic bone.
  The degree of cervical dilatation and effacement and level at which presenting part impacted are depended for fistula site. This results in an incidence rate of obstetric fistula of 2.15% of neglected obstructed labor cases.
  Broad area of injury during obstructed labor results in multiple injuries along with VVF and RVF, i.e. total urethral loss, stress incontinence, hydroureteronephrosis, renal failure, rectal atresia, anal sphincter incompetence, amenorrhea, cervical destruction, vaginal stenosis, osteitis pubis, and foot drop.[9]
- *Ketoacidosis*: Increased and prolonged myometrial contraction leads to accumulation of lactic acid resulting in metabolic acidosis. Inadequate caloric intake leads to breakdown of fat and endogenous tissue breakdown leads to production of ketones leading to acidosis. Oliguria due to dehydration increases acidemia
- *Stress incontinence*: It is due to multigravida, large baby and forceps delivery are responsible for a ten times increase of the risk of postpartum stress incontinence in a developed country
- Shock—Hypovolemic/septic
- *Paralytic ileus*: Bowel distension due to hypokalemia

- *Maternal morbidity and mortality*: Morbidity is due to secondary infertility, vaginal scarring and stenosis, severe anemia, musculoskeletal injury, urinary incontinence, obstetric fistula, and mortality is due to rupture uterus, PPH, and puerperal sepsis.[13]

Fetal Complications

- *Fetal asphyxia*: Prolonged uterine contraction may lead to reduced intervillous blood flow and reduce exchange of gases between mother and fetus.
- *Fetal death*: Early rupture of membranes and amniotic fluid, fetus is forced into lower uterine segment, excessive pressure on placenta and umbilical cord leads to fetal distress and death and cord prolapse in shoulder presentation
- Fetal trauma due to operative vaginal delivery
- Intracranial hemorrhage
- *Acidosis*: Due to fetal hypoxia and maternal acidosis
- Neonatal sepsis B
- Contusion
- Facial injury.

MANAGEMENT[14]

Investigations

- CBC, blood grouping, and Rh typing.
- Blood urea and serum creatinine
- Urine routine for protein, ketone, and sugar
- High vaginal swab for culture and sensitivity
- Serum electrolytes
- Obstetric scan.

Treatment

Preliminary treatment:
- Correction of dehydration and acidosis with 1–3 liter of normal saline (NS) or Ringer's lactate (RL) solution.
- *Arrange blood*: In case of suspected or diagnosed rupture uterus, atonic or traumatic PPH or septic shock.
- Broad spectrum antibiotic to combat sepsis.
- Abdominal examination to rule out rupture uterus and FHR monitoring.

Intact Uterus

- Fetus is alive:
    - *Unengaged head*
        - Seen in severe cephalopelvic disproportion (CPD) and malpresentations. Pelvic tumor, vesical calculus emergency lower segment cesarean-section (LSCS) is done.
    - *Engaged head*:
        - Vacuum extraction with fully dilated cervix—mild CPD
        - Forceps delivery—midcavity forceps by trained personnel
        - Symphysiotomy—borderline CPD where very long duration of transport or facilities of LSCS is not available.
- *Dead fetus*: Destructive procedures are considered when the maternal condition is morbid. Resuscitation of the mother is a prerequisite to destructive surgeries, i.e. antibiotic to combat infection, measures for prevention and treatment of PPH.
    - Cervix fully dilated with unengaged head—craniotomy using axis traction forceps to steady the head and craniotomy with Oldham's or Simpson's perforator
    - Contracted pelvis—LSCS if fetus is dead
        - *Neglected shoulder presentation*: Internal podalic version is contraindicated. Decapitation procedure is done, applying traction on the prolapsed hand using the decapitating hook and embryotomy scissors, the neck of the fetus is

reached easily and severed, delivering the headless trunk by traction on the prolapsed hand and fetal head delivered by forceps or manually by suprapubis pressure.
- Lower segment cesarean section—midline vertical incision or inverted T-shaped incision is preferred compared to destructive procedures in modern obstetrics due to nonexpertise of destructive procedures
- Placenta removal by spontaneous or manually and uterus and cervix is explored to rule out rupture uterus and trauma to cervix.

Rupture Uterus
- Management of hypovolemia
- *Laparotomy*:
  – *To remove fetus and placenta*:
    - The surgical management of the rupture uterus depends on the various factors like condition of the patient, type of rupture, facilities available, and surgeon's experience.
    - Laceration repair and tubal ligation
    - Laceration repair alone
    - Total hysterectomy
    - Subtotal hysterectomy.

CONCLUSION

- In the 21st century obstructed labor is a life-threatening complication that increases maternal and perinatal mortality
- Identification of risk factors and early diagnosis helps in preventing sequelae of obstructed labor
- Continuous support during labor will lead to good maternal and fetal outcome with no harm[15]
- Most common complications of obstructed labor is PPH, puerperal sepsis, and uterine rupture
- Cesarean section (68%) is the most common surgery in obstructed labor, it may decrease the poor outcome followed by, destructive surgeries (7%), repair of rupture uterus with bilateral tubal ligation (5%), obstetric hysterectomy (20%).[16]

REFERENCES

1. EL-Hamamy E, Arulkumaran A. Poor progress of labour. Current Obstet Gynecol. 2005;15:1-8.
2. Hofmeyr GJ. Obstructed labor: using better technologies to reduce mortality. Int J Gynaecol Obstet.2004;85(Suppl 1):S62-72.
3. Cron J, Medscape General Medicine. (2003). Lessons from the developing world: obstructed labor and the vesico-vaginal fistula. [online] Available from: https://www.medscape.com/viewarticle/455965_4 [Last accessed September, 2019].
4. Melah GS, Massa AA, Yahaya UR, et al. Risk factors for obstetric fistulae in north-eastern Nigeria. J Obstet Gynaecol. 2007;27:819-23.
5. Ould El Joud D, Bouvier-Colle MH. Dystocia: frequency and risk factors in seven areas in West Africa. J Gynecol Obstet Biol Reprod. 2002;31:51-62.
6. Chabra S, Gandhi D, Jaiswal M. Obstructed labor-a preventable entity. J Obstet Gynaecol. 2000;20(2):151-3.
7. Adhikari SM, Dasgupta M. Management of obstructed labour: a retrospective study. J Obstet Gynaecol India. 2005;55(1):48-51.
8. Cruickshank EK, Lawson JB, Stewart D. Nutrition in pregnancy and lactation. Obstetrics and gynaecology in the tropics and developing countries. London: Edward Arnold Press; 1967. pp. 11-28.
9. Bhatt RV, Modi NS, Acharya PT. Height and reproductive performance. J Obstet Gynaecol India 1967;17:75-9.
10. Neilson JP, Lavender T, Quenby S. Obstructed labour: reducing maternal death and disability during pregnancy. Br Med Bull. 2003;67(1):191-204.
11. Justin CK, Oladapo AL. Nutrition and obstructed labor. Am J Clin Nutri. 2000;72(1):291-7.
12. Dolea C, Zahr CA. Global burden of obstructed labour in the year 2000. Evidence and Information for Policy (EIP). Geneva: World Health Organization; 2003. pp. 1-17.

13. Wall LL, Arrowsmith SD, Briggs ND, et al. The obstetric vesicovaginal fistula in the developing world. Obstet Gynecol Surv. 2005;60(7):3-51.
14. Fourth Edition of the ALARM International Program. Chapter 4: Management of labour and obstructed labour. [online] Available form: https://www.glowm.com/pdf/AIP%20Chap4%20Management%20of%20Labour.pdf [Last accessed September, 2019].
15. Hodnett ED, Gates S, Hofmeyr GJ, et al. Continuous support for women during childbirth. Cochrane Database Syst Rev. 2011(2):CD003766.
16. Sabyasachi M, Arunima C, Gourisankar K, et al. Fetomaternal outcome in obstructed labor in a peripheral tertiary care hospital. Medical Journal of Dr. D.Y. Patil University. 2013;6(2):146-50.

42
Retained Mop in Abdomen/ Gossypiboma in Abdomen

Shashikala KT

DEFINITION

Retained foreign object (RFO) is a generic term usually denoting any object retained unintentionally following a surgical or other intervention, inside the patient's body.[1] "Gossypiboma" is in particular used to describe a mass of cotton material, ranging from gauze, sponges, and towels, accidentally retained in any body cavity following a surgical procedure. The word, gossypiboma, originated from the Latin word "gossypium", which means textile or cotton, combined with a Swahili word "boma" which means place of concealment. Wilson in 1884[2] had used the word gossypiboma, which is also referred to as textiloma and gauzoma in literature.

BURDEN OF GOSSYPIBOMA

This is more common especially following surgeries involving body cavities such as the abdomen, pelvis, and retroperitoneal space. The incidence of RFO is between 0.3 and 1.0 per 1,000 abdominal operations.[3] Any material used during a surgical procedure, ranging from artery forceps, small pieces of broken instruments or irrigation sets, scissors, needles and rubber material, etc. can be retained accidentally after a surgery.[4] But sponges are reported to be the most common foreign bodies retained in the human body after surgery accounting for as high as 68% of RFO.[1]

MEDICAL AND LEGAL IMPLICATIONS

Medical Implications

Gossypiboma may lead serious negative consequences, not only to the patient, but also to the involved surgeon and the healthcare institution. For patient, it can cause serious morbidity, often may lead to mortality. Affected patients may incur heavy expenditure on evaluation and management. For a healthcare provider, it poses a major diagnostic challenge. Delayed presentation often months or even years after the surgical intervention responsible for, often leads to low levels of suspicion. Since gossypiboma mimics wide variety of clinical conditions depending on its size, location, and the host response to it, it is often misdiagnosed. Performance of unnecessary radical surgical procedures due to misdiagnosis of gossypiboma is also reported frequently in literature.

Legal Implications

Gossypiboma or any other RFO is considered as medical negligence, according to doctrine of *res ipsa loquitur*. It may lead to serious medicolegal consequences including mental agony, humiliation, huge monetary compensation, and imprisonment on the part of the surgeon.

Hence, it is important for surgical practitioner to have a high index of suspicion, and to have a thorough understanding of the common clinical and radiological features, to be able to diagnose and treat it effectively.

RISK FACTORS FOR GOSSYPIBOMA

Landmark work by Gawande et al.[5] had reported high body mass index (BMI), unplanned changes in operation and emergency nature of surgery as the independent risk factors for gossypiboma.

CLINICAL PRESENTATION

The consequence of foreign bodies after surgery may manifest in different forms immediately after the operation, months or even years after the surgical procedure. It should be considered in the differential diagnosis of any postoperative case with unresolved or unusual problems.[6] Hence, it poses a serious diagnostic dilemma to the clinician.[7]

The immediate consequences are usually caused by foreign body or inflammatory reaction generated by the gauze or due to infection. Patients develop symptoms of abdominal pain, nausea, vomiting, anorexia, and weight loss, resulting from obstruction or a malabsorption-type syndrome caused by multiple intestinal fistulas or intraluminal bacterial overgrowth. The timing of presentation may rage from immediate postoperative period to few days and weeks following surgery. There are few cases reported where there was transmural migration of the gauze, presenting as acute intestinal obstruction or hollow viscus perforation.[8,9]

Choric presentation may include nonspecific findings like, vague abdominal discomfort, unexplained weight loss,[10] malabsorption syndrome, etc.[11] Most common presentation is mass per abdomen in different segments of the abdomen, mimicking wide range of intra-abdominal and pelvic tumors. Most often the diagnosis of gossypiboma is made after extensive investigation of the patient and in majority of the cases only after laparotomy.[12] There are various case studies reporting gossypiboma mimicking ovarian teratoma[13] mesenchymal tumor,[14] dermoid cyst of ovary,[15] ovarian maliganancy,[16] and wide range of other tumors. There were also reports of uterine wound dehiscence caused by retained gauze following myomectomy[17] and urinary retention.[18] Some studies have reported actual development of malignant conditions like malignant fibrous histiocytoma, induce by retained gauze.[19]

Transmural migration of the foreign body into the lumen of hollow viscera and presentation as various intraluminal conditions has also been widely reported. The presentation may range from intractable duodenal ulcer,[20] chronic intestinal obstruction,[21] colonic mass,[22] etc. Migration of the gossypiboma can occur across different segments of the body, i.e. from abdomen to thorax or vice versa.

A recent systematic review[23] conducted on gossypibomas in India has reported average time to discovery was 1225.62 days and only 49% of cases were diagnosed within 1 year of primary surgery. The most common reported symptom was pain in 73.8% of cases, followed by palpable mass in 47.6% and vomiting 35% of cases. The other common symptoms were abdominal distention and fever. Spontaneous expulsion of the gossypiboma was also noted in minor proportion of patients. Transmural migration was observed in about 30% of cases.

Considering the wide variation in clinical presentation, often mimicking of various other pathological conditions and due to the delayed presentation, it is often least anticipated by the clinicians. The probability of missed diagnosis, delayed diagnosis inadvertent, and often invasive workup is high and inappropriate management is very high. High index of suspicion and knowledge regarding common imaging features of gossypiboma may minimize this.

IMAGING FEATURES OF GOSSYPIBOMA

Even though they are nonspecific and considerable overlap with other pathological conditions, few radiological features are consistent with gossypibomas.

Conventional Radiology

In the postoperative period, it usual practice to use conventional radiology to screen for presence of retained sponges or swabs (gossypiboma). Usually, the diagnosis is made appearance of radiopaque markers incorporated in their composition. The reported sensitivity of conventional radiographs by some studies exceeds 90%. But there are many limitation also reported regarding the conventional radiography. The key issues to address are the poor quality of the radiographs obtained in the surgery room, by means of bedside apparatuses due to various technical restrictions. Appropriate manipulation and postprocessing of the images may be able to address this problem to some extent.

Clinicians evaluating the postoperative radiographs must give due consideration to the appropriateness of the field of view and also careful evaluation of the periphery of the obtained image, may significantly enhance the chances of detecting gossypiboma in doubtful cases.

The most common presentation reported in plain radiography includes radio dense irregular linear images, some of them serpiginous, sometimes with increased volume, and density of adjoining soft tissues.

In few cases, amorphous radiolucent images may be noted, attributed to gas entrapment or secondary infection by gas-forming microbes. But there are multiple studies reporting a missed diagnosis, especially small fragments of surgical material by conventional X-ray. In such cases, advanced imaging modalities like ultrasonography (US) and magnetic resonance imaging (MRI) may play a vital role.[24]

Ultrasonography

The most common ultrasound finding is "well-delineated mass with whorl like, hyperreflective echo, with a hypoechoic rim and strong posterior acoustic shadowing".[25] Ultrasound characteristics can be classified into two types, (1) a cystic type and (2) a solid type. The cystic type usually presents as a cystic lesion with a wavy echogenic structure with in. The solid type may be visible as a complex mass containing hyper- and hypoechoic regions. The acoustic shadowing is usually caused by the retained material itself or sometimes can be caused by calcified are as inside the gossypiboma or sometimes due to pocket so fair inside it.[26]

Computed Tomography Scan

The computed tomography (CT) findings may be quite variable. It often shows shallow-density, heterogeneous mass surrounded by a thick peripheral rim. The presence of "mottled", bubbly gas shadows should prompt high index of suspicion. The spongiform pattern with gas bubbles "is often regarded as the most characteristic CT finding".[27] The mass usually may contain wavy, striped, and high-density zones. Some of the CT features may aid in suspecting the type of materials, albeit with low certainty. For instance, "linear densities with a peculiar infolding/whorled configuration may suggest a retained towel". Sponges and gel foam tablets may appear as low-attenuation masses with multiple gas bubbles. Dense peripheral ring on CT may indicate calcification of the wall.[28,29]

Magnetic Resonance Imaging

Magnetic resonance imaging is suggested to be used only in those cases, when more easily available imaging modalities could not identify direct or indirect signs suggestive of gossypibomas and inconclusive.[30] MRI appearance of gossypiboma may be quite varied. The most commonly reported MRI finding is a heterogeneous mass, with a mixed solid-cystic component, often having well-defined contours, with surrounding well-delimited capsule. Hyposignal and hypersignal predominate respectively on T1-weighted and T2-weighted images, with internal serpiginous and irregular images having intermediate signal on both T1- and T2-weighted imaging.[31]

PREVENTION OF GOSSYPIBOMA

Perceived by majority as essentially a medical negligence, meticulous analysis of possible causes of retained gauze shows that this notion is over simplification of a complex entity. It can occur in spite of the best possible efforts by the entire team involved in planning and execution of surgery to prevent it. But certain standard operating procedures can grossly minimize the chance of its occurrence. Despite best intentions and precaution like radiographic screening, there will still be some cases, where sponges would get retained and escape detection, till they cause diagnostic dilemma.[32]

Probably, standard drills need to be observed to minimize chances of retained foreign body (RFB), such as, exclusive use of sponges with radiopaque marker, avoiding use of small gauze pieces in large cavities, taking some dedicated time off at the end of surgery, and "play around in abdomen", i.e. thoroughly inspect and reinspect the abdomen for inadvertent mistakes, such as, overlooked sponge/foreign body, unclosed rents in mesentery, unevacuated blood clots, needles, loose strips of suture, internal hernia, etc. despite a correct count call by scrub nurse. Newer modalities such as tagging with electronic surveillance, bar coding of sponges with sponge counting using bar code scanner and radiofrequency identification have been proposed to prevent and detect RFB. However, they do not seem to have been widely adopted. Systematic methodical sponge and instrument count is the cornerstone of prevention of gossypiboma. Introducing surgical safety protocols, such as the World Health Organization (WHO) recommended "safe surgery saves lives" checklist, can be effective in preventing its occurrence. Safety-focused institutional policies, including never event reporting system, elaboration of prevention strategies and their regular monitoring and evaluation, are highly essential for any healthcare setting.[33]

MANAGEMENT AND OUTCOMES

Successful treatment of gossypiboma through laparotomy, laparoscopy,[34] endoscopic removal[35] of intraluminal gossypiboma, etc. have been described methods in the literature. Many studies have reported performing diagnostic laparotomy with uncertain diagnosis, turning out to be gossypiboma and treated successfully (Figs. 1A to D) Few other studies have reported performing excision of gossypiboma assuming some other diagnosis, alter confirmed as gossypiboma

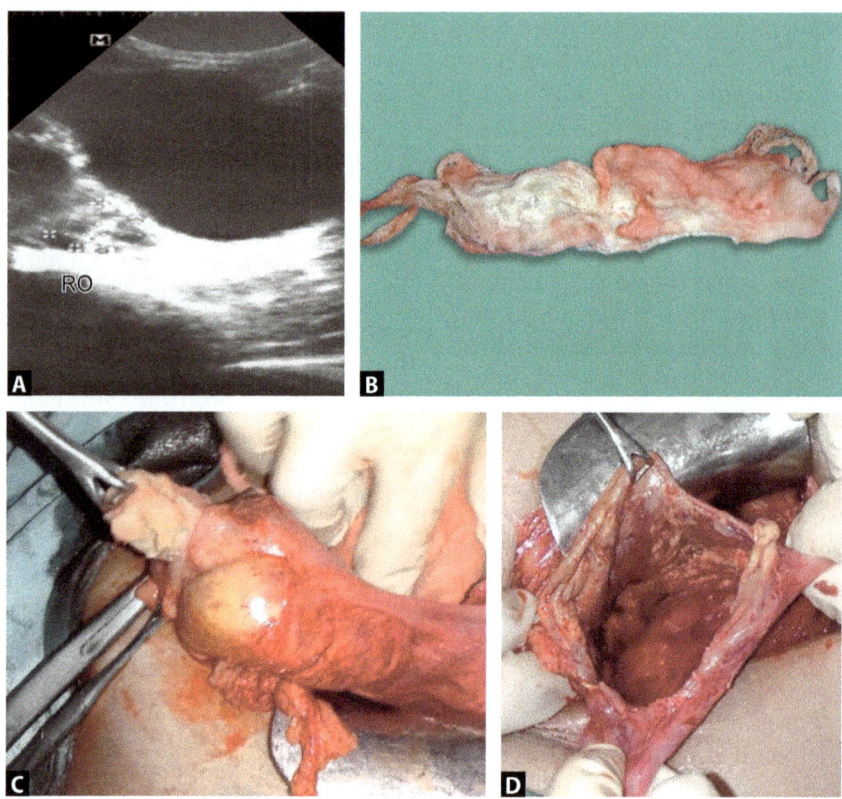

Figs. 1A to D: (A) Sonographic appearance of retained gauze mimicking dermoid cyst of ovary; (B) Intraoperative appearance of gossypiboma; (C) Retained surgical gauze 6 × 3 cm in size; (D) Thick-walled cavity after removal of gauze.

by histopathological examination. Hence there cannot be any generalization about the most appropriate way of management of gossypiboma of abdomen. The treatment may depend on factors the location, size, and associated clinical features. Patient-related parameters like, age, comorbidities, etc. may also play a vital role in deciding the most appropriate management. But in majority of the reported case studies, the treatment was successful, without any major untoward complications and mortality. But few authors have also highlighted the possibility of gross under reporting of gossypiboma, especially where the treatment outcomes are poor, considering the medicolegal implications of the same.

CONCLUSION

It is essential for surgeons and gynecologists to have a good understanding of varied clinical presentation and common imaging findings of retained mop in the abdomen. The most essential aspect is always to keep it as one of the differential diagnosis, eliciting meticulous history regarding previous surgeries, mode of delivery, etc. This may help in avoiding inadvertent and often invasive evaluation of the patients and effective management. Even most important is to make all possible efforts to prevent the occurrence of retained mop abdomen, by means of establishing and meticulously following standard operating protocols in all surgical procedures.

REFERENCES

1. Cima RR, Kollengode A, Garnatz J, et al. Incidence and characteristics of potential and actual retained foreign object events in surgical patients. J Am Coll Surg. 2008;207(1):80-7.
2. Wilson CP. Foreign bodies left in the abdomen after laparotomy. Gynecol Tr. 1884;9:109-12.
3. Zejnullahu VA, Bicaj BX, Zejnullahu VA, et al. Retained Surgical Foreign Bodies after Surgery. Open Access Maced J Med Sci. 2017;5(1):97-100.
4. Gibbs VC, Coakley FD, Reines HD. Preventable errors in the operating room: retained foreign bodies after surgery—Part I. Curr Probl Surg. 2007;44(5):281-337.
5. Gawande AA, Studdert DM, Orav EJ, et al. Risk factors for retained instruments and sponges after surgery. N Engl J Med. 2003;348(3):229-35.
6. Chopra S, Suri V, Sikka P, et al. A case series on gossypiboma-varied clinical presentations and their management. J Clin Diagn Res. 2015;9(12):Qr01-3.
7. Srivastava KN, Agarwal A. Gossypiboma posing as a diagnostic dilemma: a case report and review of the literature. Case Rep Surg. 2014;2014:713428.
8. Agrawal H, Gupta N, Krishengowda U, et al. Transmural migration of gossypiboma: a rare cause of acute abdomen. Indian J Surg. 2018;80(1):84-6.
9. Colak T, Olmez T, Turkmenoglu O, et al. Small bowel perforation due to gossypiboma caused acute abdomen. Case Rep Surg. 2013;2013:219354.
10. Tanrikulu Y, Tanrikulu CS, Yilmaz G, et al. Idiopathic weight loss due to an entero-enteric fistula from a gossypiboma retained for 27 years. Turk J Surg. 2018;34(1):65-7.
11. Rehman A, Baloch NU, Awais M. Gossypiboma diagnosed fifteen years after a cesarean section: A case report. Qatar Med J. 2014;2014(2):65-9.
12. Oran E, Yetkin G, Aygun N, et al. Intra-abdominal gossypiboma: report of two cases. Turk J Surg. 2018;34(1):77-9.
13. Zhang H, Jiang Y, Wang Q, et al. Lower abdominal gossypiboma mimics ovarian teratoma: a case report and review of the literature. World J Surg Oncol. 2017;15(1):6.
14. Eken H, Soyturk M, Balci G, et al. Gossypiboma mimicking a mesenchymal tumor: a report of a rare case. Am J Case Rep. 2016;17:27-30.
15. Rafat D, Hakim S, Sabzposh NA, et al. Gossypiboma mimicking as dermoid cyst of ovary: a case report. J Clin Diagn Res. 2015;9(3): Qd01-2.
16. Cengiz H, Kaya C, Deniztas C, et al. Gossypiboma: after 13 years of a gynecologic procedure-masquerading as an ovarian tumor. J Obstet Gynaecol India. 2014;64(Suppl 1):81-2.
17. Usta TA, Yildirim D, Ozyurek SE, et al. Conservative treatment of a gossypiboma causing uterine wound dehiscence. Case Rep Obstet Gynecol. 2013;2013:578027.
18. Konstantinidis C, Vlachos S. Urinary Retention as the Only Symptom of Retained Surgical Sponge (Gossypiboma), 29 Years After Cesarean Procedure. Urol Case Rep. 2017;11:9-10.
19. Kaplan M, Iyikosker HI. A new complication of retained surgical gauze: development of malignant fibrous histiocytoma—report of a case with a literature review. World J Surg Oncol. 2012;10:139.
20. Lv YX, Yu CC, Tung CF, et al. Intractable duodenal ulcer caused by transmural migration of gossypiboma into the duodenum--a case report and literature review. BMC Surg. 2014;14: 36.
21. Khan HS, Malik AA, Ali S, et al. Gossypiboma as a cause of intestinal obstruction. J Coll Physicians Surg Pak. 2014;24(Suppl 3):S188-9.
22. Tchangai B, Alassani F, Tchaou M. Unusual complication following a myomectomy: colic migration of a forgotten abdominal swab. Case Rep Surg. 2017;2017:3962506.
23. Patial T, Thakur V, Vijhay Ganesun N, et al. Gossypibomas in India—a systematic literature review. J Postgrad Med. 2017;63(1):36-41.
24. O'Connor AR, Coakley FV, Meng MV, et al. Imaging of retained surgical sponges in the abdomen and pelvis. Am J Roentgenol. 2003;180(2):481-9.
25. Barriga P, Garcia C. Ultrasonography in the detection of intra-abdominal retained surgical sponges. J Ultrasound Med. 1984;3(4):173-6.
26. Pole G, Thomas B. A Pictorial review of the many faces of gossypiboma—observations in 6 Cases. Pol J Radiol. 2017;82:418-21.
27. Rabie ME, Hosni MH, Al Safty A, et al. Gossypiboma revisited: a never ending issue. Int J Surg Case Rep. 2016;19:87-91.

28. Sheward SE, Williams JA, Mettler JF, et al. CT appearance of a surgically retained towel (gossypiboma). J Comput Assist Tomogr. 1986;10(2):343-5.
29. Parienty R, Pradel J, Lepreux J, et al. Computed tomography of sponges retained after laparotomy. J Comput Assist Tomogr. 1981;5(2):187-9.
30. Silva C, Caetano M, Silva E, et al. Complete migration of retained surgical sponge into ileum without sign of open intestinal wall. Arch Gynecol Obstet. 2001;265(2):103-4.
31. Bani-Hani KE, Gharaibeh KA, Yagha RJ. Retained surgical sponges (gossypiboma). Asian J Surg. 2005;28(2):109-15.
32. McIntyre LK, Jurkovich GJ, Gunn ML, et al. Gossypiboma: tales of lost sponges and lessons learned. Arch Surg. 2010;145(8):770-5.
33. Tchangai B, Tchaou M, Kassegne I, et al. Incidence, root cause, and outcomes of unintentionally retained intraabdominal surgical sponges: a retrospective case series from two hospitals in Togo. Patient Saf Surg. 2017;11:25.
34. Ozsoy Z, Okan I, Daldal E, et al. Laparoscopic removal of gossypiboma. Case Rep Surg. 2015;2015:317240.
35. Karasaki T, Nomura Y, Nakagawa T, et al. Beware of gossypibomas. BMJ Case Rep. 2013; 2013:bcr2013010059.

CHAPTER 43

Malpresentations

Sneha

■ DEFINITION OF MALPRESENTATION

When the presenting part of the fetus over the internal os is anything other than vertex of the fetal head, it is labeled as *malpresentation*.[1]

The various malpresentations encountered in clinical practice are:
- *Occiput posterior*: 1/19 deliveries
- *Breech*: 1/33 deliveries
- *Face*: 1/600–1/800 deliveries
- *Brow*: 1/1,000–1/2,000 deliveries
- *Transverse lie*: 1/500 deliveries
- *Compound*: 1/1,500 deliveries.

The comparison of the characteristics of face and brow presentation has been shown in Table 1.

The diameters of fetal skull have been shown in Figure 1.

■ DIAGNOSIS OF FACE PRESENTATION

Diagnosis is usually made in the intrapartum period during the first or second stage of labor by per vaginal examination. The orbits and orbital ridge, saddle of the nose, mouth, and chin are palpated on per vaginam examination.

The various positions of face presentation are:
- Mentoanterior (60%)—left or right
- Mentoposterior (25%)—left or right
- Mentotransverse (15%)—left or right.

Diagnosis of face presentation before the onset of labor is rare. It may be suspected if, on abdominal palpation, there is a marked depression between the back and occiput due to the hyperextended neck.

TABLE 1: Comparison of the characteristics of face and brow presentation.

Characteristics	Face presentation	Brow presentation
Presenting part	Fetal face from forehead to chin	Anterior fontanelle to the brow (orbital ridge), but does not include the mouth and chin
Degree of flexion of fetal neck	Sharply deflexed and the occiput may touch the back	Partially deflexed, not to the degree of a face presentation
Causes	<ul><li>*Fetal malformations*: 15% of face presentations (anencephaly, severe hydrocephalus with cephalomegaly, anterior neck mass, multiple nuchal cords)</li><li>Cephalopelvic disproportion (most common cause in brow presentation)</li><li>Prematurity/low birth weight</li><li>Multiparity</li><li>Polyhydramnios</li></ul>	
Denominator	Chin	Brow
Presenting diameter	Submentobregmatic—9.5 cm	Mentovertical—13.5 cm

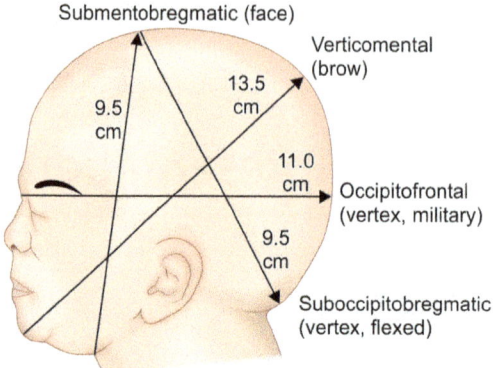

Fig. 1: Diameters of fetal skull.

Hyperextended fetal neck will be visible on sonography. However, sonography is neither diagnostic nor predictive of the course of labor in face presentation.

Occasionally, it may be confused with a frank breech presentation due to palpable soft parts. The mouth and anus can be distinguished by inserting the fingers into the orifice and feeling for the hard bony gum ridges in face presentation.

Course of Labor

Mentoanterior Face Presentation

There is increasing extension of the fetal neck as it descends in the pelvis, making chin as the presenting part. Internal rotation occurs at a level of ischial spine. Further descent presents the chin below the pubic symphysis. Head is delivered by flexion with maternal expulsive forces. It is estimated that about 75% of face presentation is delivered vaginally.[2]

Mentoposterior Face Presentation

Fetal face, neck and shoulder have to pass through the pelvis simultaneously in this presentation. The pelvis is not roomy enough to accommodate this in an average sized baby. The face can reach the perineum only if the fetal neck extends the whole length of the sacrum, i.e. 12 cm. Descent of the face is hindered by the fetal mouth which acts as a fulcrum against the sacrum. Hence, delivery is not possible if spontaneous rotation to mentoanterior does not occur.

Management

If the diagnosis of face presentation is confirmed in antepartum period and all fetal anomalies have been ruled out, elective cesarean must be planned.

Mentoanterior

If diagnosis is done intrapartum, continuous external fetal heart monitoring is advisable due to the increased risk of variable decelerations (29%) and late decelerations (24%).

Fetal anomalies must be ruled out, size of the fetus assessed and clinical pelvimetry done to assess the feasibility of vaginal delivery.

Partogram must be used. The parturient must be monitored for signs of obstructed labor. Oxytocin must be used for augmentation of labor in case of abnormal labor progression. Cesarean is reserved for obstetric indications. Outlet forceps should be applied by an experienced clinician. Descent of the face is delayed in this presentation and forceps must be applied only when the face distends the perineum (+2 station).

Midforceps delivery, version and extraction should not be attempted as they are associated with increased risk of maternal injury, neonatal mortality and morbidity.[3]

An increased risk of facial ecchymosis, bruising, edema and skull molding is noted in these neonates. There will be problems in ventilation during resuscitation, if required, due to the associated laryngeal and tracheal edema.

Mentoposterior

If spontaneous rotation to mentoanterior does not occur, cesarean delivery must be planned.

In the past, forceps was used to rotate to mentoanterior and allow for vaginal delivery. However, due to the increased risk of uterine rupture, fetal asphyxia due to cord prolapse and spinal cord injury, this is no longer advocated.

DIAGNOSIS OF BROW PRESENTATION

It is generally diagnosed intrapartum by vaginal examination. Palpation of the following parts confirms brow presentation: anterior fontanelle, supraorbital ridges and root of nose. If this is missed initially, it is difficult to identify the landmarks in late labor due to considerable molding and caput formation. However, the bony supraorbital ridge and root of the nose may still be identified.

Course of Labor

During the descent of the fetus in brow presentation in the pelvis, due to the combined effects of uterine contractions and maternal pushing efforts, it gets converted into face-mentoanterior in 30% of cases. In 20% of cases, neck gets flexed and gets converted into occipitoposterior. However, flexion of the neck to become occipitoanterior is rare.

If brow presentation persists, the largest presenting diameter being mentovertical (13.5 cm) cannot pass through the pelvis and vaginal delivery is not possible.[1]

Management

If diagnosed early in labor and clinical pelvimetry confirms adequate pelvis, trial of vaginal delivery can be given with the observation for spontaneous conversion to face or vertex presentation. Partogram must be used. Continuous external fetal heart monitoring is recommended. The diagnosis of persistent brow presentation and abnormal progression of labor warrants cesarean delivery.

If maternal pelvis is not adequate, spontaneous conversion is unlikely. In such cases, cesarean delivery in early labor is recommended.

TRANSVERSE LIE

It is a malpresentation in which the longitudinal axis of the fetus is at right angles to the longitudinal axis of the uterus (Fig. 2). It is the most unfavorable lie. It may be:
- *Dorsoanterior*: When the curvature of the fetal spine is oriented upward.
- *Dorsoposterior*: When the curvature of the fetal spine is oriented downward.

Commonly oblique lie may be encountered when the head or breech occupies one of the iliac fossa.

Presenting part is the shoulder. Arm may prolapse through the cervix in this presentation.

Causes

- Placenta previa—must be considered when transverse lie is diagnosed
- Prematurity
- Multiparity—due to the poor tone of uterine and abdominal muscles
- Uterine anomaly—septate uterus (version not possible)

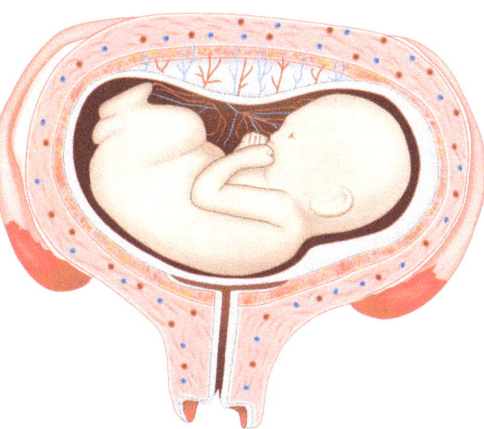

Fig. 2: Transverse lie.

- Fetal anomaly
- Large pelvic mass—fibroid in lower segment of uterus, ovarian tumor
- Multiple pregnancy.

Diagnosis

Transverse lie is suspected on inspection of the abdomen when the uterus is enlarged transversely and shorter vertically. In 70% of cases, it is diagnosed by abdominal palpation using Leopold's maneuver. The lower pole above the symphysis pubis is empty. The fetal head and breech can be felt in the flanks on each side connected by the fetal back.

Role of Ultrasonography

- To diagnose transverse lie and position of the fetal back in obese patients
- To rule out placenta previa
- To diagnose structural fetal anomaly.

If placental localization is not previously done on scan, vaginal examination must be avoided.

Diagnosis during labor is by palpation of the presenting part—shoulder, which is felt as a small rounded body with clavicle and ribs on one side. In neglected cases of shoulder presentation, the arm, foot or cord prolapse into the cervix.

Management

A fetus in transverse lie is usually delivered by a cesarean section.

Factors which determine the mode of delivery include:
- Position of placenta and umbilical cord
- Fetal viability and period of gestation
- Whether patient is in labor
- Whether membranes have ruptured
- Transverse lie in second twin.

Transverse Lie, Viable Fetus with Intact Membranes (Flowchart 1)

To reduce the risk of cord prolapse with rupture of membranes, a 20 gauge needle (spinal needle) is used. This avoids the sudden gush of fluid and cord prolapse which occurs when membranes are ruptured with an amniohook.

In early labor:
- Tocolysis followed by external cephalic version and membrane rupture is preferred.
- In a study by Phelan JP et al.,[4] 83% had a successful version and 50% delivered vaginally when external cephalic version (ECV) was done in early labor.
- If ECV is unsuccessful, cesarean delivery should be performed.

In active labor:
Emergency cesarean is performed.

Transverse Lie with Ruptured Membranes

Management depends on the period of gestation. If >34 weeks, emergency lower segment cesarean section (LSCS) is performed. If between 28 weeks and 34 weeks, a course of antenatal corticosteroids with continuous monitoring of fetus and mother for 48 hours is preferred. Intervention is indicated if:
- Cervix dilated
- Cord presentation
- Facility for emergency LSCS is not available.

Version must be avoided in these patients as it is more likely to fail and is associated with multiple maternal and fetal complications.[5]

Transverse Lie of Second Twin after Delivery of the First Twin

After the first twin is delivered, the second twin occasionally assumes a transverse lie regardless of the initial position. Internal podalic version (Fig. 3) with breech extraction must be done in the following circumstances:
- Cervix fully dilated
- Under general anesthesia
- By an obstetrician with adequate experience in this maneuver.

The other option is cesarean delivery if the operator is not adequately trained, due to the increased risk of fetal trauma.

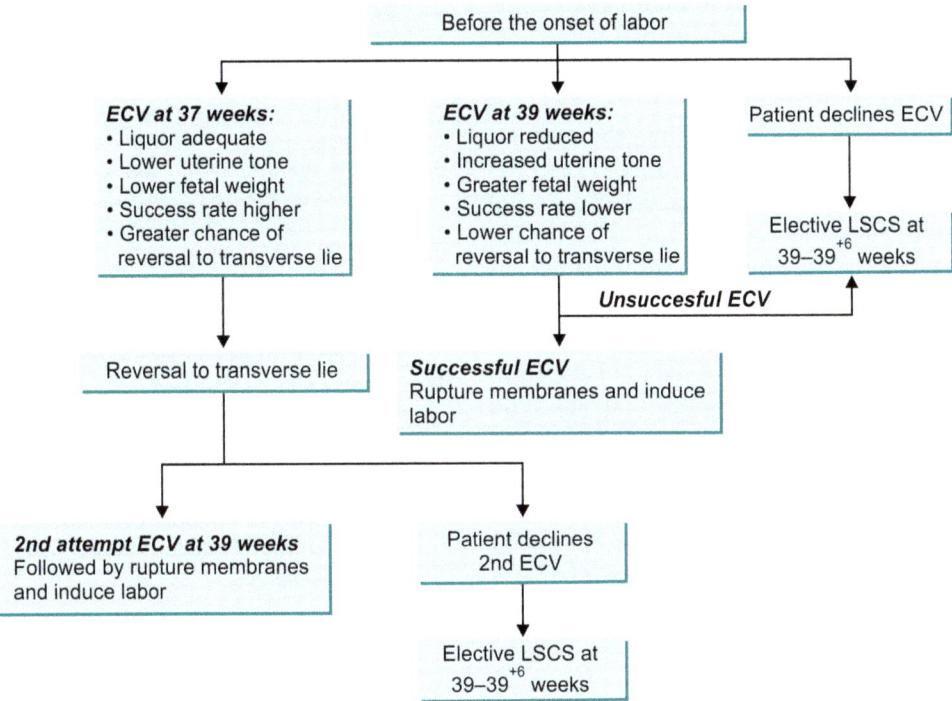

Flowchart 1: Transverse lie, viable fetus with intact membranes.

(ECV: external cephalic version; LSCS: lower segment cesarean section)

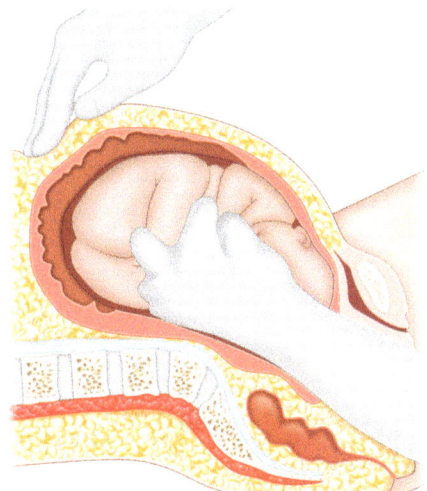

Fig. 3: Internal podalic version.

Transverse Lie with Fetal Demise or Nonviable Fetus

External version into cephalic or breech presentation can be done in early labor or before labor. This is followed by augmentation or induction of labor. If it is not feasible for external version or dystocia is present, cesarean delivery must be carried out.

If the fetus is too small or macerated, it will double upon itself and be delivered vaginally. In such cases, the head and thorax will simultaneously be delivered.[6]

CONCLUSION

- *Malpresentation*: When the presenting part of the fetus over the internal os is anything other than vertex of the fetal head.

- Face presentation is when the fetal face from forehead to chin lies over the internal os. Vaginal delivery is possible in mentoanterior but not in mentoposterior position.
- Brow presentation is when the anterior fontanelle to the brow (orbital ridge) lies over the internal os. Vaginal delivery is not possible.
- When the longitudinal axis of the fetus is perpendicular to long axis of uterus, it is labeled as transverse lie.
- The complications associated with transverse lie are cord prolapsed, fetal trauma, prematurity, obstructed labor and fetal demise in neglected cases.
- External cephalic version or cesarean delivery must be performed in transverse lie depending on the circumstances.

REFERENCES

1. Gardberg M, Leonova Y, Laakkonen E. Malpresentations—impact on mode of delivery. Acta Obstet Gynecol Scand. 2011;90:540-2.
2. Ducarme G, Ceccaldi PF, Chesnoy V, et al. Face presentation: retrospective study of 32 cases at term. Gynecol Obstet Fertil. 2006;34:393-6.
3. Vialle R, Piétin-Vialle C, Ilharreborde B, et al. Spinal cord injuries at birth: a multicenter review of nine cases. J Matern Fetal Neonatal Med. 2007;20:435-40.
4. Phelan JP, Stine LE, Edwards NB, et al. The role of external version in the intrapartum management of the transverse lie presentation. Am J Obstet Gynecol. 1985;151:724-6.
5. Quist-Nelson J, Landers K, McCurdy R, et al. External cephalic version in premature rupture of membranes: a systematic review. J Matern Fetal Neonatal Med. 2017;30:2257-61.
6. Digonnet L, Le Goff J. Observation of spontaneous delivery in conduplicato corpore with living infant. Bull Fed Soc Gynecol Obstet Lang Fr. 1950;2:563-4.

44

Acute Asthma in Pregnancy

A Shilpa Reddy

INTRODUCTION

Asthma is a common condition that affects around 10% of pregnant women, making it the most common chronic condition in pregnancy. The severity of asthma during pregnancy remains unchanged, worsens or improves in equal proportions. Asthma exacerbations are a significant clinical problem during pregnancy. Up to 45% of pregnant women with asthma have moderate to severe exacerbations requiring medical intervention during pregnancy.[1] For women with severe asthma, control is more likely to deteriorate (around 60% of cases), compared to women with mild asthma (around 10% of cases). However, all pregnant women with asthma need to be closely reviewed throughout pregnancy, irrespective of severity. Exacerbations during pregnancy occur primarily in the late second trimester.[2] Management and treatment of asthma in pregnant women should be generally the same as for nonpregnant women and men, with the intensity of antenatal maternal and fetal surveillance to be based on the severity of their condition.

DEFINITION: ASTHMA FLARE-UPS (EXACERBATION)

A flare-up or exacerbation is an acute or subacute worsening in symptoms and lung function from the patient's usual status, occasionally it may be the initial presentation of asthma.

ETIOLOGY AND TRIGGERING FACTORS

The major triggers are viral infection[2] and the nonadherence to inhaled corticosteroid medication.[3] Pregnant women may be more susceptible to viral infection because of changes in cell-mediated exacerbations[4] of asthma. Severe asthma appears to be the biggest risk factor for exacerbations during pregnancy. Atopy does not appear to be a risk factor for exacerbations during pregnancy. It has been shown that exacerbation rate increases with increasing asthma severity.[5]

ADVERSE EFFECTS ON ASTHMA EXACERBATIONS IN PREGNANCY

In addition to the adverse effects on maternal health, exacerbations are a key contributor to adverse perinatal outcomes in asthma. No significant association was found between asthma exacerbations during pregnancy and pre-eclampsia. Women with exacerbations of asthma are three times more likely to have a low birth weight baby compared to asthmatic women without exacerbations, suggesting that prevention of exacerbations during pregnancy may also lead to improvements in perinatal outcome.[6]

SYMPTOMS

Breathlessness, cough, wheezy breathing and chest tightness.

SIGNS

Increased respiratory rate, wheeze, use of accessory muscles and tachycardia.

DIFFERENTIAL DIAGNOSIS

Differential diagnosis of acute asthma during pregnancy should include other conditions that may complicate pregnancy, such as pulmonary edema, cardiomyopathy, pulmonary embolism, and amniotic fluid embolism.

Home Management

Home management of asthma exacerbations during pregnancy and lactation has been shown in Flowchart 1.

Patient should be referred to a consultant immediately worsening of day time symptoms i.e. asthma is uncontrolled.

Flowchart 1: Home management of asthma exacerbations.

Assess Severity
Measure PEF: Value <50% personal best or predicted suggests severe exacerbation, suggest referral
Note signs and symptoms: Degrees of cough, breathlessness, wheeze, and chest tightness correlate imperfectly with severity of exacerbation
Note presence of fetal activity*

↓

Initial Treatment
Short-acting inhaled beta2-agonist: Up to 3 treatments of 2–4 puffs by MDI at 20 minutes intervals or single nebulizer treatment

↓

Good response
Mild Exacerbation
PEF >80% predicted or personal best. No wheezing or shortness of breath. Response to short-acting inhaled beta2–agonist sustained for 4 hours
Appropriate fetal activity*

Treatment:
*Many continue short-acting inhaled beta2–agonist every 3–4 hours for 24–48 hours
*For patients on inhaled corticosteroid double dose for 7–10 days

↓

Contact clinician for follow-up instructions

Incomplete response
Moderate exacerbation
PEF 50–80% predicted or personal best
Persistent wheezing and shortness of breath
Decreased fetal activity*

Treatment:
• Add oral corticosteroid
• Continue short-acting inhaled beta2-agonist

↓

Contact clinician urgently (this day) for instructions

Poor response
Severe exacerbation
PEF <50% predicted or personal best.
Marked wheezing and shortness of breath
Decreased fetal activity*

Treatment:
• Add oral corticosteroid
• Repeat short-acting inhaled beta2-agonist immediately
• If distress is severe and non-responsive, proceed to emergency department

↓

Proceed to emergency department

*Fetal activity is monitored by observing whether fetal kick counts decrease over time. (MDI: metered-dose inhaler; PEF: peak expiratory flow)

- Need to rescue medication—patients required add on therapy beyond inhaled short-acting beta-agonist and inhaled steroids and patients with persistent poor control
- Asthma attacks/exacerbations
- Limitation of daily activity
- PER <80% of expected.

EMERGENCY DEPARTMENT EVALUATION

Emergency department evaluation and treatment of the pregnant asthmatic are the same as in nonpregnant state, with some modifications. Peak flows should be compared with usual predicted values or personal best if available. If arterial blood gases are obtained, it should be remembered that a pregnant woman usually has a baseline compensated respiratory alkalosis.

Asthma exacerbations can be classified into three types: acute severe asthma, life-threatening asthma, and near-fatal asthma.

Features of asthma exacerbations have been shown in Table 1.

Worsening of the alkalosis as a result of asthma exacerbation may lead to fetal hypoxia. Conversely, acute respiratory acidosis may be present when $PaCO_2$ is above the normal 28–32 mm Hg. Maternal acidosis can lead to inability of the fetus to unload CO_2 if maternal venous and fetal umbilical artery CO_2 gradient is diminished. The hemodynamic effects of enlarging uterus on maternal circulation in supine position should always be kept in mind during the assessment of a pregnant woman in the third trimester of pregnancy and the patient should be examined in a sitting position, if possible, or in a supine position with a left or right tilt and the uterus displaced to avoid the supine hypotensive syndrome.[7]

TREATMENT OF ACUTE ASTHMA IN PREGNANCY

It is of paramount importance to initiate treatment for acute asthma exacerbation as early as possible. All patients with moderate to severe exacerbation should be treated in a monitored setting. The well-being of the fetus should also be monitored. It is very important to identify potential patients who may be at risk for fatal asthma, such as those with history of intubation and those with frequent emergency department (ED) visits, hospitalization, or previous intensive care unit (ICU) admission for asthma. Even in the absence of acute severe asthma, there should be a very low threshold for admission because pregnant patients can deteriorate very rapidly. Prevention of maternal hypoxia or hypercarbia, reversal of bronchospasm, and prevention of exhaustion are overarching

TABLE 1: Features of acute severe asthma, life-threatening asthma and near-fatal asthma.

Acute severe asthma	Life-threatening asthma	Near-fatal asthma
PEF 33–50% best or predicted Respiratory rate ≥ 25/min Heart rate ≥110/minute Inability to complete sentences in one breath	PEF <33% best or predicted SpO_2 <92% PaO_2 <8 kPa Normal or raised $PaCO_2$ (4.6–6.0 kPa) Silent chest Cyanosis Poor respiratory effort Arrhythmia Exhaustion Hypotension Altered consciousness	Features of life-threatening asthma Plus Raised $PaCO_2$ and/or requiring mechanical ventilation with raised inflation pressures

concerns during the management of acute asthma in a pregnant woman. Treatment of severe asthma in pregnant women is not different from the nonpregnant women. Treatment should include the following:[8]

- Oxygen supplementation should be given to maintain saturation at >95%.
- Fluid status should be carefully assessed, and intravenous fluid hydration should be administered if necessary.
- The initial treatment should include the administration of inhaled albuterol every 20 minutes, up to three doses in the first hour.
- Nebulized ipratropium bromide (500 µg) may be concomitantly administered in severe cases.
- Systemic corticosteroids, either intravenously (IV hydrocortisone 100 mg) and/or orally (40–50 mg prednisolone for at least 5 days), should be given to patients who show no improvement with the initial bronchodilator therapy and to those with moderate to severe exacerbation.
- Chest radiograph should be performed (after appropriate abdominal shielding) if there is any clinical suspicion of pneumonia or pneumothorax or if the woman fails to improve.
- Patients should be reassessed closely to monitor response to therapy. This includes continuous fetal heart rate monitoring if fetus is >23 weeks. The decision to hospitalize the patient or discharge home is based on the response achieved in the first 4 hours in the ED.
- If oral steroids are required for asthma control, prednisolone and methylprednisolone are the preferred preparations since they cross the placenta poorly. Prednisolone is extensively metabolized by placental enzymes so only 10% reaches to the fetus, making this the oral steroid of choice to treat maternal asthma in pregnancy. There is much published literature showing that steroid tablets are not teratogenic, but there is a slight concern that they may be associated with oral clefts, the association is not definite and even if it is real, the benefit to the mother and fetus of steroids for treating a life-threatening disease justifies the use of steroids in pregnancy. It was noticed that pregnant women with acute asthma attacks are less likely to be treated with steroid tablets than nonpregnant women. Failure to administer steroid tablets when indicated increases the risk of ongoing asthma attacks and therefore the risk to the mother and her fetus.[9]

EMERGENCY DEPARTMENT AND HOSPITAL-BASED CARE

No advantage has been found for higher dose corticosteroid in severe asthma exacerbations, nor is there any advantage for intravenous administration over oral therapy provided gastrointestinal transit time or absorption is not impaired. The usual regimen is to continue the frequent multiple daily dose until the patients achieve an FEV_1 or PEF of 50% of predicted or personal best and then lower the dose to twice daily. This usually takes place within 48 hours. Therapy following a hospitalization or ED visit may last from 3 days to 10 days. If patients are then started on inhaled corticosteroids, studies indicate there is no need to taper the systemic corticosteroid dose. If the follow-up systemic corticosteroid therapy is to be given once daily, one study indicates that it may be more clinically effective to give the dose in the afternoon at 3 PM, with no increase in adrenal suppression.

Intensive care management of acute, life-threatening asthma exacerbations during pregnancy has the immediate goals (Flowchart 2).

Acute Asthma in Pregnancy

Flowchart 2: Emergency department management.

Initial assessment
History, physical examination (auscultation, use of accessory muscles, heart rate, respiratory rate), PET or FEV_1, oxygen saturation, and other tests as indicated. Initiate fetal assessment (consider continuous electronic fetal monitoring and/or biophysical profile if pregnancy has reached fetal viability)

FEV_1 or PEF >50%
- Short-acting inhaled beta2-agonist by MDI or nebulizer, up to three doses in first hour
- Oxygen inhalation
- Oral systemic corticosteroid if no immediate response or if patient recently took oral systemic corticosteroid

FEV_1 or PEF <50% (severe exacerbation)
- High-dose short-acting inhaled beta2-agonist by nebulization every 20 minutes or continuously for 1 hour plus inhaled ipratropium bromide
- Oxygen to achieve O_2 saturation >95%
- Oral systemic corticosteroid

Impending or actual respiratory arrest
- Intubation and mechanical ventilation with 100% O_2
- Nebulized short-acting inhaled beta2-agonist plus inhaled ipratropium bromide
- Intravenous corticosteroid

Admit to hospital intensive care (see box below)

Repeat assessment
Symptoms, physical examination, PEF, O_2 saturation, other tests as needed
Continue fetal assessment

Moderate exacerbation
FEV_1 or PEF 50–80% predicted/personal best.
Physical examination: moderate symptoms
- Short-acting inhaled beta2-agonist every 60 minutes
- Systemic corticosteroid
- Oxygen to maintain O_2 saturation >95%
- Continue treatment 1–3 hours, provided there is improvement

Severe exacerbation
FEV_1 or PEF <50% predicted/personal best.
Physical examination: severe symptoms at rest. Accessory muscle use, chest retraction
History: High-risk patient
No improvement after initial treatment
- Short-acting inhaled beta2-agonist hourly or continuously plus inhaled ipratropium bromide
- Oxygen
- Systemic corticosteroid

Good response
- FEV_1 or PEF ≥70%
- Response sustained 60 minutes after last treatment
- No distress
- Physical examination: Normal
- Reassuring fetal status

Incomplete response
- FEV_1 or PEF ≥50% but <70%
- Mild or moderate symptoms
- Continue fetal assessment

Poor response
- FEV1 or PEF <50%
- PCO_2 >42 mm Hg
- Physical exam: symptoms severe, drowsiness, confusion
- Continue fetal assessment

Admit to hospital ward
- Short-acting inhaled beta2-agonist plus inhaled ipratropium bromide
- Systemic (oral or intravenous) corticosteroid
- Oxygen
- Monitor FEV_1 or PEF, O_2 saturation, pulse
- Continue fetal assessment until patient stabilized

Admit to hospital intensive care
- Short-acting inhaled beta2-agonist hourly or continuously plus inhaled ipratropium bromide
- Intravenous corticosteroid
- Oxygen
- Possible intubation and mechanical ventilation
- Continue fetal assessment until patient stabilized

Improve

Discharge home
- Continue treatment with short-acting inhaled beta2-agonist
- Continue course of oral systemic corticosteroid
- Initiate or continue inhaled corticosteroid until review at medical follow-up
- Recommend close medical follow-up

TABLE 2: Medications and dosages for asthma exacerbations during pregnancy and lactation.

Medications	Dosages Adult dose	Comments
Short-acting inhaled beta 2-agonists		
Albuterol		
Nebulizer solution (5.0 mg/mL, 2.5 mg/3 mL, 0.63 mg/3 mL)	2.5–5 mg every 20 minutes for 3 doses, then 2.5–10 mg every 1–4 hours as needed, or 10–15 mg/hour continuously	Only selective beta2-agonists are recommended. For optimal delivery, dilute aerosols to minimum of 3 mL at gas flow of 6–8 L/minute
MDI (90 µg/puff)	4–8 puffs every 20 minutes up to 4 hours, then every 1–4 hours as needed	As effective as nebulized therapy if patient is able to coordinate
Bitolterol		
Nebulizer solution (2 mg/mL)	See albuterol dose	Has not been studied in severe asthma exacerbations. Do not mix with other drugs
MDI (370 µg/puff)	See albuterol dose	Has not been studied in severe asthma exacerbations
Levalbuterol (R-albuterol)		
Nebulizer solution (0.63 mg/3 mL, 1.25 mg/3 mL)	1.25–2.5 mg every 20 minutes for 3 doses, then 1.25–5 mg every 1–4 hours as needed, or 5–7.5 mg/hour continuously	0.63 mg of levalbuterol is equivalent to 1.25 mg of racemic albuterol for both efficacy any side effects
Pirbuterol		
MDI (200 µg/puff)	See albuterol dose	Has not been studied in severe asthma exacerbations
Systemic (injected) beta2-agonists		
Epinephrine		
1:1,000 (1 mg/mL)	0.3–0.5 mg every 20 minutes for 3 doses SQ	No proven advantage of systemic therapy over aerosol
Terbutaline		
(1 mg/mL)	0.25 mg every 20 minutes for 3 doses SQ	No proven advantage of systemic therapy over aerosol
Anticholinergics		
Ipratropium bromide		
Nebulizer solution (0.25 mg/mL)	0.5 mg every 30 minutes for 3 doses, then every 2–4 hours as needed	May mix in same nebulizer with albuterol. Should not be used as first-line therapy; should be added to beta2-agonist therapy
MDI (18 µg/puff)	4–8 puffs as needed	Dose delivered from MDI is low and has not been studied in asthma exacerbations
Ipratropium with albuterol		
Nebulizer solution (Each 3 mL vial contains 0.5 mg ipratropium bromide and 2.5 mg albuterol)	3 mL every 30 minutes for 3 doses, then every 2–4 hours as needed	Contains EDTA to prevent discoloration. This additive does not induce bronchospasm
MDI (Each puff contains 18 µg ipratropium bromide and 90 µg albuterol)	4–8 puffs as needed	

Contd...

Contd...

Medications	Dosages Adult dose	Comments
Systemic corticosteroids (dosages and comments apply to all three corticosteroids)		
Prednisone Methylprednisolone Prednisolone	120–180 mg/day in 3 or 4 divided doses for 48 hours, then 60–80 mg/day until PEF reaches 70% of predicted or personal best	For outpatients "burst" use 40–60 mg in single or 2 divided doses for adult [children: 1–2 mg/kg/day (maximum 60 mg/day) for 3–10 days]

Notes: The most important determinant of appropriate dosing is the clinician's judgment of the patient's response to therapy.

Preventing and correcting hypoxemia (PaO_2 <60) and reducing hypercarbia ($PaCO_2$ >40) with supplemental oxygen or mechanical ventilation.

Reducing and reversing bronchospasm with bronchodilators—inhaled beta2-agonists remain the most important bronchodilators in this setting. Intravenous or subcutaneous administration of beta2-agonists such as terbutaline may be considered in some cases.

Systemic administration of epinephrine should be avoided (if possible) during pregnancy because of its vasoconstrictive effect on uteroplacental vasculature. When used in ICU setting close monitoring is needed to avoid maternal and fetal complications.

Intravenous infusion of $MgSO_4$ has an added bronchodilator effect in patients with acute severe asthma. Blood levels of $MgSO_4$ can be safely maintained at 4-6 mmol/L in pregnant women (infusion of 2 g/hour), but there is the potential for respiratory depression and the patient should be monitored for this complication.[10]

MECHANICAL VENTILATION IN ACUTE ASTHMA

Intubation and mechanical ventilation are often needed in pregnant women with life-threatening asthma, especially in those who develop severe hypercapnia ($PaCO_2$ >40–45 mm Hg), respiratory acidosis, maternal exhaustion, altered consciousness, and fetal distress.

ACUTE ASTHMA EXACERBATION DURING LABOR AND DELIVERY

Asthma does not usually affect labor or delivery with less than a fifth of women experiencing an exacerbation during labor and severe or life-threatening exacerbations are very rare.[11] Exacerbation during labor is uncommon due to endogenous steroid production, but if it occurs, it may cause substantial maternal and fetal distress (Table 2). In women receiving oral steroid (at a dose exceeding 7.5 mg/day) for more than 2 weeks prior to delivery, there is a theoretical risk of maternal hypothalamic-pituitary-adrenal axis suppression should receive parenteral hydrocortisone 100 mg 6-8 hourly during labor.

POSTPARTUM ASTHMA EXACERBATIONS

Postpartum asthma exacerbations are increased in women having cesarean sections. This may be related to several factors such as postoperative pain with diaphragmatic splinting, hypoventilation and atelectasis.

CONCLUSION

The mechanisms which lead to asthma exacerbations during pregnancy are poorly understood; however, viral infections and discontinuation of anti-inflammatory medications may play a role. Asthma exacerbations require appropriate treatment in order to protect mother and fetus as far as possible from adverse outcome. In particular, the fetus is at risk of being born of low birth weight, which may predispose to diseases in later life. Advances in the pharmacotherapy and ICU management of asthma during pregnancy have the potential to improve health outcomes for both mother and baby.

REFERENCES

1. Murphy VE, Gibson PG. Asthma in pregnancy. Clin Chest Med. 2011;32:93-110.
2. Hartert TV, Neuzil KM, Shintani AK, et al. Maternal morbidity and perinatal outcomes among pregnant women with respiratory hospitalizations during influenza season. Am J Obstet Gynecol. 2003;189:1705-12.
3. Stenius-Aarniala BS, Hedman J, Teramo KA. Acute asthma during pregnancy. Thorax. 1996;51:411-4.
4. Gluck JC, Gluck P. The effects of pregnancy on asthma: a prospective study. Ann Allergy. 1976;37:164-8.
5. Stenius-Aarniala B, Piirila P, Teramo K. Asthma and pregnancy: a prospective study of 198 pregnancies. Thorax. 1988;43:12-8.
6. Namazy JA, Murphy VE, Powell H, et al. Effects of asthma severity, exacerbations and oral corticosteroids on perinatal outcomes. Eur Respir J. 2013;41:1082-90.
7. Hanania NA, Belfort MA. Acute asthma in pregnancy. Crit Care Med. 2005;33(10 Suppl):S319-24.
8. Nelson-Piercy C. Asthma in pregnancy. Thorax. 2001;56:325-8.
9. Murphy VE, Gibson P, Talbot PI, et al. Severe asthma exacerbations during pregnancy. Obstet Gynecol. 2005;106:1046-54.
10. Rowe BH, Camargo CA Jr. The role of magnesium sulfate in the acute and chronic management of asthma. Curr Opin Pulm Med. 2008;14(1):70-6.
11. Goldie MH, Brightling CE. Asthma in pregnancy. Obstet Gynaecol. 2013;15:241-5.

CHAPTER 45

Scar Dehiscence

Sumi Maria

INTRODUCTION

Uterine scar dehiscence is an important complication in modern obstetric practice due to a rise in the cesarean section rates both in developed and developing countries. It is a notable complication that can arise in a scarred uterus which if left unidentified can lead to complete uterine rupture with a high incidence of fetal and maternal morbidity and mortality. The incidence ranges between 6.6% and 69% with variations mostly due to absence of criteria to define scar dehiscence.[1-3] Worldwide the incidence irrespective of cause is around 0.6%.[4]

DEFINITION

Uterine scar dehiscence is defined as an incomplete uterine rupture with disruption of the uterine muscle with intact serosa and visceral peritoneum.[5] The uterine contents are confined to the uterine cavity and the incidence of serious maternal and neonatal morbidity and mortality is low.

CAUSES AND RISK FACTORS

Pre-existing uterine injury from:
- Cesarean section/hysterotomy
- Myomectomy
- Metroplasty, septoplasty for uterine anomalies
- Uterine curettage
- Cornual resection of ectopic pregnancy.

Scar Dehiscence in Previous Cesarean Section

This is the most common cause of scar dehiscence. The incidence of scar rupture is greater with classical incision when compared to lower segment cesarean section. With a classical incision, the incidence of rupture is 2-9% when compared to low transverse incision which has only about 0.2-0.9% estimated rupture rate. The rupture with a classical cesarean scar occurs mostly before the onset of labor while the lower segment scar tends to rupture in labor. Estimated rupture rate in various types of uterine incision is given in Table 1.

TABLE 1: Estimated rupture rate in various types of uterine incision.

Prior incision	Estimated rupture rate (%)
Classical	2-9
T-shaped	4-9
Low-vertical	1-7
One low transverse	0.2-0.9
Multiple low transverse	0.9-1.8
Prior preterm cesarean	Increased
Prior uterine rupture:	
Lower segment	2-6
Upper uterus	9-32

Source: Data from American College of Obstetricians and Gynecologists, 2013a; Cahill, 2010b; Chauhan 2002; Landon 2006; Macones 2005; Martin 1997; Miller 1994; Sciscione 2008; Society of Maternal-Fetal Medicine 2012; Tahseen, 2010.

Other risk factors are:
- Interpregnancy interval less than 18 months—threefold increase in rupture rate (Shipp et al.)
- Poor wound healing due to postpartum fever, hematoma, sepsis, poor general health, obesity
- *Number of previous cesarean sections*: Incidence of uterine rupture was thrice more common when there was a history of two or more scars (OR, 3.06; 95% CI, 1.95-4.79; $P <0.001$)[6]
- *Closure of prior uterine incision*: There is no consensus regarding the type of uterine closure (single or double layer) that can best prevent scar dehiscence or rupture. In spite of many studies, the data are mostly conflicting or have not found any correlation between single or double layer suturing and the risk of subsequent uterine rupture[7,8]
- Retroflexed uterus (stretch on the scar is more leading to poor wound healing and inappropriate apposition)
- Advanced maternal age
- Macrosomia
- Multiple gestation
- Abnormal placentation.

Why is the scar dehiscence rate more with classical cesarean section?

The classical scar is in the upper uterine segment which keeps contracting even during puerperium resulting in defective healing. The wound approximation is usually less effective compared to a lower segment scar which leads to myometrial thinning and subsequent development of scar dehiscence.

■ SIGNS AND SYMPTOMS

Intrapartum

Maternal

- Sharp pain in between contractions
- Staircase sign—a stepwise gradual decrease in contraction amplitude which is followed by sudden onset of profound and prolonged fetal bradycardia[9]
- Suprapubic discomfort
- Scar tenderness
- Sudden cessation of uterine activity which was previously efficient
- Maternal tachycardia due to concealed hemorrhage and hypovolemia
- Shoulder pain due to hemoperitoneum causing diaphragmatic irritation
- Vaginal bleeding
- Hot and dry vagina
- Blood-stained urine
- Uterus palpable separately as a globular mass in case of complete rupture.

Fetal

- Nonreassuring fetal heart rate pattern—earliest sign (variable decelerations evolving to late decelerations and fetal bradycardia)
- Meconium staining of amniotic fluid
- Loss of station of presenting part
- Easily palpable fetal parts.

Postpartum

Immediately postpartum or after 2-4 weeks of delivery.
- Postpartum hemorrhage
- Endometritis
- Peritonitis.

Before Pregnancy

- Dysmenorrhea
- Intermenstrual spotting (most common symptom)
- Chronic pelvic pain
- Dyspareunia
- Secondary infertility.

■ PREDICTION

Early Pregnancy Predictors

Risk factors identified early in pregnancy are assigned numerical scores ranging from –1 to 2. 2 points for ≥2 prior cesarean scars, 1 point for interdelivery interval ≤18 months, 1 point for maternal age of 30–39 years, 2 points for maternal age ≥40 years, –1 point for women with prior vaginal delivery and one prior cesarean.[10] Rate of uterine rupture with predictive score using early pregnancy predictors is given in Table 2.

Scar thickness measuring <3.5 mm on transvaginal ultrasound in labor or at 36 weeks is a good predictor for scar dehiscence with a specificity of 91%.[11]

▌ INVESTIGATIONS

The simplest and the first-line investigation in a case of suspected scar dehiscence is transvaginal ultrasonography (TVUS).[12,13] In TVUS, the scar dehiscence appears as a defect which is triangular or dome-shaped echo-free space. This was called a "niche" by Monteagudo et al. It was referred to as "isthmocele" by Gubbini et al.[14] and as "dehiscence" by Regnard et al if the niche had a depth 80% or more of the anterior uterine musculature. Saline sonohysterography can also be used to identify the scar defect with more clarity.[15-19]

Magnetic resonance imaging (MRI) is the most definitive modality to evaluate uterine scars after cesarean deliveries.[20] Due to superior contrast resolution, a detailed analysis of tissue planes is possible and better assessment of scar defect. It also has the advantage of not being impeded by body habitus or bowel gas. It also helps in identifying posterior wall dehiscence which is difficult to estimate with ultrasonography. MRI can be used for expectant management of scar dehiscence once the diagnosis is made which can be further followed up with ultrasonography.

▌ PROGNOSIS

It depends on the type on the extent of scar dehiscence; with incomplete scar dehiscence the incidence of fetal and maternal morbidity and mortality being quite low.

▌ MANAGEMENT

The treatment of scar dehiscence in women desiring childbirth is surgical repair. In the past, surgical treatment required an exploratory laparotomy; conservative resuturing after debridement was the preferred treatment but in presence of marked wound infection, endomyometritis and/or intra-abdominal abscess, hysterectomy had been considered.[21-24] Recently, minimally invasive modalities like laparoscopic, laparoscopic-assisted vaginal, hysteroscopic, and robotic surgical repair are being done worldwide.[23-28]

In women who do not desire to bear children, the treatment choices have involved either low doses of monophasic contraceptives or total hysterectomies. There are also reports of resectoscopic surgery for removal of the flap-shaped fibrous tissue at the site of the scar and symptomatic improvement.[29-33] Based on the current report and technological advancements, a more conservative treatment seems to be possible.

When scar dehiscence is suspected in labor or before labor, immediate cesarean section has to be done and all intrauterine manipulations avoided to prevent the risk of progression into a complete uterine rupture. The dehiscent scar has to be managed with expertise so as to prevent the extension of the

TABLE 2: Rate of uterine rupture with predictive score using early pregnancy predictors.

$P = 0.001$.

Score	Rate of uterine rupture (%)
–1	0.26
0	0.25
1	1.11
2	2.43
3	3.70
4	14.29

tear into the bladder or parametrium. There are a few case reports of expectant management of scar dehiscence diagnosed in second trimester followed up with close monitoring.[21]

PREVENTION

- Use of electric clippers, rather than a razor, to remove the hair at the site of the surgical incision to reduce the incidence of abdominal wound infections.
- Washing the skin with a chlorhexidine solution.
- Administering broad-spectrum antibiotic prophylaxis at the onset of surgery.
- Avoid manual extraction of placenta to minimize postpartum endometritis.
- Meticulous repair of uterine wound.
- Closure of the deep subcutaneous layer in patients whose subcutaneous tissue is greater than 2 cm in thickness to reduce the risk of seroma, hematoma, and subsequent wound disruption.[34]
- Improved general health to promote wound healing.
- Identify risk factors and early screening and diagnosis in suspected cases using ultrasound or MRI.

CONCLUSION

Cesarean section remains the most common surgery performed in modern obstetrics, hence the importance of scar dehiscence in future pregnancies and in the nonpregnant state cannot be over emphasized. Identification of risk factors and early detection of myometrial thinning in suspected cases is the key to prevent catastrophic uterine rupture in labor and also to prevent long-term complications in women presenting in nonpregnant state. Transvaginal ultrasound can be the first-line screening tool for diagnosing suspected cases and MRI for confirmation. Early detection leads to significant reduction in fetal and maternal mortality and morbidity as the surgeon can proceed with a more conservative approach to repair the uterus. Also newer advances in microsurgical techniques have facilitated correction in prepregnant state using hysteroscopic, laparoscopic and robotic surgeries. As prevention is better than cure, it is of utmost importance to reduce the number of cesarean sections globally so as to prevent the rising incidence of this complication in future for a woman of childbearing age.

REFERENCES

1. Thurmond AS, Harvey WJ, Smith SS. Cesarean section scar as a cause of abnormal vaginal bleeding: diagnosis by sonohysterography. J Ultrasound Med. 1999;18:13-6.
2. Bromley B, Pitcher BL, Klapholz H, et al. Sonographic appearance of uterine scar dehiscence. Int J Gynaecol Obstet. 1995;51:53-6.
3. Ofili-Yebovi D, Ben-Nagi J, Sawyer E, et al. Deficient low-segment cesarean section scars: prevalence and risk factors. Ultrasound Obstet Gynecol. 2008;31:72-7.
4. Diaz SD, Jones JE, Seryakov M, et al. Uterine rupture and dehiscence: ten-year review and case-control study. South Med J. 2002;95:431-5.
5. Kore S, Pandole A, Akolekar R, et al. Rupture of the left horn of bicornuate uterus at twenty weeks of gestation. J Postgrad Med. 2000;46:39-40.
6. Miller DA, Diaz FG, Paul RH. Vaginal birth after cesarean: a 10-year experience. Obstet Gynecol. 1994;84(2):255-8.
7. Bujold E, Bujold C, Hamilton EF, et al. The impact of a single-layer or double-layer closure on uterine rupture. Am J Obstet Gynecol. 2002;186:1326-30.
8. Reed WC. Large uterine defect found at caesarean section. A case report. J Reprod Med. 2003;48:60-2.
9. Matsuo K, Scanlon JT, Atlas RO, et al. Staircase sign: a newly described utcrine contraction pattern seen in rupture of unscarred gravid uterus. J Obstet Gynecol Res. 2008;34:100-4.
10. Shipp TD, Zelop C, Lieberman E. Assessment of the rate of uterine rupture at the first prenatal visit: a preliminary evaluation. J Matern Fetal Neonatal Med. 2008;21:129-33.
11. Rozenberg P, Goffinet F, Phillippe HJ, et al. Echographic measurement of the inferior

uterine segment for assessing the risk of uterine rupture. J Gynecol Obstet Biol Reprod (Paris). 1997;26:513-9.
12. Royo P, Manero MG, Olartecoechea B, et al. Two-dimensional power Doppler-three-dimensional ultrasound imaging of a cesarean section dehiscence with utero-peritoneal fistula: a case report. J Med Case Rep. 2009;3:42.
13. Gubbini G., Casadio P., Marra E. Resectoscopic correction of the "isthmocele" in women with postmenstrual abnormal uterine bleeding and secondary infertility. J Minim Invasive Gynecol. 2008;15:172-5.
14. Gotoh H, Masuzaki H, Yoshida A, et al. Predicting incomplete uterine rupture with vaginal sonography during the late second trimester in women with prior cesarean. Obstet Gynecol. 2000;95:596-600.
15. Osser OV, Jokubkiene L, Valentin L. Cesarean section scar defects: agreement between transvaginal sonographic findings with and without saline contrast enhancement. Ultrasound Obstet Gynecol. 2010;35:75-83.
16. Monteagudo A, Carreno C, Timor-Tritsch IE. Saline infusion sonohysterography in nonpregnant women with previous cesarean delivery: the "niche" in the scar. J Ultrasound Med. 2001;20(10):1105-15.
17. Regnard C, Nosbusch M, Fellemans C, et al. Cesarean section scar evaluation by saline contrast sonohysterography. Ultrasound Obstet Gynecol. 2004;23:289-92.
18. Ida A, Kubota Y, Nosaka M, et al. Successful management of a cesarean scar defect with dehiscence of the uterine incision by using wound lavage. Case Rep Obstet Gynecol. 2014;2014:421014.
19. Woo GM, Twickler DM, Stettler RW, et al. The pelvis after cesarean section and vaginal delivery: normal MR findings. AJR Am J Roentgenol. 1993;161:1249-52.
20. Dicle O, Kucukler C, Pirnar T, et al. Magnetic resonance imaging evaluation of incision healing after cesarean sections. Eur Radiol. 1997;7:31-4.
21. Humar BD, Levine D, Katz NL, et al. Expectant management of uterine dehiscence in the second trimester of pregnancy. Obstet Gynecol. 2003;102(5 Pt 2):1139-42.
22. Maldjian C, Adam R, Maldjian J, et al. MRI appearance of the pelvis in the post cesarean-section patient. Magn Reson Imaging. 1999;17:223-7.
23. Larsen JV, Janowski K, Krolilowski A. Secondary postpartum hemorrhage due to uterine wound dehiscence. Cent Afr J Med. 1995;41: 294-6.
24. Rivlin ME, Patel RB, Carroll CS, et al. Diagnostic imaging in uterine incisional necrosis/dehiscence complicating cesarean section. J Reprod Med. 2005;50:928-32.
25. Donnez O, Jadoul P, Squifflet J, et al. Laparoscopic repair of wide and deep uterine scar dehiscence after cesarean section. Fertil Steril. 2008;89:974-80.
26. Klemm P, Koehler C, Mangler M, et al. Laparoscopic and vaginal repair of uterine scar dehiscence following cesarean section as detected by ultrasound. J Perinat Med. 2005;33:324-31.
27. Yalcinkaya TM, Akar ME, Kammire LD, et al. Robotic-assisted laparoscopic repair of symptomatic cesarean scar defect: a report of two cases. J Reprod Med. 2011;56:265-70.
28. Fabres C, Arriagada P, Fernández C, et al. Surgical treatment and follow-up of women with intermenstrual bleeding due to cesarean section scar defect. J Minim Invasive Gynecol. 2005;12:25-8.
29. Shih CL, Chang YY, Ho M, et al. Hysteroscopic transcervical resection. A straightforward method corrects bleeding related to cesarean section scar defects. Am J Obstet Gynecol. 2011;204:278.e1-2.
30. Marra E, Casadio P, Armilotta F, et al. Resectoscopic treatment of "isthmocele": "isthmoplasty". Gynaecol Surg. 2009;6(Suppl 1):S1-31.
31. Li C, Guo Y, Liu Y, et al. Hysteroscopic and laparoscopic management of uterine defects on previous cesarean delivery scars. J Perinat Med. 2014;42:363-70.
32. Raimondo G, Grifone G, Raimondo D, et al. Hysteroscopic treatment of symptomatic cesarean-induced isthmocele: a prospective study. J Minim Invasive Gynecol. 2015;22: 297-301.
33. Vervoort AJ, Van der Voet LF, Witmer M, et al. The HysNiche trial: hysteroscopic resection of uterine caesarean scar defect (niche) in patients with abnormal bleeding, a randomised controlled trial. BMC Womens Health. 2015;15:103.
34. Duff P. A simple checklist for preventing major complications associated with cesarean delivery. Obstet Gynecol. 2010;116:1393-6.

CHAPTER 46

Disseminated Intravascular Coagulation in Obstetrics

Vinay Kumar, Harleen Kour, Anju Dogra

INTRODUCTION

Disseminated intravascular coagulation (DIC) is an acquired clinicopathological syndrome characterized by disturbance in hemostatic balance due to widespread intravascular fibrin deposition. It is also known as consumptive coagulopathy. DIC is a process or complication of some diseases and not an independent disease.[1] As a result, coagulation responses that may be naturally protective to the host can change into maladaptive response with pathological consequences. DIC is thus associated with increased morbidity and mortality.

NORMAL HEMOSTASIS

Normal hemostasis depends upon a number of interrelated systems which are:
- Coagulation system
- Coagulation inhibitory system
- Fibrinolytic system.

Intravascular coagulation results from pathological disturbances in any of these systems.[2,3]

Coagulation system involves two different pathways, i.e. intrinsic and extrinsic pathway of blood coagulation (Flowchart 1). Initiation of both pathways is by different stimuli but ultimately they culminate into common pathway of conversion of prothrombin into thrombin.[4]

Coagulation inhibitory systems include anticoagulants like antithrombin III (main inhibitor of thrombin and factor Xa), protein C, protein S and thrombomodulin.

Fibrinolytic system leads to lysis of fibrinogen.

PATHOGENESIS OF DISSEMINATED INTRAVASCULAR COAGULATION

Disseminated intravascular coagulation results from continuous fibrin generation and procoagulants and platelets consumption.[5] This results from:
- Initiation of thrombin generation by activation of coagulation cascade by procoagulants
- Inhibition of anticoagulant pathway
- Inhibition of fibrinolytics resulting in fibrin deposition and thrombus formation leading to ischemic tissue damage and multiple organ dysfunction syndrome (MODS)
- Endothelial injury
- Diffuse bleeding resulting from consumption of platelets and coagulation factors.

Flowchart 2 explains the pathogenesis of disseminated intravascular coagulation.

Pregnancy is a hypercoagulable state.

Fetal trophoblast cells which are present in the vascular bed of the placenta have the ability to regulate hemostasis like the endothelial cells. Several distinct hemostatic properties that help in homeostatic maintenance in normal pregnancy include the (1) tissue factor expression, (2) altered anticoagulant function, (3) suppression of fibrinolysis, and (4) exposure of anionic phospholipids.[6]

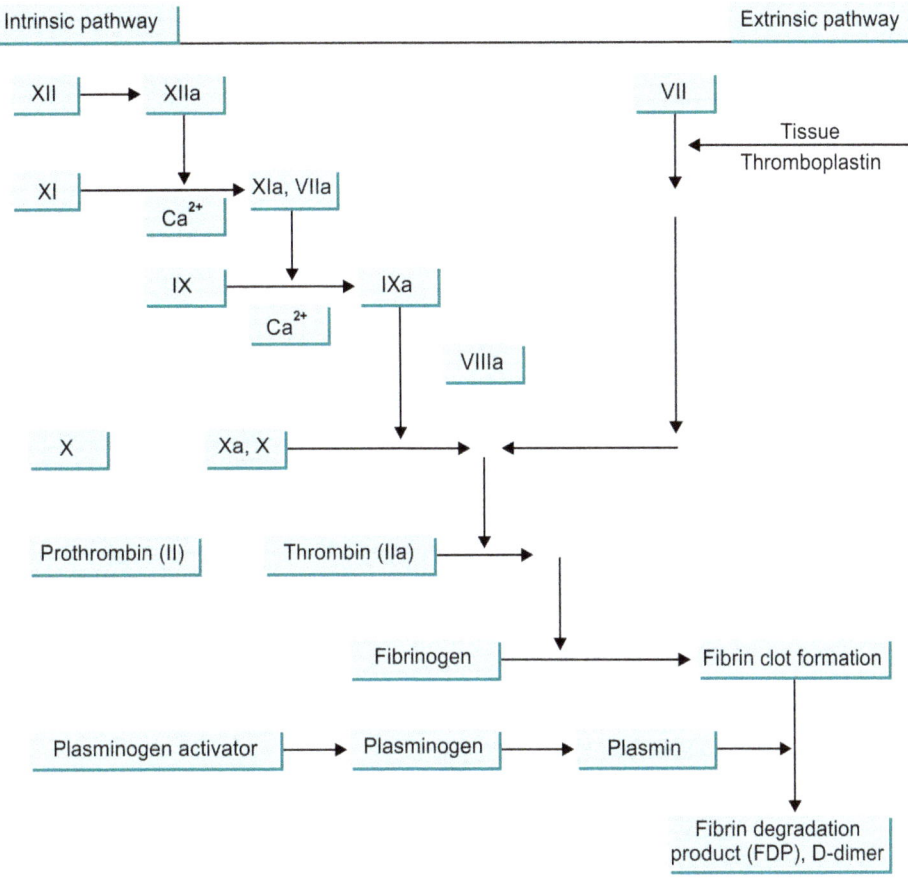

Flowchart 1: Normal coagulation cascade.

Procoagulant factors are increased in pregnancy including factor II, V, VII, VIII, IX, X, XII. Plasma fibrinogen is markedly increased.[7]

Platelet count is slightly decreased during pregnancy and labor.

Obstetrical Causes of Disseminated Intravascular Coagulation

- Abruptio placentae
- Amniotic fluid embolism
- Preeclampsia, eclampsia
- HELLP (hemolysis, elevated liver enzymes, and low platelet count) syndrome
- Intrauterine fetal demise
- Septicemia—septic abortion, chorioamnionitis, pyelonephritis, infections
- Postpartum hemorrhage (PPH), hypovolemia
- Shock
- Hydatidiform mole
- Cesarean section
- Intra-amniotic hypertonic saline infusion
- Incompatible blood transfusion
- Massive intravascular hemolysis.

Nonobstetrical Causes of Disseminated Intravascular Coagulation[8]

- Trauma
- Sepsis
- Organ damage
- Malignancies—leukemia, ovarian malignancies

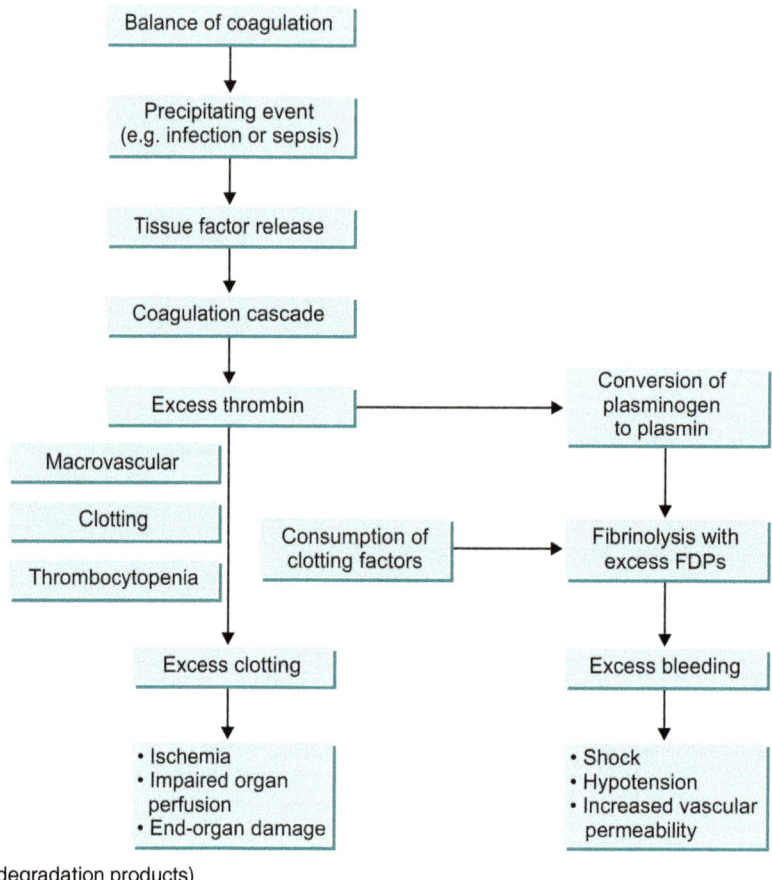

Flowchart 2: Pathogenesis of disseminated intravascular coagulation.

(FDPs: fibrin degradation products)

- Acute liver failure
- Toxic and immunological causes
- Transplant rejection
- ABO incompatibility.

Mechanism of Acquired Coagulopathy in Common Obstetrical Causes

Abruptio Placentae[9,10]

Mechanism of acquired coagulopathy in abruptio placentae has been shown in Flowchart 3.

Amniotic Fluid Embolism[11]

Mechanism of acquired coagulopathy in amniotic fluid embolism has been shown in Flowchart 4.

Intrauterine Fetal Demise[12]

Mechanism of acquired coagulopathy in intrauterine fetal demise has been shown in Flowchart 5.

Preeclampsia[13]

A maternal inflammatory response formed against the trophoblasts results in a systemic endothelial dysfunction. Thus, uteroplacental ischemia increases as a result of decrease in vasodilator prostaglandins and thrombocyte aggregation. Hence, preeclampsia is a predisposing factor for DIC.

Septic Abortion[14]

Septic abortion triggers the release of inflammatory substances (tissue thromboplastin or

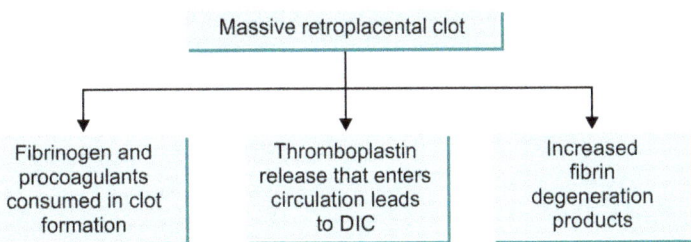

Flowchart 3: Abruptio placentae.

(DIC: disseminated intravascular coagulation)

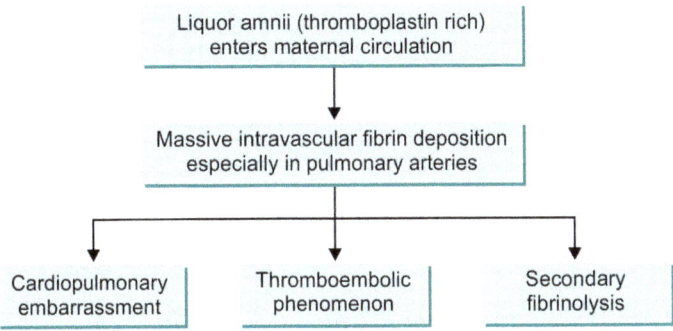

Flowchart 4: Amniotic fluid embolism.

bacterial endotoxin) which eventually disrupt the coagulation mechanisms.

Postpartum Hemorrhage[15]

In cases of severe PPH, increased consumption of coagulation factors as a consequence of severe amount of blood loss may result in DIC.

■ CLINICAL FEATURES

The overall clinical picture of DIC is often dominated by the cause of DIC. Hemorrhage from various sites is the most common manifestation (Fig. 1).[16,17]

Acute Disseminated Intravascular Coagulation

- Bleeding including petechiae, ecchymosis, blood oozing from injection sites, catheters, mucosal surface, gastrointestinal tract (GIT), lungs or central nervous system (CNS)
- Renal dysfunction
- Hepatic dysfunction

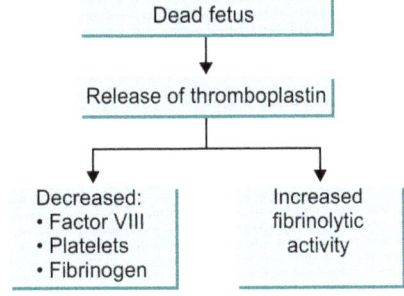

Flowchart 5: Intrauterine fetal demise.

- Respiratory dysfunction
- Shock
- Thromboembolism
- Multiple organ dysfunction syndrome.

Chronic Disseminated Intravascular Coagulation

- Venous or arterial thromboembolism
- Superficial migrating thrombophlebitis (Trousseau's syndrome)
- Nonbacterial thrombotic endocarditis (Libman-Sacks endocarditis).

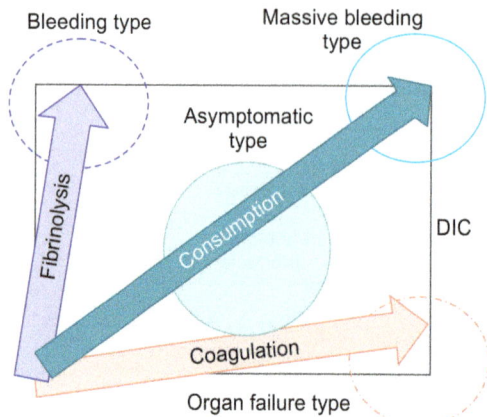

Fig. 1: Manifestations of disseminated intravascular coagulation.
(DIC: disseminated intravascular coagulation)

Postpartum Risks in Disseminated Intravascular Coagulation

- Postpartum hemorrhage
- Bleeding from episiotomy site or stitch line
- Hematoma formation
- Collection of blood in serous cavities.

■ INVESTIGATIONS

The diagnosis of DIC is not based on any isolated test rather it is an interpretation of several hemostatic parameters taken together.[18,19]

Commonly Available Tests of Hemostasis

- Bleeding time (BT)—increased
- Clotting time (CT)—increased
- Peripheral blood film (PBF)—in DIC, red blood cell (RBC) morphology is altered helmet-shaped or fragmented cells seen. Thrombocytopenia [<4 platelets/HPF (high-power field)]
- Platelet count—decreased (normal value—146,000-429,000)*
- Activated partial thromboplastin time (aPTT)—prolonged. It is marker of intrinsic coagulation pathway (normal value—22.6-35 seconds)*

*Reference values from Williams Obstetrics.[20]

- Prothrombin time (PT)—prolonged. It is marker of extrinsic coagulation pathway (normal value—9.6-12.9 seconds)*
- Thrombin time (TT) (normal value— 16.5 ± 2.4 seconds)*
- Fibrinogen—decreased (normal value— 301-696 mg/dL)*
- Fibrin degradation products (FDPs)—increased
- D-dimer—increased
- Protamine test.

Single time testing of the above is not so helpful rather it is the serial coagulation tests which guide us in the proper diagnosis and management.

Specialized Tests

- Prothrombin activation fragments 1 and 2
- Protein C—decreased
- Fibrinopeptide A
- D-dimer monoclonal antibody test
- Thrombin-antithrombin (TAT) complexes.

Imaging Studies

Thromboelastography (TEG).

Subcommittee of International Society of Thrombosis and Haemostasis (ISTH), Scientific and Standardization Committee (SCC) has devised a scoring system for DIC as described in Box 1.[21]

■ DIFFERENTIAL DIAGNOSIS

- HELLP syndrome—presents with elevated liver enzymes, low platelets, hemolysis and normal FDP and negative D-dimer and Coombs test
- Coagulopathy associated with severe liver disease—in this there is known source of liver injury
- Coagulopathy associated with vaso-occlusive diseases like sickle cell anemia
- Thrombotic thrombocytopenic purpura.

Box 1: Diagnostic algorithm for the diagnosis of overt DIC.

1. *Risk assessment:* Dose the patient have a underlying disorder known to be associated with overt DIC? If yes: proceed; If no: do not use this algorithm
2. Order global coagulation tests [platelet count, prothrombin time (PT), fibrinogen, soluble fibrin monomers of fibrin degradation products]
3. Score global coagulation test results
   Platelet count (>100 = 0; <100 = 1; <50 = 2)
   Elevated fibrin-related marker (e.g. soluble fibrin monomers/fibrin degradation products) (no increase: 0; moderate increase: 2; strong increase: 3)
   Prolonged PT (<3 sec = 0; >3sec but <6 sec = 1; >6 sec = 2)
   Fibrinogen level (>1.0 g/L = 0; <1.0 g/L = 1)
4. *Calculate score:* If >5: compatible with overt DIC; repeat scoring daily
   If <5: suggestive (not affirmative) for nonovert DIC; repeat next 1–2 days

Source: Bedside critical care 2012.

TREATMENT

The management of disseminated intravascular coagulopathy includes the following:
- Identify and treat the cause
- Supportive measures
- Actual management.

First priority in managing DIC is to identify and treat the cause of DIC.[22] In most cases, delivery of the fetus brings the resolution of coagulopathy. Once the underlying disorder is properly managed DIC resolves spontaneously in many cases.

Supportive measures include volume replacement, administration of antibiotics, respiratory support and intense monitoring of vital parameters.

Actual treatment includes:
- Blood component therapy
- Heparin
- Antifibrinolytic therapy
- Anti-Xa
- Activated factor VII
- Synthetic protease inhibitor
- Vitamin K.

Treatment of DIC varies according to the manifestations in a particular patient.[6]

Blood Component Therapy

- To control bleeding using surgical and/or radiological interventions.
- Using fluids and blood products to restore circulating blood volume.
- Preventing factors like hypothermia and acidosis which act as exacerbating factors for abnormal coagulation.
- *Blood product support as follows:*
  - *Red cells:* To maintain circulating blood volume, red cells are required. Use blood that is cross-matched or use O negative red cells. Hypothermia should be avoided by warming the blood before use.
  - Fresh frozen plasma—for every one unit of red cell, transfuse one unit of plasma.
  - Platelet transfusion—may be done. After at the rate of blood volume replacements, one to two adult doses can be given.
  - Fibrinogen cryoprecipitate (dose = two donation pools). Fibrinogen concentrates (4 g) aim for fibrinogen level over 1 g/L.
  - Autotransfusion—blood is collected from the operative field, filtered and the blood is then transfused back.

Heparin

Disseminated intravascular coagulation is characterized by extensive activation of coagulation, but still there is some difference of opinion in administration of anticoagulant therapy. In cases where thrombosis predominates, therapeutic doses of heparin should be considered. Studies suggest that use of low-molecular-weight heparin (LMWH) is superior to unfractionated heparin (UFH) in cases of DIC.[23] Using heparin is useful in patients of DIC as it provides venous thromboembolism (VTE) prophylaxis.[24,25] Patients who are having bleeding manifestation, in such patients heparin is not recommended as it will increase risk of bleeding.

Antifibrinolytic Therapy

Fibrinolysis may be protective phenomenon. So, use of antifibrinolytic treatment is very limited. In patients with organ failure or nonsymptomatic type of DIC, use of antifibrinolytic therapy is not recommended,[26] exception is case of massive bleeding.

Fibrinolytic inhibitors include:
- Epsilon aminocaproic acid (EACA)—inhibits plasminogen and plasmin
- Trasylol—inhibits plasmin
- Aprotinin—nonspecific enzyme inhibitor.

Anti-Xa Agents

These agents are used primarily for prevention of DVT.[27-29] Agents include:
- Fondaparinux
- Danaparoid sodium.

Some studies suggest use of danaparoid sodium in DIC in countries like Japan.

Synthetic Protease Inhibitor

These drugs have mild anticoagulant and antifibrinolytic effect. These include gabexate mesilate and nafamostat.

Recombinant Activated Factor VIIa[30,31]

Recombinant factor VIIa can directly activate factor X on the surface of locally activated platelets at supraphysiological concentrations. It can reverse DIC by being a precursor for the extrinsic clotting cascade. Dose 15–120 µg/kg.

Vitamin K

Many of the coagulation factors like factor II, VII, IX and X are vitamin K dependent. So vitamin K helps replenish these factors.

Emerging Therapies[32]

- Recombinant human soluble thrombomodulin (ART-123)[33]—anticoagulant and anti-inflammatory
- Recombinant hirudin
- Recombinant nematode anticoagulant protein c2 (NAPc2)[34]
- Recombinant interleukin 10 (IL)-10—anti-inflammatory cytokine.

PROGNOSIS[35,36]

Disseminated intravascular coagulation resolution requires synthesis of coagulation factors and FDPs from circulation which can take several days even after management of the cause of DIC.

Morbidity and mortality rates are very high.

REFERENCES

1. Bick RL. Disseminated intravascular coagulation current concepts of etiology, pathophysiology, diagnosis, and treatment. Hematol Oncol Clin North Am. 2003;17(1):149-76.
2. Lillicrap D, Key N, Makris M, O'Shaughnessy D (Eds). Practical Hemostasis and Thrombosis, 2 edition. Chapel Hill, NC: Wiley-Blackwell; 2009. pp. 1-5.
3. Chris H. Haematology: Lecture Notes. Cambridge: Blackwell Publishers; 2008. pp. 145-66.
4. Hoffbrand AV, Pettit JE, Moss PA. Essential Haematology, 4th edition. Oxford: Blackwell Science; 2002. pp. 241-3.
5. Saxena P, Sharma A, Agarwal M, et al. Disseminated intravascular coagulation: management updates. In: Gupta P. Medicine Update. New Delhi, India: Evangel; 2018.
6. Wada H, Matsumoto T, Yamashita Y. Diagnosis and treatment of disseminated intravascular coagulation (DIC) according to four DIC guidelines. J Intensive Care. 2014;2:15.

7. Bremme KA. Haemostatic changes in pregnancy. Best Pract Res Clin Haematol. 2003;16(2):153-68.
8. Sahin S, Eroglu M, Tetik S, et al. Disseminated intravascular coagulation in obstetrics: etiopathogenesis and up to date management strategies. J Turk Soc Obstet Gynecol. 2014; 11(1):42-51.
9. Ananth CV, Getahun D, Peltier MR, et al. Placental abruption in term and preterm gestations: evidence of heterogeneity in clinical pathways. Obstet Gynecol. 2006;107(4):785-92.
10. Oyelese Y, Ananth CV. Placental abruption. Obstet Gynecol. 2006;108(4):1005-16.
11. Sultana S, Begum A, Khan MA. Disseminated intravascular coagulation (DIC) in obstetric practice. J Dhaka Med Coll. 2011;20(1):68-74.
12. Kobayashi T, Terao T, Maki M, et al. Diagnosis and management of acute obstetrical DIC. Semin Thromb Hemost. 2001;27(2):161-7.
13. Redman CW, Sacks GP, Sargent IL. Pre-eclampsia: an excessive maternal inflammatory response to pregnancy. Am J Obstet Gynecol. 1999;180(2 Pt 1):499-506.
14. Boisrame-Helms J, Kremer H, Schini-Kerth V, et al. Endothelial dysfunction in sepsis. Curr Vasc Pharmacol. 2013;11(2):50-60.
15. Hess JR. Blood and coagulation support in trauma care. Hematology Am Soc Hematol Educ Program. 2007:187-91.
16. NHLBI, NIH. Disseminated intravascular coagulation. [online] Available from: www.nhlbi.nih.gov [Last accessed September, 2019].
17. Moake JL. Disseminated intravascular coagulation (DIC). Hematology and Oncology. Merck Manuals. Professional edition. September 2016.
18. Hoffman R, Benz E, Heslop H, Weitz J (Eds). Hematology: Basic Principles and Practice, 6th edition. Philadelphia: Elsevier Saunders; 2012.
19. Levi M, Toh CH, Thachil J, et al. Guidelines for the diagnosis and management of disseminated intravascular coagulation. British Committee for Standards in Haematology. Br J Haematol. 2009;145(1):24-33.
20. Cunningham FG, Leveno KJ, Bloom SL, Spong CY, Dashe JS, Hoffman BL, Casey BM, Sheffield JS (Eds). Williams Obstetrics, 24th edition. New York: McGraw-Hill Education; 2014. pp. 1287-93.
21. Taylor FB Jr, Toh CH, Hoots WK, et al. Towards definition, clinical and laboratory criteria, and a scoring system for disseminated intravascular coagulation. Thromb Haemost. 2001;86:1327-30.
22. Levi M. Disseminated intravascular coagulation. Crit Care Med. 2007;38(9):2191-5.
23. Sakuragawa N, Hasegawa H, Maki M, et al. Clinical evaluation of low-molecular-weight heparin (FR-860) on disseminated intravascular coagulation (DIC): a multicenter co-operative double-blind trial in comparison with heparin. Thromb Res. 1993;72:475-500.
24. Patel R, Cook DJ, Meade MO, et al. Burden of illness in venous thromboembolism in critical care: a multicenter observational study. J Crit Care. 2005;20:341-7.
25. Samama MM, Cohen AT, Darmon JY, et al. A comparison of enoxaparin with placebo for the prevention of venous thromboembolism in acutely ill medical patients. Prophylaxis in Medical Patients with Enoxaparin Study Group. N Engl J Med. 1999;341:793-800.
26. Mannucci PM, Levi M. Prevention and treatment of major blood loss. N Engl J Med. 2007;356:2301-11.
27. Beyer-Westendorf J, Lützner J, Donath L, et al. Efficacy and safety of rivaroxaban or fondaparinux thromboprophylaxis in major orthopedic surgery: findings from the ORTHO-TEP registry. J Thromb Haemost. 2012;10: 2045-52.
28. Girard P, Demaria J, Lillo-Le Louët A, et al. Transfusions, major bleeding, and prevention of venous thromboembolism with enoxaparin or fondaparinux in thoracic surgery. Thromb Haemost. 2011;106:1109-16.
29. Soff CA. A new generation of oral direct anticoagulants. Arterioscler Thromb Vasc Biol. 2012;32(3):569-74.
30. Franchini M, Manzato F, Salvango GL, et al. Potential role of recombinant activated factor VII for treatment of severe bleeding associated with disseminated intravascular coagulation: a systematic review. Blood Coagul Fibrinolysis. 2007;18:589-93.
31. Gabriel A, Li X, Monroe DM 3rd, et al. Recombinant human factor VIIa (rFVIIa) can activate FIX on activated platelets. J Thromb Haemost. 2004;2:1816-22.

32. Levi M, de Jonge E, van der Poll T. New treatment strategies for disseminated intravascular coagulation based on current understanding of the pathophysiology. Ann Med. 2004;36:41-9.
33. Vincent JL, Ramesh MK, Ernest D, et al. A randomized, double blind, placebo-controlled, phase IIb study to evaluate the safety of recombinant human soluble thrombomodulin, ART-123, in patients with sepsis and suspected disseminated intravascular coagulation. Crit Care Med. 2013;41:2069-79.
34. Moons AH, Peters RJ, Cate Ht, et al. Recombinant nematode anticoagulant protein c2, a novel inhibitor of tissue factor-factor VIIa activity, abrogates endotoxin-induced coagulation in chimpanzees. Thromb Haemost. 2002;88:627-31.
35. Franchini M, Lippi G, Manzato F. Recent acquisitions in the pathophysiology, diagnosis and treatment of disseminated intravascular coagulation. Thromb J. 2006;4:4.
36. Gando S, Levi M, Toh CH. Disseminated intravascular coagulation. Nat Rev Dis Primers. 2016;2:16037.

CHAPTER 47

In Utero Transfer

Vinay Kumar, Anju Dogra, Harleen Kour

INTRODUCTION

Emergency in utero transfers (IUTs) of pregnant women is required when delivery of either a preterm or other compromised baby is anticipated as a result of spontaneous preterm labor or when obstetric complications have arisen which demand immediate delivery. These may be maternal complications like pre-eclampsia or fetal complications like severe intrauterine growth restriction (IUGR) with fetal compromise.[1]

Maternal safety is paramount in all cases, particularly in the situation where maternal disease and deterioration in maternal condition are the precipitating factors as transfer in these situations could put the mother's life at risk. Therefore, good communication between midwifery, obstetric and neonatal staff on both sides of the proposed transfer is essential.

It is seen that even 96 hours after IUT about 25% women remain undelivered and the number may be even higher in women presenting with spontaneous labor with intact membranes. The rationale for transfer should be clear and the final decision should be taken by consultant obstetric as multiple IUT of the mother causes significant stress and anxiety to the parents.[2]

With regard to IUT for the management of patients, consultant obstetric and senior neonatal staff along with most senior midwife must be available, at both the hospitals, i.e. referring and receiving. And the relative benefits and risks of transfer to both maternal and fetal health must be assessed.

Communication between all is very important at both hospitals including the mother. There must be clear and agreed instructions as to who is responsible for care of mother during different stages of the transfer process. The receiving unit should clarify their on-going care plans as soon as after the woman has been transferred.

In recent years, significant developments have been made in order to improve the management of high-risk obstetric patients at local, regional and national level.[3] Still during emergency IUT, there remains the risk of an adverse or fatal outcome of either mother and/or baby.

INCIDENCE

The data regarding exact incidence of IUT and neonatal outcomes in recent years is limited. The Perinatal Emergency Transfer Study conducted in 1999 recorded that about 309 mothers or infants were transferred out of the 37 largest perinatal centers in the United Kingdom (UK) during a 3-month census which equates to 1,236 episodes per year.[4] Due to lack of neonatal cots, most perinatal centers were unable to meet in-house demands for neonatal intensive care and as a result there were a large number of inappropriate and unplanned neonatal transfers.[5] There was a wide geographical variation in the extent to which supply met demand.[5] The National Perinatal Epidemiology Unit Survey conducted in 2006 in England including over 2,500 women, showed in their report that about 0.5% of women were transfer from one hospital to another during labor, with 1.7% being transferred from separate birth centers or maternity units to hospitals.[6] A regional annual acute IUT rate of 3.7/1,000 deliveries was reported by Fenton et al. with fetal reasons as the primary indications.[7]

For babies <32 weeks' gestational age, IUT patterns over 10 years (1995-2004) were recorded which showed a gradual decline from 2.1/1,000 births to 1.8/1,000 births with the overall average about 2.1.[8] The average rate of IUT/1,000 births <32 weeks of gestation however was 87.8 over 10 years, indicating the increased risk of transfer being done for preterm delivery.[8]

DEFINITION

In utero transfer is defined as safe transfer of a woman from one clinical care setting to another to provide care in specialist area or center.

Transfer may be made for maternal or fetal reasons and can occur at any stage of antenatal, intrapartum or postnatal period.

Emergency IUT is defined as: *"the unplanned, acute transfer of a mother to other units or, designated tertiary centers for specialist care which cannot be provided locally"*.[9]

INDICATIONS FOR TRANSFER

- Suspected or actual preterm labor <34 weeks' gestation when no neonatal intensive care unit (NICU) cot available.
- Women <34 weeks' gestation requiring delivery for fetal or maternal reasons when no NICU cot available.
- Unit unable to safely facilitate management of high-risk cases due to delivery suite activity, e.g. pre-eclampsia, eclampsia, antepartum hemorrhage (APH).
- Specialist neonatal care not available at local unit, e.g. elective early postnatal surgery indicated for neonate.
- Requirement of enhanced care for mother, fetus or neonate.
- Lack of availability of the appropriate level neonatal cot.
- Neonatal team request.
- Delivery suite capacity.

CONTRAINDICATIONS FOR TRANSFER

- Obstetric or neonatal staff are unable to accept transfer.
- Mother is unstable.
- There is significant risk of delivery occurring during transfer, e.g. patient in advanced labor.
- Known fetal compromise which requires immediate delivery.
- If mother refuses transfer.

BACKGROUND

NICU Cot Provision

One of the primary aims of the development of networks for the provision of neonatal intensive care is to ensure an adequate provision of neonatal intensive care cots within the local regions, thereby reducing the need for long distance transfers of mothers and their babies as well as ensuring availability of cots and appropriate staff. Ability to accurately predict those pregnant women who will deliver an infant requiring neonatal intensive care is limited. In those obstetric units where neonatal intensive care is not available, there is the need to consider transfer of expectant mothers during pregnancy. This can be elective, e.g. in the situation of an antenatally diagnosed congenital malformation which will require NICU admission such as congenital diaphragmatic hernia, or, more commonly, in the emergency situation of an obstetric complication which renders the pregnancy at risk of premature delivery.

Emergency In Utero Transfer

In the emergency situation, it is clearly recognized that the outcome following delivery of a sick, preterm infant is improved if that delivery occurs in the same unit that provides the neonatal intensive care, particularly for infants of low and very low birth weight.[10-12]

Studies on the outcome following IUTs have shown no adverse events from transfers[13] but a significant number of women transferred to a tertiary center remain undelivered. It has been estimated to be between 25% and 35%.[13,14]

Considering the costs of antenatal transfers, and the disruption to the life of the mother and her family, it is important that unnecessary transfers are kept to a minimum, while those transfers where delivery within a few days of transfer is likely are maximized.

Emergency Transfers

Emergency antenatal transfers are required when delivery of either a very preterm or other sick baby is anticipated because of spontaneous preterm labor or when obstetric complications have arisen which indicate a need for preterm delivery. These may be maternal complications like severe pre-eclampsia or fetal complications like severe IUGR with fetal compromise. In all cases, maternal safety is paramount, particularly in the situation where maternal disease and deterioration in maternal condition are the precipitating factors. It is therefore evident that good communication between midwifery, obstetric and neonatal staff on both sides of the proposed transfer is essential.

Decision to Request Transfer

The decision to request a transfer will be made after discussion between the referring obstetric team and their local neonatal team. There is considerable debate as to whose responsibility it is to find a neonatal cot and obstetric bed, but considering the fact that the referral will be made on obstetric grounds, the referring obstetric team will have the overall responsibility. Decisions to request a transfer must only be made after consultation with, and with the agreement of, the duty consultant or responsible consultant obstetrician at the referring hospital. If the referring consultant obstetrician is of the opinion that antenatal transfer is inappropriate for reasons of maternal or fetal safety, then the referring neonatologists will be required to arrange postnatal transfer. Accurate assessment of need for transfer is essential to minimize both unnecessary and repeat transfers (i.e. a mother who is transferred from her booked unit to the tertiary unit on more than one occasion which can account of up to 15% of transfers).[15]

NICU and Labor Ward Availability

The referring team will contact the NICU for cot availability. If a cot is available, the referring team will then inquire the labor ward coordinator about availability of a suitable bed for the mother. If the labor ward coordinator can accommodate the mother, then the referring team must speak to the on-call obstetric senior resident (SR) before booking transport, etc. If the receiving obstetric SR or labor ward coordinator is concerned about the advisability of accepting a transfer (e.g. concerns over safety, capacity issues) then they must discuss the case with the duty receiving consultant obstetrician who may speak to the referring consultant if required. The receiving unit must ensure that all three points of contact (NICU, labor ward coordinator and duty obstetric SR) have agreed to the transfer. The receiving on call consultant should be informed by the receiving duty obstetric SR and the transfer sanctioned (Flowchart 1).

Documentation

The referring team must send, as a minimum, a photocopy of the mother's obstetric notes. Ideally, the referring hospital notes and the mother's hand held notes should accompany the other at transfer. These notes must be returned after delivery, and this is the responsibility of the receiving obstetric team.

Threatened Preterm Labor

The diagnosis of preterm labor is difficult and inaccurate. While the definition of labor is clear (regular painful uterine contractions with progressive effacement and dilatation of the cervix with descent of the presenting part), preterm labor can be extremely rapid and silent. Therefore, there is a tendency to treat all women who complain of uterine tightening before term as being in preterm labor.

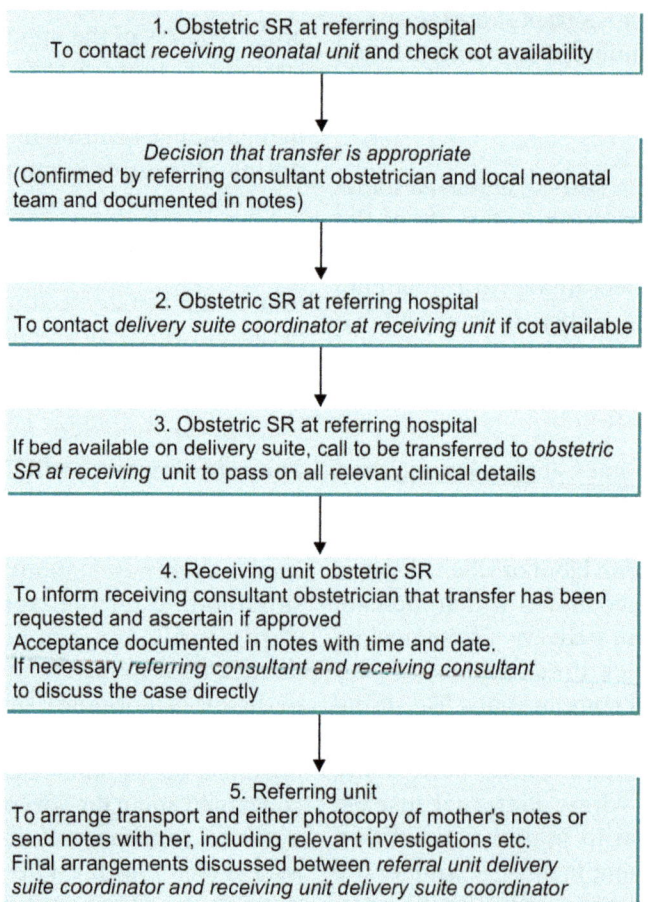

Flowchart 1: In utero transfer roles and responsibilities.

Not only does this lead to unnecessary administration of corticosteroids and tocolytics, but it also accounts for a significant proportion of unnecessary transfer of women who undergo antenatal transfer but do not deliver.

Accurate Tests for Preterm Labor

There are, however, well-established tests to help differentiate between those women who appear to be in threatened preterm labor and who will deliver and those who will not deliver in the immediate future. These include measurement of cervical length using transvaginal ultrasound,[16-18] cervical fetal fibronectin (fFN)[19] and cervical insulin-like growth factor (IgF)-binding protein (Actim Partus).[20] In order for a test to be of clinical value in screening women who are potentially in preterm labor, it must have not only good sensitivity, specificity and positive predictive value, it should be simple to use as a bedside test. Ideally, it should also be inexpensive but as it is to be used to minimize the use of more expensive options (tocolysis and IUT); the cost can be offset to some degree. The use of cervical length measurement using transvaginal ultrasound would be inappropriate as a screening test in this circumstance. However, the Hologic fFN test is a simple objective bedside test which could be performed by either a doctor or midwife.

Preterm Labor

For women who are suspected to be in preterm labor, fFN should be used and, if positive, referral made. Maternal corticosteroids should be administered with tocolysis cover. Considering the high negative predictive values for fFN for delivery within 7 days (99.5% and 94.1% respectively), a negative result would indicate that transfer was not appropriate in the absence of any other complicating factors and indeed the role for steroids carefully considered.

Antepartum Hemorrhage

Vaginal bleeding during pregnancy is a recognized risk factor for premature labor and delivery. However, in the absence of maternal or fetal compromise, management will usually be directed to reach maximum gestation before delivery. In the presence of acute maternal or fetal compromise, transfer to a tertiary unit will usually be inappropriate. Therefore, the indications for IUTs for women experiencing this complication of pregnancy are relatively few. Although no mother should be transferred if there is significant active bleeding, it may be appropriate to transfer some cases of symptomatic placenta previa as long as it is safe to do so. Careful assessment of the suitability for transfer is essential and sanctioning at consultant level.

Maternal Disease

Pre-existing medical conditions and some pregnancy complications, e.g. pre-eclampsia may require urgent or semielective preterm delivery. Such transfers will often be possible during the working day. If delivery out-of-hours is contemplated because of maternal compromise, very careful consideration must be given to the safety of both mother and fetus before IUT. If such a transfer is indicated, it is essential that all information relating to the maternal and fetal assessment is made available to the receiving unit to prevent unnecessary duplication of investigations and sanctioning at consultant level.

Fetal Compromise

Intrauterine growth restriction accounts for a significant number of referrals. Decisions about timing of delivery will usually be made on the basis of a number of factors like estimated fetal weight, evidence of central redistribution of blood flow, changes in venous Doppler, fetal activity, liquor volume and cardiotocogram. A more detailed assessment by fetomaternal specialists will allow prolongation of the gestation by a number of days, and weeks in some circumstances. Referring obstetricians are encouraged to utilize the fetal medicine service in order to gain additional information about fetal well-being if this is feasible. It is not uncommon for a mother to be transferred for delivery, but receiving unit assesses the need for delivery as less urgent. Therefore, in circumstances where there is any uncertainty about the need for urgent delivery (which will be in the majority of cases where delivery is contemplated before 34 weeks or where the estimated fetal weight is <1.5 kg) outpatient referral can be done. Mother should be informed that, while delivery is likely to be effected soon, the decision about timing of delivery will lie with the receiving unit. This approach can reduce the distress and anxiety caused by a transfer for delivery when the need to deliver is not urgent.

FEASIBILITY OF IN UTERO TRANSFER

It depends upon:
- Before anticipated delivery or an intervention (not available locally) is required, how much time is available?
- What is the travel time for reaching the nearest available appropriately staffed and resourced facility?
- Calculating the likely timing of delivery.

Factors to consider while determining the likely timing of delivery in a patient of spontaneous preterm labor in an otherwise uncomplicated pregnancy might include: preterm labor and prelabor preterm rupture of membranes (PPROM).

Preterm Labor (Flowchart 2)
- Lesser than 50% of women will deliver during the current episode who present with suspected preterm labor.

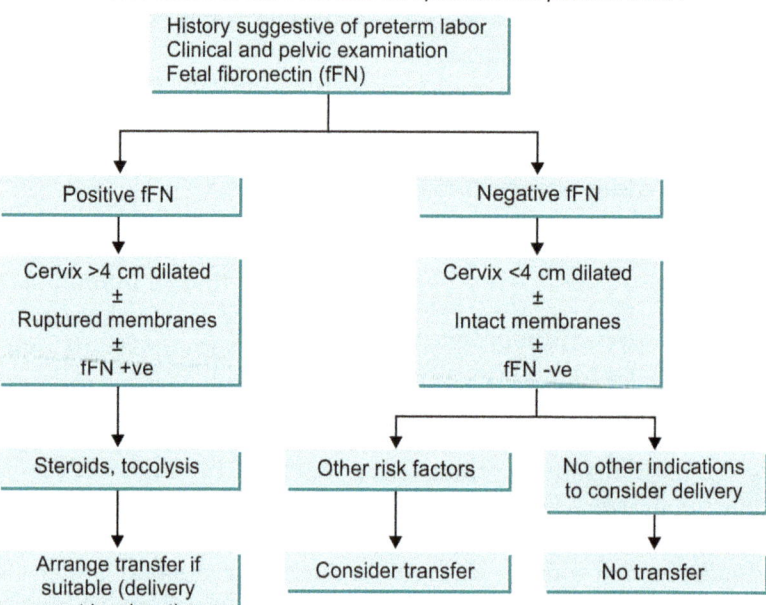

Flowchart 2: In utero transfer for spontaneous preterm labor.

- Cervical fibronectin appears to be an efficient short-term marker of preterm delivery, especially in women with symptoms of preterm labor.[21]
  - Meta-analysis shows that sensitivity of fibronectin is 77% and specificity is 87% in predicting delivery within 7 days in symptomatic women.
- Cervical length is best measured by vaginal ultrasound.
  - It is seen that about 50% of women with a cervical length of ≤15 mm deliver within 7 days.
  - Women with a cervical length of 16 mm or more, only 1% deliver within 7 days despite symptoms of preterm labor.[22]
- Cervical length of ≤15 mm, positive fibronectin level and history of preterm delivery are independent predictors of preterm delivery.
- Transfer must be considered in women with symptoms of preterm labor associated with one or more of the following: cervical length <15 mm, positive fibronectin, history of prior preterm delivery or PPROM.[23,24]

Prelabor Preterm Rupture of Membranes

- At 25–31 weeks' gestation, the median interval between rupture of membranes and delivery is 10 days and 30% of women will not have delivered by 20 days. Following PPROM transfer should be considered if there is any evidence of uterine activity or clinical chorioamnionitis (one or more of following signs: maternal pyrexia, maternal or fetal tachycardia, uterine tenderness, offensive liquor, leukocytosis).[25]
- Uterine contractions in case of PPROM are associated with a shorter interval to delivery than with intact membranes.

MANAGEMENT PRIOR TO IN UTERO TRANSFER

- The referring unit is responsible for safe, efficient and rapid transfer.
- If woman in labor cervical assessment should be done immediately prior to transfer (either digitally or using translabial/transvaginal ultrasound).
- Women in preterm labor (or threatened preterm labor) between 23 + 0 and 35 + 6 weeks of *gestation should be given betamethasone 12 mg by intramuscular injection, two doses, 12 hours apart. If this is unavailable then dexamethasone is a suitable alternative.*

MANAGEMENT DURING IN UTERO TRANSFER

- Tocolysis—to ensure safe transfer, tocolysis can be used to delay delivery. It is not required if there is no uterine activity. The efficacy of tocolysis must be assessed before transfer, i.e. complete cessation of uterine activity for at least 1 hour and no cervical change during this time.
- If delivery appears imminent during transfer, the woman will be taken to the nearest hospital with maternity facilities.

STAFFING NEEDS FOR IN UTERO TRANSFER

- Midwife—an experienced midwife should accompany the women during transfer.
- Pediatric presence is not indicated, if delivery that likely, does not consider transfer.

The following administrative conditions must be fulfilled prior to IUT being initiated:[26]
- Availability of neonatal intensive care cot in the receiving hospital
- Confirmation with the obstetric and midwifery staff that the delivery suite in the receiving hospital can accommodate the woman
- Availability of a midwife to escort the woman
- Availability of a paramedic ambulance to facilitate the transfer.

In addition, the following clinical criteria must be met immediately before patient is put in ambulance:[26]

- Mother not shocked or bleeding
- No fetal distress
- Cervix closed at internal os
- Not obviously in established labor
- Pr-labor, preterm rupture of membranes or
- Threatened preterm labor
- Stable maternal complication of pregnancy, e.g. severe IUGR + preeclamptic toxemia (PET).

PREPARATION FOR ALL TRANSFERS

- Good preparation reduces risk of deterioration in woman's condition during transfer.
- Inform clinical staff and woman of reason for transfer.
- Document events leading up to decision to transfer, together with a provisional diagnosis.
- Before transfer, provide receiving unit with written and verbal summary of woman's condition and provisional diagnosis.
- Woman and baby's medical record must accompany them when they transfer.
- Local agreements should be made with the ambulance service regarding availability at emergencies or when transfer required.
- Urgency of transfer will determine personnel required and mode of transport.
- Midwife allocated to woman should identify fetal well-being if applicable.

Accept Transfer Tool (If Used Locally)[27]

- ACCEPT transfer tool ensures structured assessment and procedure.
- Person making decision to transfer woman indicates which transfer categories apply on the ACCEPT checklist (if used locally).
  A—Assessment
  C—Control
  C—Communication
  E—Evaluation
  P—Preparation and packaging
  T—Transportation.

Equipment

- Ensure accompanying equipment functioning
- Supply sufficient drugs and fluids for entire journey
- Secure lines (e.g. IV, CVP, CBD).

Woman

- Explain reason for transfer to woman and partner and document discussion in healthcare record
- Obtain and record consent (where able)
- Stabilize woman for transfer.

Fetus

- Assess fetal well-being if appropriate.

Documentation (Requirements for Each Staff Group)

Midwife

- Documentation and handover responsibility, to include: summary of maternal transfer documented in woman's healthcare record and continue to complete appropriate tool (e.g. ACCEPT) for handover.
- Ensure full photocopy of maternal healthcare record (including EFM traces, drug charts, investigation results, etc.) accompanying woman; if not available at time of transfer, is telephoned as soon as available.

Medical Staff

- If transferring to another hospital, obstetric registrar to write detailed letter containing patient history and treatment, including:
  - Drugs prescribed and administered

- Investigation reports/results
- Fetal heart rate (FHR) trace
- Anesthetic chart (if applicable).

Prepare for Transportation

Personnel

- Qualified midwife must accompany woman.
- Specialist personnel may be required to accompany woman, depending on her condition and current condition of fetus after assessment by person(s) making decision to transfer.

Monitoring during Transportation

- Continue appropriate monitoring during ambulance transfer until handover at receiving unit.
- Both the maternal and fetal condition should be monitored safely during transfer.
- Observations should be recorded every 15 minutes or more frequently depending on the clinical situation.
- At the receiving hospital, a formal handover should take place with the obstetric team—medical and midwifery.
- The handover should be documented in the transfer proforma at receiving hospital. Only after that the mother becomes the responsibility of the receiving hospital.

Audit

In utero transfer should be subjected to close audit. The following items should be considered where possible:

- Number of deliveries occurred during transfer
- Delivery within 30 minutes of arrival at the delivery unit
- Maternal mortality or morbidity on route (like hypertensive crisis, eclampsia, hemorrhage and/or requirement for resuscitation)
- Fetal mortality en route
- Numbers of transfers occurring outside of the network
- The outcome following transfer—like the time of delivery, hospital where delivery occurred, neonatal and maternal outcome
- Maternal and neonatal outcomes in cases where requested IUT could not take place

Maternal Refusal to be Transferred

- If the mother refuses transfer, we cannot transfer her against her wishes.
- If acute IUT is considered as most appropriate course of action the senior staff can reduce the likelihood of her refusal by compassionately communicating with her.
- The mother must understand that, if IUT being declined, ex utero transfer may need to be arranged if this is in the baby's best interest.
- If the mother refuses an IUT, there should be clear documentation that the risks and benefits both to her and subsequently to her baby have been explained and understood.

REFERENCES

1. Beattie B, Bell C, Doherty C, et al. All Wales In Utero Transfer Guideline. 2011.
2. Fenton A, Peebles D, Ahluwalia J. Management of acute in utero transfers: a framework for practice. Report for the British Association of Perinatal Medicine. 2008.
3. GAIN guideline. Management of pre-eclampsia and severe eclampsia. 2012.
4. Paramanum J, Field D, Rennie J, et al. National census of availability of neonatal intensive care. British Association for Perinatal Medicine. BMJ. 2000;321:727-9.
5. Department of Health, Social Services and Public Safety (DHSSPS). Supporting Safer Services. A summary of key themes and learning from Serious Adverse Incidents reported to DHSSPSNI between 1st April 2007 and 30th April 2010. DHSSPSN; 2011.
6. National Perinatal Epidemiology Unit. Recorded delivery: a national survey of

women's experience of maternity care 2006. Oxford University Press. 2007.
7. Fenton AC, Ainsworth SB, Sturgiss SN. Population-based outcomes after acute antenatal transfer. Paed Perinatal Epid. 2002; 16(3):278-85.
8. Cusack J, Field D, Manktelow B. Impact of service changes on neonatal transfer patterns over 10 years. Arch Dis Child Fetal Neonatal Ed. 2007;92:181-4.
9. Department of Health. (2009). Toolkit for high quality neonatal services. [online] Available from: http://webarchive.nationalarchives.gov.uk/20130107105354/http:/www.dh.gov.uk/en/Publicationsandstatistics/Publications PolicyAndGuidance/DH107845 [Last accessed September, 2019].
10. Watkinson M, Mcintosh N. Outcome of neonatal intensive care: obstetric implications for a regional service. BJOG. 1986;93:711-6.
11. Chien LY, Whyte R, Aziz K, et al. Improved outcome of preterm infants when delivered in tertiary care centers. Obstet Gynecol. 2001;98:247-52.
12. Hohlagschwandtner M, Husslein P, Klebermaß-Schrehof K, et al. Perinatal mortality and morbidity. Comparison between maternal transport, neonatal transport and inpatient antenatal treatment. Arch Gynecol Obstet. 2001;265:113-8.
13. Fenton AC, Ainsworth SB, Sturgiss SN. Population-based outcomes after antenatal transfer. Paediatr Perinat Epidemiol. 2002;16:278-85.
14. Roberts CL, Smart DH, Ellwood DA. Antenatal transfer of rural women to perinatal centres. Aust N Z J Obstet Gynaecol. 2000;40:377-84.
15. Gill AB, Bottomley L, Chatfield S, et al. Perinatal transport: problems in neonatal intensive care capacity. Arch Dis Child Fetal Neonatal Ed. 2004;89:F220-3.
16. Sanin-Blair J, Palacio M, Delgado J, et al. Impact of ultrasound cervical length assessment on duration of hospital stay in the clinical management of threatened preterm labor. Ultrasound Obstet Gynecol. 2004;24:756-60.
17. Daskalakis G, Thomakos N, Hatziioannou L, et al. Cervical assessment in women with threatened preterm labor. J Matern Fetal Neonatal Med. 2005;17:309-12.
18. Tekesin I, Wallwiener D, Schmidt S. The value of quantitative ultrasound tissue characterization of the cervix and rapid fetal fibronectin in predicting preterm delivery. J Perinat Med. 2005;33:383-91.
19. Peaceman AM, Andrews WW, Thorp JM, et al. Fetal fibronectin as a predictor of preterm birth in patients with symptoms: a multicenter trial. Am J Obstet Gynecol. 1997;177:13-8.
20. Lembet A, Eroglu D, Ergin T, et al. New rapid bed-side test to predict preterm delivery: phosphorylated insulin-like growth factor binding protein-1 in cervical secretions. Acta Obstet Gynecol Scand. 2002;81:706-12.
21. Leitich H, Kaider A. Fetal fibronectin—how useful is it in the prediction of preterm birth? BJOG. 2003;110 Suppl 20:66-70.
22. Nicolaides KH, Tsoi E, To MS, et al. Sonographic measurement of cervical length and preterm delivery. In: Critchley HO, Bennett PR, Thornton S (Eds). Preterm Birth. London: RCOG Press; 2004. pp. 124-39.
23. Goldenberg RL, Iams JD, Mercer BM, et al. The Preterm Prediction Study: toward a multiple-marker test for spontaneous preterm birth. Am J Obstet Gynecol. 2001;185:643-51.
24. Tekesin I, Eberhart LH, Schaefer V, et al. Evaluation and validation of a new risk score (CLEOPATRA score) to predict the probability of premature delivery for patients with threatened preterm labor. Ultrasound Obstet Gynecol. 2005;26:699-706.
25. Farooqi A, Holmgren PA, Engberg S, et al. Survival and 2-year outcome with expectant management of second-trimester rupture of membranes. Obstet Gynecol. 1998;92:895-901.
26. Royal Berkshire NHS Foundation Trust. (2018). Annual Report and Accounts 2017 to 2018. [online] Available from: www.royalberkshire.nhs.uk [Last accessed September, 2019].
27. Maternal transfer. (2013-15). [online] Available from: http://www.networks.nhs.uk [Last accessed September, 2019].

Delivery in Emergency Department

Sowmya Davuluri

INTRODUCTION

Labor and delivery in the emergency department (ED) is rare and when required the emergency physician has to take the role of an obstetrician. Pregnancy-related problems are the fifth common reason for presentation to the ED.[1] The preparation and management of an unexpected delivery in the ED can be anxiety provoking. The ED physician must possess the basic skills for intrapartum management of both normal and abnormal deliveries. The obstetrician has to be informed immediately. In an emergent situation, the ED personnel should be able to recognize labor and its complications, followed by an assessment of the maternal and the fetal status and reassurance to the family.

ASSESSMENT OF THE PREGNANT MOTHER ON ARRIVAL IN THE EMERGENCY DEPARTMENT

Assessment of the pregnant mother on arrival in the emergency department has been labeled in Tables 1 and 2.

While assessing the fetus and the pregnant mother arrange for delivery or the operating theater for emergency cesarean.

What to Expect When a Pregnant Lady Comes to ER (Table 3)?

If considering to transfer the patient to a labor room at a tertiary center, the clinician has to consider certain factors like—the transit time to the hospital, the maternal status (parity and stage of labor), if labor is imminent, and availability of obstetrician. Informed consent must be taken before shifting the patient and before taking the patient for delivery.

If the placental location is unknown—avoid per vaginal examination.

Blood and blood products: If there is an ongoing massive obstetric hemorrhage, the need for initiating a massive transfusion protocol with group and type-specific blood/O negative-packed cells and fresh frozen plasma (FFP).

- Informed consent (written/video consent)
- Debriefing the attenders about the patients' condition and need for delivery in the ED
- *Need for emergency interventions*: Instrumental delivery, perimortem cesarean section, and blood transfusion
- Need for surgical intervention specific to the associated morbidities
- Need for intensive care unit/high dependency unit (ICU/HDU) for the mother and neonatal intensive care unit (NICU) for the neonate
- Risk of infection to the mother and the neonate due to delivery in the ED
- Risk of maternal mortality and neonatal morbidity/mortality.

CONTENTS OF EMERGENCY DELIVERY TRAY

Contents of emergency delivery tray have been given in Box 1.

Obstetric Emergencies

TABLE 1: Assessment of the pregnant mother on arrival in the emergency department.

History	• Presenting complaint • Period of amenorrheas • Prior obstetric history • Significant antepartum, intrapartum and postpartum events in the previous pregnancy/present pregnancy • Bleeding/leak per vagina/convulsions • History of fall or trauma • History relevant to cardiac/renal diseases/anemia/fever/loss of consciousness
Clinical examination	• Pallor/icterus/cyanosis/edema/petechiae/rashes • Temperature–hypothermia (evidence of shock), hyperthermia (evidence of infection) • Tachypnea, dyspnea • Tachycardia (Hemorrhage), Bradycardia (septic shock) • Altered sensorium (dyselectrolytemia, hypoglycemia, profound hypoxia • Oliguria, anuria (AKI secondary to hemorrhage), hematuria • *Obstetric examination:* Per abdominal—to assess the frequency, duration, location and the intensity of contractions • *Digital examination:* True labor or false labor—pelvic assessment • Assessment of stage labour, dilatation effacement of the cervix, station of the head/presenting part • Presence or absence of the membranes • Meconium stain—yes or no?
Lab investigations	• Complete hemogram, blood group and Rh type • Blood urea and S. creatinine • Liver function tests • Serum electrolytes • In hemorrhagic patient/DIC-coagulation profile, fibrinogen, FDP, D-Dimer in suspected sepsis—septic work up including cultures, markers like CRP and procalcitonin imaging modalities—USG/MR/Conventional X-rays

(DIC: disseminated intravascular coagulation; FDP: fibrin degradation product; CRP: C-reactive protein; USG: ultrasonography; MR: magnetic resonance imaging)

TABLE 2: Assessment of pregnant women on arrival in the emergency department.

A-Airway: Secure airway

B-Breathing: O_2 by mask or higher levels of respiratory support as indicated

C-Circulation: Secure an 18G cannula, crystalloids/Volume expanders if required

D-Drugs: Adrenaline, Atropine, Efcorlin

E-Ecbolics: Oxytocin, prostaglandins, ergot alkaloids

F-Fetal parameters: Cardiotocography, Doppler's, growth assessment, modified BPP score if feasible

Box 1: Contents of emergency delivery tray.

- Sterile gloves
- Gown, towels, and drapes
- Povidone-iodine—to clean the perineum
- Sponges-1
- Allis and Kochers clamps—to rupture the membranes
- Cord clamp—for cord
- 1 sterile curved scissors and 1 straight scissors, episiotomy scissors
- Towel for the infant
- Obstetric forceps, vacuum
- Suction catheter and tubing
- Bag valve mask device, laryngeal mask, and ET tube
- Oxygen source, oxygen saturation probe, and monitor
- Radiant warmer, warm blankets, and towels
- Drugs—oxytocin, prostaglandins, methergin, misoprostol, adrenaline, atropine, volume expanders like hemocele and steroid
- Defibrillator

PRECIPITOUS DELIVERY

It is a common scenario in multiparous women.

Risk of perineal tears, lacerations, and atonicity is common. Prompt identification of tear and repair is important. Use of uterotonics to correct the uterine atony is suggested.

After delivery, the neonate should be vigorously dried, and placed in a warmer and the nose and mouth should be suctioned.

SPECIAL SITUATIONS

Cardiopulmonary Resuscitation

Maternal resuscitation includes management of the airway, cardiopulmonary resuscitation (CPR), fluids, and advanced life support protocols (Flowchart 1).

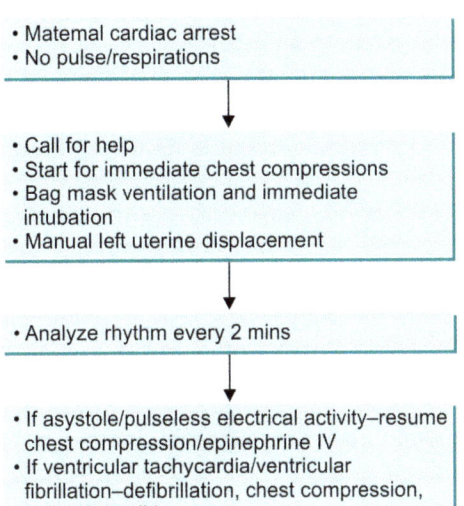

Flowchart 1: Maternal resuscitation.

Perimortem Cesarean Section

Perimortem cesarean is done primarily to save the mother, as delivery of the fetus relieves the aortocaval compression and helps to restore the hemodynamic stability by increasing the venous return and cardiac output.[2]

The incidence of perimortem cesarean delivery (PMCS) is 1 in 30,000 cases.[3]

This procedure if done at the right time can yield up to 15% of viable infants.

Indications (Flowchart 2)

Cardiac arrest accounts for 1 in 30,000[4] cases, while the incidence of a significant trauma complicating a pregnancy is 6–8%. All these conditions increase the risk of preterm labor, abruptio placenta, and fetomaternal hemorrhages. CPR has to be continued throughout the procedure (Table 3).

Contraindications of Perimortem Cesarean

- Return to spontaneous circulation after resuscitation
- Gestational age <24 weeks
- If no fetal cardiac activity.

ANTICIPATED COMPLICATIONS DURING DELIVERY

Shoulder dystocia:
- Call for help
- Episiotomy

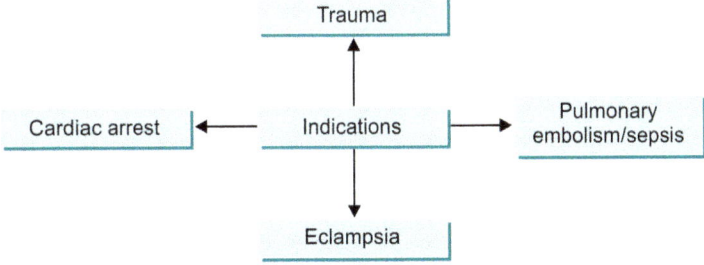

Flowchart 2: Indications for perimortem cesarean.

Obstetric Emergencies

TABLE 3: What to expect when a pregnant lady comes to emergency department.

Systems involved	Symptoms	Signs	Differential diagnosis	Indication	Management
Cardiovascular system	Palpitations, shortness of breath, swelling of the extremities	Pedal edema, basal crepts, tender hepatomegaly, and raised JVP	Cardiac failure and peripartum cardiomyopathy	Cardiac arrest	• When resuscitation fails and with fetal viability (>28 weeks)—perform cesarean section • When fetus <23 weeks—delivering the fetus does not help in improving the venous return as the cardiovascular changes are not profound, aggressive resuscitation to be performed[5] • If no return to spontaneous circulation within 4 minutes—emergency cesarean should be performed[6] • The possibility of a neurologically intact fetus increases when the interval between the arrest and resuscitation is short[7]
Respiratory system	Shortness of breath and productive cough	Wheeze and rhonchi	Pneumonia, bronchial asthma, H1N1 virus, and pulmonary embolism	Trauma	• Blunt trauma accounts for 70% of the cases—car accidents • Penetrating injuries—gunshot wounds and knives • Management depends on the location of the injury and the amount of blood loss • If gestational is beyond viability (>28 weeks)—consider delivering the fetus • If below viability and if the fetus is not compromised—continue with fetal surveillance • If maternal health is jeopardized—consider terminating the pregnancy in maternal interest
Genitourinary	Anuria, oliguria, hematuria, and dysuria	Pedal edema, facial puffiness, secondary hypertension, and renal angle tenderness	Acute/chronic renal failure, pyelonephritis, glomerulonephritis, and renal colic	Eclampsia	• Can also be due to magnesium sulfate toxicity
Hepatobiliary	Nausea, vomiting, pain abdomen, and itching	Icterus, tenderness in the right upper quadrant	Acute cholecystitis, acute pancreatitis, and intrahepatic cholecystitis		
Gastrointestinal	Pain in the upper quadrant of abdomen, vomiting	Tenderness in epigastric region	Gastric ulcer and duodenal ulcer/perforation		

- McRoberts maneuver to flex the legs
- Application of suprapubic pressure and pressure on the shoulder
- Rotational and interval maneuvers, delivery of the posterior arm.

Prolapsed Umbilical Cord

This condition results in 8–49% of perinatal mortality. Usually presents in the second stage of labor associated with a malpresentation. Also follows the rupture of membranes and in cases of polyhydramnios (Flowchart 3).[8]

After delivery—collect the cord blood samples for pH.

Cord entanglement—could result due to excess fetal movements in the early pregnancy. Immediate delivery and prevention of further traction are important.

Breech presentation—call the obstetrician immediately and allow the delivery to happen spontaneously till the umbilicus is visible or shift immediately to the operating room.

NEONATAL CARE AFTER THE DELIVERY

- Keep the baby dry and warm to maintain the temperature
- Establish airway, suction the secretions
- Stimulate the baby to cry
- *Establish effective ventilation*: Bag mask—valve/endotracheal intubation
- Chest compressions
- *Drugs*: Vitamin K injection.

LIMITATIONS OF DELIVERY IN THE EMERGENCY DEPARTMENT

- Limitations of delivery in the emergency department
- No experienced personnel
- *Unavailability of monitoring instruments*:
  - Tocodynamometry
  - Ultrasound
  - NST machine

Improper equipment and set up:
- Vacuum extractors
- Forceps
- Lack of instruments
- No prenatal history
- Increased maternal morbidity
- Increased risk of unexpected complications
- Increased risk of injuries to the bladder and ureters
- Increased risk of needle pricks and injuries.

CONCLUSION

Delivery in the ED is a challenge in itself. However, delivering a healthy baby with

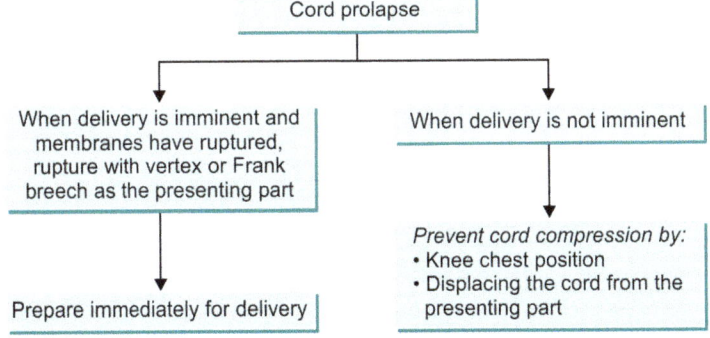

Flowchart 3: Management of cord prolapse in the emergency department.

a healthy mother would be a feasibility, if executed by a trained medical personnel. Lack of competence is the most important limiting factor rather than lack of relevant drugs and equipment. Hence training of healthcare personnel in the ED should be the priority. Checking clinical competence through vignettes,[9] could contribute to a more comprehensive approach to handle this complex problem.

REFERENCES

1. Centre of disease control and prevention. (2011). National hospital ambulatory medical care survey. [online] Available from: https://www.cdc.gov/nchs/data/ahcd/nhamcs_emergency/2011_ed_web_tables.pdf [Last accessed September, 2019].
2. DePace NL, Betesh JL, Kotler MN. Post mortem cesarean section with recovery of both mother and the offspring. JAMA. 1982;248:971-3.
3. Blackham J. Perimortem Caesarean section for the nonobstetrician. [online] Available from: https://www.rcem.ac.uk//docs/CPDConference/3.4.17%20-%2012.15-12.35%20-%20Jules%20Blackham%20-%20Perimortem%20Caesarean%20section%20for%20the%20non-obstetrician.pdf [Last accessed September, 2019].
4. Mallampalli A, Powner DJ, Gardner MO. Cardiopulmonary resuscitation and somatic support of the pregnant patient. Crit Care Clin. 2004;20(4):747-61.
5. Muench MV, Canterino JC. Trauma in pregnancy. Obstet Gynecol Clin North Am. 2007;34(3):555-83.
6. Vanden Hoek TL, Morrison LJ, Shuster M, et al. Part 12: cardiac arrest in special situations: 2010 American Heart Association Guidelines for Cardiopulmonary Resuscitation and Emergency Cardiovascular Care. Circulation. 2010;122(18 Suppl 3):S829-61.
7. Gunevsel O, Yesil O, Ozturk TC, et al. Perimortem caesarean section following maternal gunshot wounds. J Res Med Sci. 2011;16(8):1089-91.
8. Anderson GV Jr, Anderson GV Sr. Umbilical cord prolapse in the emergency department. J Emergency Department. 1989(7)(2):207.
9. Lohela TJ, Nesbitt RC, Manu A, et al. Competence of health workers in emergency obstetric care: an assessment using clinical vignettes in Brong Ahafo region, Ghana. BMJ Open. 2006;6(6): e010963.

CHAPTER 49

Induction of Labor

Karthigayeni Rathinam

INTRODUCTION

Induction of labor (IOL) is the initiation of labor artificially before its spontaneous onset in order to deliver the fetoplacental unit.

Over the past decades, the IOL incidence has raised. It is one of the most commonly practiced interventions in the era of modern obstetrics. The infants delivered by IOL are found to be as high as one in five deliveries.[1,2]

The goal of IOL is to achieve a vaginal delivery in a more natural way successfully.

DEFINITION

Induction of labor is defined as the process of stimulating the uterus artificially to start labor.[3]

Augmentation of labor is defined as the process of stimulating the uterus after the spontaneous onset of labor in order to increase the duration, frequency, and intensity of uterine contractions.[4]

RECOMMENDATIONS FOR IOL[3]

- Performed only if there is a clear indication and the expected benefits are more compared to its potential harm.
- Consider the women's wish and preferences along with the emphasis on cervical status, method of IOL, and associated conditions like rupture of membrane and parity.
- Since the procedure is associated with the risk of uterine hyperstimulation and rupture, and fetal distress, it should be performed with caution.
- Should be carried out in a center where facilities for assessing maternal and fetal well-being are available.
- Never leave a woman unattended, if she was induced with oxytocin or prostaglandins.
- Failed IOL does not indicate cesarean section necessarily.
- Better to carry out IOL in centers where facilities for cesarean section are available.

COUNSELING THE COUPLE PRIOR TO INDUCTION

The following should be discussed during the counseling:[5]
- Indication for IOL, more specific about the risk of continuing the pregnancy
- Method and time of IOL
- Pain relief measures
- Close monitoring of the fetal heart rate (FHR)
- Risk associated with IOL
- Available alternative options, if she refuses IOL
- The chance of failure and available options in such cases.

EVALUATION BEFORE IOL

Before proceeding with IOL evaluate both maternal and fetal conditions (Table 1).

TABLE 1: Evaluation before induction of labor (IOL).	
Maternal	Fetal
• Confirm the indication • Rule out contraindication for normal delivery or labor • Clinical pelvimetry to assess pelvis adequacy • Cervical assessment (Assign Bishop score) • Review the benefit, risk, and alternatives of IOL	• Confirm gestational age • Ensure the fetal lung maturity status • Estimated fetal weight • Fetal presentation and lie • Confirm fetal well-being

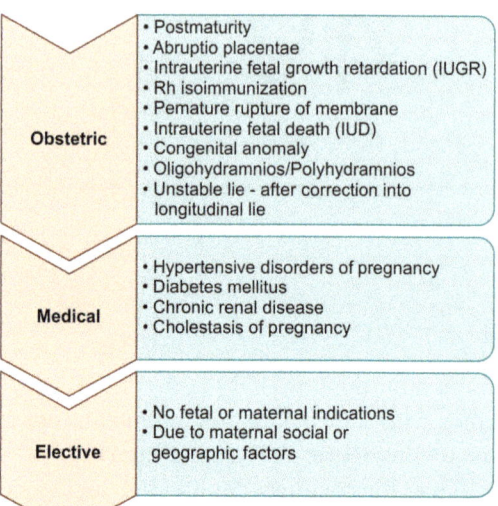

Flowchart 1: Indications for labor induction.

INDICATIONS OF IOL (FLOWCHART 1 AND TABLE 2)

Elective Induction of Labor

- In spite of overall increase, the IOL in clinically indicated cases is lower suggesting a rise in elective IOL[19]
- With elective IOL modest increase in operative vaginal delivery has been observed, might be due to higher usage of epidural analgesia[20]
- Twofold increased risk of cesarean delivery in nulliparous women undergoing elective IOL at term[21]
- But there is no increased risk of cesarean delivery in multiparous women undergoing elective IOL at term with favorable cervix[20]
- Elective IOL in women with appropriately calculated gestational age had no significant change in terms of perinatal outcome.[22]

CONTRAINDICATIONS FOR IOL

The contraindications for induction of labor are listed in Table 3.

Induction of labor includes two components as shown in Figure 1.

CERVICAL RIPENING

Before the labor onset the cervix becomes complaint and soft allowing the cervix to be thinned out (effaced) and starting to open (dilate). It occurs either naturally or by physical or pharmacological interventions.[5]

Cervical ripening occurs due to following factors (Fig. 2):

- Cervical examination is essential before IOL since the condition of the cervix influences the success of IOL.
- Bishop in 1964 developed a scoring system to assess the multiparous women undergoing elective IOL at term (Table 4).
- Later it was modified by Calder in 1974 (Table 5):
  - Score 3 or less has an increased chance of cesarean section
  - Score 6 or more has a higher probability of vaginal delivery.

METHODS OF INDUCTION OF LABOR (FLOWCHART 2)

Mechanical Methods

Stripping of Membrane

- Sweeping of the membrane involves separation of the chorion from decidua so there is an increase in prostaglandin F2 (PGF2) secretion leading to initiation of labor.[23] Exploration of cervix manually

TABLE 2: Indications for induction of labor (IOL).

Indication	Evidence
Post-term pregnancy	• Two systematic reviews are in favor of IOL after 41 or 42 completed gestational weeks[6,7] • IOL compared to expectant management had less perinatal deaths and cesarean sections. Meconium aspiration syndrome was found to be reduced in IOL group, but no significant difference in terms of NICU admission[6] • In uncomplicated singleton pregnancies, IOL reduces the rate of cesarean deliveries without affecting perinatal outcomes[7]
Prelabor rupture of membranes (PROM) at term	Planned management either with oxytocin or prostaglandin compared to expectant management is associated with lesser maternal infections and fewer neonatal intensive care admissions without increasing operative vaginal delivery or cesarean section[8]
Preterm prelabor rupture of membranes (PPROM)	A systematic review analyzed four randomized controlled trial (RCT) in women with PPROM between 30 and 36 weeks of gestation comparing immediate IOL with expectant management. They concluded that immediate IOL is associated with significantly lesser incidence of chorioamnionitis and reduced duration of maternal hospital stay[9]
Suspected macrosomia	• IOL is associated with increased cesarean section rate with no improvement in terms of perinatal outcome[10] • The maternal or neonatal morbidity risk is not altered by IOL in nondiabetic women[11]
Suspected intrauterine fetal growth restriction (IUGR)	• A randomized trial compared immediate delivery versus delayed delivery in women with fetal compromise between 24 and 36 weeks and was found to have insufficient evidence to prove which is better over other[12] • No significant difference was found between the induction and expectant management group in terms of neonatal morbidity rate and obstetric intervention in clinically suspected IUGR at term[13]
Oligohydramnios	No significant difference was found between IOL group and expectant management group in terms of neonatal or maternal outcome[14]
Diabetes mellitus requiring insulin	Limited evidence to suggest either elective delivery or expectant management at term is effective[15]
Hypertension/pre-eclampsia/eclampsia	In severe preeclampsia with preterm, elective cesarean section was found to have better perinatal outcome compared to vaginal delivery or emergency cesarean section following IOL[16]
Intrahepatic cholestasis of pregnancy	In addition to monitoring of fetal wellbeing, elective delivery at 37 weeks is associated with reduced stillbirth rate significantly without increasing the cesarean delivery rate[17]
Congenital anomaly	No significant benefit was found by elective preterm delivery in a RCT done in fetus with gastroschisis[18]

TABLE 3: Contraindications for induction of labor (IOL).

Absolute	Relative
• Cephalopelvic disproportion • Major placenta previa • Vasa previa • Cord prolapse • Transverse lie • Active primary genital herpes • Previous classical cesarean section	• Breech presentation • Triplet or higher order pregnancy • Two or more previous low transverse cesarean sections

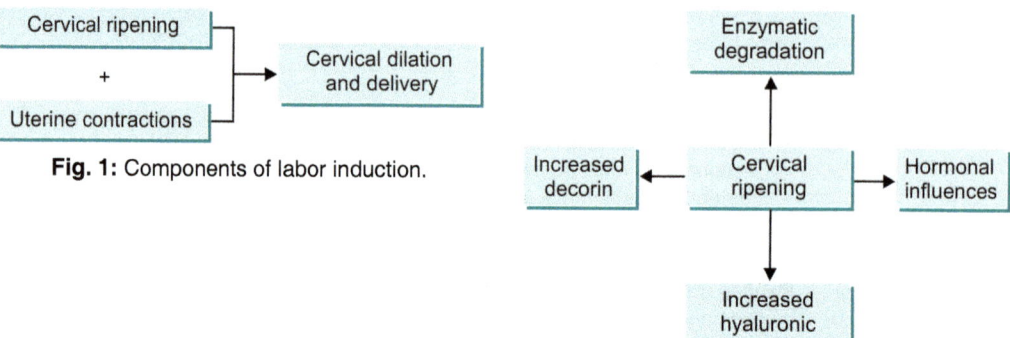

Fig. 1: Components of labor induction.

Fig. 2: Factors causing cervical ripening.

TABLE 4: Bishop score (1964).

	0	1	2	3
Dilatation (cm)	0	1–2	3–4	5–6
Effacement (%)	0–30	40–60	60–70	80+
Station (cm)	−3	−2	−1/0	+1/+2
Consistency	Firm	Medium	Soft	
Position	Posterior	Mid position	Anterior	

TABLE 5: Modified Bishop score (1974).

	0	1	2	3
Dilatation (cm)	<1	1–2	2–4	>4
Length (cm)	>4	2–4	1–2	<1
Station	−3	−2	−1/0	+1/+2
Consistency	Firm	Average	Soft	
Position	Posterior	Middle or anterior		

triggers the Ferguson reflex hence promoting the release of oxytocin from maternal pituitary.
- Technically, for doing the procedure the cervical scoring should be at least more than 4.[24]
- Cochrane review has suggested that routine use of membrane stripping from 38 weeks of gestation does not have any clinical benefits, although it was associated with reduced pregnancy duration and reduced chance to continue pregnancy beyond 41 weeks.[25]
- There was observed a reduced proportion of women with postdated pregnancy, if membrane stripping was performed at 41 weeks of pregnancy.[26]
- Membrane sweeping can be offered to all women (nullipara at 40 and 41 weeks, multipara at 41 weeks) before the formal IOL.[5]

Transcervical Catheter and Extra-amniotic Saline Instillation

First described in 1967, it is cheap and safer method:

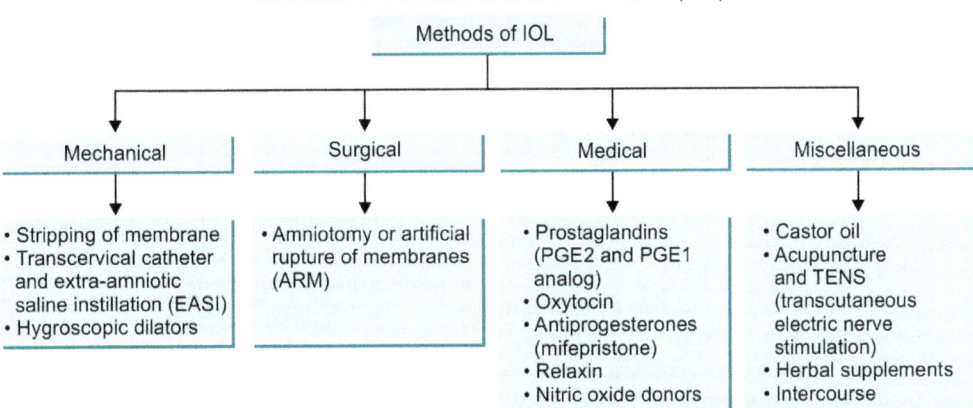

Flowchart 2: Methods of induction of labor (IOL).

- *Advantage*:
  - Combination of balloon catheter with oxytocin is an alternative method when prostaglandins are not available or contraindicated (previous cesarean)
  - Useful for outpatient ripening
  - Inserted irrespective of presence or absence of membranes
  - Associated with favorable Bishop scores
  - No additional side effects.
- *Mechanism of action*:
  - Foley catheter improves the cervical score by its mechanical effect and also it strips the fetal membranes from the lower segment of the uterus causing release of phospholipase A, causing prostaglandin formation.
- *Methodology and evidences*:
  - Foley's catheter or designer balloon devices inserted intracervically
  - Once placed beyond the internal os of cervix, the catheter or balloon is inflated with 30–50 mL saline
  - To the catheter end, attach either a defined weight [1 liter of intravenous (IV) fluid] or "gentle tugs" are used at a count of 2–4 every hour until the balloon or the catheter passes out
  - Extra-amniotic saline infusion at the rate of 1 cc/minute is also recommended. But there are conflicting reports regarding the addition of extra-amniotic saline instillation (EASI) to the balloon catheter[27]
  - Preinduction cervical ripening with EASI along with oxytocin was found to be better than Foley and prostaglandins E2 (PGE2) in terms of Bishop score and labor outcomes[28]
  - There is no evidence of infection associated with this method
  - Cochrane review has concluded that mechanical methods of IOL results in similar cesarean rates compared to prostaglandins with lower risk of uterine hyperstimulation and with reduced risk of cesarean deliveries compared to oxytocin.[29]

Hygroscopic Dilators

- Natural or synthetic rods are inserted through the cervical os and left in situ for a particular time. Natural dilators are obtained from the *Laminaria japonica* (seaweed)
- They absorb local tissue fluid and endocervical fluid due to their osmotic properties. This causing swelling of the dilator hence leading to dilatation of the cervix with release of prostaglandins due to stripping of fetal membranes from the lower segment of the uterus.[5]

Surgical Methods

Amniotomy or Artificial Rupture of Membranes

Ideally, artificial rupture of membranes (ARM) should be performed, if the cervix is effaced and at least 2 cm dilated but can be done with minimal cervical dilatation also:

- *Methodology of ARM*:
  - First auscultate the FHR
  - Cervix and station of the fetal head should be evaluated. The cervix should be well applied to the fetal head
  - Introduce two fingers into the cervix, sweep the membranes away from the cervix
  - Between the groove of your two fingers, pass an Kocher's or Allis forceps, hook the membranes and rupture them
  - Look for the clarity of liquor.
- *Risks*:
  - Cord prolapse
  - Fetal heart rate deceleration
  - Bleeding through vasa previa
  - Fetal injury
  - Maternal and fetal infection.
- *Advantages*:
  - It shortens duration of labor
  - Allows for early diagnosis of meconium staining of amniotic fluid,
  - Specially in high-risk pregnancy
  - Facilitates invasive fetal monitoring.

As primary method of IOL amniotomy alone is not recommended unless other pharmacological methods of IOL are contraindicated.[5]

As primary method of IOL amniotomy with oxytocin is not recommended unless there is specific contraindication for vaginal PGE2 usage.[5]

Medical Methods

Prostaglandins (PGE2 and PGE1 Analog)

Prostaglandin E2 analog:
- Prostaglandin E2 gel is widely used method of IOL

- *Mechanism of action*:
  - Alters the cervical extracellular grounds substance (by increasing elastase, glycosaminoglycans, collagenase, hyaluronic acid, and dermatan sulfate levels)
  - Smooth muscle of the cervix are relaxed
  - Formation of gap junction leading to uterine contractions.
- *Preparation and dosage*:
  - *Prostaglandin E2 gel*:
    - Contains 0.5 mg of PGE2
    - Before using the gel bring it to room temperature and instill the gel in the cervical canal below the internal os
    - After insertion the woman should lie in the supine position for 15–30 minutes
    - Repeat the gel insertion, if no response after 6 hours
    - Over a period of 24 hours maximum of three insertions or 1.5 mg are allowed.
  - *Intravaginal PGE2 gel*:
    - Vaginal PGE2 gel—contains 2.5 mg PGE2
    - Two doses are recommended 6 hours apart
    - Vaginal controlled release insert (Cervidil)—10 mg insert releases 0.3 mg/hours of the prostaglandin. No need to prewarm the insert. The patient should lie supine for 2 hours following the insertion. The insert is to be removed after 12 hours or when active labor begins or in case of hyperstimulation
    - Oral prostaglandin (PGE2) has no clear advantage over other methods of IOL with higher gastrointestinal side effects[30]
    - Intravaginal PGE2 are preferred to intracervical preparations as they are equally effective and

intravaginal PGE 2 administration is less invasive. Tablets are recommended to use than gels as they are equally effective and cheaper as well.[5]

- *Contraindications*:
  - Established uterine activity
  - Glaucoma
  - Asthma
  - Severe hepatic or renal impairment
  - Known hypersensitivity to prostaglandins
  - Active vaginal bleeding:
    - For administration of PGE2, Bishop's score should ideally be less than 4. Administer the drug near the delivery suite. After instillation women should lie recumbent for 30 minutes[1]
    - Uterine activity and FHR should be monitored once in 30 minutes for 2 hours. If FHR is normal and no increase in uterine activity the women may be transferred elsewhere[1]
    - The controlled release insert should be removed at labor onset. Oxytocin must be avoided for initial 6-12 hours.[1]

PGE1 analog:
- Misoprostol is a synthetic PGE1 analog initially used in treatment of peptic ulcer. Further studies showed that intravaginal misoprostol causes abortion in first and second trimester and recently was found to cause cervical ripening and hence used in labor induction.
- *Pharmacokinetics*:
  - After an oral administration, peak plasma concentration is achieved earlier and higher
  - But after vaginal administration, the peak levels attained slowly but sustained for longer time compared to oral route
  - Systemic bioavailability of the drug was found to be three times higher with the vaginal route.
- *Advantages*:
  - Cheaper drug
  - Does not require storage conditions
  - Can be given by oral, buccal, or vaginal routes, although vaginal route is the most commonly used.
- *Dosage and usage*:
  - Tablets are available as either 100 µg or 200 µg
  - *Dosage*: 25-50 µg is administered 4-6 hourly
  - The tablet is inserted into the posterior vaginal fornix, prior to insertion one may or may not wet the tablet with saline
  - At term 25 µg should be the initial dose for IOL and frequency of administration should not be more than 3-6 hours. Within 4 hours after the last dose of PGE1 tablet oxytocin should not be administered[1]
  - Drug should not be used in women with major uterine surgery or with previous cesarean delivery[1]
  - Higher dosage 50 µg might be of use in some situations but with an increased risk of uterine hyperstimulation and rupture.[1]
- There is insufficient evidence regarding the safety of misoprostol in women with suspected fetal macrosomia and multiple gestations.[1]
- In presence of ruptured membranes for IOL, misoprostol is found to be more effective compared to oxytocin or vaginal PGE2. Compared to vaginal route, oral misoprostol appears to be less effective. However, oral route has lesser incidence of uterine hypercontractility with higher incidence of meconium stained amniotic liquor.[5]

- Insufficient data regarding the buccal and sublingual misoprostol for IOL.[31]
- The safety issues surrounding the use of misoprostol have not been clearly evaluated.[5]

Oxytocin

- It is a polypeptide hormone, which acts as potent uterotonic and it is secreted from the posterior pituitary gland. The drug was first used intravenously for IOL in 1948. Since then it is one of the most commonly used drug for IOL.
- *Pharmacokinetics and mechanism of action*:
  - Half-life is about 3–5 minutes
  - Act on oxytocin receptors (OTR) present on the myometrium
  - Oxytocin once it gets bind to OTR, it causes increase in the concentration of intracellular calcium which leads to myometrial cell contraction
  - Prostaglandin are increased during oxytocin administration and uterine contractions are stimulated via calcium-independent mechanism
  - It is considered that prostaglandin release due to oxytocin is needed to establish full efficient uterine contractions.
- *Routes of administration*:
  - By any parenteral route, oxytocin can be administered, but IV route is the most widely used route
  - Also absorbed from the buccal or nasal mucosa, however, gets inactivated by trypsin, if used orally.
- *Dosing and usage*:
  - About 10–20 units are dissolved in 1,000 mL of balanced salt solution (ringer lactate solution or normal saline) making it as 10–20 mU/mL and it is preferable to give it through an infusion pump
  - Further increments are made according to the low-dose or high-dose protocol given below (Table 6)
  - After IV infusion, within 3–5 minutes of administration uterine response happens and in about 40 minutes a steady plasma level is reached
  - The endpoint should be to obtain uterine contractions in every 2–3 minutes each lasting for 60–90 seconds and a uterine pressure of 50–60 mm Hg or 150 Montevideo units.
- *Risks of oxytocin*:
  - Uterine hyper stimulation, with or without FHR changes
  - Failed induction with need for repeat induction or possibly cesarean
  - Increased risk for uterine rupture in some studies
  - Hypotension if administered by IV bolus
  - Hyponatremia if administered with large amounts of sodium poor fluids

TABLE 6: Protocol for oxytocin dosage.

Regimen	Starting dose (mU/min)	Incremental dose (mU/min)	Dosage interval (min)
Low dose	0.5–1	1	30–40
	1–2	2	15
High dose	6	6	15
	6	6, 3*, and 1*	20–40

Note:* The incremental increase in dose is reduced to 3 mU/min in case of hyperstimulation and further reduced to 1 mU/min in case of recurrent hyperstimulation

- Antidiuretic hormone like effect if administered at high dose[32]
- Increased risk for neonatal hyperbilirubinemia.
- *Contraindications*:
  - Unfavorable fetal positions
  - Uterine tachysystole
  - Hypersensitivity to the drug
  - Cases where vaginal delivery is contraindicated, such as complete placenta previa, vasa previa, and cord prolapse.
- There are no data regarding safety and efficacy of contraction patterns in women with a prior cesarean delivery, with twins, or with an over distended uterus
- Compared to use of oxytocin alone, when it was combined with amniotomy it was found to be associated with increased vaginal deliveries in women with unfavorable cervix and also fewer instrumental deliveries. However, they had higher postpartum hemorrhage and more dissatisfaction with the treatment[33]
- Following vaginal prostaglandins administration oxytocin should not be commenced for 6 hours. If membranes are intact, it is recommended to perform amniotomy prior to oxytocin infusion if feasible[5]
- Recommended to use minimal dose of oxytocin and it should be titrated against uterine contractions. Maximum-licensed dose for usage is 20 mU/min and it should not be more than 32 mU/min.[5]

Mifepristone (RU 486)

- It is a progesterone receptor antagonist
- Rational for its use is that fall in progesterone was found to be associated with labor
- 200 mg misoprostol for 2 days has been recently used for cervical priming
- However, this method had insufficient evidence so as to recommend its usage for IOL.[34]

Relaxin

- Relaxin was found to cause changes in the collagen, which results in cervical softening
- Both purified porcine and DNA-produced human relaxin have been studied regarding cervical ripening and it had no adverse maternal and fetal outcomes. But it is not yet commercially available.

Nitric Oxide

Animal studies regarding its use as cervical ripening agent were performed but unless its safety in late pregnancy is established, it is unlikely to be used in humans' studies.

Combined Methods

Combined method (medical and surgical) is often required in some cases, it yields higher success rate of about 80%.

Miscellaneous

Castor Oil

- Extract from "*Ricinus communis*" and a crude ricinoleic acid
- Due to prostaglandins release, it stimulates gut peristalsis and labor
- This is no longer used. One study has found a higher incidence of meconium staining liquor with this method.

Acupuncture and Transcutaneous Electric Nerve Stimulation

Fewer studies have reported successful IOL but further trials are needed before its use.

Herbal Supplements

- Commonly used agents are evening primrose oil, black cohosh, and raspberry leaves.
- The liquid of black cohosh is used as 10 drops sublingually hourly till we see changes in cervix.

- Evening primrose oil is administered orally as 3 capsules daily for 1 week, can be repeated the same as three courses.

Intercourse

Results in increased cervical mucus prostaglandin by 10-50 fold 2-4 hours later and it remains at the same level for more than 12 hours. Hence, associated with an increase in the uterine activity.

■ COMPLICATIONS OF IOL

The complications of induction of labor are enlisted in Table 7.

■ INDUCTION OF LABOR IN SPECIAL SITUATIONS

Previous Cesarean Section

- One or more previous cesarean section are not a contraindication to the induction of labor

TABLE 7: Complications of induction of labor (IOL).

Maternal	Fetal
• Failure leading to cesarean section • Uterine hyperstimulation • Rupture uterus • Intrauterine infection and chorioamnionitis • Amniotic fluid embolism • Precipitate labor and dysfunctional labor • Increased risk of operative vaginal delivery • Increased risk of postpartum hemorrhage • Abruptio placentae • APH from undiagnosed placenta previa • Water intoxication	• Fetal distress • Fetal death • Neonatal sepsis • Iatrogenic delivery of a preterm infant • Cord prolapse • Neonatal jaundice • Increased risk of birth trauma

- Consider woman wishes and decides on individual basis
- Cervical ripening can be done in these situations with PGE2 gel—either intravaginal or intracervical
- Misoprostol is an absolute contraindication
- Oxytocin can be safely used in low doses with close monitoring of uterine contractions and FHR
- It is preferable to have continuous electronic fetal monitoring
- Inform women regarding increased risk of uterine rupture and increased need for emergency cesarean sections with IOL.

Preterm Prelabor Rupture of Membranes

- Carries risk of infection, cord compression, oligohydramnios, and fetal pneumonia
- About <34 weeks—expectant management
- About >34 weeks—intravaginal PGE2
- Beware of hyperstimulation
- Continuous electronic fetal monitoring is recommended.

Prelabor Rupture of Membrane at Term

- Induction of labor is recommended 24 hours later after prelabor rupture of membrane (PROM)
- Choice of IOL is with vaginal PGE2.

Intrauterine Fetal Growth Restriction

Severe intrauterine fetal growth restriction (IUGR) with fetal compromise—IOL is not recommended.

Intrauterine Fetal Death

- Offer support to the couple to cope with the emotional consequence
- If intact membranes and no evidence of bleeding or infection offer the choice of expectant management or immediate IOL
- In case ruptured membranes, bleeding, or infection, prefer immediate IOL

- Induction of labor is done with oral mifepristone followed by vaginal PGE2 or misoprostol
- Intrauterine insemination (IUI) in women with previous cesarean section, offer IOL with reduced dose of prostaglandin. Explain regarding the risk of uterine rupture.

Unstable Lie: Stabilizing Induction

- Stabilizing induction is sometimes recommended in a multipara
- Cervix is made favorable by any ripening agent and the oxytocin is commenced
- artificial rupture of membranes is done once contraction is established and fetal head is fixed
- Stabilizing induction may affect vaginal delivery and avoid a cesarean section
- Carries some risk of PROM and cord prolapse.

FAILED INDUCTION

- Failed induction is considered when cervix failed to dilate up to 3–4 cm in 24 hours of induction. It occurs in about 15% cases in the presence of unfavorable cervix[5]
- Defined as failure to induce labor after one cycle of IOL, which included insertion of two vaginal PGE2 gel (1–2 mg) or tablet (3 mg) keep at 6 hours[5]
- Review the woman's status and fetal well-being, discuss with the patient, and decide the further management options[5]
- The options for subsequent management include:[5]
  - Cesarean section
  - Further attempt for IOL.

CONCLUSION

- Women should be informed regarding the indication for IOL, when and how IOL could be performed, the risks and benefits of IOL and the alternative options available
- Benefits of IOL must be weighed against the risk both maternal and fetal
- If IOL is indicated and Bishop score is unfavorable, agents for cervical induction are used
- IOL should be offered between 41 and 42 completed weeks in women with uncomplicated pregnancies to avoid the risk of prolonged pregnancy
- IOL should not be routinely offered on maternal request alone
- In women with previous cesarean section, prefer IOL with vaginal PGE2 than misoprostol. However, they should be informed about increased risk of uterine rupture and about chance of emergency cesarean section
- If there is severe IUGR with fetal compromise, do not offer IOL
- In case of intrauterine fetal death (IUD), proceed for IOL with oral mifepristone followed by vaginal PGE1 or PGE2
- Vaginal PGE2 is the preferred method of IOL unless there are specific reasons for not using the drug such as risk of uterine hyperstimulation
- Facilities for continuous electronic FHR and uterine contractions are mandatory in IOL
- If IOL fails, the next management options include either for further attempt to induce labor or delivery by cesarean section.

REFERENCES

1. ACOG Committee on Practice Bulletins—Obstetrics. ACOG Practice Bulletin no 107: induction of labor. Obstet Gynecol. 2009;114: 386-97.
2. National Institute for Health and Clinical Excellence. (2008) Induction of labour [clinical guideline 70]. [online] Available from: https://www.nice.org.uk/guidance/cg70 [Last accessed September, 2019].

3. WHO. Managing complication in pregnancy and childbirth: a guide for midwives and doctors. Geneva: World Health Organization; 2000.
4. WHO. WHO recommendations for Augmentation of Labour. Geneva: World Health Organization; 2014.
5. RCOG. (2008). Induction of labour (NICE guidelines 70). [online] Available from: https://www.rcog.org.uk/en/guidelines-research-services/guidelines/induction-of-labour/ [Last accessed September, 2019].
6. Gulmezoglu AM, Crowther CA, Middleton P. Induction of labour for improving birth outcomes for women at or beyond term. Cochrane Database Syst Rev. 2006;5:CD004945
7. Sanchez-Ramos L, Olivier F, Delke I, et al. Labor induction versus expectant management for post-term pregnancies: a systematic review with meta-analysis. Obstet Gynecol. 2003;101:1312-8
8. Dare MR, Middleton P, Crowther CA, et al. Planned early birth versus expectant management (waiting) for prelabour rupture of membranes at term (37 weeks or more). Cochrane Database Syst Rev. 2006;1:CD005302
9. Hartling L, Chari R, Friesen C, et al. A systematic review of intentional delivery in women with preterm prelabor rupture of membranes. J Matern Fetal Neonatal Med. 2006;19:177-87
10. Sanchez-Ramos L, Bernstein S, Kaunitz AM. Expectant management versus labour induction for suspected fetal macrosomia: a systematic review. Obstet Gynecol. 2002;100: 997-1002.
11. Irion O, Boulvain M. Induction of labour for suspected fetal macrosomia. Cochrane Database Syst Rev. 2000;(2):CD000938.
12. GRIT Study Group. A randomised trial of timed delivery for the compromised preterm fetus: short term outcomes and Bayesian interpretation. BJOG. 2003;110:27-32.
13. Van den Hove MM, Willekes C, Roumen FJ, et al. Intrauterine growth restriction at term: induction or spontaneous labour? Disproportionate intrauterine growth intervention trial at term (DIGITAT): a pilot study. Eur J Obstet Gynecol Reprod Biol. 2006;125:54-8.
14. Ek S, Andersson A, Johansson A, et al. Oligohydramnios in uncomplicated pregnancies beyond 40 completed weeks. A prospective, randomised, pilot study on maternal and neonatal outcomes. Fetal Diagn Ther. 2005;20: 182-5.
15. Boulvain M, Stan C, Irion O. Elective delivery in diabetic pregnant women. Cochrane Database Syst Rev. 2001;(2):CD001997
16. Mashiloane CD, Moodley J. Induction or caesarean section for preterm pre-eclampsia? J Obstet Gynaecol. 2002;22:353-6.
17. Roncaglia N, Arreghini A, Locatelli A, et al. Obstetric cholestasis: outcome with active management. Eur J Obstet Gynecol Reprod Biol. 2002;100:167-70.
18. Logghe HL, Mason GC, Thornton JG, et al. A randomized controlled trial of elective preterm delivery of fetuses with gastroschisis. J Pediatr Surg. 2005;40(11):1726-31.
19. Rayburn WF, Zhang J. Rising rates of labor induction: present concerns and future strategies. Obstet Gynecol. 2002;100(1):164-7.
20. Crowley P. Interventions for preventing or improving the outcome of delivery at or beyond term. Cochrane Database Syst Rev. 2000;(2):CD000170.
21. Luthy DA, Malmgren JA, Zingheim RW. Cesarean delivery after elective induction in nulliparous women: the physician effect. Am J Obstet Gynecol. 2004;191(5):1511-5.
22. Glantz JC. Elective induction vs. spontaneous labor associations and outcomes. J Reprod Med. 2005;50(4):235-40.
23. McColgin SW, Bennett WA, Roach H, et al. Parturitional factors associated with membrane stripping. Am J Obstet Gynecol. 1993;169(1):71-7.
24. Cammu H, Haitsma V. Sweeping of the membranes at 39 weeks in nulliparous women: a randomised controlled trial. Br J Obstet Gynaecol. 1998;105(1):41-4.
25. Boulvain M, Stan C, Irion O. Membrane sweeping for induction of labour. Cochrane Database Syst Rev. 2001;(2):CD000451.
26. De Miranda E, van der Bom JG, Bonsel GJ, et al. Membrane sweeping and prevention of post-term pregnancy in low-risk pregnancies: a randomised controlled trial. BJOG. 2006;113(4): 402-8.
27. Karjane NW, Brock EL, Walsh SW. Induction of labor using a Foley balloon, with and without extra-amniotic saline infusion. Obstet Gynecol. 2006;107:234-9.

28. Ghanaie MM, Jafarabadi M, Milani F. A randomized controlled trial of foley catheter, extra-amniotic saline infusion and prostaglandin E2 suppository for labor induction. J Family Reprod Health. 2013;7(2): 49-55.
29. Jozwiak M, Bloemenkamp KW, Kelly AJ, et al. Mechanical methods for induction of labour. Cochrane Database Syst Rev. 2012;(3): CD001233.
30. French L. Oral prostaglandin E2 for induction of labour. Cochrane Database Syst Rev. 2001;(2):CD003098.
31. Muzonzini G, Hofmeyr GJ. Buccal or sublingual misoprostol for cervical ripening and induction of labour. Cochrane Database Syst Rev. 2004; (4):CD004221.
32. Theobald GW. The separate release of oxytocin and antidiuretic hormone. J Physiol. 1959;149(3):443-61.
33. Howarth GR, Botha DJ. Amniotomy plus intravenous oxytocin for induction of labour. Cochrane Database Syst Rev. 2001;(3): CD003250.
34. Hapangama D, Neilson JP. Mifepristone for induction of labour. Cochrane Database Syst Rev. 2009;(3):CD002865.

CHAPTER 50

Abnormal Progress of Labor

Komal Unadkat

INTRODUCTION

Prolonged labor or dystocia is a common birth complication and constitutes the major indication of instrumental deliveries and delivery by emergency cesarean section (CS).[1,2] Very often it causes suffering from difficulties that may have lifelong complications. Careful management of interventions is crucial in order to keep normal births normal and avoid mistreatment.

DEFINITION

Dystocia is defined as abnormal labor that results from what have been categorized classically as abnormalities of the power (uterine contractions or maternal expulsive forces), the passenger (position and size or presentation of the fetus) or the passage (pelvis or soft tissues).[3]

Because dystocia can rarely be diagnosed with certainty, the relatively imprecise term "failure to progress" has been used, which includes lack of progressive cervical dilation or lack of descent of the fetal head or both. The diagnosis of dystocia should not be made before an adequate trial of labor has been achieved.[3]

Prolonged Labor

It is when the combined duration of the first and second stage of labor is more than the arbitrary time limit of 18 hours. Labor is considered prolonged when the cervical dilatation rate is less than 1 cm/hour and descent of the presenting part is less than 1 cm/hour for a period of minimum 4 hours observation (WHO, 1994).[4]

TYPES OF LABOR ABNORMALITIES

- Prolonged latent phase
- Protraction disorders
- Arrest disorders
- Precipitate labor.

CLASSIFICATIONS

- *Friedman (1989)*:[5]
  - Prolonged latent phase
  - *Protraction disorders*:
    - Protracted active phase
    - Protracted descent
  - *Arrest disorders*:
    - Secondary arrest of cervical dilatation
    - Prolonged deceleration phase
    - Arrest of descent
    - Failure of descent.
- *ACOG (1995)*:
  - Protraction disorders (slower-than-normal progress)
  - Arrest disorders (complete cessation of progress)

CAUSES OF PROLONGED LABOR

Any one or combination of the factors in labor could be responsible.[3]

First Stage

Failure of cervical dilation is due to:
- *Fault in power*: Abnormal uterine contraction such as uterine inertia (common) or incoordinate uterine contraction.
- *Fault in the passage*: Contracted pelvis, cervical dystocia, pelvic tumor or even full bladder.
- *Fault in the passenger*: Malposition [occipitoposterior (OP)], malpresentation (face and brow), congenital anomalies of the fetus (hydrocephalus), too often deflexed head, minor degrees of pelvic contraction, and disordered uterine action have got sinister effects in causing nondilatation of the cervix.
- *Others*: Injudicious (early) administration of sedatives and analgesics before the active labor begins.

Second Stage

Sluggish or nondescent of the presenting part in the second stage is due to:
- *Fault in the power*: (1) Uterine inertia, (2) Inability to bear down, (3) Regional (epidural) analgesia, and (4) Constriction ring.
- *Fault in the passage*: (1) Cephalopelvic disproportion (CPD), android pelvis, and contracted pelvis, (2) Undue resistance of the pelvic floor or perineum due to spasm or old scarring, and (3) Soft-tissue pelvic tumor.
- *Fault in the passenger*: (1) Malposition (OP), (2) Malpresentation, (3) Big baby, and (4) Congenital malformation of the baby.

DIAGNOSIS

Evaluation Index

- Cervical dilatation
- Descent of presenting part
- Use of Friedman's curve/partograph.[6]

The labor process is divided into:

First stage: Its average duration is 12 hours in primigravidae and 6 hours in multiparae. First stage of labor is considered prolonged when the duration is more than 12 hours.

	Cervical dilatation rate	Descent of presenting part rate
Nulliparas	<1 cm/hr	<1 cm/hr
Multiparas	<1.5 cm/hr	<2 cm/hr

In partogram (WHO, 1994) the labor process is divided into:
- Latent phase that ends when the cervix is 4 cm dilated.
- Active phase—starts with cervical dilatation of 4 cm or more.
  - Cervix should dilate at least 1 cm/hour in active phase. Cervical dilatation rate (cervicograph) is plotted in relation to alert line and action line.
  - Alert line starts at the end of latent phase (4 cm cervical dilatation) and ends with full dilatation of the cervix (10 cm) in 6 hours (1 cm/hour dilatation rate).
  - The action line is drawn 4 hours to the right of the alert line.
  - An interval of 4 hours is allowed to diagnose delay in active phase to allow appropriate intervention to be done.
  - Labor is considered abnormal when cervicograph crosses the alert line and falls on zone 2 and intervention is required when it crosses the action line and falls on zone 3. Partograph can diagnose any dysfunctional labor early and help to initiate correct management.

Prolonged Latent Phase

Latent phase is the preparatory phase of the uterus and the cervix before the actual onset of labor. Prolonged latent phase may be worrisome to the patient but does not endanger the mother or fetus. It is not an indication for cesarean delivery.

	Normal (average duration)	Prolonged
Nulliparas	8 hr	>20 hr
Multiparas	4 hr	>14 hr

The causes of which are depicted in Box 1.

Management

- Expectant management is usually done unless there is any indication for expediting the delivery.
- Rest and analgesia.
- When augmentation is decided, medical methods (oxytocin or prostaglandins) are preferred.
- Amniotomy is usually avoided.

Table 1 showing evidence-based diagnostic criteria on labor dystocia.

Active Phase Disorders

- Protraction disorders

Box 1: Causes of prolonged latent phase of labor.
- Unripe cervix
- Malpresentation and malposition
- Cephalopelvic disproportion
- Premature rupture of the membranes
- Induction of labor
- Early onset of regional anesthetic

	Cervical dilatation rate
Nulliparas	<1.2 cm/hr
Multiparas	<1.5 cm/hr

Causes:
- Inadequate uterine contractions
- Cephalopelvic disproportion
- Malposition (OP) or malpresentation (brow)
- Regional (epidural) anesthesia.

- *Arrest disorders*:
  - Arrest of dilatation is defined when no cervical dilatation occurs after 2 hours in the active phase of labor (most common cause is uterine inertia).
  - No descent for a period of more than 2 hours is called arrest of descent (most common cause is CPD).

Secondary arrest: It is defined when the active phase of labor (cervical dilatation) commences normally but stops or slows significantly for 2 hours or more prior to full dilatation of the cervix. It is commonly due to malposition or CPD.

Second stage: Mean duration of second stage is 50 minutes for nullipara and 20 minutes in multipara.[7]

	Protraction of descent	Arrest of descent
Nulliparas	<1 cm/hr	No descent for 2 hours
Multiparas	<2 cm/hr	No descent for 2 hours

TABLE 1: Evidence-based diagnostic criteria on labor dystocia.

	First stage		Second stage	
	Nulliparous	Multiparous	Nulliparous	Multiparous
NICE: Intrapartum Care, 2007	After cx 4 cm dilated, cx dilation <2 cm in 4 hours	After cx 4 cm dilated, <2 cm in 4 hours or a slowing in the progress of labor	Active second stage >2 hours and birth not imminent	Active second stage >1 hour and birth not imminent
ACOG: Practice Bulletin, 2003	An adequate trial of labor	An adequate trial of labor	>3 hours with regional anesthesia or 2 hours without	>2 hours with regional anesthesia or 1 hour without

(ACOG: American College of Obstetricians and Gynecologists; NICE: National Institute for Health and Care Excellence)

RISKS

- *Fetal*: Increased due to the combined effects of:
  - Hypoxia due to diminished uteroplacental circulation, especially after rupture of the membranes
  - Intrauterine infection
  - Intracranial stress or hemorrhage following prolonged stay in the perineum and/or supermolding of the head
  - Increased operative delivery.

  All these result in increased perinatal morbidity and mortality.

  Monitoring:
  - Cardiotocography (often associated with variable and delayed decelerations)[8]
  - Scalp blood pH estimations (fetal acidosis).

- *Maternal*: There is increased incidence of:
  - Distress
  - Chorioamnionitis
  - Postpartum hemorrhage
  - Trauma to the genital tract—concealed (undue stretching of the perineal muscles which may be the cause of prolapse at a later period) or revealed such as cervical tear, rupture uterus
  - Increased operative delivery (vaginal instrumental or difficult cesarean)
  - Puerperal sepsis
  - Subinvolution.

  The sum effects of all these lead to increased maternal morbidity and also increased maternal deaths.

MANAGEMENT

Prevention

- Anticipation of the factors likely to produce prolonged labor (antenatal or early intranatal detection)
- Monitoring of uterine activity (palpation, external tocodynamometry or internal pressure catheters)[8]
- Use of partograph helps early detection
- Selective and judicious augmentation of labor
- Ambulation/change of posture in labor other than supine to increase uterine contractions
- Emotional support
- Careful monitoring of vitals
- Avoidance of dehydration in labor
- Use of adequate analgesia for pain relief.

Actual Treatment

- *Careful evaluation is to be done to find out*: (1) cause of prolonged labor (2) effect on the mother, and (3) effect on the fetus.
- Correction of ketoacidosis.

Definitive Treatment

- *First stage delay*:
  - Per vaginal examination to verify the fetal presentation, position, and station. Clinical pelvimetry.
  - Amniotomy and/or oxytocin infusion is adequate[9]
  - Effective pain relief injection/regional (epidural) analgesia.
  - *Secondary arrest, especially in multipara*:
    - Careful use of oxytocin
    - Cesarean section when vaginal delivery is unsafe.
- *Second stage delay*:
  - Expectant management is reasonable provided the FHR (electronic monitoring) is reassuring and vaginal delivery is imminent.
  - If not, appropriate assisted delivery, vaginal (forceps, ventouse) or abdominal (cesarean) should be done.
  - Avoid difficult instrumental delivery.

PRECIPITATE LABOR

Definition

A labor is called precipitate when the combined duration of the first and second stage is less than 3 hours. Labor is short as the rate of cervical dilatation is 5 cm/hour or more for the nulliparous women. It is common in multiparae and may be repetitive.

Prevalence is about 2%. Short labors may be associated with placental abruption and uterine tachysystole.

Causes

Rapid expulsion is due to the combined effect of hyperactive uterine contractions associated with diminished soft tissue resistance.

Maternal Risks

- Injury to the cervix, vagina, and perineum (to the extent of complete perineal tear)
- Postpartum hemorrhage due to uterine hypotonia that develops subsequent to unusual vigorous contractions
- Inversion
- Uterine rupture
- Infection
- Amniotic fluid embolism.

Fetal Risks

- Intracranial stress and hemorrhage because of rapid expulsion without time for molding of the head.
- Serious injuries if delivery occurs in standing position; bleeding from the torn cord and direct hit on the skull.
- Brachial plexus injury.[10]

Treatment

- Anticipation with past history of precipitate labor should be hospitalized prior to labor.
- During labor, use of ether or magnesium sulfate during contractions as a uterine relaxant.
- Controlled delivery of the fetal head.
- Liberal use of episiotomy.
- Elective induction of labor by low rupture of membranes and conduction of controlled delivery.
- Avoid oxytocin augmentation.

CONCLUSION

Abnormal progress of labor increases both fetal and maternal morbidity and mortality, identification and initiation of appropriate management reduces the risks associated with emergencies. Early detection of abnormal progress helps obstetrician to consider alternate methods of delivery.

REFERENCES

1. Lowe NK. A review of factors associated with dystocia and e section in nulliparous women. J Midwifery Womens Health. 2007;52(3):216-28.
2. Shields SG, Ratcliffe SD, Fontaine P, et al. Dystocia in nulliparous women. Am Fam Physician. 2007;75(11):1671-8.
3. American College of Obstetrics and Gynecology Committee on Practice Bulletins-Obstetrics. ACOG Practice Bulletin Number 49, December 2003: Dystocia and augmentation of labor. Obstet Gynecol. 2003;102(6):1445-54.
4. World Health Organization partograph in management of labour. World Health Organization Maternal Health and Safe Motherhood Programme. Lancet. 1994;343(8910):1399-404.
5. Friedman E. The graphic analysis of labor. Am J Obstet Gynecol. 1954;68(6):1568-75.
6. Duncan GR, Costello E. The partogram: a graphic guide to progress in labour. N Z Med J. 1975;82(548):193-5.
7. Kilpatrick SJ, Laros RK Jr. Characteristics of normal labor. Obstet Gynecol. 1989;74:85-7.
8. ACOG technical bulletin. Fetal heart rate patterns: Monitoring, interpretation and management. Number 207—July 1995 (replaces No. 132, September 1989). Int J Gynaecol Obstet. 1995;51(1):65-74.
9. Fraser WD, Marcoux S, Moutquin JM, et al. Effect of early amniotomy on the risk of dystocia in nulliparous women. The Canadian Early Amniotomy Study Group. N Eng J Med. 1993;328(16):1145-9.
10. Ouzounian JG, Korst LM, Miller DA, et al. Brachial plexus palsy and shoulder dystocia: obstetric risk factors remain elusive. Am J Perinatol. 2013;30:303-7.

CHAPTER 51

Transfusion Reactions

Rekha Viswanath

WHAT IS A TRANSFUSION REACTION?

The adverse event associated with the transfusion of whole blood or one of its components is called a transfusion reaction.

Components of blood:
- Packed red blood cells
- Leukocyte reduced red blood cells
- Fresh frozen plasma
- Platelet concentrate
- Cryoprecipitate.

Transfusion reactions can occur during the transfusion which is known as *acute transfusion reaction* or after few days or weeks after transfusion which is known as *delayed transfusion reaction*.

Transfusion reactions may be *immunogenic or nonimmunogenic*.

ETIOLOGY

- Immune-mediated transfusion reactions
  - Antibodies in the recipient, e.g. anti-A and anti-B
  - Alloantibodies (Alloantibodies)
  - Antibodies in the donor [transfusion-related acute lung injury (TRALI)]
- Nonimmune-mediated transfusion reactions
  - Physical effects of blood components, e.g. septic transfusion reactions
  - Transmission of disease
- Transfusion reactions unrelated to intrinsic factors of blood
  - Transfusion-associated circulatory overload (TACO)
  - Hypothermia

PATHOPHYSIOLOGY (TABLE 1)

Mild allergic: Hypersensitivity to foreign protein in the donor product.

Anaphylactic: More severe hypersensitivity reaction. E.g. in immunoglobulin A (IgA) deficient patients who have alloantibodies against IgA and receive blood products containing IgA.

Febrile nonhemolytic: Caused due to cytokines released from blood donor leukocytes.

Septic: Caused by bacteria or bacterial products which may contaminate the blood.

Acute hemolytic: Due to intravascular or extravascular hemolysis, depending on the

TABLE 1: Pathophysiology of acute transfusion reactions and delayed transfusion reactions.

Acute transfusion reactions	Delayed transfusion reactions
- Mild allergic - Anaphylactic - Febrile nonhemolytic - Septic - Acute hemolytic - Transfusion-associated circulatory overload (TACO) - Transfusion-associated acute lung injury (TRALI)	- Delayed hemolytic transfusion reaction - Transfusion-associated graft-versus-host disease

specific cause. They may be immune due to recipient antibodies present to blood donor antigens or may be nonimmune due to red blood cells that are damaged before transfusion.

Transfusion-associated circulatory overload (TACO): Caused as a result of hypervolemia resulting from transfusion.

Transfusion-associated acute lung injury (TRALI): Caused as a result of antibodies in the donor product human leukocyte antigen (HLA) reacting with antigens in the recipient. The recipient immune system releases mediators that lead to pulmonary edema. Predisposing factors include infection, recent surgery, and inflammation.

Delayed hemolytic reaction: It is an anamnestic response to a foreign antigen that the patient was previously exposed to (e.g. prior transfusion and pregnancy).

Transfusion-associated graft-versus-host disease: Caused by the engraftment of donor lymphocytes into an immunocompromised recipients' bone marrow. The donor lymphocytes recognize the recipient as foreign and react against the recipients' body. The recipient immune system, however, is not able to clear the foreign lymphocytes. This is rare but fatal.

SYMPTOMS AND SIGNS

Prerequisites before Starting a Transfusion

- Patients medical history.
- Blood sample of patient to be sent for crossmatching.
- Extra caution to be taken in confirming and reconfirming patient name, identification, blood group, and Rh typing on the blood packet received from the blood bank before starting the transfusion.
- Vital signs to be monitored and recorded every 15 minutes. Small changes during transfusion may be considered "normal", e.g. 0.5°C rise or fall of temperature, rise or fall of five respirations per minute, rise or fall of 10 beats per minute in heart rate, and rise or fall of 20 mm Hg in the blood pressure.
- The bedside nurse should be extra vigilant in monitoring for a reaction.

Abnormal Responses Include

- Itching
- Fever more than 1°C above the temperature at the start of transfusion
- Chills
- Hypotension
- Dyspnea.

DIAGNOSIS

Diagnosis begins with the recognition of common signs and symptoms by the bedside.

Urticaria (or itching): It can occur as a result of a mild allergic reaction or with the life-threatening anaphylactic reaction. The transfusion has to be stopped immediately and patient monitored for the progress of symptoms.

Fever/chills: Commonly associated with febrile nonhemolytic reaction. They can also be the sign of more serious acute hemolytic reaction, TRALI, or septic transfusion reaction. If there is a temperature rise of 1°C or higher, the transfusion should be stopped immediately, acute hemolytic reaction or bacterial contamination should be suspected if there is a higher rise of temperature, or more serious symptoms like rigors.

Respiratory distress/dyspnea: They are seen in more serious reactions like anaphylactic, TRALI, and TACO.

Hypotension: May be associated with acute hemolytic reaction, septic transfusion reactions, anaphylaxis, and TRALI.

Hypothermia: May be seen with large volume transfusions of refrigerated products. Here the only intervention required is warming the patient and/or the blood product.

TREATMENT/MANAGEMENT

- Transfusion to be stopped immediately.
- *Intravenous line to be kept open with appropriate fluids*: 0.9% saline.
- Examine the blood product and confirming the patient's identification.
- Monitor patient's vitals every 15 minutes.
- A post-transfusion sample should be drawn and sent to the laboratory, in addition to sending the bag and tubing.
- The blood bank should conduct additional checks to rule out an incompatible transfusion.
- Supportive treatment for specific transfusion reactions, e.g. antihistaminics for mild allergic reactions or antipyretics for nonhemolytic febrile transfusion reaction.

CONCLUSION

- Blood transfusion is extremely safe, but deaths and morbidity do occur.
- Errors in patient identification and blood sampling are the root causes of many preventable serious adverse reactions.
- Monitoring of the patient and avoiding inappropriate and unnecessary transfusions are hence extremely important.

SUGGESTED READING

1. Crookston KP, Koenig SC, Reyes MD. Transfusion reaction identification and management at bedside. J Infus Nurs. 2015;38(2):104-13.
2. DeLisle J. Is this a blood transfusion reaction? Don't hesitate; check it out. J Infus Nurs. 2018;41(1):43-51.
3. Gehrie EA, Roubinian NH, Chowdhury D, et al. A multicentre study investigating vital sign changes occurring in complicated and uncomplicated transfusions. Vox Sang. 2018;113(2):160-9.
4. Harvey AR, Basavaraju SV, Chung KW, et al. Transfusion-related adverse reactions reported to the National Healthcare Safety Network Hemovigilance Module, United States, 2010 to 2012. Transfusion. 2015;55(4):709-18.
5. Saadah NH, van der Bom JG, Wiersum-Osselton JC, et al. Comparing transfusion reaction risks for various plasma products—an analysis of 7 years of ISTARE haemovigilance data. Br J Haematol. 2018;180(5):727-34.

52

Anaphylaxis

Neha Tyagi

INTRODUCTION

The term *aphylaxis* was coined by Charles Richet in 1902, which was later changed to *anaphylaxis*. Sir Richet described the phenomenon of anaphylaxis though his experiments of injecting sea anemone (Actinia) toxin into a dog, which developed fatal reaction on further exposure of the allergen. He was subsequently awarded the Nobel Prize in Physiology or Medicine for his work on anaphylaxis in 1913.[1]

The Greek word "*ana*" means without, "*phylaxis*" means protection—anaphylaxis is a rare, life-threatening medical emergency that can be encountered by a pregnant woman, and can cause potential increase in fetal morbidity and mortality.[2] It is a systemic type I hypersensitivity reaction, which is rapid in onset and can lead to sudden collapse of the cardiovascular system resulting in maternal and often fetal death.

PREVALENCE

The lifetime prevalence of anaphylaxis in the general population is estimated as 0.05–2%.[3-6] Although, the exact incidence of anaphylaxis in pregnancy is not known, there is a gradual crescendo in various case reports of anaphylaxis in pregnancy being published in the indexed peer-reviewed journals.

ETIOLOGY

During pregnancy, the etiological factors of anaphylaxis are similar to those of the general population. Various factors (Fig. 1) that were found to be involved were certain foods, medications [most commonly beta-lactams and nonsteroidal anti-inflammatory drugs (NSAIDs)], stinging insect venoms, natural latex rubber, intravenous iron, radiocontrast media, and exercise.[7-13]

During labor and delivery, agents associated are antibiotics, neuromuscular blockers, local anesthetics, natural latex rubber, oxytocin, and transfusion of blood and blood products.

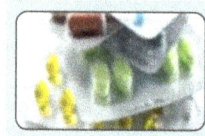
Pharmlogic agents
- Antibiotics (penicillin)
- Nonsteroidal anti-inflammatory drugs (Asprin)
- Intravenous (IV) contrast agents

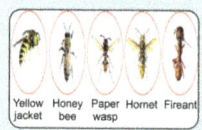
Stinging insects
- Ants, bees, hornets, wasps, and yellow jackets

Yellow jacket   Honey bee   Paper wasp   Hornet   Fireant

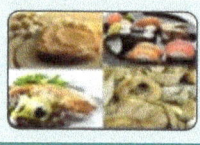
Food
- Peanuts, seafood, and wheat

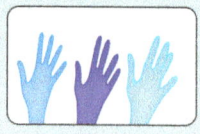
Latex
- Rare
- No latex-associated deaths

Fig. 1: Etiological factors of anaphylaxis.

Rare Types of Anaphylaxis Seen in Pregnant and Postpartum Women

Almost anything can trigger anaphylactic reaction in a susceptible individual. We, at our center, have witnessed a case of anaphylaxis in a pregnant woman following intake of grapes. The actual culprit was later found to be the insecticide sprayed over the fruit. Few other examples are:

- *Exercise-induced anaphylaxis:*[14] Can be seen during labor, although it is rare.
- *During breastfeeding:*[15] Usually occurs in first 3 days postpartum, mainly due to rapid decrease in serum progesterone. Concurrent use of NSAIDs can amplify its incidence.

PATHOGENESIS

Immunoglobulin E (IgE) isotype is found in much higher concentration in patients with allergic diseases. IgE binds to the high affinity receptor FcεRI present on blood basophils and tissue-resident mast cells, other cell types like neutrophils, monocytes, macrophages, dendritic, and platelets. Following exposure to a bivalent or multivalent allergen, there is cross-linking of IgE-FcεRI, resulting in activation of mast cells and basophils with subsequent release of potential mediators such as histamine, prostaglandins, cytokines, and certain leukotrienes (Fig. 2).[16]

Immunoglobulin E-independent Anaphylaxis

It is also referred to as anaphylactoid reaction and is clinically indistinguishable from anaphylactic reaction. It has been observed that few people developed anaphylactic reactions, despite having low circulating levels of IgE, suggesting the IgE-independent pathways of developing anaphylaxis. More convincing evidence has been obtained using mouse models.[17]

Role of Immunoglobulin G and FcYRs

It has been shown that IgG antibodies with its specific receptors can mediate anaphylaxis in mouse, a condition known as *passive systemic anaphylaxis,* with a similar clinical presentation as that seen in IgE-mediated

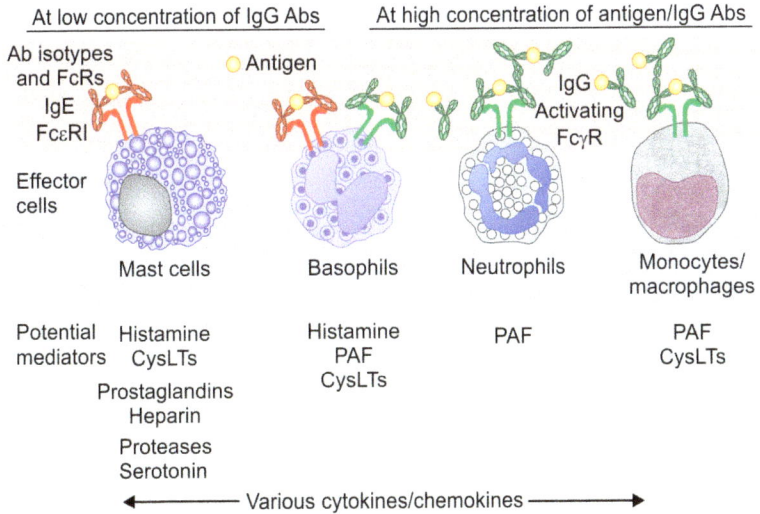

Fig. 2: Pathogenesis of anaphylaxis (Abs: antibodies; CysLTs: cysteinyl leukotrienes; FcRs: Fc receptors; IgG: immunoglobulin G; PAF: platelet-activating factor)

prostate-specific antigen (PSA) in humans.[18-20] IgG-mediated anaphylaxis requires a much higher dose of antigen than does IgE antibodies.[21,22] Role of IgG in humans is still a topic for more research.

DIAGNOSIS

The term *"anaphylactoid"* is no longer recommended and does not need to be distinguished from anaphylaxis as long as diagnosis and management is concerned.[2] The diagnosis is mostly clinical; detailed history of the episode, sudden onset and rapid progression, within minutes to few hours, of signs and symptoms following exposure to the allergen, favor an anaphylactic episode.

There is usually a multisystem involvement (Table 1).[2,9]

The clinical criteria for diagnosis of anaphylaxis as given by Simons et al. is as follows (Box 1).[23]

The severity of manifestations differs from one patient to another and even from one episode to the other in the same patient.

Various mediators are responsible for the pathophysiological manifestations seen during an anaphylactic episode, as illustrated in Figure 3.[16]

Clinical Features Specific to Pregnancy (Fig. 4)[23]

- Pain abdomen and uterine cramps
- Lower backache
- Vulval and vaginal itching
- Decreased fetal movements.

Pathophysiology of Fetal Hypoxemia

The amount of oxygen reaching the fetal circulation is based on *Fick's principle*, i.e. fetal oxygenation is a direct function of the difference between the partial pressure of oxygen (PO_2) between fetal and maternal

TABLE 1: Multisystem involvement in anaphylaxis.[2]

Organ system	Involvement (%)
Skin and mucosa	80–90
Respiratory tract	70
Gastrointestinal tract	45
Cardiovascular system	45
Central nervous system	15

Box 1: Clinical criteria for diagnosis of anaphylaxis during pregnancy.

Anaphylaxis is highly likely when any one of the following three criteria is fulfilled:

1. Acute onset of an illness (minutes to several hours) with involvement of the skin, mucosal tissue, or both (e.g. generalized urticaria, itching or flushing, swollen lips-tongue-uvula)
   And at least one of the following:
   a. Respiratory compromise (e.g. dyspnea, wheeze-bronchospasm, stridor, reduced peak expiratory flow, hypoxemia)
   b. Reduced blood pressure or associated symptoms of end-organ dysfunction (e.g. hypotonia [collapse], syncope, incontinence)

   OR

2. Two or more of the following that occur rapidly after exposure to *a likely allergen for that patient* (minutes to several hours):
   a. Involvement of the skin-mucosal tissue (e.g. generalized urticaria, itch-flush, swollen lips-tongue-uvula)
   b. Respiratory compromise (e.g. dyspnea, wheeze-bronchospasm, stridor, hypoxemia)
   c. Reduced blood pressure or associated symptoms [e.g. hypotonia (collapse), syncope, incontinence]
   d. Persistent gastrointestinal symptoms (e.g. crampy abdominal pain, vomiting)

   OR

3. Reduced blood pressure after exposure to *known allergen for that person* (minutes to several hours) defined as systolic blood pressure of < 90 mm Hg or > 30% decrease from that person's basel line value

circulation. As the period of gestation increases, the volume of blood flow across the placenta increases in order to compensate for the increased fetal demand and placental

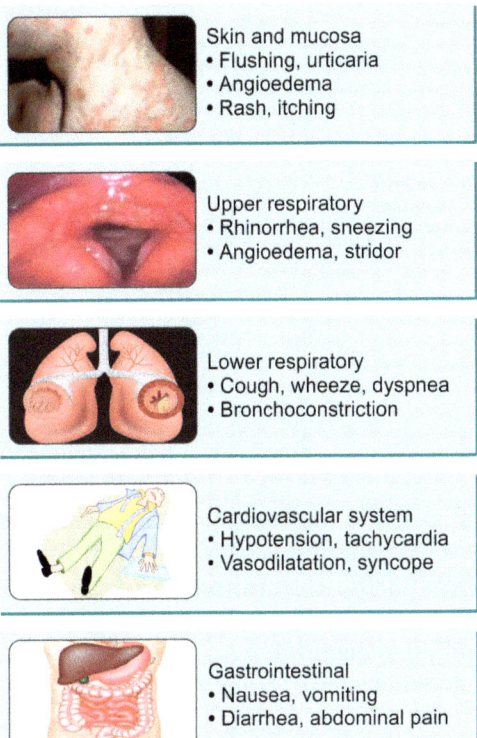

Fig. 3: Clinical manifestations of anaphylaxis with role of mediators. (CysLTs: cysteinyl leukotrienes; PAF: platelet-activating factor)

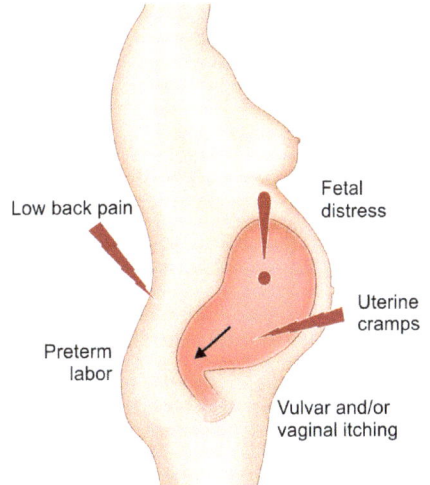

Fig. 4: Potential symptoms and signs of anaphylaxis during pregnancy.

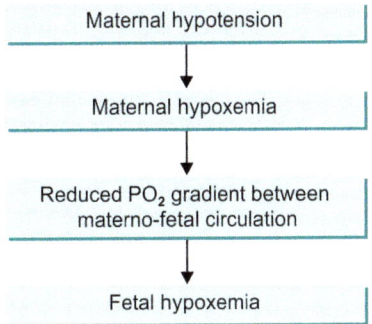

Flowchart 1: Pathophysiology of fetal hypoxemia during maternal anaphylaxis. (PO$_2$: partial pressure of oxygen)

insufficiency. There is systemic vasodilatation in anaphylaxis causing maternal hypotension and hypoxemia. This, in turn, causes fetal hypoxemia (Flowchart 1).[24]

The compensatory mechanisms occurring in the fetus following maternal anaphylaxis are described in the Figure 5. A prompt decision regarding immediate cesarean delivery must be taken to ensure a neurologically healthy newborn. Around 90% of the neonates born within 5 minutes of maternal cardiac arrest are neurologically intact, as against less than 60%, if delivered within 15 minutes.[25,26]

Maternal outcomes include:
- Acute kidney injury (AKI)
- Acute hepatic failure
- Acute respiratory distress syndrome (ARDS)
- Disseminated intravascular coagulopathy (DIC)
- Maternal mortality.

MANAGEMENT OF ANAPHYLAXIS IN PREGNANCY

The basic management of anaphylaxis in a pregnant woman is same as in any other individual. It is a medical emergency, therefore, any delay in diagnosis or prompt treatment could have fatal implications, both for mother

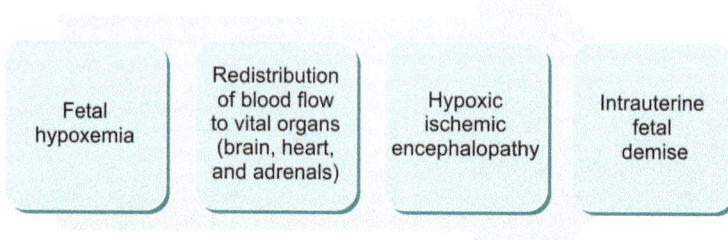

Fig. 5: Fetal outcome in case of maternal anaphylaxis.

and the fetus. The algorithm provided in Figure 6 gives an overview of the management of anaphylaxis in pregnancy.[23]

Anaphylaxis Refractory to Basic Initial Treatment

Airway Support

Endotracheal intubation or tracheostomy, if required, should be performed if oxygen saturation is inadequate. It should be performed by an experienced doctor, as difficult airway entry can be anticipated owing to the swollen tongue, mucus secretions, and pregnancy associated laryngeal edema.

Blood Pressure Support

Transfusion of large volumes of intravenous fluid preferably crystalloids (isotonic normal saline) with the aim of maintaining the systolic pressure at a minimum of 90 mm Hg so as to ensure adequate placental perfusion. Glucose containing fluids are best avoided, as they can cause a glucose overload leading to decreased umbilical cord pH and eventually neonatal hypoglycemia.

Vasopressors during Labor and Delivery

Intravenous administration of vasopressors using an infusion pump with frequent titration according to the blood pressure, heart rate, and oxygenation is required. Intravenous epinephrine is vasopressor of choice at present, although intravenous ephedrine and phenylephrine have also been used to maintain maternal blood pressure.

Adjuvant Treatment

This is an add-on symptomatic approach, rather than the first-line management of anaphylaxis. Various adjunctive treatments that have been practiced are mentioned in Figure 7.[27-29]

Fetal Monitoring

In addition to managing maternal hemodynamic status, it is equally important to perform continuous fetal heart rate (FHR) monitoring of potentially viable fetus that could be severely affected by anaphylactic episode during pregnancy. A reassuring FHR pattern is a sensitive of stable cardiorespiratory status of the pregnant female.

Nonreassuring FHR patterns require prompt intervention to correct maternal hypotension and hypoxemia. If there is no improvement in FHR pattern, emergency cesarean section should be performed to salvage the pregnancy, and have a neurologically

Anaphylaxis

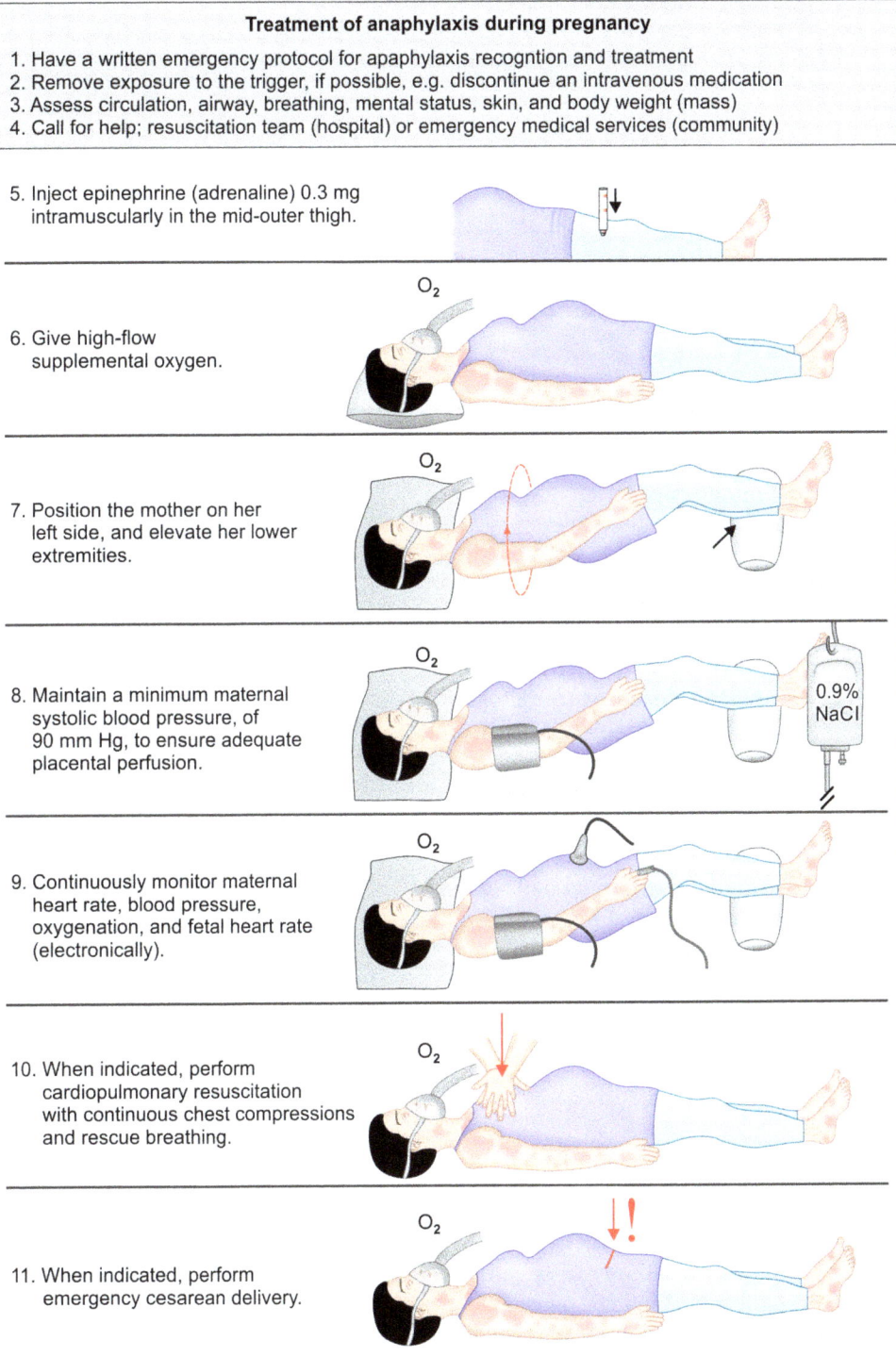

Treatment of anaphylaxis during pregnancy

1. Have a written emergency protocol for apaphylaxis recogntion and treatment
2. Remove exposure to the trigger, if possible, e.g. discontinue an intravenous medication
3. Assess circulation, airway, breathing, mental status, skin, and body weight (mass)
4. Call for help; resuscitation team (hospital) or emergency medical services (community)
5. Inject epinephrine (adrenaline) 0.3 mg intramuscularly in the mid-outer thigh.
6. Give high-flow supplemental oxygen.
7. Position the mother on her left side, and elevate her lower extremities.
8. Maintain a minimum maternal systolic blood pressure, of 90 mm Hg, to ensure adequate placental perfusion.
9. Continuously monitor maternal heart rate, blood pressure, oxygenation, and fetal heart rate (electronically).
10. When indicated, perform cardiopulmonary resuscitation with continuous chest compressions and rescue breathing.
11. When indicated, perform emergency cesarean delivery.

Fig. 6: Basic initial management of anaphylaxis in pregnancy.[23]

Bronchodilators
- Selective β2-agonist (albuterol) using nebulizer if cough and wheezing are prominent

H1-antihistamines
- Parenteral: Diphenhydramine 50 mg intravenous to relieve itching and hives
- Oral: Cetirizine and Loratadine, safe in pregnancy, nonsedating, minimally secreted in breast milk

Glucocorticoids
- Methylprednisolone: 1 mg/kg intravenous every 8 hours up to 3 doses, in cases of severe anaphylaxis, to reduce the risk of protracted anaphylaxis

Fig. 7: Adjunctive treatment in anaphylaxis.[27-29]

sound newborn.[30] If the abnormal pattern resolves, it is still advisable to continue electronic FHR monitoring for 48–72 hours postanaphylaxis.[31]

Emergency Cesarean Delivery

It is considered in the setting of continuous nonreassuring FHR pattern, despite all resuscitative medical measures to restore fetomaternal hemodynamic stability. The aim should be to deliver the baby within 5 minutes of maternal cardiac arrest. Cesarean delivery can have beneficial effect on the maternal cardiac status (Flowchart 2).

The decision for delivery should be taken with high risk consent for both mother and fetus. The potential benefit of prompt delivery should be calculated against possible neonatal morbidity and mortality in case of extreme prematurity.[23]

■ PREVENTION

The prophylactic management involves a detailed history taking so as to find out the culprit allergen and prevention of the exposure to the specific allergen trigger. Patients with history of allergy to specific agents like drugs or latex should be referred to an allergy specialist, ideally before pregnancy, so as to perform noncritical skin testing

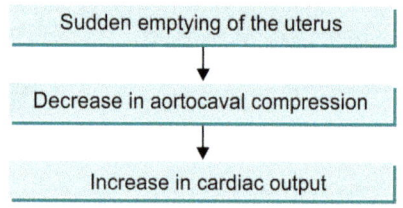

Flowchart 2: Effect of cesarean delivery on maternal cardiac status.

of required. It is best deferred until after pregnancy due to the possibility of a systemic allergic reaction during the procedure. Various aspects of emergency preparedness for anaphylactic reaction during pregnancy have been summarized in Figure 8.[23]

■ DIFFERENTIAL DIAGNOSIS OF ANAPHYLAXIS

There are many medical conditions,[32-34] as given in Table 2 and Box 2, which can be confused with anaphylaxis. The major differentiating point is a history of exposure to a specific allergen.

■ CONCLUSION

- Anaphylaxis is a very rare life-threatening medical emergency encountered during pregnancy.
- The presentation could include a combination of various signs and symptoms

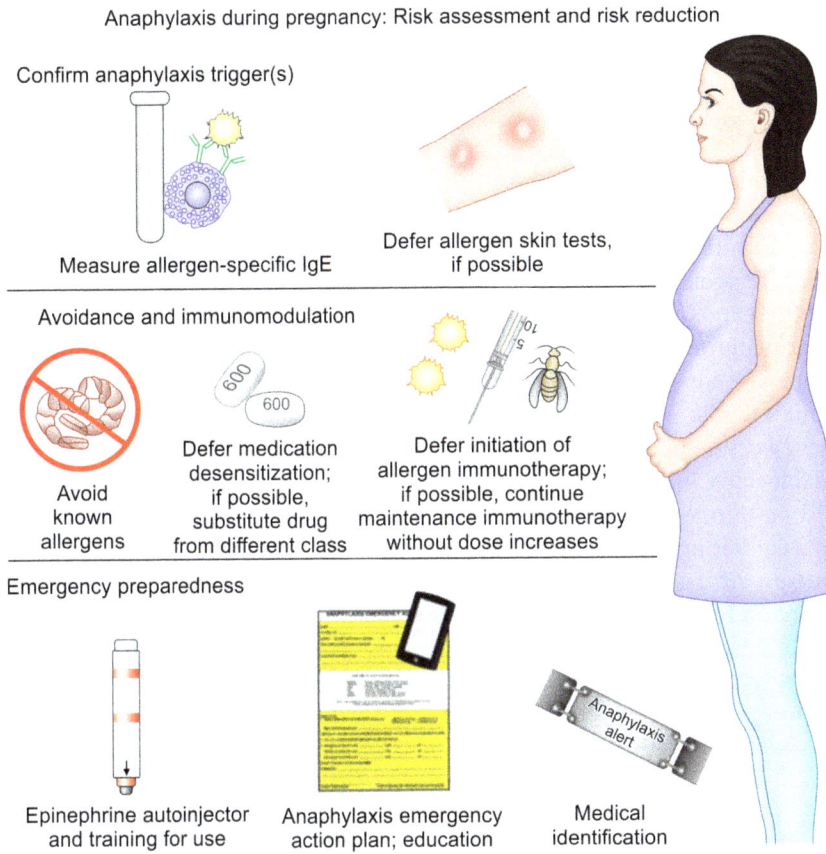

Fig. 8: Prophylactic management of anaphylaxis in pregnancy.

TABLE 2: During antenatal period.

Category	Example
Common dilemmas	Acute asthma, panic attack, acute angioedema, acute urticaria, and syncope
Upper airway obstruction	Pre-eclampsia, hereditary angioedema, and laryngopathia gravidarum
Shock	Hypovolemic, septic, and cardiogenic
Others	Mastocytosis, carcinoid syndrome, and Munchausen stridor

such as pruritus, urticaria, bronchospasm, angioedema, hypotension, and tachycardia.

Box 2: During labor and delivery.

- Pulmonary embolism and pulmonary edema
- Cardiac conditions (acquired and congenital)
- Hypotension (spinal block, local anesthetic, and postpartum hemorrhage)
- Cerebrovascular accident
- Amniotic fluid embolism
- Pre-eclampsia/eclampsia

- The features specific to pregnancy are uterine contractions, vulval itching, lower backache, fetal distress, and preterm labor.
- Anything could be a trigger to anaphylaxis, be it a drug, food, insect bite in the community setting, or latex, oxytocin or neuromuscular blockers during labor or delivery.

- The diagnosis is based mostly on clinical history and physical diagnosis, after excluding the possible differential diagnoses.
- Sudden cardiorespiratory collapse of the pregnant mother could lead to catastrophic events for the fetus as well, like hypoxic ischemic encephalopathy or fetal demise.
- Medical management includes discontinuing the exposure to allergen, intramuscular or intravenous administration of epinephrine, airway management, and intravenous fluids.
- Emergency cesarean delivery of a potentially viable fetus, in case of a nonreassuring FHR pattern, or within 5 minutes of maternal cardiac arrest.
- Prevention of anaphylaxis includes recognition and avoidance of the concerned allergen, emergency preparedness using epinephrine autoinjector, anaphylaxis emergency action plan, and medical identification.

REFERENCES

1. John M. Rosen's Emergency Medicine: Concepts and Clinical Practice, 7th edition. Philadelphia, PA: Mosby/Elsevier; 2010.
2. Sampson HA, Muñoz-Furlong A, Campbell RL, et al. Second symposium on the definition and management of anaphylaxis: summary report—Second National Institute of Allergy and Infectious Disease/Food Allergy and Anaphylaxis Network symposium. J Allergy Clin Immunol. 2006;117:391-7.
3. Wood RA, Camargo CA Jr, Lieberman P, et al. Anaphylaxis in America: the prevalence and characteristics of anaphylaxis in the United States. J Allergy Clin Immunol. 2014;133:461-7.
4. Decker WW, Campbell RL, Manivannan V, et al. The etiology and incidence of anaphylaxis in Rochester, Minnesota: a report from the Rochester Epidemiology Project. J Allergy Clin Immunol. 2008;122:1161-5.
5. Lieberman P, Camargo CA Jr, Bohlke K, et al. Epidemiology of anaphylaxis: findings of the American College of Allergy, Asthma and Immunology Epidemiology of Anaphylaxis Working Group. Ann Allergy Asthma Immunol. 2006;97:596-602.
6. Simons FE. Anaphylaxis. J Allergy Clin Immunol. 2010;125:S161-81.
7. Chaudhuri K, Gonzales J, Jesurun CA, et al. Anaphylactic shock in pregnancy: a case study and review of the literature. Int J Obstet Anesth. 2008;17:350-7.
8. Mulla ZD, Ebrahim MS, Gonzalez JL. Anaphylaxis in the obstetric patient: analysis of a statewide hospital discharge database. Ann Allergy Asthma Immunol. 2010;104:55-9.
9. Simons FE, Ardusso LRF, Bilo MB, et al. World Allergy Organization Guidelines for the Assessment and Management of Anaphylaxis. J Allergy Clin Immunol. 2011;127:593. e1-22.
10. Cox L, Nelson H, Lockey R, et al. Allergen immunotherapy: a practice parameter third update. J Allergy Clin Immunol. 2011;127(1 Suppl):S1-55.
11. Romero R, Kusanovic JP, Munoz H, et al. Allergy-induced preterm labor after the ingestion of shellfish. J Matern Fetal Neonatal Med. 2010;23:351-9.
12. Sengupta A, Kohli JK. Antibiotic prophylaxis in cesarean section causing anaphylaxis and intrauterine fetal death. J Obstet Gynaecol Res. 2008;34:252-4.
13. Khan R, Anastasakis E, Kadir RA. Anaphylactic reaction to ceftriaxone in labour. An emerging complication. J Obstet Gynaecol. 2008;28:751-3.
14. Smith HS, Hare MJ, Hoggarth CE, et al. Delivery as a cause of exercise induced anaphylactoid reaction: case report. Br J Obstet Gynaecol. 1985;92:1196-8.
15. Shank JJ, Olney SC, Lin FL, et al. Recurrent postpartum anaphylaxis with breast-feeding. Obstet Gynecol. 2009;114:415-6.
16. Reber L, Hernandez J, Galli S. The pathophysiology of anaphylaxis. J Allergy Clin Immunol. 2017;140:335-48.
17. Simons FE, Frew AJ, Ansotegui IJ, et al. Risk assessment in anaphylaxis: current and future approaches. J Allergy Clin Immunol. 2007;120(1 Suppl):S2-24.
18. Beutier H, Gillis CM, Iannascoli B, et al. IgG subclasses determine pathways of anaphylaxis in mice. J Allergy Clin Immunol. 2017;139:269-80.

19. Jonsson F, Mancardi DA, Kita Y, et al. Mouse and human neutrophils induce anaphylaxis. J Clin Invest. 2011;121:1484-96.
20. Brown SG, Stone SF, Fatovich DM, et al. Anaphylaxis: clinical patterns, mediator release, and severity. J Allergy Clin Immunol. 2013;132:1141-9.
21. Strait RT, Morris SC, Finkelman FD. IgG-blocking antibodies inhibit IgE-mediated anaphylaxis in vivo through both antigen interception and Fc gamma RIIb cross-linking. J Clin Invest. 2006;116:833-41.
22. Strait RT, Mahler A, Hogan S, et al. Ingested allergens must be absorbed systemically to induce systemic anaphylaxis. J Allergy Clin Immunol. 2011;127:982-9.
23. Simons FE, Schatz M. Anaphylaxis during pregnancy. J Allergy Clin Immunol. 2012; 130(3):597-606.
24. Cousins L. Fetal oxygenation, assessment of fetal well-being, and obstetric management of the pregnant patient with asthma. J Allergy Clin Immunol. 1999;103(2 Pt 2):S343-9.
25. Lombaard H, Soma-Pillay P, Farrell el-M. Managing acute collapse in pregnant women. Best Pract Res Clin Obstet Gynecol. 2009; 23:339-55.
26. Suresh MS, LaToya Mason C, Munnur U. Cardiopulmonary resuscitation and the parturient. Best Pract Res Clin Obstet Gynecol. 2010;24:383-400.
27. Perel P, Roberts I, Ker K. Colloids versus crystalloids for fluid resuscitation in critically ill patients. Cochrane Database Syst Rev. 2013;(2):CD000567.
28. Sheikh A, Ten Broek V, Brown SG, et al. H1-antihistamines for the treatment of anaphylaxis: Cochrane systematic review. Allergy. 2007;62:830-7.
29. Choo KJ, Simons FE, Sheikh A. Glucocorticoids for the treatment of anaphylaxis. Cochrane Database Syst Rev. 2012;(4):CD007596.
30. Hepner DL, Castells M, Mouton-Faivre C, et al. Anaphylaxis in the clinical setting of obstetric anesthesia: a literature review. Anesth Analg. 2013;117:1357-67.
31. Berenguer A, Couto A, Brites V, et al. Anaphylaxis in pregnancy: a rare cause of neonatal mortality. BMJ Case Rep. 2013;2013. pii:bcr2012007055.
32. Fontaine C, Mayorga C, Bousquet PJ, et al. Relevance of the determination of serum-specific IgE antibodies in the diagnosis of immediate beta-lactam allergy. Allergy. 2007;62:47-52.
33. Antico A, Pagani M, Compalati E, et al. Risk assessment of immediate systemic reactions from skin tests with beta-lactam antibiotics. Int Arch Allergy Immunol. 2011;156:427-33.
34. Accetta Pedersen DJ, Klancnik M, et al. Analysis of available diagnostic tests for latex sensitization in an at-risk population. Ann Allergy Asthma Immunol. 2012;108:94-7.

CHAPTER 53

Sickle Cell Crisis

Priyanka Yadav

◼ OBJECTIVES

- Improve the management of sickle cell crisis and its related complications during pregnancy.
- Prevent mortality and morbidity associated with the disease.

◼ DEFINITION AND INTRODUCTION

Sickle cell disease is a hemoglobinopathy which includes group of inherited single gene autosomal recessive disorders caused by sickle gene, which affects hemoglobin (Hb) structure. It is typical Mendelian disorder which includes sickle hemoglobin (HbS) interaction with Hb variants other than normal HbA.[1,2] The pregnancies are at increased risk of obstetrical and fetal complications as well as medical complication of sickle cell disease. These risks are due to metabolic demands, hypercoagulable state, and vascular stasis associated with pregnancy.[3,4]

◼ INCIDENCE

Sickle cell crisis is most frequent complication of sickle cell disease during pregnancy with 27–50% women having painful crisis during pregnancy.[4]

◼ PATHOPHYSIOLOGY

Sickle hemoglobin is formed as the result of a single gene defect causing substitution of valine for glutamic acid in position 6 of the beta chain of adult hemoglobin [sickle cell anemia (HbSS)]. Structurally abnormal (deoxyhemoglobin) HbS polymerization is primarily indispensable initiating event in sickle cell disease in which HbS molecule undergoes "hypoxia-induced polymerization" followed by red blood cell injury and sickling with resultant microvascular occlusion. Clinically manifested most often as an acute painful episode or crisis.

◼ COMPLICATIONS[5,6]

Complications of sickle cell crisis are given in Table 1.

◼ PRECIPITATING FACTORS[4]

- Infection
- Hypoxia

TABLE 1: Complications of sickle cell crisis.

Maternal risk	Fetal risk
Painful crisis (>50%)	Miscarriage
Acute chest syndrome	Perinatal mortality
Urinary tract infection (UTI)	Intrauterine growth restriction (IUGR)
Pregnancy induced hypertension	Low birth weight (LBW)
Severe anemia	Premature delivery
Antepartum hemorrhage (APH)	
Thrombosis and acute stroke	
Increased cholecystitis	
Increased cesarean rate	
Increased maternal mortality	

- Hypothermia
- Hypotension
- Severe dehydration
- Venous stasis
- Pregnancy (because of hypercoagulable state).

INVESTIGATION[7,8]

Complete blood count (CBC), reticulocyte count, liver function test, renal function test, blood group, viral markers, and arterial blood gas (ABG).

Microbiological tests: Urine c/s and blood c/s.

Radiological tests: Chest X-ray (if chest is involved).

MANAGEMENT

The management of painful crisis in pregnant female with sickle cell disease does not have any randomized controlled trials. So, treatment of acute pain in pregnant female is usually the same as applicable to nonpregnant women.[9-11]

General Measures

- Pregnant women with sickle cell disease who is not well should have sickle cell crisis excluded as matter of urgency.
- A multidisciplinary team (senior obstetrician, anesthesiologist, hematologist, and pediatrician) should assess women.[8]
- Maintain circulation, airway, and breathing.
- Adequate rest and warmth, avoid precipitants.
- Assess and maintain airway patency (give oxygen if hypoxic on monitoring of O_2 saturation).
- Attach pulse oximeter, electrocardiogram (ECG) monitor, and assess vitals [pulse rate (PR), blood pressure (BP), respiratory rate (RR), temperature, and hydration)].
- Ensure adequate hydration, at least 60 mL/kg/24 h should be ensured either orally or intravenous (IV). Strict input output charting.
- Continuous fetal monitoring for viable fetus.

Pain Management (Box 1)

Aim

Analgesia to be given with 30 minutes of arriving hospital and effective analgesia should be achieved with in 1 hour.

- Antibiotics are not routinely required unless evidence of infection is there; low grade fever—38°C is in painful crisis even in absence of infection.
- Thromboprophylaxis including low-molecular-weight heparin (LMWH) and compression stocking should be given.
- Fetal well-being assessed regularly with cardiotocography (CTG).

Blood Transfusion (Box 2)

Although transfusion in pregnancy is well tolerated, it carries a risk of alloimmunization, iron overload, and transfusion-transmitted infection.

Box 1: Acute pain management.[11]

- *Nonopioid analgesia*: Paracetamol (PCM) for mild pain, nonsteroidal anti-inflammatory drug (NSAID) for mild-to-moderate pain between 12 weeks and 28 weeks of gestation
- *Strong opioids for severe pain*: Morphine, diamorphine or oxycodone
- Patient-controlled analgesia or subcutaneous pumps are occasionally required
- Monitor pain, sedation, vitals, respiratory rate (RR), O_2 saturation every 30 minutes until pain is controlled and signs are stable, then monitor every 2 hours (hourly if on intravenous opiates)
- Give rescue dose of analgesia, if required
- If RR is less than 10 breaths per minute, omit maintenance analgesia; consider naloxone
- Consider reducing analgesia after 2–3 days and replacing injections with equivalent dose of oral analgesia
- Prescribe antiemetic and laxatives, if required

> **Box 2:** Indications for blood transfusion.[4,8]
> - Hemoglobin (Hb) <6 g/dL
> - Fall of Hb by 2–3 g/dL
> - Anemia with cardio or respiratory compromise
> - History of sickle cell disease related complication
> - Patient already on a chronic transfusion program
> - Hemorrhage
> - Acute stroke
> - High output cardiac failure
> - Acute folate deficiency
> - Splenic or hepatic sequestration
> - Aplastic crisis

> **Box 3:** Indications for exchange transfusion.
> - Eclampsia and severe pre-eclampsia
> - Acute chest syndrome
> - Severe jaundice
> - Repeated stroke
> - Polycythemia
> - History of cerebrovascular accident

Exchange Transfusion (Box 3)

Its aim is to reduce the maternal Hb to less than 30% to reduce the chances of sickling. Transfusion is done to maintain normal Hb.

ACUTE CHEST SYNDROME

It is a leading cause of death in sickle cell disease in pregnancy.

Incidence

Acute chest syndrome is the most common complication after acute pain with incidence of 7-20% of pregnancies.[6,12]

PATHOPHYSIOLOGY[13-15]

Pathophysiology of acute chest syndrome (ACS) is described in Figure 1.

Causes

- Infection
- Fat embolism
- *Lung infection*: Pneumonia and pulmonary embolism
- Asthma.

Clinical Features

Acute onset of fever, respiratory symptoms, pleuritic chest pain, breathlessness, dry cough, and tachypnea.
- *On auscultation*: Basal crepps, signs of congestion, and pleural effusion.
- *On X-ray*: New infiltrate.

Treatment

- Hospitalize
- Antibiotics
- Oxygen
- Analgesics
- Bronchodilators
- Blood transfusion to maintain hematocrit >30
- Continuous monitoring of hydration is required to prevent pulmonary edema
- Exchange transfusion can be considered if arterial saturation drops to <90%.

ACUTE STROKE

Stroke is medical emergency. It is a devastating manifestation of sickle cell disease, both infarctive and hemorrhagic are associated with sickle cell disease and this diagnosis should be considered in pregnant women with sickle cell disease who presents with neurological impairment.[16]

Clinical Features

- Severe headache
- Speech abnormalities
- Weakness
- Numbness
- Visual disturbances
- Altered mental status.

Management

- Brain imaging
- Rapid exchange transfusion.

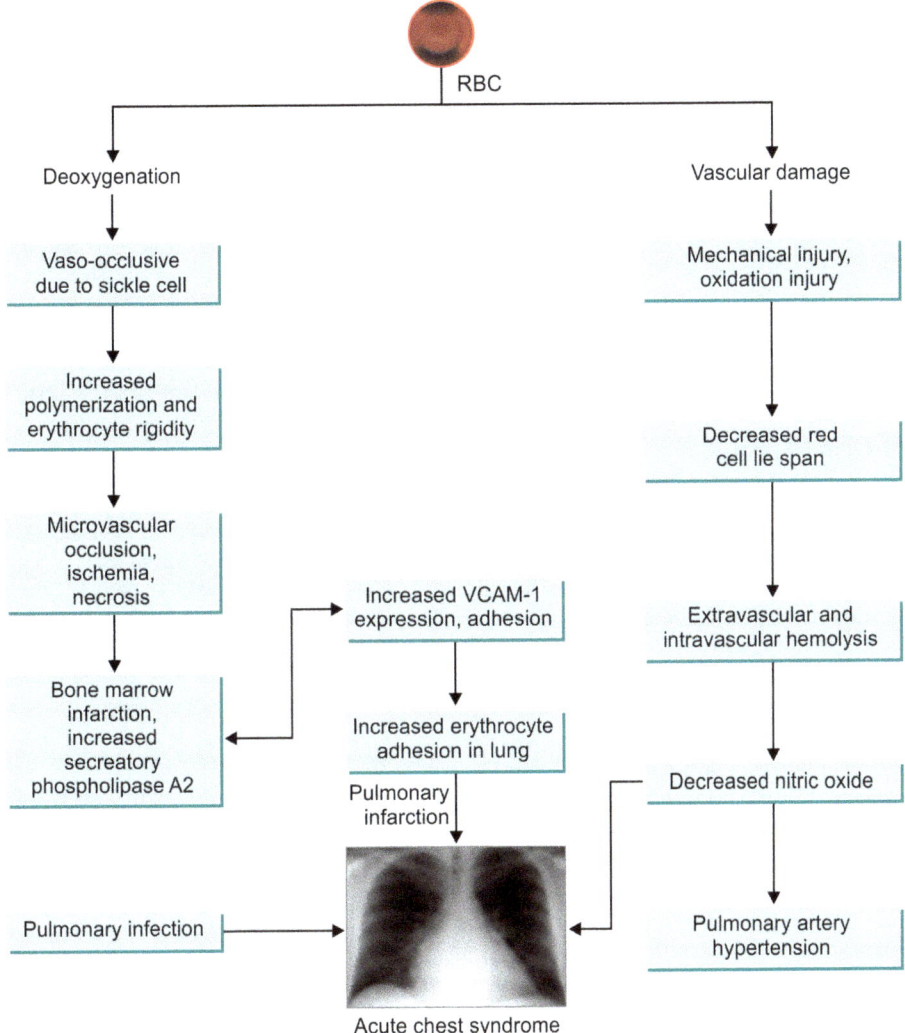

Fig. 1: Pathophysiology of acute chest syndrome.
(RBC: red blood cell; VCAM-1: vascular cell adhesion protein)

Differential Diagnosis

- Valvular heart disease
- Sepsis
- Upper respiratory tract infection
- Lupus erythematosus
- Rheumatic fever
- *Obstetrical emergencies*: Pre-eclampsia, abruption, acute anemia, intrahepatic cholestasis of pregnancy, and acute fatty liver of pregnancy
- *Surgical emergencies*: Pancreatitis, splenic infarction, deep vein thrombosis, cholecystitis, and appendicitis.

All the above conditions can present with same symptoms of pain, fever, and anemia, so need to be cautiously differentiated from sickle cell crisis during pregnancy.

CONCLUSION

Sickle cell crisis in pregnancy is an obstetrical emergency. This includes high-risk maternofetal complications which need multidisciplinary approach to deliver optimal care, which is crucial for both maternal and fetal well-being. A high index of suspicion, good judgment, and quick decision are necessary to obtain optimal results in the pregnant patient affected by sickle cell crisis and significantly decrease morbidity and mortality.

REFERENCES

1. Pauling L, Itano HA, Singer SJ, et al. Sickle cell anemia a molecular disease. Science. 1949;110(2865):543-8.
2. Weatherall D, Akinyanju O, Fucharoen S, et al. Inherited disorders of hemoglobin. Disease Control Priorities in Developing Countries, 2nd edition. Washington, DC: World Bank; 2006. pp. 663-80.
3. ACOG Committee on Obstetrics. ACOG practice bulletin no. 78: hemoglobinopathies in pregnancy. Obstet Gynecol. 2007;109(1):229-37.
4. Royal College of Obstetricians and Gynaecologists. (2011) Management of sickle cell disease in pregnancy. [online] Available from: https://www.guidelinecentral.com/summaries/management-of-sickle-cell-disease-in-pregnancy/#section-society [Last accessed September, 2019].
5. Al Jama FE, Gasem T, Burshaid S, et al. Pregnancy outcome in patients with homozygous sickle cell disease in a university hospital, Eastern Saudi Arabia. Arch Gynecol Obstet. 2009;280(5):793-7.
6. Serjeant GR, Loy LL, Crowther M, et al. Outcome of pregnancy in homozygous sickle cell disease. Obstet Gynecol. 2004;103(6):1278-85.
7. Sickle Cell Society. Standards for the Clinical Care of Adults with Sickle Cell Disease in the UK. London: Sickle Cell Society; 2008.
8. Parrish MR, Morrison JC. Sickle cell crisis and pregnancy. Semin Perinatol. 2013;37(4):274-9.
9. Martin JN Jr, Martin RW, Morrison JC. Acute management of sickle cell crisis in pregnancy. Clin Perinatol. 1986;13(4):853-68.
10. Marti-Carvajal AJ, Peña-Marti GE, Comunián-Carrasco G, et al. Interventions for treating painful sickle cell crisis during pregnancy. Cochrane Database Syst Rev. 2009;(1): CD006786.
11. Rees DC, Olujohungbe AD, Parker NE, et al. Guidelines for the management of acute painful crisis in sickle cell disease. Br J Haematol. 2003;120(5):744-52.
12. Howard RJ, Tuck SM, Pearson TC. Pregnancy in sickle cell disease in the UK: results of a multicentre survey of the effect of prophylactic blood transfusion on maternal and fetal outcome. Br J Obstet Gynaecol. 1995;102(12); 947-51.
13. Styles LA, Abboud M, Larkin S, et al. Transfusion prevents acute chest syndrome predicted by elevated secretory phospholipase A2. Br J Haematol. 2007;136(2):343-4.
14. Nomura RM, Igai AM, Tosta K, et al. Acute chest syndrome in pregnant women with hemoglobin SC disease. Clinics (Sao Paulo). 2009;64(9):927-8.
15. Elsayegh D, Shapiro JM. Sickle cell vasoocclusive crisis and acute chest syndrome at term pregnancy. South Med J. 2007;100(1):77-9.
16. Ohene-Frempong K, Weiner SJ, Sleeper LA, et al. Cerebrovascular accidents in sickle cell disease: rates and risk factors. Blood. 1998;91(1):288-94.

CHAPTER 54

Severe Anemia in Pregnancy and Labor

Jyothirmayi Kunam

INTRODUCTION

Anemia in pregnancy requires more attention than it is currently receiving. Estimates of the World Health Organization (WHO) report that around 35-75% of antenatal women in developing countries and 18% of antenatal women in developed countries are anemic.[1] In India, anemia is often severe and contributes to mortality in pregnancy and also reproductive health morbidity. A lot of programs have been implemented for safety of motherhood but still maternal anemia remains a problem of major concern.

DEFINITION

The WHO defines anemia in pregnancy as hemoglobin (Hb) content below 11 g/dL and also hematocrit below 0.33.[2] The Centers for Disease Control (1990) has definition of anemia is Hb below 11 g/dL in the 1st, 3rd trimesters and below 10.5 g/dL in the 2nd trimester. In India anemia is defined as Hb <10 g/dL as given by the Federation of Obstetric and Gynaecological Societies of India (Mudaliar).

This difference between the cutoff values based on gestational age is explained by the fact that the drop in Hb level in pregnancy is very much higher in the 2nd trimester due to a relatively higher increase of the plasma volume compared with the Hb mass and red blood cell (RBC) volume. Late in pregnancy, plasma expansion ceases while Hb content continues to rise.

PHYSIOLOGICAL ANEMIA DURING PREGNANCY

The progressive increase in circulating blood volume in pregnancy is due to increase in plasma and RBC volume. These changes start at 7-8 weeks and reach maximum by 32 weeks of gestation and the Hb level does not usually go below 11 g% (Figs. 1 and 2).

CLASSIFICATION OF ANEMIAS

The WHO classification has been shown in Table 1.

Although Hb of 11 g% is taken as cutoff point as per WHO definition, in developing countries and India, cutoff point is taken as 10.5 g%. According to the guidelines by WHO (1999), Hb percentage is represented in g/L, instead of g/dL.

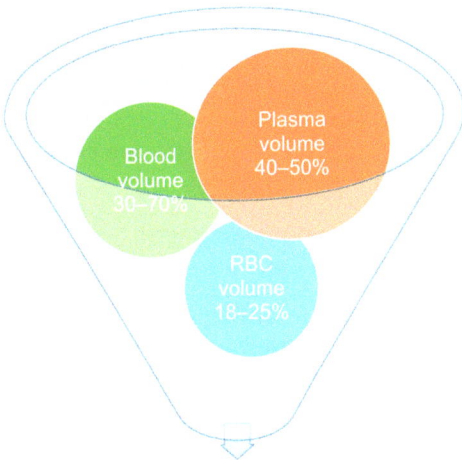

Physiological anemia in pregnancy

Fig. 1: Representation of hemodynamic changes in pregnancy.

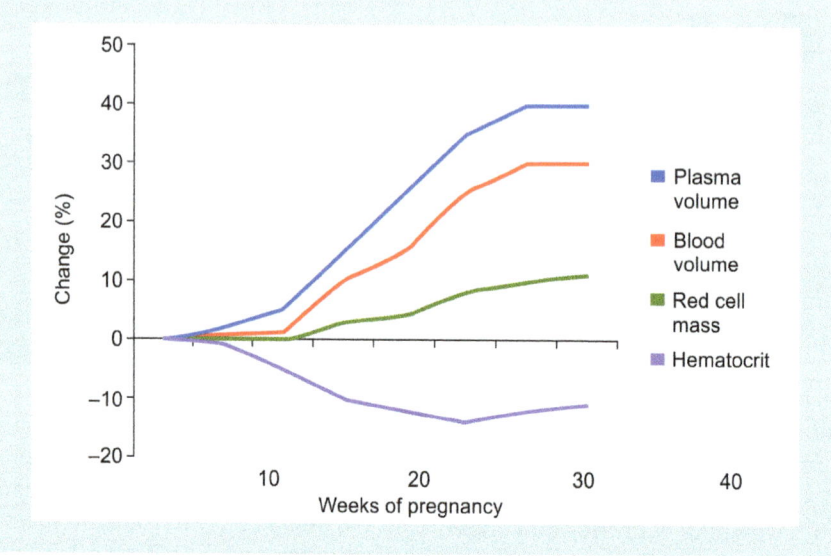

Fig. 2: Graphical representation of the hemodynamic changes in pregnancy.[3]

TABLE 1: The WHO classification.		
Mild anemia	Moderate anemia	Severe anemia
9.1–11 g/dL	7.1–9 g/dL	<7–11 g/dL

TABLE 2: Indian Council of Medical Research (ICMR) classification.			
Category 1	Category 2	Category 3	Category 4
• Mild • 10–10.9 g/dL	• Moderate • 7–10 g/dL	• Severe • <7 g/dL	• Very severe • <4 g/dL

Recent Classification

According to WHO 2002, recent classification of anemia is as follows:
- Mild/moderate anemia—7.0–10.9 g/dL
- Severe anemia—7 g/dL.

Indian Council of Medical Research classification has been shown in Table 2.

Modern classification—kinetic has been shown in Flowchart 1.

Different types of anemia are shown in Flowchart 2.

ETIOLOGY OF ANEMIA IN PREGNANCY

Anemia may be both physiological and pathological. Pathological anemia is the common complication in pregnancy (Table 3).

DETERMINANTS OF ANEMIA

Many factors like nutrition, pregnancy, menstruation, lactation, gender, age, ethnicity and race influence anemia. Anemia occurs in conditions where the production of RBCs is exceeded by their destruction. Hence the factors that lead to anemia act by reducing production of RBCs or by increasing their damage or both.[4]

Iron Deficiency Anemia

The most common type of anemia in pregnancy is iron deficiency anemia.[5] Iron deficiency anemia in pregnancy occurs primarily due to plasma volume expansion without normal Hb mass expansion.

Iron requirement in a singleton pregnancy is around 1,000 mg[6]. Fetus and placenta require 300 mg whereas growing RBCs of mother require 500 mg, 200 mg are shed through

Severe Anemia in Pregnancy and Labor

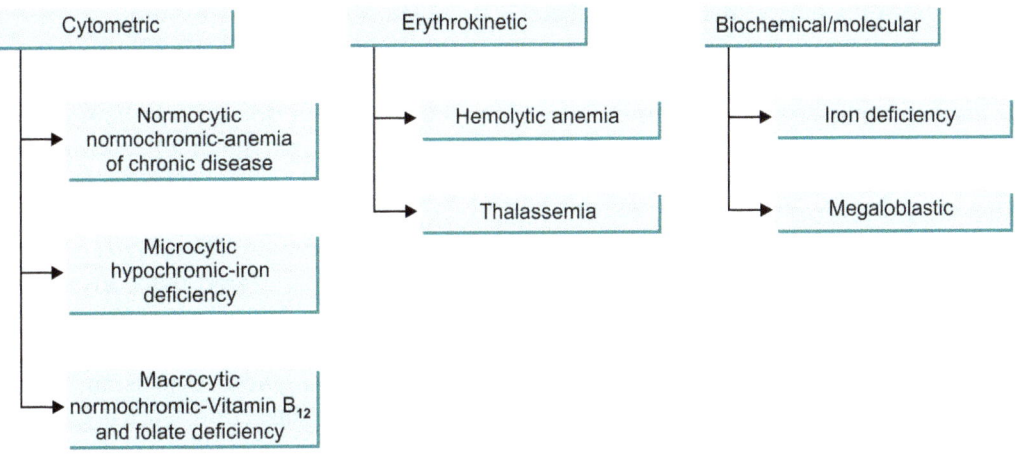

Flowchart 1: Modern classification—kinetic.

Flowchart 2: Types of anemia.

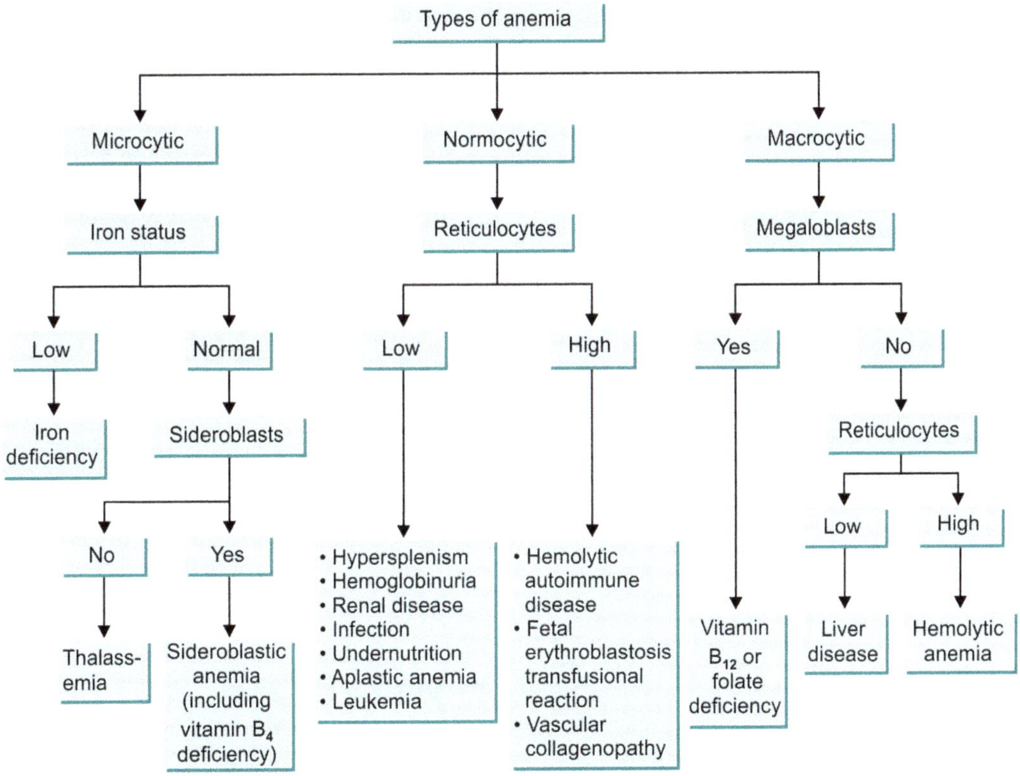

Source: Adapted from De Regl LM, Peha-Rosas JP, Garcia-Casal MN. Anemias de origen nutricio. In: Kaufer-Horwitz M, Perez-Lizaur AB, Arroyo P (Eds). Nutriologia Medica, 4th edition. Mexico City: Panamericana; 2014. pp. 401-33.

gut, skin, and urine. There is additional loss of 200 mg at the time of delivery. 300 mg of iron is saved due to amenorrhea. The total amount (1,000 mg) surpasses the iron stores in maximum women and hence results in iron deficiency anemia. This implies approximately 900–1,000 mg is required during pregnancy, i.e. 4–6 mg of iron per day.

Diagnosis

- *Hemoglobin estimation*: It is the most practical, cost-effective and one of the easiest method of diagnosis. The most commonly used method of Hb estimation is Sahil's method whereas Taliquist's method is simple and easy but is inaccurate. Cyanmethemoglobin method is apparently more accurate but not commonly used.
- *Peripheral blood film*: Iron deficiency, megaloblastic and hemolytic anemia can be differentiated with this simple bedside test. Microcytic, hypochromic blood picture indicates iron deficiency. Anisocytosis, poikilocytosis and target cells are also noted. Iron deficiency anemia must be differentiated from thalassemia.

Comparison of red cell indices in thalassemia and iron deficiency anemia has been shown in Table 4.

- *Serum ferritin*: It is an accurate reflection of the iron stores. Recent iron intake does not affect the stable iron stores but it is the first parameter to fall in iron deficiency. Serum ferritin is estimated by sensitive immunoradiometric assay. Anemic mothers have low serum cord ferritin. Serum ferritin <12 µg/L indicates iron deficiency.
- *Serum iron*: A healthy adult woman has serum iron between 60 mg/dL and 120 mg/dL. It shows significant diurnal

TABLE 3: Pathological anemia of pregnancy.

Deficiency anemia (isolated or combined)	- Iron deficiency - Folic acid deficiency - Vitamin B$_{12}$ deficiency - Protein deficiency
Hemorrhagic	- Acute following bleeding in early months or APH - Chronic—Hookworm infestation, bleeding piles
Hereditary	- Thalassemias - Sickle cell hemoglobinopathies - Other hemoglobinopathies - Hereditary hemolytic anemias - RBC membrane defects - Spherocytosis
Bone marrow insufficiency	Hypoplasia or aplasia due to irradiation
Chronic renal disease or neoplasm	

TABLE 4: Comparison of red cell indices in thalassemia and iron deficiency anemia.[7,8]

Characteristics	Calculation	Normal range	Iron deficiency	Thalassemia
MCV* (fL)	PCV/RBC	75–96	Reduced	Very reduced
MCH (pg)	Hb/RBC	27–33	Reduced	Very reduced
MCHC** (g/dL)	Hb/PCV	32–35	Reduced	Normal or slightly receded
Hb (%)	HbF/HbA × 100	<2%	Normal	Raised
HbA$_2$ (%)	HbA$_2$ × 100	2–3%	Normal or reduced	Raised
FEB (µg/dL)		<35	>50	Normal
Red cell width		High		Normal

*Mean corpuscular volume (MCV) is the first to get reduced and is the most sensitive indicator of iron deficiency.
**Mean corpuscular hemoglobin concentration (MCHC) is reduced in more severe cases of iron depteiction.

variation, even with hourly fluctuations. Serum iron even in combination with total iron-binding capacity (TIBC) is not a reliable indicator of iron stores due to wide fluctuations with oral iron, infections, etc.

- *Total iron binding capacity*: In the nonpregnant state, TIBC lies in the range of 300–350 mg/dL (increased to 300–400 mg/dL in pregnancy) and is approximately one-third saturated with iron in nonanemic person. It is raised in iron deficiency and low in chronic inflammatory states.
- *Serum iron*: Indicators of iron deficiency during pregnancy include serum iron levels <60 mg/dL, transferring saturation <15% and TIBC >350 mg/dL.

Hematological changes according to stages of anemia have been shown in Figure 3.

- *Free erythrocyte protoporphyrin (FEP)*: It rises with iron deficiency and becomes evident 2–3 weeks after iron depletion. Iron deficiency anemia and thalassemia can be differentiated by FEP.[7]
- *Serum transferrin receptor (TfR)*: It is a transmembrane protein that attaches to transferrin iron and transports it to the cell interior. Serum TfR is a good indicator of iron deficiency in pregnancy with high sensitivity and specificity and is a reliable indicator of cellular iron status. TfR will give a true reflection of iron deficit in the tissues in pregnancy when ferritin may be low because of mobilization and in chronic inflammatory disease when ferritin is inappropriately elevated because of release from cells. Its levels are increased in iron deficiency anemia.

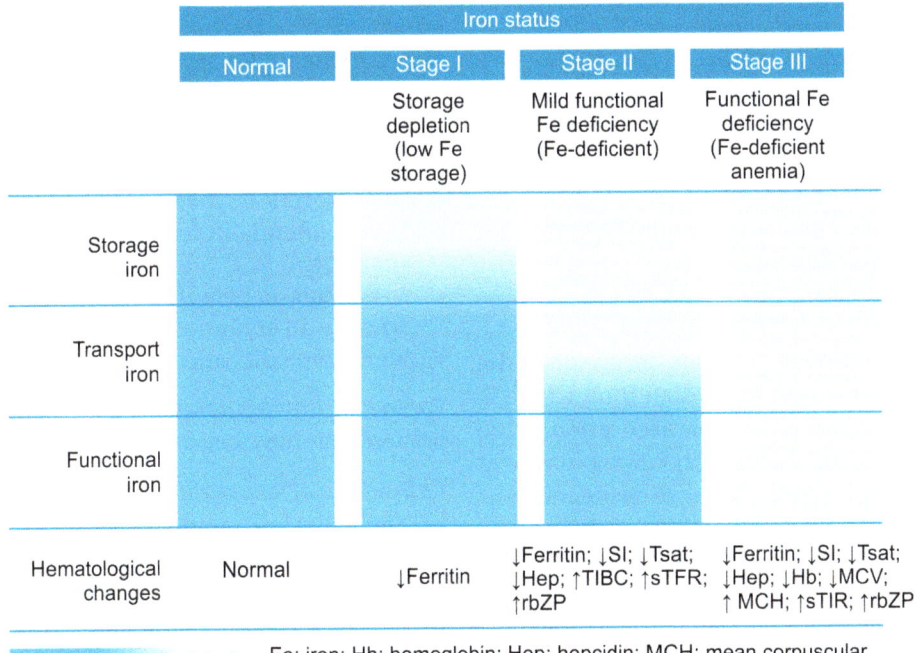

Fe: iron; Hb: hemoglobin; Hep: hepcidin; MCH: mean corpuscular hemoglobin; MCV: mean corpuscular volume; rbZP: red blood cell zinc protoporphyrin; SI: serum iron; sTfR: serum transferrin receptor; TIBC: total iron-binding capacity; Tsat: transferrin saturation

Fig. 3: Hematological changes according to stages of anemia.[4]

- *Marrow iron*: Blue granules of stainable iron with potassium ferrocyanide are the characteristic finding in bone marrow examination. It is the test with good accuracy for iron stores but as it is an invasive test and is not practical. Bone marrow examination is done very rarely. If anemia does not improve after 4 weeks of iron therapy, in suspected aplastic anemia and in diagnosis of kala-azar bone marrow examination helps in easy diagnosis.[9]
- *Stool examination*: One of the common causes of anemia in developing countries is worm infestation. Hence stool examination for ova and cysts should be done in all cases.
- *Urine examination*: Testing for occult blood and parasites like schistosomes is indicated in prevalent areas. Bacteriuria should also be ruled out.
- *Peripheral blood smear* reveals the presence of malarial parasites.
- *Other tests*:
  - Sputum examination
  - Chest X-ray posteroanterior (PA) view for pulmonary tuberculosis (with abdominal shield)
  - Blood urea and serum creatinine
  - Liver function tests.[7]

Management of Iron Deficiency Anemia

Oral iron therapy: Ferrous ascorbate is the best suitable iron for Indian food which is rich in inhibitors for iron absorption.[10] 100 mg of elemental iron with 0.5 mg folic acid for prophylaxis and 180 mg of elemental iron/day for treatment are the recommendations by *Ministry of Health*. Rise in reticulocyte count in 10 days and Hb concentration of 0.3–1.0 g each week is ideally expected. Oral iron must be continued for 3 months after anemia correction to replenish iron stores. Diagnostic re-evaluation is suggested if there is not much improvement in 3–4 weeks of therapy.

The *National Anemia Prophylaxis Programme* distributes folifer tablets 100 mg of elemental iron and 500 µg of folic acid to all pregnant women who are not anemic for at least last 100 days of pregnancy. For patients with Hb between 7 g/dL and 11 g/dL—2 tablets of folifer for 103 days. Patients with Hb less than 7 g/dL are referred to the first referral centers.

Oral iron is available in different salts like ferrous sulfate, ferrous gluconate, ferrous fumarate, etc. in combination with variable doses of folic acid. They release iron slowly as they pass through the digestive tract, hence not well absorbed and also does not have much gut side effects. Carbonyl iron is less toxic and has comparatively high tolerance.

New preparations of iron include complexes of iron polymaltose and polysucrose hydroxide which have more bioavailability. Sulfate of ferrous glycine is easily absorbed orally and has less adverse drug reactions.

Parenteral iron therapy: Rise in Hb content after parenteral therapy is the similar to oral iron, 0.7–1 g/week.

Indications:
- Poor acceptance
- Malabsorption syndromes
- Severe anemia in the last 8–10 weeks of pregnancy
- In patients on hemo/peritoneal dialysis or who are on erythropoietin treatment
- Noncompliant patients.

Parenteral iron preparations: Parenteral iron preparations have been shown in Table 5.

Calculation of iron requirement:
- Elemental iron required in mg = Hb deficit in g/dL × Weight in kg × 2.21 + 1,000
  - Normal Hb being 14 g/dL and 2.21 is the standard coefficient. Additional 1,000 mg is given for the replenishment of stores.
- Iron requirement in mg = 0.3 × Weight (lb) × (Hb deficit). Add 500 mg for stores

Severe Anemia in Pregnancy and Labor

TABLE 5: Parenteral iron preparations.

Iron dextran complex (Imferon)	• Intramuscularly—pain at injection site, skin staining, abscess, fever, arthralgia, lymphadenopathy • Intravenously—severe anaphylaxis • If the iron requirement is >2,500 mg, divided dose therapy is to be administered
Iron sorbitol citrate (Jactofer)	• Intramuscularly • Elemental iron with folic acid and B_{12}
Iron sucrose complex (Venofer)	• 200–300 mg/dose to maximum 600 mg/week at intravenous rate of 20 mg/minute • Or 200 mg in 200 mL NS infusion
Iron gluconate	Also called Ferrlecit which contains sodium ferric gluconate
Iron carboxymaltose (FCM)	• Slow IV at 100 mg/minute or infusion 1,000 mg over 15 minutes (2 mg/mL) • No test dose required

- 4.4 × Body weight (kg) × Hb deficit (g/dL), this formula includes iron needed for replenishment of stores
- 250 mg of elemental iron for each g% of Hb deficit.

Technique of giving parenteral iron:
Intravenous route:
- All the necessary resuscitation equipment and drugs are to be kept ready.
- Test dose is to be given.
- Extra vigilance for any signs of adverse reaction like chest discomfort, dyspnea, chills and rigors, hypotension and anaphylactic response.[7]
- Stop the infusion in case of reaction.
- Antihistaminics, corticoids and epinephrine to be administered.

Intramuscular route:
- Oral iron is not given concurrently to avoid adverse reaction.
- To test for hypersensitivity.
- Deep intramuscular injections are given on alternate buttocks (Z technique).
- Side effects include pain, injection abscess, lymphadenopathy and very rarely anaphylactic reactions.

Blood transfusion:
- Pregnancy after 36 weeks with severe anemia
- Concomitant infection
- Blood loss due to antepartum or postpartum hemorrhage (PPH)
- Refractory anemia
- Side effects include transfusion reaction, preterm labor and rarely cardiac failure.[7,11]

Recombinant erythropoietin: Extremely useful substitute to blood transfusion.

Injection erythropoietin/Epofer:
- Preliminary subcutaneous sensitivity test is to be done.
- Adrenaline, hydrocortisone and oxygen should be kept ready.
- It can be administered either by subcutaneous or intravenous route.
- *Dose:* 100–150 IU/kg on days 1, 3 and 5 along with intravenous iron or 6,000 units of subcutaneous erythropoietin on days 1, 3 and 5 and 100 mg of iron dextran deep intramuscular every day for 5 days.

Folic Acid Deficiency

It was called pernicious anemia of pregnancy. Folic acid requirement is 400 µg/day in the pregnant women.

Investigations (Figs. 4 and 5)

Other Investigations: Deoxyuridine suppression test differentiates between folic acid and B_{12} deficit.

Additional folic acid dose is recommended in:
- Hemolytic anemia
- Previous baby had neural tube defects

- Multifetal pregnancy
- Alcoholism
- Inflammatory skin disorders
- Crohn's disease.

Prophylaxis

Though 300–500 μg in most iron preparations is sufficient for prophylaxis,[8,12] WHO recommends an everyday folate consumption of 800 μg in the pregnancy period and 600 μg throughout lactation.

Treatment

Folic acid, 5 mg/day, must be continued for a minimum of 4 weeks in puerperium. By 4–7 days of treatment the reticulocyte count is noticeably improved.

Vitamin B_{12} Deficiency

Addisonian pernicious anemia due to intrinsic factor deficiency results in absence of absorption of vitamin B_{12}. It is uncommon in pregnancy as it generally results in childlessness. Females with partial/total gastrectomy, Crohn's disease, ileal illness, *Diphyllobothrium latum* infestation and bacterial overgrowth in small bowel may lead to vitamin B_{12} deficiency. Acquired vitamin B_{12} deficiency resulting in megaloblastic anemia is equally infrequent, as the day-to-day necessity of vitamin B_{12} is 3.0 μg in pregnancy which is certainly met through a regular diet.[13]

Signs and Symptoms

Onset of anemia is usually insidious and is gradually progressive. Clinical features include weakness, easy fatigability, tiredness, gastrointestinal symptoms like vomiting, anorexia, loose stools and glossitis. Skin and oral mucosal pigmentation, hepatomegaly, splenomegaly, petechial rash are likely symptoms. Megaloblastic anemia does not have nail changes. It arises more frequently in multiple gestations, appears late in pregnancy about 20–28 weeks, immediate postpartum, in oral contraceptive users or in antiepileptic drug users.[14]

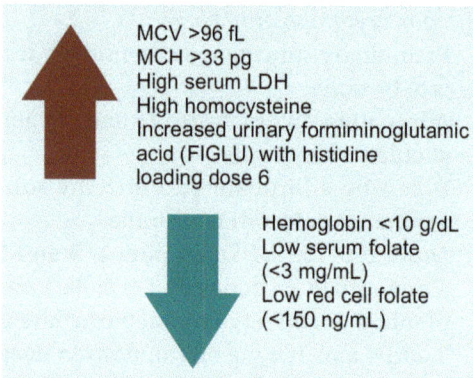

Fig. 4: Blood indices in folic acid deficiency.

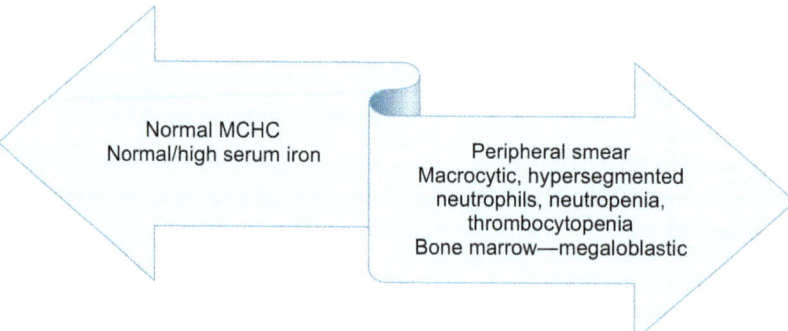

Fig. 5: Diagnostic aids for folic acid deficiency.

Investigations

Findings are similar to folate deficit. Less than 90 µg/L of vitamin B_{12} in blood is indicative of diagnosis. Serum homocysteine is raised in both folate and vitamin B_{12} deficiency. Serum methylmalonic acid is raised in vitamin B_{12} shortage. Schilling test is also diagnostic of pernicious anemia.

Treatment

Cyanocobalamin (250 µg) is prescribed intramuscularly every month before pregnancy.

Anemia due to Blood Loss

- In tropical countries hookworm infestation is the common cause of anemia. *Ancylostoma duodenale* draws 0.25 mL of blood/worm/day and *Necator americanus* 0.03 mL/worm/day. Those with worm infestation are given tablet albendazole 400 mg stat.
- Antepartum hemorrhage is also a cause for anemia and may also aggravate the pre-existing anemia.

Anemia due to Hemolysis

Intravascular microangiopathic hemolysis, which occurs in HELLP syndrome, is the most common form of hemolytic anemia seen during pregnancy. Thrombotic thrombocytopenic purpura (TTP) and hemolytic uremic syndrome (HUS) along with HELLP syndrome show burr cells, schistocytes and fragmented red cells.

Sickle Cell Disease

The most common hemoglobinopathy encountered in pregnancy is sickle cell disease (SCD) which is an autosomal recessive disorder triggered by point mutation in the beta-globin chain on chromosome 2 resulting in substitution of glutamic acid by valine in 6th position.

Sickle Cell Trait

Sickle cell trait is due to heterozygous inheritance of the Hb S gene.

In conditions where there is deoxygenation, hyperpyrexia, dehydration, acidosis, sustained capillary stasis sickling is triggered resulting in the occlusion of the microvasculature, producing a *painful sickle cell crisis*.

The greatest common reason for mortality in sickle cell patients is *acute chest syndrome*. It is characterized by chest discomfort, breathlessness, cough, hyperpyrexia. Infection is the most common reason for sickle cell crisis. High temperature, leukocytosis, raised bilirubin, and lactate dehydrogenase (LDH) are some of the markers of crisis (Flowchart 3).

Thalassemia in Pregnancy

- Globin gene point mutations are the root cause of thalassemia.
- Naked eye single tube red cell osmotic fragility test (NESTROFT) is a screening test. The definitive test is estimation of HbA2 by liquid performance chromatography.
- Rise in HbA2 above 3.5%.
- Fetal hemoglobin (HbF) is typically greater than 2%.
- Microcytic hypochromic peripheral smear picture, and also basophilic stippling of the RBCs.
- Hemoglobin content falls in the range of 8–10 g/dL.
- Mean cell volume (MCV) is lower than 75 fL and the RBC count is above 4.5–5.0 million cells/µL.
- Serum ferritin and iron simplify the diagnosis.

Beta Thalassemia Major

This is a grave illness in which both beta chains remain defective. Hence these females are frequently infertile and have short life period. It is highly difficult for the women to have successful pregnancy even with extensive

Flowchart 3: Management of sickle cell anemia.

Prenatal:
- Preconception counseling
- The male partner
- Early prenatal genetic diagnosis of (PCR), amniocentesis or chorionic villus sampling

↓

Antepartum:
- Folic acid supplementation, 5 mg
- sickle cell crisis—good hydration
- Screening, treatment of UTI
- Fetal health assessment—antenatal fetal surveillance every week beginning at 32–34 weeks, serial USG
- Prophylactic transfusions
- Routine iron supplementation is not needed unless lab evidence of iron deficiency

↓

Intrapartum:
- Epidural analgesia is ideal
- IV fluids
- Oxygen inhalation
- Antibiotics
- Thromboprophylaxis
- Incentive spirometry
- Bronchodilators
- Transfusion therapy—prophylactic red cell transfusion (if hematocrit <20%,HbS <60%) before crisis helps decreasing the severity of crisis
- Avoid overloading of circulatory system and pulmonary oedema

↓

Postpartum management:
- Ambulate early to avoid VTE
- good hydration
- Analgesics for pain relief
- Cord blood for electrophoresis
- Contraception
- Progesterone-based contraception like DMPA—stabilizes of red blood cell membrane
- Permanent contraception after completing family

(PCR: polymerase chain reaction; VTE: venous thromboembolism; DMPA: depotmedroxy progesterone acetate: USG: ultrasonography; HbS: hemoglobin S)

maternal and fetal care by a multidisciplinary approach from obstetrician and hematologist.
- Cardiac evaluation.
- Blood transfusion and folate supplementation is needed.
- Regular iron supplementation is not advised.
- Chelation with desferrioxamine might be helpful.

Hemolytic Anemia

Hemolysis due to *Plasmodium falciparum* malarial infections in addition to all the hemolytic anemias of genetic origin.

Immune Hemolytic Anemia

- Autoimmune condition is the most common cause for this anemia in pregnancy. Premature damage of the red cells occurs due to formation of warm antibodies or immunoglobulin G (IgG). RBCs are sensitized with IgG antibody and also complement C3.
- It is also evident in leukemias, lymphomas, viral toxicities, immunological response to medications like penicillin, sulfa drugs, and quinidine. It can also be idiopathic with no cause noticeable.

Direct Coombs test helps in the diagnosis of immune-mediated hemolytic anemia (IHA).

Anemia Associated with Infections

Urinary tract infection (UTI) and pancytopenia due to human immunodeficiency virus (HIV) infection have been reported.

Chronic Renal Disease

Decreases the production of erythropoietin resulting in anemia.

Aplastic Anemia

Treatment possibilities include marrow transplantation, antilymphocyte globulin, chemotherapy with cyclosporine and steroid therapy.

■ CLINICAL FEATURES

They depend more on the degree of anemia than anything else. Majority of the patients are asymptomatic.

Symptoms

Lassitude, a feeling of exhaustion may be the earliest manifestation.

Palpitation caused by ectopic beats, dyspnea, anorexia, indigestion, giddiness and pedal edema.

On Examination

- Pallor of varying degrees
- Soft systolic murmur
- Basal crepitations due to congestion
- Glossitis, stomatitis
- Edema legs due to hypoproteinemia or associated preeclampsia.

COMPLICATIONS OF SEVERE ANEMIA (TABLE 6)

Risk Periods

- Around 30–32 weeks of gestation
- Second stage of labor
- Immediate postpartum
- In puerperium, 7–10 days following delivery due to pulmonary embolism.

TREATMENT

Identifying the reason for anemia is the initial step in the management. The identified root cause is to be treated properly or else the anemia becomes persistent. Treatment depends on the severity of anemia and the gestational age of the patient.

However, acute blood loss and features of decompensation need instant blood transfusion to replace the blood volume.

Management of anemia in pregnancy has been shown in Flowchart 4.

TABLE 6: Complications of anemia.

Pregnancy	- Pre-eclampsia - Intercurrent infection - Cardiac failure around 30–32 weeks of gestation - Premature labor pains
Labor	- *Cardiac failure:* During labor or immediately following delivery - Shock - Postpartum hemorrhage - Uterine inertia—it is not a common associate
Puerperium	- Puerperal infection - Subinvolution of uterus - Lactation failure - Peripheral vein thrombosis - Pulmonary emboli
Fetal complications	- Low birth weight - Preterm babies - Intrauterine death—due to severe maternal anoxemia

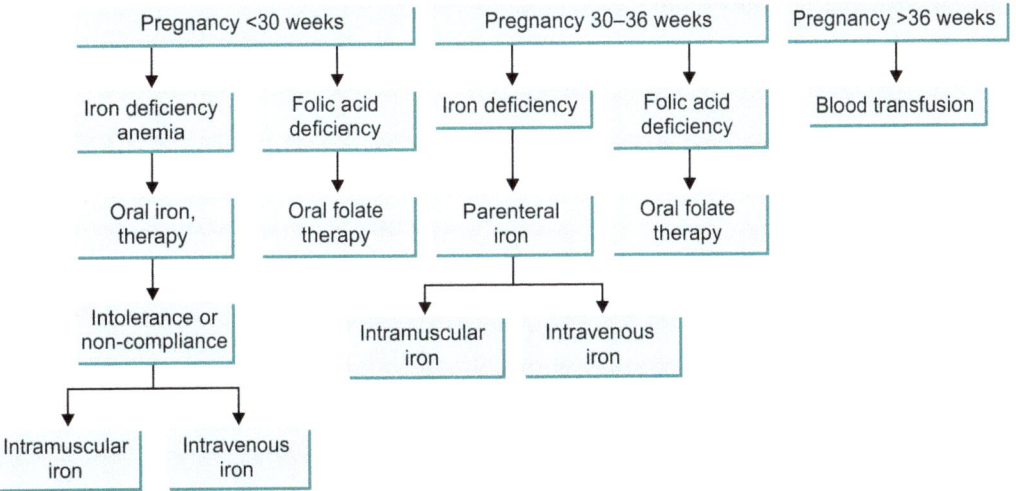

Flowchart 4: Management of anemia in pregnancy.[7]

Immediate hospitalization is required in severe and very severe anemia for the management of cardiac failure and for packed cell transfusion. Patients with severe anemia and especially those with Hb <2.5 g/dL and packed cell volume (PCV) <15% are prone to detrimental cardiac changes. Parenteral iron therapy is contraindicated in congestive cardiac failure. Rest, sedation, digitalis and diuretics to control the failure and repeated packed cell transfusion to improve anemia are useful. When the emergency is obviated, the iron supplementation can be done similar to mild and moderate anemia.

Maximum response to parenteral iron does not appear before 4–9 weeks. Hence, this method is unsuitable if 4 weeks are not available for delivery. It is most suitable between 30 weeks and 36 weeks of pregnancy.

MANAGEMENT DURING LABOR

First Stage of Labor

The patient is made to lie in a relaxed position. Puerperal infection should be avoided by maintaining strict asepsis. Antibiotic prophylaxis is preferred. Adequate analgesia and sedation is to be offered. If the patient is dyspneic, oxygen inhalation is administered. Tocolytics and prophylactic steroid therapy for the management of preterm labor pains are advised. Heart failure due to severe anemia needs treatment with digitalis. Labor must be managed with cautiousness in order to escape the danger of pulmonary edema.

Second Stage of Labor

This is the most distressing part of labor as the patient may land up in heart failure. Strict aseptic conditions should be maintained. Cut short the second stage of labor with prophylactic outlet forceps or vacuum delivery.

Third Stage of Labor

Active management of third stage of labor is mandatory but not in severe anemia patients due to the risk of heart failure. But PPH need to be treated promptly because these anemia patients tolerate blood loss very badly.[8,11] Indirect maternal death in severe anemia can occur due to heart failure or pulmonary embolism. Intravenous methergine 0.25 mg at the time of delivery of the head. Significant blood loss to be replaced but postpartum overloading of heart should be avoided.

Puerperium

Sufficient rest is to be given to the patient in puerperium. Prophylactic antibiotics are to be given to prevent infection. Iron and folic acid supplementation must be extended for a minimum of 3 months. Puerperal infection, lactation failure, uterine subinvolution and thromboembolism are frequent and must be cautiously observed.

REFERENCES

1. WHO. The global prevalence of anaemia in 2011. Geneva: World Health Organization; 2015.
2. WHO. Iron deficiency anaemia: assessment, prevention, and control. A guide for programme managers. Geneva: World Health Organization; 2001 (WHO/NHD/01.3).
3. Oliver E, Olufunto K. (2012). Management of anaemia in pregnancy. In: Silverberg D (Ed). Anemia. IntechOpen. [online] Available from: http://www.intechopen.com/books/anemia/management-of-anaemia-in-pregnancy [Last accessed September, 2019].
4. WHO. Nutritional anaemias: tools for effective prevention and control. Geneva: World Health Organization; 2017.
5. Centers for Disease Control. CDC criteria for anemia in children and childbearing-aged women. MMWR Morb Mortal Wkly Rep. 1989;38:400-4.

6. Milman N, Bergholt T, Byg KE, et al. Iron status and iron balance during pregnancy. A critical reappraisal of iron supplementation. Acta Obstet Gynecol Scand. 1999;78:749-57.
7. Sharma JB. Medical complications in pregnancy. In: Sharma JB (Ed). The Obstetric Protocol, 1st edition. New Delhi, India: Jaypee Brothers Medical Publishers (P) Ltd; 1998. pp. 78-98.
8. Letsky E. Blood volume, haematinics, anameia. In: de Swiet M (Ed). Medical Disorders in Obstetric Practice, 3rd edition. Oxford: Blackwell; 1995. pp. 33-60.
9. Lewis BJ, Laras RK. Leukemia and lymphoma in pregnancy. In: Lavos RK (Ed). Blood Disorder in Pregnancy. Philadelphia: Lea and Febriger; 1986. pp. 85-101.
10. Review of Indian clinical research with ferrous ascorbate. In Allahabadia Shroff, Agarwals 2006, Feb/Mar Issue Pg-15 (Eds). Fogs 1 Times 2006, Fab/Mar Issue P-15.
11. Sharma JB. Iron deficiency anaemia in pregnancy: still a major cause of material mortality and morbidity in India. Obs Gynae Today. 1999;IV:693-701.
12. Channarin I. Folate deficiency in pregnancy. In: Channarin I (Ed). The Megaloblastic Anaemias, 3rd edition. Oxford: Blackwell; 1990. pp. 140-8.
13. Scott JM, Weir DG. Role of folic acid/folate in pregnancy: prevention is better than cure. In: Bonnar J (Ed). Recent Advances in Obstetrics and Gynaecology. Edinburgh, UK: Churchill Livingstone; 1998. pp. 1-28.
14. Sharma JB, Shankar M. Anemia in pregnancy. JIMSA. 2010;23(4):253-60.

CHAPTER 55

Role of Imaging Modalities in Obstetric Emergencies

Roopa PS, Akhila Vasudeva

INTRODUCTION

Obstetric emergencies can occur suddenly and unexpectedly risking two lives. Two patients need to be cared for, the mother and the unborn child. Timely recognition of the risk factors and the associated complications play a major role in averting catastrophes. Imaging modalities have been increasingly used for accurate diagnosis and management plans in these situations. Ultrasonography (USG) is the recognized modality of imaging in obstetrics. In around 90% of the instances, it is the modality of choice. It is accurate, safe, easy to perform and relatively cheap. The advances in the imaging technologies have provided us with a wide range of armamentarium, to choose from, and to select the best for our patients in varying conditions. Magnetic resonance imaging (MRI) though initially accepted with skepticism, now has established its strong hold and has been accepted as one of the safer techniques which can be used in pregnancy. It has the advantage of multiplanar imaging, better soft tissue contrast, more specific characterization of tissues and fluid and lack of exposure to ionizing radiation.

The obstetric emergencies considered in this chapter are:

- Hemorrhage in pregnancy:
  - Ectopic pregnancy
  - Molar pregnancy
  - Retained products of conception (RPOC)
  - Abruption
  - Placenta previa and placenta accreta spectrum
  - Vasa previa
  - Hematomas associated with post-partum hemorrhage (PPH)
- Complications of hypertensive disorders of pregnancy:
  - Cerebral hemorrhage
  - Posterior reversible encephalopathy syndrome (PRES)
  - Hemolysis, elevated liver enzymes, and low platelets (HELLP) with subcapsular hematoma in the liver
- Thrombotic disorders of pregnancy:
  - Deep vein thrombosis (DVT)
  - Pulmonary thromboembolism (PTE)
  - Ovarian vein thrombosis
- Miscellaneous:
  - Sepsis/acute respiratory distress syndrome (ARDS) in pregnancy.

ECTOPIC PREGNANCY

It complicates 1–2% of all pregnancies and accounts for 10–15% of all maternal deaths.[1] Transvaginal sonography (TVS) findings and its correlation with beta-human chorionic gonadotropin (β-hCG) levels is the current noninvasive approach in diagnosis. The sensitivity of ultrasound has been reported to be 87–99% and specificity 94–99%.[2]

Key points in the diagnoses are:
- Presence of a normal intrauterine pregnancy *almost* excludes ectopic pregnancy

- Absence of intrauterine pregnancy—visualized as empty endometrial cavity which might be thick or thin, with or without pseudogestational sac
- Presence of adnexal mass with just an empty gestational sac, yolk sac with fetal pole and cardiac activity or presence of ring of fire in the adnexa
- Varying amount of free fluid in the pouch of Douglas (POD).

The findings on ultrasound vary with clinical presentation of the patient.

The presence of a normal intrauterine pregnancy most often rules out ectopic pregnancy. Though there are instances of both intrauterine and ectopic pregnancy, the heterotopic pregnancy, the incidence is very rare 1/30,000 pregnancies.[3] An early intrauterine pregnancy can be diagnosed by an intradecidual and double decidual sign. The intradecidual sign is described as a fluid collection with an echogenic rim located "within a markedly thickened decidua on one side of the uterine cavity".[4] The double decidual sign is described as an intrauterine fluid collection surrounded by "two concentric echogenic rings".[5]

Endometrium: There are no specific diagnostic signs in the endometrium in ectopic pregnancy. A trilaminar endometrium might be diagnostic with a specificity of 94%, but a sensitivity of only 34%.[3] The thickness of the endometrium might vary. There might be the presence of pseudogestational sac, which is a collection of fluid (hormonal induced and blood products) which conforms to the shape of an endometrial cavity, and can mimic a gestational sac (Fig. 1).

But it lacks sensitivity or specificity and might resemble the intradecidual or double decidual sign. Only 20% of ectopic pregnancies might have a pseudogestational sac.[6] Simple anechoic cysts called the decidual cysts might be nonspecific findings in ectopic pregnancy.

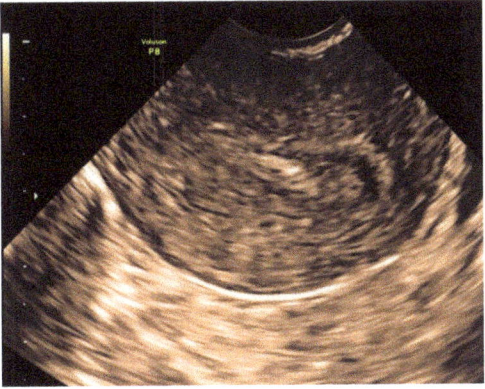

Fig. 1: Pseudogestational sac: collection of fluid which conforms to the shape of an endometrial cavity, mimicking a gestational sac.

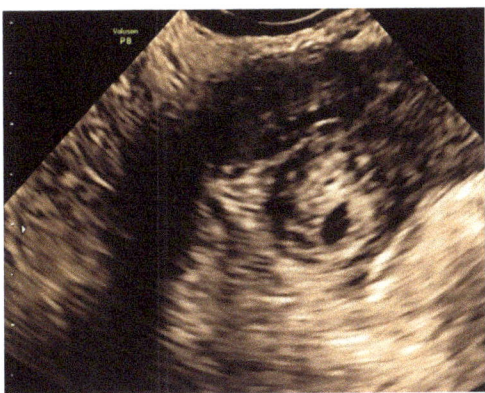

Fig. 2: Tubal ring: hyperechoic halo in the tube between the ovary and uterus.

Adnexa: The presence of an extrauterine live embryo seen in 10% of cases is diagnostic of ectopic pregnancy.[7] Commonly seen features are an inhomogeneous complex adnexal mass, anechoic sac surrounded by a hyperechoic halo or a tubal ring (Fig. 2).

Most common location of an ectopic pregnancy is in the tube, and it is important to scan between the uterus and ovaries, above and below the ovaries also to look for a dilated tube. A normal tube is not visualized in sonography and presence of any distended tube might be due to bleeding into the walls or the visualization of a gestational sac with embryo in the tube. A sliding adnexal mass independent of the ovary, between the uterus and ovary might be diagnostic of an ectopic pregnancy.[2]

Pouch of Douglas: The presence of fluid should be remarked as clear or turbid and also the amount of fluid should be quantitated. A clear fluid is unlikely to be due to blood. Turbid fluid favors ectopic pregnancy and POD being the most dependent part, is a site for collection and retention of clot. A transabdominal sonography (TAS) should also be done to evaluate the Morison's (hepatorenal) pouch. This will help in quantitating the amount of fluid, as presence of fluid in the Morison's pouch estimates to an approximate loss of 400–700 mL.[3]

Role of Doppler Sonography in the Diagnosis of Ectopic Pregnancy

Color and pulsed wave Doppler can act as an adjunct to improve the diagnosis of ectopic pregnancy when in doubt. "Ring of fire" can be seen around the adnexal mass, but it can be also seen around a corpus luteal cyst which can be confusing. The high energy output in Doppler compared to normal gray scale should be kept in mind when used in early pregnancy. The risks and benefits should be analyzed and if it betters our diagnosis and has implications on the management, then it can be used.

Also once ectopic has been confirmed, the presence of vascularity might help us in understanding if the chorionic villi are viable, and plan the management accordingly.

Criteria for Diagnosis of Rare Forms of Ectopic Pregnancy

Interstitial Pregnancy

It accounts for 2–4% of all ectopic pregnancies.

Ultrasonographic features: An eccentric gestational sac located very high up at the fundus surrounded by a mantle of myometrium measuring 5 mm is found in interstitial pregnancy. "Interstitial line sign" is the echogenic line extending onto the uterine horn and bordering the margin of the gestational sac in the intramural portion of the uterus.[1] It is found to have a sensitivity of 80% and specificity of 98%.[2] The three-dimensional (3D) USG and MRI can be used as additional modalities to prevent misdiagnosis of early intrauterine or angular pregnancy. In 3D coronal view, a connection is seen between the endometrial cavity and interstitial tube. In MRI, we can see a gestational sac like structure lateral to the cornua surrounded by myometrium. Additionally an intact junctional zone between the uterine cavity and the gestational sac might support the diagnosis.

Cornual Pregnancy

Reported incidence is 1 in 76,000 pregnancies. Many consider cornual pregnancy as a pregnancy implanted in the abnormal uterine horn.

The diagnostic criteria for cornual pregnancy are:[2]
- Visualization of a single interstitial portion of fallopian tube in the main uterine body
- Gestational sac/products of conception seen mobile and separate from the uterus and completely surrounded by myometrium
- A vascular pedicle adjoining the gestational sac to the unicornuate uterus.

Cervical Pregnancy

It accounts for <1% of pregnancies.
The ultrasound criteria for its diagnosis are:[2]
- Empty uterine cavity
- A barrel-shaped cervix
- A gestational sac present below the level of the internal os of the cervix

- The absence of sliding sign
- Blood flow around the gestational sac using color Doppler.

Sliding sign helps to differentiate cervical pregnancy from incomplete abortion, which poses a diagnostic dilemma. When pressure is applied to the cervix using a TVS probe, the gestational sac slides against endocervical canal in the latter, but it does not do so in cervical pregnancy. Another key point differentiating the two is, in cervical pregnancy the TVS shows a regular gestational sac, with an evidence of yolk sac, fetal pole with cardiac activity.[1]

Cesarean Scar Pregnancy

It accounts for 1/2,000 pregnancies. The diagnostic criteria by TVS are:
- Empty uterine cavity[8]
- Gestational sac or solid mass of trophoblast located anteriorly at the level of the internal os embedded at the site of the previous lower uterine segment cesarean section scar[9]
- Thin or absent layer of myometrium between the gestational sac and the bladder[8,10]
- Evidence of prominent trophoblastic/placental circulation on Doppler examination[11]
- Empty endocervical canal.[8]

In case of availability of an expertise in MRI, it can also add to the diagnosis of cesarean scar pregnancies.

Ovarian Pregnancy

An empty gestational sac or an anechoic area surrounded by an echogenic ring within the ovary might be seen. A corpus luteal cyst has to be seen separately for an accurate diagnosis.

Abdominal Pregnancy

Transvaginal sonography criteria included are:[2]

- Absence of an intrauterine gestational sac
- Absence of both an evident dilated tube and a complex adnexal mass
- A gestational cavity surrounded by loops of bowel and separated from them by peritoneum
- A wide mobility similar to fluctuation of the sac, particularly evident with pressure of the transvaginal probe toward the posterior cul-de-sac.

Magnetic resonance imaging is a very useful adjunct for confirmation and also identification of placental implantation over vital structures such as major blood vessels and bowel, which helps in perioperative management and also planning incision to avoid the placenta.

Heterotopic Pregnancy

An intrauterine pregnancy with ectopic pregnancy is heterotopic pregnancy. This condition should especially be looked for in assisted reproductive techniques.

Technique of ultrasound: It is always advisable to do both TAS and TVS in ectopic pregnancy as one might miss out on any pregnancy outside the plane of the vaginal transducer. In women with pelvic masses such as a fibroid, a TAS with a full bladder should be performed to evaluate the adnexa.

Role of CT and MRI in the Diagnosis of Ectopic Pregnancy

Ultrasonography is the main modality in the diagnosis of ectopic pregnancies. Computed tomography (CT) and MRI are not used in routine diagnosis of an unstable patient. In conditions where the diagnosis is indeterminate or in evaluation of other acute abdominal conditions, these might be used supplementary.

The MRI features include:
Adnexa: A heterogeneous mass, combination of hemorrhage and fetoplacental tissues

represented by a solid mass, with enhancing tree-like solid components.[12] Cystic sac-like structure (gestational sac) surrounded by thick wall exhibiting high signal intensity on T2-weighted images might be seen. Hemorrhage might show distinct low signal intensities and intermediate or high signal intensity on T2- and T1-weighted images respectively.[13] A dilated tube with wall enhancement and bloody ascites might be other features. Intrapelvic hemorrhage will be seen as collection with increased intensity on T1-weighted images.[14]

In tubal rupture, on T2-weighted images, the tubal wall enhancement is lost and the resulting acute hematoma, is shown as low signal intensity outside the implantation site.

In ovarian ectopic pregnancy, a gestational sac-like structure on or within the ovary, with low intensity signals representing acute hematoma is seen on T2-weighted images. On CT, a heterogeneous mass arising from the ovary can be seen. Considering the rarity of ovarian pregnancy as compared to other ovarian cystic structures, unless a discernible yolk sac or embryo is seen, it is inappropriate to suggest this diagnosis on the basis of imaging alone.[15]

On MRI, the cervical pregnancy may have the appearance of a lobulated mass with heterogeneous mixed signal intensity and a partial or complete dark rim on T2-weighted images. Contrast-enhanced would reveal irregular peripheral rim enhancement and densely enhancing solid components.[16] The heterogeneous signal intensity is likely due to hemorrhage of varying stages, and the enhancing solid components likely represent remnants of fetoplacental tissues.

GESTATIONAL TROPHOBLASTIC NEOPLASIA

These include a varying range of entities namely complete mole, partial mole, invasive mole, placental site trophoblastic disease (PSTD), epithelioid trophoblastic tumor and choriocarcinoma.

Transvaginal sonography forms the main modality in confirming a clinically suspected molar pregnancy. In complete molar pregnancy, ultrasound features show typical "snowstorm or granular" pattern due to multiple echogenic foci. Multiple small anechoic spaces are seen filling the endometrial cavity which represents fluid-filled molar vesicles with hydropic changes and swollen villi. These spaces grow larger as the gestation advances and are typically described as honeycomb pattern and are easier to diagnose. While imaging other than these features, the uterine volume should be measured as it represents the tumor bulk and helps in staging and giving a prognosis.

In partial mole, a severely growth restricted/malformed fetus with placenta showing vesicular changes has been described. Sometimes an empty gestational sac mimicking an anembryonic pregnancy has also been described. These imaging features have to be correlated with blood β-hCG and histopathological diagnosis. Bilateral multilocular cysts in the ovary due to hyperstimulation by the circulating β-hCG are seen in 40% of the cases.[17]

Transvaginal sonography is superior in diagnosing invasive disease. The interface between the myometrium and trophoblast needs to be examined.[17]

Doppler imaging: On insinuating color on the mass, we get a high velocity low impedance flow. Invasiveness might be demonstrated by the vascularity extending onto the myometrium. An important differential to keep in mind is RPOC which can be confirmed by β-hCG correlation.

Doppler has the potential to follow the disease response to chemotherapy and also in assessing the resistance to chemotherapeutic drugs.

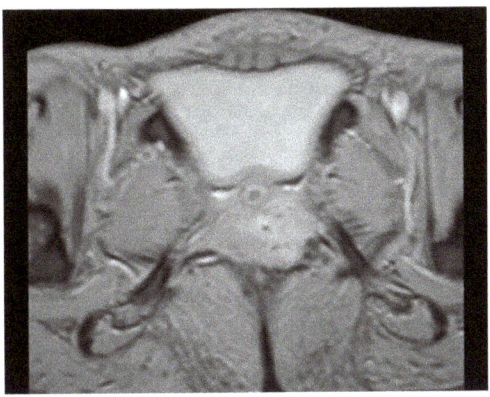

Fig. 3: Metastatic lesion from choriocarcinoma seen in the distal part of the posterior wall of the vagina on the left side abutting the left levator ani muscle.

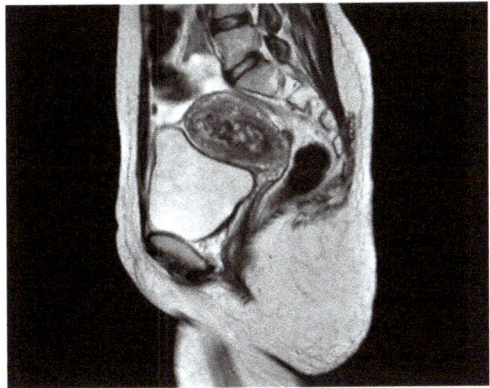

Fig. 4: Mixed echogenic mass with contrast enhancement seen in MRI representing retained products of conception (RPOC).

Role of CT and MRI: CT is the main modality to diagnose metastatic disease in choriocarcinoma. MRI is helpful mainly in second trimesters. First trimester features are nonspecific and can be confused with RPOC. It is superior to TVS in diagnosing parametrial invasion and soft tissue metastasis (Fig. 3).

RETAINED PRODUCTS OF CONCEPTION

Retained products of conception can occur after termination of pregnancy in the first trimester or in the second trimester. It more commonly occurs after the second trimester of pregnancy. Ultrasound is the main modality for diagnosis.

It will appear as mixed echogenic lesion filling the endometrial cavity. The typical description is thick endometrial echo complex (EEC) ranging from 8 mm to 13 mm.[18] An endometrial heterogeneous mass is typically described. The blood clots appear anechoic with the retained products appearing echogenic. On Doppler imaging, blood clots are avascular and the retained products appear vascular. The degree of vascularity helps in confident diagnosis of RPOC. Vascularity should be seen extending from the myometrium to the endometrium. There are four types of vascularity described.

- *Type 0*: Undetectable vascularity.[19]
- *Type 1*: Minimal vascularity—less than that of myometrium
- *Type 2*: Moderate vascularity—nearly equal flow in the endometrium and myometrium
- *Type 3*: Marked vascularity—greater than that of normal myometrium in the same image section.

Differential diagnosis includes gestational trophoblastic neoplasia (GTN) and uterine arteriovenous (AV) malformation. In AV malformation, the lesion is hypoechoic, specifically within the myometrium. On Doppler velocimetry, low resistance patterns with peak velocities of >80 cm/s have been described.[19]

Role of CT and MRI: RPOC can be diagnosed accurately with TVS with complementary Doppler imaging. CT and MRI are routinely not advisable. Only an enhancing soft tissue mass if present within the endometrial cavity can be seen and diagnosed accurately. In many cases, contrast enhancement might be required to come to an accurate diagnosis (Fig. 4).

Management in RPOC is by evacuation of the contents. With the aid of ultrasound, these products can be removed under visualization. This will ensure the completeness of the procedure and preventing complications like perforation (1.5%) associated with the procedure.

PLACENTA PREVIA

It is a condition where in the placenta implants in the lower uterine segment after the period of viability.

Diagnosis of placenta previa: Both TAS and TVS aid in the diagnosis of placenta previa. During routine anomaly scan at 18–20 weeks if the placenta is overlying the cervical os or within 2 cm from the cervical os, it is unlikely to "migrate". All the pregnant ladies with placenta as described above need to be reseen at 32 weeks and if still in doubt again at 34–36 weeks. Only 20% of the placenta persist in the lower segment at this gestation.[20]

When placenta previa is diagnosed at term, "mapping of placenta" needs to be done (Fig. 5).

Points to be noted when mapping the placenta are:
- Anterior or posterior placenta
- Laterality of the placenta—more on the right or left side of the uterus

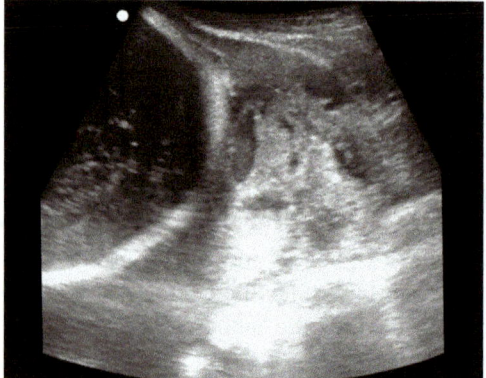

Fig. 5: Ultrasonography (USG) image of a posterior placenta covering the os and coming anteriorly.

- Accessibility of the fetal part during uterine incision (to avoid cutting through the placenta)
- Relationship of placenta to the previous uterine scar.

Around 1–5% of the placenta previa are associated with various degrees of adherence (accreta, increta and percreta).[21] So this also has to be remarked.

Signs of placenta previa—placenta accreta spectrum—have been shown in Flowchart 1.

Ultrasound imaging by a skilled operator with experience is highly accurate in diagnosing placenta accreta spectrum.[22]

Role of MRI in the diagnosis of placenta accreta: MRI has been thought to be the method of choice to rule out accreta. But there may be bias in this, as only those cases in whom there are given risk factors and suspicion of accreta by TVS are subjected to MRI. Studies quote the same sensitivity of USG with MRI. However, MRI scores over USG in demonstrating various degrees of invasion into the myometrium and also to adjacent structures mainly the bladder and also in picking up accreta in a posterior placenta. MRI can pick up percreta better than ultrasound (Fig. 6).

Magnetic resonance imaging features: Placental heterogeneity, dark intraplacental bands on T2-weighted images due to fibrin deposition, disorganized intraplacental vascularity with hypertrophied vessels, loss of retroplacental T2 dark zone, focal uteroplacental defect, uterine bulge, and direct invasion into adjacent structures. Intraplacental bands of more than 1 mm and flow voids of >6 mm increases the specificity of detection.[23]

Overall, TVS has a sensitivity of 87.5% and a specificity of 98.8%, with a positive predictive value of 93.3%, negative predictive value of 97.6% and false-negative rate of 2.33%.[24]

Flowchart 1: Signs of placenta previa—accreta spectrum.[20,22]

Presence of risk factors like previous uterine scar, placenta previa, repeated dilatation and evacuation

At the time of pregnancy confirmation in the 1st trimester
- Gestational sac implanted in the lower pole of the uterus close to the previous uterine scar

At early anomaly and 18–20 weeks anomaly scan
- Multiple irregular vascular lacunae embedded in the growing placenta bed

3rd trimester at 32 and 34–36 weeks
- Loss of normal sonolucent zone (Nitabuch's membrane) behind the placenta
- Presence of multiple vascular lacunae within the placental bed (Swiss cheese appearance or moth-eaten appearance)
- Doppler sonography showing turbulent blood flow within the lacunae
- Increased subplacental vascularity
- Extension of the villi into the myometrium, serosa, or bladder
- Retroplacental myometrial thickness of less than 1 mm
- Presence of bridging vessels from the placenta to the uterine margin
- Gaps in myometrial blood flow
- Abnormalities of the uterine serosa–bladder interface (interruption, thickening or irregularity of the line at the interface between uterine serosa and bladder with increased vascularity)

VASA PREVIA

When the fetal vessels run over the free placental membranes within 2 cm of the cervix, vasa previa occurs. Type 1 vasa previa is when the vessels are connected to a velamentous umbilical cord and type 2 when the vessels run over the free membranes while going on to insert to an accessory lobe or succenturiate lobe of the placenta.

The prevalence ranges from 1/1,200 to 1/5,000. Most of the time it is recognized when the membranes spontaneously rupture or artificial rupture of membranes are done and a blood-stained amniotic fluid is seen. Then the cardiotocograph (CTG) shows sinusoidal pattern due to the bleeding fetal vessel. It is associated with 60% fetal mortality. But when recognized antenatally and planned cesarean section undertaken the survival improved to over 95%.[25]

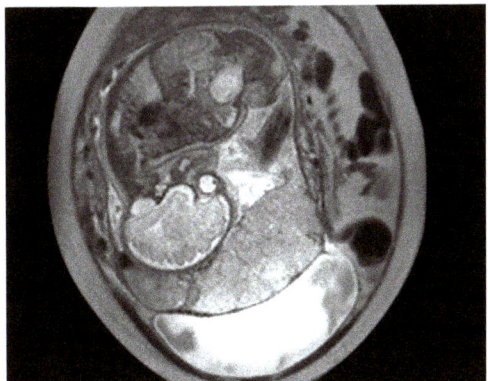

Fig. 6: MRI of a low-lying placenta completely covering the os with associated myometrial thinning and loss of distinct placental and myometrial interface.

It can be diagnosed antenatally by a combined TAS-TVS with color Doppler imaging with good accuracy.

During the 18–22 weeks scan, look for the placental location, the cord insertion, accessory lobes or succenturiate lobes of the placenta. When there is low-lying placenta, velamentous cord insertion, accessory lobes or succenturiate lobes, specifically look for vasa previa with a TVS and color Doppler imaging.

Features seen: Linear tubular echolucent body overlying the internal os. When color Doppler is insinuated, it demonstrates flow in that structure and on power Doppler, fetal vascular waveforms are picked up. This can be confused with a free loop of fetal cord overlying the cervical os. Two key points to differentiate between the two are:
1. A vessel which changes position with maternal position, i.e. a change in maternal position (Trendelenburg position) might move the vessel away from the field
2. Tracing the vessel up to its insertion might give a clearer picture.[20,26]

Vasa previa seen at 18–22 weeks has to be reconfirmed again at 32–34 weeks.

Both TAS and TVS done together might increase the accuracy. Power Doppler and MRI are additional diagnostic modalities which are being researched, but till date have not found to be superior to TAS with TVS in increasing the diagnostic accuracy. But even with all these imaging modalities cases can be missed.

ABRUPTION

Separation of a normally implanted placenta before delivery of the baby after the period of viability has crossed is termed abruption. It leads to a lot of maternal and fetal morbidity and mortality. Clinical criteria forms the basis of diagnosis. Imaging modality might help in consolidation of findings.

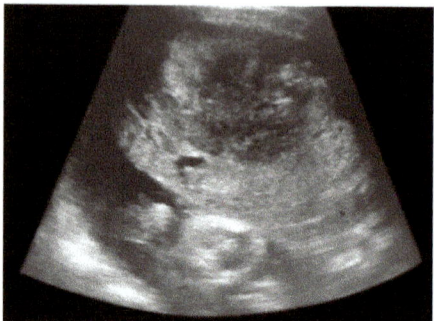

Fig. 7: USG image of an abruption with retroplacental clot.

Transabdominal sonography may show a retroplacental clot of varying size (Fig. 7). If present then the diagnosis is clinched. But an absence of retroplacental clot does not refute the diagnosis of abruption. Ultrasound has a very low sensitivity in picking up abruption and might fail to diagnose abruption in >75% of the cases. But it has a very high specificity, and when a retroplacental clot is seen the likelihood of abruption is very high.[27] The sensitivity, specificity, positive and negative predictive values of USG for a diagnosis of placental abruption are found to be 24%, 96%, 88% and 53%, respectively.[28]

The ultrasound findings in abruption might include:[29]
- Retroplacental collection/hematoma (heterogeneous lesion)
- Increased placental thickness >5 cm
- Preplacental collection under chorionic plate
- Jelly-like movement of chorionic plate with fetal activity
- Marginal hematoma, subchorionic hematoma
- Intra-amniotic hematoma.

Many a times the placenta protruding into the amniotic cavity might be another sign of abruption. USG also helps to confirm fetal viability.

RUPTURE UTERUS

It is a devastating event with a very high maternal and perinatal mortality. Diagnosis is essentially clinical. A number of ultrasound features have been proposed in predicting an integrity of the scar. An abnormal fetal position, hemoperitoneum, an absent or a thin uterine wall might be some of the features picked in uterine rupture. Cesarean scar dehiscence is more common. The uterine to bladder interface of >4.5 mm has a negative predictive value of 100% but a thickness of <3.5 mm has a poor positive predictive value of only 11.8%.[30] Postpartum CT evaluation might have a role in diagnosis varying degrees of dehiscence.

PUERPERAL HEMATOMA

Hematomas high up in the pelvis are difficult to diagnose clinically. Real-time imaging with sonography, CT and MRI help in assessing the site and extent. USG is the first line of investigation in the diagnosis. It is largely limited to only diagnosis, and the bleeder in question might not be delineated. CT is highly sensitive in the diagnosis with CT angiography able to identify the bleeder. CT images might show hyperintense lesions in the early stage, and older hematomas might become hypointense. MRI shows hypointense irregular lesions dissecting through the planes.[31]

Postcesarean hematoma and dehiscence: Ultrasound is the first step in the evaluation of suspected hematomas following cesarean. Mixed echogenic lesion of varying size at the uterine wound site might be seen. A partially full bladder with a TAS might show a presence of integrity of the uterine serosa with an elevated uterovesical flap (Fig. 8).[32]

These hematomas might dissect or get infected leading to loss of integrity of the uterine wound. Though uterine dehiscence

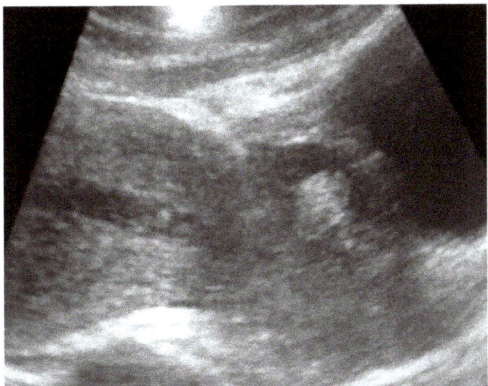

Fig. 8: Hematoma seen bulging the UV fold of peritoneum, containing mixed echogenic areas.

is picked up poorly in imaging studies, CT might show a large hematoma with a heterogeneous wound. T2-weighted MRI will show hyperintense area throughout the thickness of uterine wall along with a large size fluid collection.[33] MRI is found to be superior in picking up postcesarean scar dehiscence due to infection. Some of the features to be looked for in MRI are a lack of apposition of the endometrium and serosa at the incision site and discontinuity of the myometrium with associated fluid collection, hematoma, or regions of low signal intensity suggestive of gas.[34]

HYPERTENSIVE DISORDERS OF PREGNANCY

These disorders range from the mild gestational hypertension to the very dangerous eclampsia. The wide ranging complications associated cause severe maternal morbidity and mortality.

Liver: Subcapsular hematoma is seen in <2% of the cases with HELLP syndrome.[35] Asymptomatic hematomas are managed conservatively and are not specifically looked for. In cases with high clinical suspicion of a large hematoma or suspected intraperitoneal bleed, imaging modalities are employed. USG is the first modality of investigation. In USG, hypoechogenic area with diffuse heterogeneity is seen. Multidetector row CT (MDCT) is more accurate thus used as a first line in severely ill patient with high suspicion.[36] A hyperattenuating collection is likely to be a recent hematoma. Hematoma progressively becomes hypoattenuating relative to the adjacent hepatic parenchyma with time. Subcapsular hematoma requires follow-up with sonogram and CT to see the decrease, increase or resolution.

Brain: All eclampsias and very severe pre-eclampsia are associated with cerebral involvement and routinely do not require imaging (as they are reversible).

Following situations indicate central nervous system (CNS) imaging:[37]
- Focal neurological deficits
- Coma
- Continued deterioration 24 hours after delivery
- Eclampsia 48 hours after delivery
- Refractory eclampsia
- Eclampsia before 20 weeks.

Doppler, CT and MRI have added major insights to cerebrovascular involvements in hypertensive disorders of pregnancy (Fig. 9).

Findings may range from subtle signs of diffuse white matter or patchy low density areas, occipital white matter edema, loss of normal cortical sulci to features of intraventricular/parenchymal hemorrhage and cerebral infarction. The edema may also manifest as PRES with lesions centered mainly in the parieto-occipital lobe seen as hyperintense lesions in T2-weighted MRI. They might also be found around the basal ganglia, brain stem and cerebellum. They are reversible lesions. Cerebral infarctions also mimic these lesion but they persist (Fig. 10).

As the cerebral edema increases, the ventricles get obliterated. Summarizing, in

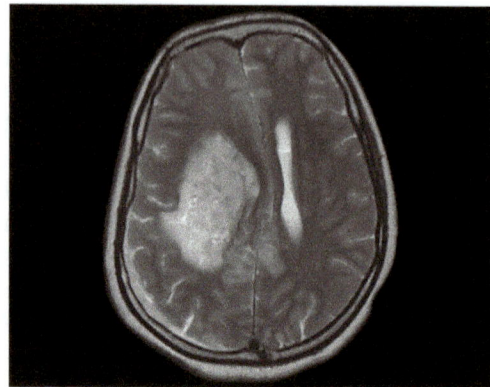

Fig. 9: MRI showing hyperintense areas in the right frontal and parietal lobes which are signs of intraparenchymal hemorrhage.

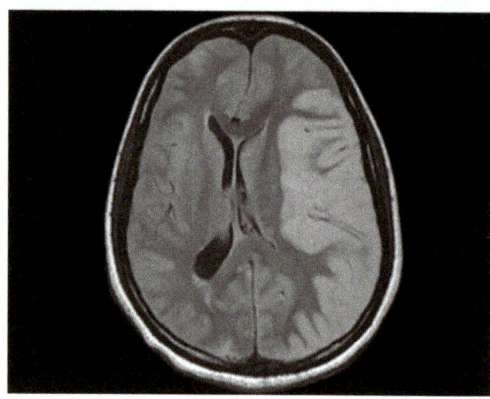

Fig. 10: MRI brain showing diffuse swelling involving the cortical and subcortical white matter of fronto-temporoparietal lobes with associated swelling and hyperintensities of the involved gyri with mass effect noted in the form of compression of frontal horn and body of left lateral ventricle with midline shift which are signs of cerebral ischemia-infarction.

cerebral imaging similar findings are found in eclampsia and in patients with hypertensive encephalopathy.[37]

THROMBOEMBOLIC DISORDERS OF PREGNANCY

They range from DVT to pulmonary embolism (PE). Compression duplex ultrasound [venous ultrasonography (VUS) with Doppler] is the first-line imaging modality in evaluation of DVT. The most accurate ultrasonic criterion for diagnosing venous thrombosis is noncompressibility of the venous lumen in a transverse plane under gentle probe pressure using duplex and color flow Doppler imaging. The sensitivity and specificity of VUS are reported to be around 90–100% for proximal veins and around 75% for distal veins.[38] MRI has been reported to be similar to VUS in it diagnostic ability with the advantage of detecting thrombosis in the more centrally placed veins like pelvic, iliac and the femoral veins.

Pulmonary Embolism

Chest radiography may be abnormal in 84% of the patients with suspected PE.[37] Nonspecific findings like pleural effusion, chest infiltrates, and elevated hemidiaphragm may point toward PE in the background of the clinical setting. It also forms a tool for selecting advanced imaging modality for confirmation which might be ventilation-perfusion scan (V/Q scan) or CT scan.

Bedside ECHO is very useful in unstable patients. Large emboli in the pulmonary artery might cause a right heart strain in around 30–80% of the patients. Classical findings include dilated and hypokinetic right ventricle with tricuspid regurgitation.

Perfusion scanning uses injection of a radioisotope-labeled macroaggregated albumin intravenously that deposits in the pulmonary capillary bed. In ventilation scanning, radiolabeled aerosols are inhaled, whose distribution is evaluated by gamma camera. The two images are compared and are interpreted for characteristic patterns that are then used to assign diagnostic probabilities (high, intermediate, or low). More than 90% of high-risk patients with high probability V/Q scans have a PE, whereas less than 6% of low-risk patients with low probability scans have a PE. The diagnostic efficacy of V/Q scanning is substantially higher in pregnancy as they are younger and have no lung pathology compared to older, nonpregnant patients.[37,38]

Computed tomography pulmonary angiography (CTPA): An intravenous contrast is injected and simultaneously a CT scanner demonstrates the distribution of contrast in the pulmonary vasculature. The diagnostic accuracy is inferior during pregnancy. Large emboli in the segmental and central vessels are easily picked up, subsegmental vessels, horizontally oriented vessels and vessels in the right middle lobe are difficult to visualize. In an abnormal chest X-ray, CTPA is a better imaging modality than V/Q scan. There is a concern of exposure to ionizing radiation with both modalities. A higher risk of childhood cancer after fetal life exposure has been reported with V/Q scan and maternal breast cancer in those exposed to CTPA. But the absolute risk is not increased.

Role of MR angiography: This is a favorable option in pregnant women in terms of fetal safety, faster image acquisition and better quality imaging with respect to respiratory and cardiac motion. Few studies have quoted a sensitivity of 100%, specificity of 95%, positive predictive value of 87% and negative predictive value of 100%.[39] But more trials involving larger sample size are required.

Algorithm of selection of imaging in acute PTE has been shown in Flowchart 2.

Ovarian Vein Thrombosis

One of the fatal conditions which can lead to the lethal PE. Myometrial veins draining an infected placental site can get thrombosed, propagate retrograde leading to PE.[1] Demonstration of dilated ovarian vein in a woman with puerperal sepsis extending onto the inferior vena cava by USG confirms the diagnosis. Care should be taken to differentiate

Flowchart 2: Algorithm of selection of imaging in acute pulmonary thromboembolism.

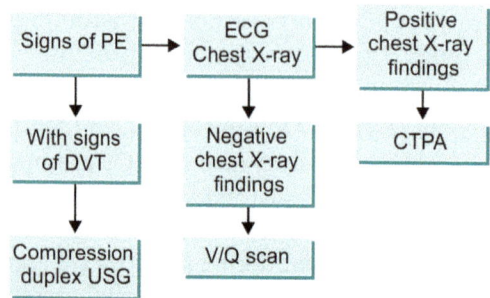

(PE: pulmonary embolism; DVT: deep vein thrombosis; USG: ultrasonography; CTPA, computed tomography pulmonary angiography)

a dilated ovarian vein from dilated ureters, bowel, tube and appendix.

Imaging modalities are useful in management of maternal sepsis, which is now the leading cause of maternal mortality all over the world. Examples include a chest X-ray for diagnosis of ARDS and a CT of abdomen/pelvis to rule out septic collections.

CONCLUSION

Imaging modalities are extremely useful adjuncts to management of obstetric emergencies in the current scenario. Ultrasound is the cheapest, safest, widely available tool helping to save lives in obstetrics. Specific circumstances warrant use of further imaging modalities like CT/MRI.

REFERENCES

1. Kaakaji Y, Nghiem HV, Nodell C, et al. Sonography of obstetric and gynecologic emergencies: Part I, Obstetric emergencies. Am J Roentgenology. 2000;174(3):641-9.
2. Elson CJ, Salim R, Potdar N, et al. on behalf of the Royal College of Obstetricians and Gynaecologists. Diagnosis and management of ectopic pregnancy. BJOG. 2016;123:e15-e55.
3. Cunningham FG, Leveno KJ, Bloom SL, et al. Williams Obstetrics, 24th edition. USA. McGraw Hill education. Chapter 19: Ectopic pregnancy, 2014 p. 377.
4. Yeh HC, Goodman JD, Carr L, et al. Intradecidual sign: a US criterion of early intrauterine pregnancy. Radiology. 1986;161:463-7.
5. Bradley WG, Fiske CE, Filly RA. The double sac sign of early intrauterine pregnancy: use in exclusion of ectopic pregnancy. Radiol. 1982;143:223-6.
6. Marks WM, Filly RA, Callen PW, et al. The decidual cast of ectopic pregnancy: a confusing ultrasonographic appearance. Radiol. 1979;133(2):451-4.
7. Callen PW. Ultrasonography in Obstetrics and Gynecology, 5th edition. Philidelphia; Elsevier Health Sciences Chapter 32 Ectopic pregnancy, 2011 p. 1020.
8. Godin PA, Bassil S, Donnez J. An ectopic pregnancy developing in a previous caesarean section scar. Fertil Steril. 1997;67:398-400.
9. Jurkovic D, Hillaby K, Woelfer B, et al. First-trimester diagnosis and management of pregnancies implanted into the lower uterine segment Cesarean section scar. Ultrasound Obstet Gynecol. 2003;21:220-7.
10. Timor-Tritsch IE, Monteagudo A, Santos R, et al. The diagnosis, treatment, and follow-up of cesarean scar pregnancy. Am J Obstet Gynecol. 2012;207:44.e1-13.
11. Seow KM, Hwang JL, Tsai YL. Ultrasound diagnosis of a pregnancy in a Cesarean section scar. Ultrasound Obstet Gynecol. 2001;18:547-9.
12. Ha HK, Jung JK, Kang SJ, et al. MR imaging in the diagnosis of rare forms of ectopic pregnancy. AJR. 1993;160:1229-32.
13. Tamai K, Koyama T, Togashi K. MR features of ectopic pregnancy. Eur Radiol. 2007;17:3236-46.
14. Kinoshita T, Ishii K, Higashiiwai H. MR appearance of ruptured tubal ectopic pregnancy. Eur J Radiol. 1999;32:144-7.
15. Kao Ly, Scheinfeld MH, Chernyak V, et al. Beyond ultrasound: CT and MRI of ectopic pregnancy. AJR. 2014;202:904-11.
16. Jung SE, Byun JY, Lee JM, et al. Characteristic MR findings of cervical pregnancy. J Magn Reson Imaging. 2001;13:918-22.
17. Dhanda S, Ramani S, Thakur M. Gestational trophoblastic disease: a multimodality imaging approach with impact on diagnosis and management. Radiol Res Pract. 2014;2014.
18. Sellmyer MA, Desser TS, Maturen KE, et al. Physiologic, histologic, and imaging features of retained products of conception. Radiographics. 2013;33(3):781-96.

19. Iraha Y, Okada M, Toguchi M, et al. Multi-modality imaging in secondary postpartum or postabortion hemorrhage: retained products of conception and related conditions. Japanese J Radiol. 2018;36(1):12-22.
20. Silver RM. Abnormal placentation: placenta previa, vasa previa, and placenta accreta. Obstetrics and Gynecology. 2015;126(3):654-68.
21. ACOG Committee on Obstetric Practice. Committee opinion# 266: placenta accreta. Obstetrics and Gynecology. 2002;99(1):169-70.
22. Jauniaux E, Alfirevic Z, Bhide AG, et al. Placenta Praevia and Placenta Accreta: Diagnosis and Management: Green-top Guideline No. 27a. BJOG: an International J Obstet Gynecol, 2018 Sep 27.
23. Gupta R, Bajaj SK, Kumar N, et al. Magnetic resonance imaging - a troubleshooter in obstetric emergencies: A pictorial review. Indian J Radiol Imaging. 2016;26:44-51.
24. Leerentveld RA, Gilberts EC, Arnold MJ, et al. Accuracy and safety of transvaginal sonographic placental localization. Obstet Gynecol. 1990;76:759-62.
25. Jauniaux ERM, Alfirevic Z, Bhide AG, et al. on behalf of the Royal College of Obstetricians and Gynaecologists. Vasa praevia: diagnosis and management. Green-top Guideline No. 27b.BJOG 2018; https://doi.org/10.1111/1471-0528.15307.
26. Sullivan EA, Javid N, Duncombe G, et al. Vasa previa diagnosis, clinical practice, and outcomes in Australia. Obstet Gynecol. 2017;130(3):591-8.
27. Haemorrhage RA. Greentop Guideline No. 63. Royal College of Obstetrics & Gynaecology, London. 2011.
28. Glantz C, Purnell L. Clinical utility of sonography in the diagnosis and treatment of placental abruption. J Ultrasound Med. 2002;21:837-40.
29. Oyeless Y, Ananth CV. Placental abruption. J Am Obstet Gynaecol. 2006;108(4):1005-16.
30. Guise JM, Eden K, Emeis C, et al. Vaginal birth after cesarean: new insights. Evidence report/technology assessment. 2010;(191):1.
31. Rooholamini SA, Au AH, Hansen GC, et al. Imaging of pregnancy-related complications. Radiographics. 1993;13(4):753-70.
32. Vasudeva A, Amin SV, Prakashini K, et al. Post-caesarean haematomas, septic collections and wound disruptions–re-laparotomy based on abdominal imaging. J Clinical and Diagnostic Research: JCDR. 2016;10(11):QJ01.
33. Paspulati RM, Dalal TA. Imaging of complications following gynecologic surgery. Radio Graphics. 2010;30(3):625-42.
34. Plunk M, Lee JH, Kani K, et al. Imaging of postpartum complications: a multimodality review. Am J Roentgenol. 2013;200(2):W143-54.
35. Wicke C, Pereira PL, Neeser E, et al. Sub-capsular liver hematoma in HELLP syndrome: evaluation of diagnostic and therapeutic options—a unicenter study. Am J Obstet Gynecol. 2004;190(1):106-12.
36. Perronne L, Dohan A, Bazeries P, et al. Hepatic involvement in HELLP syndrome: an update with emphasis on imaging features. Abdominal imaging. 2015;40(7):2839-49.
37. Gabbe SG, Niebyl JR, Simpson JL, et al. Obstetrics: normal and problem pregnancies e-book. Elsevier Health Sciences; 2016; Chapter 31, 661-70.
38. Royal College of Obstetricians and Gynaecologists. Thromboembolic disease in pregnancy and the puerperium: acute management. London: RCOG. 2015 April.
39. Meaney J, Weg J, Chenevert T, et al. Diagnosis of pulmonary embolism with magnetic resonance angiography. N Engl J Med. 1997; 336:1422-7.

CHAPTER 56

Uterine Rupture

Sudeepti Mummadi

INTRODUCTION

Uterine rupture is a life-threatening pregnancy complication for both mother and fetus. Most uterine ruptures in resource-rich countries are associated with a trial of labor after cesarean (TOLAC) delivery. In resource-limited countries, many uterine ruptures are related to obstructed labor and lack of access to operative delivery.

TERMINOLOGY

- *Uterine dehiscence* represents an occult scar separation observed at laparotomy in women with a prior cesarean delivery. With uterine dehiscence, the serosa of the uterus is intact and hemorrhage, with its potential for fetal and maternal sequelae, is absent.
- In contrast, *uterine rupture* is a through-and-through disruption of all uterine layers, with potential consequences of no reassuring fetal status and perinatal mortality along with severe maternal morbidity, hemorrhage, and mortality.

INCIDENCE

The overall incidence of uterine rupture (scarred and unscarred uteri) is 1 in 2,000 deliveries. Uterine rupture is most common in women with a scarred uterus, including those with prior cesarean delivery and myomectomy. The incidence of uterine rupture in women with prior cesarean delivery varies from 0.3% to 1%.[1]

FACTORS THAT INCREASE RISK OF UTERINE RUPTURE

Previous Uterine Rupture

Previous Cesarean Section[2]

Risk for uterine rupture based on incision type has been shown in Table 1.

In counseling women with an unknown scar, the physician should attempt to understand whether a prior cesarean delivery had been performed under circumstances in which it was more likely that a different type of incision had been used. For example, a history of preterm cesarean delivery should warrant caution, especially in the setting of malpresentation, because the incision may have involved an undeveloped muscular portion of the uterus, or it may have been a classical incision. For these reasons, if the clinician suspects that the prior delivery occurred under circumstances in which an incision that extended into the muscular

TABLE 1: Risk for uterine rupture based on incision type.

Prior incision type	Rupture rate (%)
Low transverse	0.5–1.0
Low vertical	0.8–1.1
Classic or T-shaped	4–9

TABLE 2: Risk of perinatal death related to uterine rupture.

Study		Perinatal deaths/ ruptures with TOLAC
Guise et al.[3] (pooled data)	74	0.14/1,000
Landon et al.[4]	123	0.11/1,000
Chauhan et al.[5] (pooled data)	880	0.40/1,000

(TOLAC: trial of labor after cesarean)

portion of the uterus was used, we generally proceed with repeat cesarean delivery.

Risk of perinatal death related to uterine rupture has been shown in Table 2.

Previous Fundal or High Vertical Hysterotomy

Induction

The incidence of rupture is higher in women with a prior cesarean who undergo induction trial than in women who experience spontaneous onset labor [NIH state-of-the science statement 2010: 1.5% vs 0.8%;[6] systematic review 2015: rupture/dehiscence odds ratio (OR) 1.62, 95% CI 1.13–2.31].

The risk of rupture with use of prostaglandins is sufficiently high (2.45%) that the American College of Obstetricians and Gynecologists (ACOG) has advised against misoprostol use for induction of labor in women with a previous cesarean delivery.[7]

Labor

The incidence of rupture is higher in women who undergo a TOLAC than in women who undergo planned repeat cesarean delivery. A low Bishop score on admission and dystocia, particularly at advanced dilation (>7 cm) may increase the risk of rupture in laboring women. Slower cervical dilation in the first stage of labor and a longer second stage also appear to increase the risk for rupture.[8]

Obstructed Labor

Trauma

- External cephalic version
- Breech extraction
- Instrumental delivery (forceps)
- Manual removal of placenta in adherent placenta
- Manipulations in shoulder dystocia.

Müllerian Duct Anomalies

Possible risk factors—factors inconsistently reported to be associated with an increased risk of rupture include:[9]
- Increasing maternal age
- Gestational age > 40 weeks
- Birth weight > 4,000 g
- Interdelivery interval < 18–24 months
- Single-layer uterine closure, especially if locked
- More than one previous cesarean deliveries.

FACTORS THAT DECREASE THE RISK OF RUPTURE

A prior vaginal delivery, either before or after the prior cesarean delivery, significantly reduces, but does not eliminate the risk of uterine rupture.[10]

PREDICTING UTERINE RUPTURE

Antepartum Imaging

Ultrasound measurement of both the thickness of the residual myometrium in the lower segment of uterus and the width, depth, and length of the hypoechoic uterine defect at the site of the previous cesarean is the method most studied to predict risk of rupture and counsel women contemplating a trial of labor. These measurements change with increasing gestational age.

Some authors consider a full lower uterine segment thickness <2.0 mm predictive of an increased risk of rupture or dehiscence.[11]

CLINICAL FINDINGS OF UTERINE RUPTURE

Intrapartum

- *Abnormal fetal heart rate (FHR)*: The most common FHR abnormality is fetal bradycardia, which may be sudden or preceded by variable or prolonged decelerations.[12]
- *Abdominal pain*: Rupture may be associated with sudden onset of abdominal pain, but pain may be partially masked by neuraxial analgesia administered for management of labor pain.
- *Vaginal bleeding*: Vaginal bleeding may occur but is not a cardinal symptom.
- Loss of station of the fetal presenting part.
- Uterine tenderness, cessation of contractions, change in uterine shape.
- Hematuria if the rupture extends into the bladder.
- *Hemodynamic instability*: Intra-abdominal hemorrhage can lead to rapid maternal hemodynamic deterioration (hypotension and tachycardia).
- Over 90% of uterine ruptures occur in the anterior lower uterine segment, but the corpus, cervix, vaginal wall, posterior uterus, or parametrium may be involved.[13]

Postpartum

In postpartum women, occult uterine rupture that occurred during delivery is characterized by pain and persistent vaginal bleeding despite use of uterotonic agents. Hematuria may occur if the rupture extends into the bladder.

Intraoperative Findings

A uterine rupture is usually immediately recognized upon opening the abdomen. Hemoperitoneum is usually present and fetal parts or membranes are often visible.

DIFFERENTIAL DIAGNOSIS

- Abruption is one of the main diagnoses in pregnant women with acute pain abdomen, bleeding per vagina (PV), and category II or III FHR tracings.
- Maternal markers of hemodynamic instability occur with intra-abdominal bleeding from any source, including rupture of the liver, which can occur in severe pre-eclampsia or hemolysis elevated liver enzymes, low platelet count (HELLP) syndrome. In contrast to uterine rupture, these disorders do not have an acute onset and are often associated with hypertension, proteinuria, epigastric or right upper quadrant pain, and low platelets.
- Inversion.
- Broad ligament hematoma.
- *Surgical causes*: Appendicitis, biliary colic, pancreatitis, peptic ulcer disease, intestinal obstruction, and ovarian torsion.

MANAGEMENT

- The patient should be prepared for laparotomy at the earliest suspicion of rupture. Resuscitation is carried out simultaneously.
- The anesthesia staff should be notified for assistance with patient management and to provide anesthetic support for delivery. Epidural and spinal anesthesia are generally contraindicated in patients who require urgent delivery because of the time required to achieve an adequate level, and are contraindicated in patients with a severe bleeding diathesis because of the risk of epidural or spinal hematoma.
- *Choice of incision*: A Pfannenstiel incision provides good exposure of the lower uterine segment and pelvis. A midline incision is better for abdominal

exploration, including the uterine fundus, which extends above the umbilicus by the late second trimester.[14]
- *Repair versus hysterectomy*:[15] A clean rupture of the previous scar requires surgical repair, with or without tubal ligation. Following delivery of the fetus and placenta, primary single- or double-layered closure with a delayed absorbable suture is a rapid technique for repairing the rupture and closing the incision.[16]

Indications for hysterectomy in uterine rupture:
  - Ragged tears
  - Rupture involving broad ligament or the uterine artery
  - Extension to the cervix
  - Broad fundal rupture.

Care should be taken to identify the ureters (especially when the tears have extended to the lower segment) and avoid injury to them. Anterior wall rupture is more common. Posterior wall rupture is more difficult to repair.

- *Management of bladder injury*: Uterine rupture may lead to bladder injury. If the uterine laceration extends to the bladder or a ureteral injury is suspected, we suggest an intraoperative consultation with an experienced urologic surgeon. Large anterior ruptures that extend into the bladder are repaired in two layers followed by urethral and/or suprapubic catheter placement for up to 14 days.[17]

MATERNAL AND PERINATAL COMPLICATIONS

Perinatal Complications

- Intrapartum stillbirth
- Hypoxic ischemic encephalopathy
- Neonatal death
- Admission to the neonatal intensive care unit
- Acidosis in fetus at birth.

Maternal Complications

- Need for hysterectomy
- Complications of blood component therapy
- Genitourinary tract injury
- Risk of recurrence.

PREVENTION

- Fundal pressure in the second stage of labor should be avoided because it can rupture the uterus and is not an effective approach to dystocia.[18]
- Procedures that involve uterine manipulation, such as external cephalic version for malpresentation in a woman with a significant uterine anomaly, should be performed gently or not at all.
- Judicious use of uterotonic agents for induction and augmentation of labor and appropriate use of cesarean delivery for management of protraction or arrest should reduce the risk of rupture of the unscarred normal uterus.

MANAGEMENT OF SUBSEQUENT PREGNANCIES

- Frequent antenatal checkups
- Prophylactic steroids for pulmonary maturity
- Elective cesarean section
- Admission to hospital at least 1 week before the gestational age at which labor started in the previous pregnancy is advised
- Timing for delivery is individualized based on data about the gestational age at which the woman went into labor in previous pregnancies, type of scar and the gestational age at which the rupture occurred.

REFERENCES

1. National Institutes of Health Consensus Development Conference Panel. National

Institutes of Health Consensus Development conference statement: vaginal birth after cesarean: new insights March 8-10, 2010. Obstet Gynecol. 2010;115(06):1279-95.
2. Gabbe SG, Niebyl JR, Simpson JL, Landon MB, Galan HL, Jauniaux ER, Driscoll DA, Berghella V, Grobman WA (Eds). Obstetrics: Normal and Problem Pregnancies, 7th edition. Philadelphia, PA: Elsevier Health Sciences; 2017.
3. Guise JM, Berlin M, McDonagh M, et al. Safety of vaginal birth after cesarean: a systematic review. Obstet Gynecol. 2004;103(3):420-9.
4. Silver RM, Landon MB, Rouse DJ, et al. Maternal morbidity associated with multiple repeat cesarean deliveries. Obstet Gynecol. 2006;107(6):1226-32.
5. Chauhan SP, Martin JN Jr, Henrichs CE, et al. Maternal and perinatal complications with uterine rupture in 142,075 patients who attempted vaginal birth after cesarean delivery: a review of the literature. Am J Obstet Gynecol. 2003;189(2):408-17.
6. Rossi AC, Prefumo F. Pregnancy outcomes of induced labor in women with previous cesarean section: a systematic review and meta-analysis. Arch Gynecol Obstet. 2015;291(2):273-80.
7. Committee on Practice Bulletins-Obstetrics. Practice Bulletin No. 184: vaginal birth after cesarean delivery. Obstet Gynecol. 2017;130:e217-33.
8. Vachon-Marceau C, Demers S, Goyet M, et al. Labor dystocia and the risk of uterine rupture in women with prior cesarean. Am J Perinatol. 2016;33(06):577-83.
9. Roberge S, Demers S, Berghella V, et al. Impact of single- vs double-layer closure on adverse outcomes and uterine scar defect: a systematic review and meta-analysis. Am J Obstet Gynecol. 2014;211(5):453-60.
10. Guise JM, Eden K, Emeis C, et al. Vaginal birth after cesarean: new insights. Evid Rep Technol Assess. 2010;191:1-397.
11. Jastrow N, Vikhareva O, Gauthier RJ, et al. Can third-trimester assessment of uterine scar in women with prior cesarean section predict uterine rupture? Ultrasound Obstet Gynecol. 2016;47(4):410-4.
12. Ridgeway JJ, Weyrich DL, Benedetti TJ. Fetal heart rate changes associated with uterine rupture. Obstet Gynecol. 2004;103(3):506-12.
13. Ofir K, Sheiner E, Levy A, et al. Uterine rupture: differences between a scarred and an unscarred uterus. Am J Obstet Gynecol. 2004;191(2):425-9.
14. Wylie BJ, Gilbert S, Landon MB, et al. Comparison of transverse and vertical skin incision for emergency cesarean delivery. Obstet Gynecol. 2010;115(6):1134-40.
15. Arulkumaran S, Arjun G, Penna LK. The Management of Labour, 3rd edition. Hyderabad, India: Universities Press; 2011.
16. Majumdar S, Warren R, Ifaturoti O. Fetal survival following posterior uterine wall rupture during labour with intact previous caesarean section scar. Arch Gynecol Obstet. 2007;276(5):537-40.
17. Yang B. Bladder rupture associated with uterine rupture at delivery. Int Urogynecol J. 2011;22(5):625-7.
18. Dow M, Wax JR, Pinette MG, et al. Third-trimester uterine rupture without previous cesarean: a case series and review of the literature. Am J Perinatol. 2009;26(10):739-44.

Index

Page numbers followed by *b* refer to box, *f* refer to figure, *fc* refer to flowchart, and *t* refer to table.

A

Abdomen 234
　blunt injury 73
　lower 300
　X-ray 61
Abdominal circumference 174, 177
Abdominal examination 23, 200, 289, 367
Abdominal trauma, penetrating 75, 79, 82*fc*
Abdominovaginal examination 66
Abortion 4, 12, 53
　complete 6
　　tubal 22
　incomplete 7
　　tubal 22
　induced 10
　inevitable 7
　medical 11
　missed 8
　　tubal 22
　septic 8, 9, 399, 400
　spontaneous 329
　threatened 6
Abruptio placenta 73, 146, 218, 399, 400, 401*fc*
Abruption 6, 480*f*
Accelerations 210
Acetaminophen 275
Acidosis 369
Acquired immunodeficiency syndrome 12, 332
Activated partial thromboplastin time 115, 117, 187
Active phase disorders 438
Acupuncture and transcutaneous electric nerve stimulation 431
Acute abdomen 24, 297
　differential diagnosis of 298
　incidence of 297
Acute asthma 385, 386, 391
　exacerbation 391
　treatment of 387
Acute chest syndrome 456
　causes 456
　clinical features 456
　incidence 456
　pathophysiology of 456, 457*f*
　treatment 456
Acute disseminated intravascular coagulation 401
Acute pain 300
　abdomen 488
　management 455*b*
Acute polyhydramnios 188
　diagnosis of 184
　management of 185
Acute respiratory distress syndrome 196, 447, 472
Acute stroke 456
　clinical features 456
　differential diagnosis 457
　management 456
Acute transfusion reaction 441
　pathophysiology of 441*t*
Addison's disease 17
Additional obstetric
　maneuvers 226
　procedures 86
Adenosine 274
　triphosphate 366
Adherent placenta 163*f*, 342, 487
　accreta 262
　diagnosis of 162
Adhesions 52
Adnexa 25, 473
Adnexal mass 327
　presence of 473
Advanced life support in obstetrics 242
Air
　bags, deployment of 83
　embolism 186
Airway 240, 295
　assessment of 157, 218, 227
　difficulties 75
　obstruction, upper 75, 451
　support 448
Alanine transaminase 115
Albuminuria 2
Albuterol 275, 390
Alkaline phosphatase 116, 117
Alkalosis, worsening of 387
Allergy 78, 142
Alloantibodies 441
Allograft rejection 143
Alloimmune thrombocytopenia 190
Amenorrhea 41, 49
American Academy of Pediatrics 259
American College of Obstetricians and Gynecologists 145, 230, 258, 273, 293, 363
Aminoglycoside 273
Amiodarone 274
Amniocentesis 142
Amnioinfusion 304, 308
　role of 184
Amniotic fluid
　embolism 158, 185, 186*fc*, 188, 193, 196, 226, 294, 347, 354, 399, 400, 401*fc*, 451
　　clinical features of 193, 194*t*
　　diagnosis of 194, 195*t*
　　incidence 193
　　management 195
　　pathogenesis of 193, 194*fc*
　　pathophysiology 193
　　prognosis 196
　emergency, management of 181, 183
　index 178, 181, 182, 201
　methods of sonographic measurement of 181
　physiology of 181
　sources of 181
　volume 77, 179
　　severe reduction in 188
Amniotomy 262, 428
Ampicillin 152, 362
Ampullary lumen, normal 21*f*
Anal sphincter 254
　external 254
　injuries, obstetrical 255
　internal 254
Anal triangle 253
Analgesia 236, 317
　epidural 208, 224
　nonopioid 455
Anaphylactoid reaction hypothesis 193
Anaphylaxis 444
　clinical manifestations of 447*f*
　diagnosis of 446, 446*b*
　differential diagnosis of 450
　etiology 444

exercise induced 445
management of 447, 449f, 451f
multisystem involvement in 446t
pathogenesis of 445, 445f
prevalence 444
prevention of 450, 452
refractory 448
signs of 447f
symptoms of 447f
treatment in 450f
types of 445
Anechoic fluid collections 25
Anemia 76, 459, 467, 468
aplastic 468
classification of 459
complications of 469t
determinants of 460
etiology of 460
hemolytic 468
hereditary hemolytic 462
immune hemolytic 468
management of 469, 469fc
pathological 462t
physiological 459
rule out 2
severe 459, 469
stages of 463f
types of 461fc
Anesthesia 225, 231, 241
epidural 286
general 217, 223, 225
high spinal 186
local 232
Anesthetic complications 216
Anesthetic management 217, 218, 220, 222
Aneurysm, abdominal aortic 299
Angiogenesis imbalance 279
Angiography, pulmonary 131
Angiotensin receptor blocker 111, 283, 284
Angiotensin-converting enzyme 284
inhibitor 111, 283
Anhydramnios 183, 183f
diagnosis of 183
etiology of 183
management of severe 183
Anorexia 333
Antacids 275
Antenatal care 1
components of 1
mental preparation 3
objectives of 1
physical examination 2
Antenatal monitoring 316

Antenatal visits, protocols of 1
Anterior sacculation 53
management of 54
Antibiotics 148, 236, 241
prophylaxis 152, 230
intrapartum 121fc
regimens 362t
Antibodies 441, 445
Anticoagulant 273
drugs 273t
therapy 133
initial 132
Anticoagulation 282, 285
postnatal 134
Anti-D
administration 64
immunoglobulin 64
Antidepressants 274
Antiemetics, low dose 16
Antiepileptic drugs 316
adverse effects of 315
common 314t
dose modification, postpartum 317
effect of 313, 318
monitoring of 315
Antifibrinolytic 196
therapy 404
Antifungal agents 275, 275t
Antihistamine H1 receptor blocker 16
Antihypertensive 105t
category of 105
treatment 103
Antimicrobial therapy 361
Antioxidants 101, 102
Antishock garment, nonpneumatic 246
Antithrombin concentrates 196
Antithrombotic agents 102
Antiviral agents 275, 275t
Anxiety 141, 333
Anxiolytics 328
Appellant's arguments 345, 350
Appendicitis 17, 300, 327, 488
Arrest disorders 436, 438
Arrhythmia 194
management 112, 282, 285
Arterial balloon occlusion 250
Arterial blood gas 455
Arteriovenous malformation 298
ablation of 185
Artery
ligation, ovarian 250
thromboembolectomy, pulmonary 196

utero-ovarian 32
uteroplacental 173
Asherman's syndrome 250
Aspartate
aminotransferase 223
transaminase 115
Asphyxia 90
perinatal 175
Assisted reproductive technology
pregnancies 297
Asthma 385, 387
acute severe 387, 387t
attacks 387
exacerbations 385, 387
dosages for 390t
features of 387
home management of 386, 386fc
life-threatening 388
postpartum 391
flare-ups 385
life-threatening 387, 387t
near-fatal 387, 387t
Atopy 385
Atosiban 147
Autoimmune disease 190
Azithromycin 335

B

Bacterial infection 119
tests 190
Bacterial vaginosis 360
Bagel sign 25
Ballooning cervical pregnancy,
ultrasound appearance
of 42f
Bandl's ring 366
Barker hypothesis 175fc
Basic life support 295
Benzodiazepines 316, 317
Beta-adrenergic receptor agonists 147
Beta-blockers 111
Beta-hemolytic streptococcus 359
Beta-human chorionic gonadotropin
surveillance 65
Beta-lactams 444
Betamimetics 146
Beta-thalassemia major 467
Biochemical tests 152, 176
pathophysiological basis of 101t
Biophysical tests 152
Biopsy
endometrial 27
endomyocardial 281

Index

Bipolar cautery 45
Birth weight, low 133, 164, 173, 173f, 304
Bishop score 426t, 487
Bitolterol 390
Bladder
   displace 242
   drainage 236
   filling 306
   injury 91
      management of 489
Bleeding 340
   abdominal 49
   abnormal 23
   implantation 4
   intraoperative 62
   neonatal 133
   per vagina 488
   torrential 49
Blood 72
   and blood products 417
   component
      physical effects of 441
      therapy 403
   components of 441
   flow, renal 323
   for cross matching 218
   glucose values 324
   group 57, 230
   indices 477f
   loss 216, 467
      minimize 234
      severity of 155
   pressure 283, 297
      diastolic 95
      monitoring 2
      reduce 103
      regular 2
      support 448
      systolic 72, 95, 359
   product
      support 403
      transfusion 217
   stained urine 394
   sugar 230
   supply, reduction of 42
   tests 280
   transfusion 9, 39, 354, 455, 465
      incompatible 399
      indications for 456b
   urea nitrogen 15, 280
   volume 100
Blunt trauma 72, 73, 79
   obstetric consequences of 74
B-lynch suture 187, 248f

Body mass index 114, 231, 363
Bolam test 340
Bone marrow insufficiency 462
Bony pelvis 366
Bowel
   disorders 300
   segment of 38f
Brachial plexus injury 88, 90
Bradycardia 209
Brain 100
   growth 174
   type natriuretic peptide 108, 280
Brandt-Andrews method, modified 170
Breast examination 2
Breastfeeding 113, 134, 445
Breathing 240, 290, 295
   assessment of 157, 227
   shortness of 109
   wheezy 386
Breathlessness 58, 66, 386
Breech
   complete 198
   delivery
      documentation of 206
      types of 202
   diagnosis of 200
   extraction, reverse 235
   footling 198
   frank 198
   incomplete 198
   labor in 201
   nonengaged 201
   positions, incomplete 199f
   presentation 198, 236, 421
      external version of 201f
      management of 200
      positions of 198, 199f
Broad ligament hematoma 488
Bromocriptine 285
Brow presentation 379t, 384
   diagnosis of 381
Burn injuries 75
Buttocks 202

C

Calcium
   channel blocker 146, 147
   serum 244
Carbamazepine 272, 314
Carbon
   dioxide 327
      partial pressures of 221
   monoxide 297

Carboperitoneum 328
Carboprost 63, 221
Cardiac arrest 194, 196
   reversible causes of 227
Cardiac disease 109
Cardiac failure 108
Cardiac index 328
Cardiac magnetic resonance imaging 280, 281
Cardiac medications 274, 274t
Cardiac resynchronization therapy 282
Cardiomyopathy
   drugs induced 109
   familial dilated 282
   hereditary 109
   idiopathic dilated 278
Cardiorespiratory systems 293
Cardiotocography 208, 329
   characteristics 209
   limitations of 214
   monitoring 189, 208
   nonreassuring 165
   recording, prerequisites for 208
Cardiovascular collapse 194
Cardiovascular support 195
Cardiovascular system 72, 420
Caregivers blame victim 331
Castor oil 431
Catheter placement 354
Ceftriaxone 10
Cells of Cajal 20
Central nervous system 274
Central venous pressure 10
Cephalic version, role of external 267
Cephalosporins 273
Cerebellar atrophy, midline 274
Cerebral
   artery Doppler, middle 177
   venous thrombosis 294
Cerebrovascular accident 195, 451
   history of 456
Cerebrovascular pathophysiology 100
Cervical
   canal 289
   changes 142
   dilatation, advanced 146
   encerclage 149
   fetal fibronectin 411
   fibronectin 413
   finding 367
   incompetence 141, 142
   insufficiency 143
   lacerations 91

length 145, 413
  assessment 144
  transvaginal 144, 145
pregnancy 41, 43f, 474
  management of 41
pretreatment 62
ripening 424, 426f
spine injury 75
vaginal swabs 359
Cervix 51, 62
  barrel-shaped 474
  examination of 217
  laceration of 91
  lower fibrous 51
  unfavorable 102
Cesarean delivery 133, 229, 230, 258, 384
  complications of 235, 235t
  effect of 450fc
  indications for 229b
  number of prior 266
  pregnancy with prior 258
Cesarean scar
  ectopic pregnancy 50
    ruptured 44f
  pregnancy 43, 44f, 475
Cesarean section 115, 217, 219, 229, 263, 264fc, 308, 370, 393, 399, 433
  anesthesia for 225
  complicated 235
  consent for 230
  elective repeat 266
  lower segment 260, 340, 383
  planned 201
  urgency of 230b
Cetirizine 275
Chemotherapy
  prophylactic 66
  single-agent 68
  systemic 42
Chest
  compressions 187
  radiograph 280, 388
  tightness 386
Chlamydia trachomatis 124
  diagnosis 124
  management 124
  maternal and fetal risks 124
Chloramphenicol 273
Chlorpheniramine 275
Chlorpromazine 271
Cho suture 249, 249f
Cholecystitis 17, 327
  management of acute 299

Cholesterol, total 297
Chorioamnionitis 146, 155, 221, 399
  signs of 150b
Choriocarcinoma 66, 67, 477f
Chorionic plate, movement of 480
Chorionic villi 21f, 43f, 55, 96
  absence of 27
  immature 41f
Chorionic villus sampling 142
Chromosomal anomalies, detection of 178
Chromosome 98
Chronic disseminated intravascular coagulation 401
Circulation 240, 290, 295
  assessment of 157, 227
  pulmonary 193
Classical segment scar 263t
Cleidotomy 89
Clindamycin 273, 362
Clobazam 316
Clotrimazole 275
Coagulation 218
  inhibitory system 398
  profile 244
  system 398
Coagulopathy 196, 218, 220, 244
  management of 187
  mechanism of acquired 400
  prevention of 196
  treatment of 196
Cobweb appearance 26f
Cocaine 155
Cochrane review 201
Coitus 21
Colles' fascia, superficial space 253
Color flow Doppler 262
Complement activation hypothesis 193
Complete blood count 62, 117, 280, 335
Complete mole 57f, 60, 60f
Compression
  duplex ultrasound 130
  sutures
    advantages of 250, 250t
    disadvantages of 250, 250t
  uterocaval 79
Computed tomography 77, 131, 374
  scan 61, 374
Conception
  products of 7
  retained products of 472, 477
Congenital anomaly 200, 425

Congenital malformations
  reducing risk of 314
  risk of major 311
Congestion, hepatic 279
Consciousness 75
Contraception 65, 318
  advice 12
  emergency 5, 335
  methods of 318
  reversible 7
Contraceptive
  combined oral 65
  device, intrauterine 65
  oral hormonal 318
Convulsions, control of 104
Copper intrauterine devices 318
Cord
  abnormalities 304
  accidents 200
  entanglement 421
  multiple loops of 185
  prolapse 225, 304
  types of 303fc, 304t
Corpus
  callosum, agenesis of 274
  luteum 26f
Cortisol 323
Cough 66, 386
Couvelaire uterus 155
Crackles, pulmonary 279
C-reactive protein 279, 418
Creatine kinase 25
Crede's method 169, 170
Crohn's disease 466
Cryoprecipitate 217, 441
Culdocentesis 25
Cullen's sign 23
Customized symphyseal-fundal distance charts 177
Cyclizine 271
Cyclooxygenase inhibitors 147
Cyclophosphamide 68
Cyst, ovarian 39
Cysteinyl leukotrienes 445
Cytomegalovirus 174

D

Dalteparin, initial dose of 133t
Dandy-Walker malformation 274
D-antigen 64
D-dimer 131
Dead fetus 369
Death
  causes of 196

maternal 73
neonatal 201, 327, 489
sudden unexpected 311
Decelerations 210
Decidua basalis 97
Deep vein thrombosis 73, 129, 472, 484
Defibrillation 187
Dehydration, severe 455
Delivery 240, 286
decision for 158
expected date of 2
in emergency department, limitations of 421
indications for 103, 165
instrumental 88
vaginal 88
method of 73
mode of 113, 316
placental 233
precipitous 418
preterm 327
route of 166
timing of 179*fc*
Deoxyhemoglobin 454
Deoxyribonucleic acid 34
Deoxyuridine monophosphate 34
Depotmedroxy progesterone acetate 468
Diabetes mellitus
gestational 2, 87, 190, 322
pregestational 323
requiring insulin 425
treatment of 273*t*
type 1 137, 322
type 2 322
Diabetic ketoacidosis 17, 298, 325
management of 325
prevention of 325
risk factors of 324
Diarrhea 17
Digoxin 274
Dihydroergotamine 275
Dinoprostone 261
Diphenhydramine 275
Diphtheria 3
Diphyllobothrium latum infestation 466
Disseminated gonococcal infection 124
Disseminated intravascular coagulation 8, 76, 103, 116, 155, 158, 196, 218, 398, 401, 402, 418, 447
causes of 399

manifestations of 402*f*
nonobstetrical causes of 399
pathogenesis of 398, 400*fc*
postpartum risks in 402
Diuretics 104, 110
Doppler sonography, role of 474
Doxycycline 273
Drugs 221, 240
antiarrhythmic 187
antibiotics 273*t*
antiepileptic 316
antithrombotic 101
antituberculous 274, 275*t*
cardiovascular 101
categorization of 270
immunosuppressive 285
therapy 110, 224, 269
usage 269
Dysmenorrhea 333, 394
Dyspareunia 394
Dyspnea 442
acute 194
exertional 279
paroxysmal nocturnal 279
Dystocia 436

E

Early pregnancy 54
discomforts 23
loss 4
predictors 394
Echocardiogram, transthoracic 280
Echocardiography 281
parameters 278
Eclampsia 96, 103, 104, 195, 223, 342, 399, 408, 425, 451, 456
clinical features in 103
management of 104
severe 58, 146
syndrome 95
treatment 342
Ectopic pregnancy 19, 21, 25, 26*f*, 27*f*, 30, 31, 35, 40, 41, 41*f*, 49, 49*f*, 327, 472, 474
acute 21, 22, 49
chronic 21, 22, 24
classification 19
clinical manifestations 22
cornual resection of 393
diagnosis of 19, 49, 474, 475
diaphragmatic 49
epidemiology 19
etiology 20
incidence of 297

interstitial 46*f*
management 19, 29
pathophysiology 20
persistent 36
postoperative plan 33
preparation 29
procedures 30
recurrent 36, 50
risk factors for 20
ruptured 26*f*
sites of 19*f*
splenic 47*f*
technique 29
tubal 23, 31*f*
Eczema 134
Edema 2
interstitial alveolar 75
leg 279
pathological 2
physiological 2
pulmonary 103, 451
Electrocardiogram 280
Electrolytes 325
serum 244
Emboli, pulmonary 469
Embolism, pulmonary 129, 186, 195, 226, 451, 483, 484
Embryofetal malformations 313
Emergency
cesarean
delivery 450, 452
section 436
delivery tray, contents of 417, 418*b*
department
and hospital-based care 388
delivery in 417
evaluation 387
management 389*fc*
hypertensive 95
in utero transfer 407, 409
interventions 417
laparotomy 30
transfers 409
treatment 340
Emphysema, subcutaneous 329
Empty uterine cavity 474
Encephalopathy
hepatic 114
syndrome, posterior reversible 472
Endocrine disorders 143
Endometrial cavity 25, 473*f*
Endometrial echo complex 477
Endometriosis 52

Endometritis 360, 394
    puerperal 362t
Endometrium 20, 473
    trilaminar pattern of 26f
Endothelial cell
    activation 98, 99fc
    injury 99
Endothelial damage 129
Enoxaparin, dose of 132t
Enterocolitis, necrotizing 175
Entonox 317
Eosinophilia 363
Epilepsy 71, 311, 315-317
    diagnosis of 311
    during pregnancy, management of 319
    juvenile myoclonic 312
Epinephrine 275, 390
    systemic administration of 391
Epsilon aminocaproic acid 404
Ergot alkaloids 221
Ergotamine tartrate 275
Erythrocyte sedimentation rate 6
Erythromycin 152
Erythropoietin, injection 465
Escherichia coli 8, 142, 360
Esophageal rupture 17
Estimated gestational age 82
Estrogen, levels of 323
Ethambutol 275
Etomidate 219
European Society of Cardiology 284
    Guidelines 282
Exchange transfusion, indications for 456b
External cephalic version 155, 200, 304, 383, 384, 487
Extra-amniotic saline instillation 426
Extracorporeal membrane oxygenation 196

F

Face presentation 379t, 384
    diagnosis of 379
    mentoanterior 380
    mentoposterior 380
Fallopian tube 21f, 40
Family planning 3
Fatigue 109, 279
Feeding difficulties 175
Femur length 174
Ferritin, serum 462
Fetal
    abnormalities, screening for 315

acidosis, early 72
activity 386
    maternal perception of 152
anemia 78
anomalies 304
asphyxia 369
assessment 166, 306, 329
bleeding 133
bradycardia 200, 201, 209
chest 89
chimerism 279
complications 150t, 174, 369
component 141
compromise 103, 411
condition, assessment of 158
death 369
demise 103, 218, 383
distress 73, 146, 194, 218, 219, 225
fibronectin 25, 144, 145
genes 98
growth
    abnormal 208
    restriction 110
    retardation 17
head
    extended 200
    manual delivery of 234f
    palpable 201
heart rate 208, 309, 329, 367
    abnormal 488
    external monitoring of 208
    monitoring 152, 218
heart tone 81, 82
hypoxemia, pathophysiology of 446, 447fc
hypoxia 200
infections 190
injury 76
    common 73
invasive procedures 304
laser therapy 185
loss 4
lung maturity assessment 152
monitoring 316, 448
    electronic 81
    intraoperative 329
morbidity 76
    majority of 155
movements 179, 210
neck, hyperextended 380
risks 440
skull, diameters of 380f
surveillance, antepartum 178

survival 241
tachycardia 209, 209f
tone 179
weight 87t
well-being, assessment of 77
Feticide, intra-amniotic 42
Fetus 414
    and placenta, microbiological examination of 190
    delivery of 196
    low profile 173
    minimizing radiation exposure to 301
    neuroprotective for 147
    nonviable 383
    placenta 340
    prompt delivery of 306
Fever
    persistent puerperal 362, 363t
    rheumatic 457
Fexofenadine 275
Fibrin degradation product 402, 418
Fibrinogen 244, 402
Fibrinolytic system 398
Fibroblast proliferation 266
Fibroid 52
    polyp 291
Fick's principle 446
Fire, ring of 26f
Fistula 368
Flank pain 300
Flecainide 274
Flu vaccination 3
Fluconazole 275
Fluid
    status 388
    therapy 9, 217, 325
Foley's catheter 427
Folic acid
    deficiency 462, 465, 466f
    supplementation 3
Folinic acid 42
Food and Drug Administration 270t
Forceful violent Act 331
Forceps 235
Fractures 90
Free erythrocyte protoporphyrin 463
Free fatty acids 324
Fresh frozen plasma 196, 417, 441
Functional residual capacity 297
Fundal fibroid, posterior wall 52
Fundal pressure 90, 489
    excessive 288
Fusobacterium species 142

G

Gallbladder 299
  disease 299
Gamma glutamyl transpeptidase 116, 117
Gardnerella vaginalis 142
Gas insufflation 327
Gastric emptying, prolonged 72
Gastroenteritis 299
Gastrointestinal medications 275, 275t
Gastrointestinal system 72
Genital infections, female 360b
Genital trauma 220, 221
  anesthetic management of 222
Gentamicin 362
Gestation
  ectopic 33
  multiple 221, 394
  period of 181
  singleton 213f
  tubal ectopic 27f
Gestational age 103
  for termination of pregnancy 337
  pregnancy of 11
  small for 173, 173f
Gestational sac 42f, 48f, 60, 473f
Gestational trophoblastic disease 55, 56
  classification of 56f
Glands, endocervical 43f
Glipizide 273
Glomerular filtration rate 139
Gluconeogenesis, ketones stimulating 324
Glucose tolerance, normal 323
Glyburide 273
Glycogenolysis 324
Gonorrhea 124
  diagnosis 124
  management 124
  maternal and fetal risks 124
  uncomplicated 124
Gossypiboma 372, 374
  burden of 372
  imaging features of 374
  intraoperative appearance of 376f
  prevention of 375
  risk factors for 373
Grand multipara 304
Group B *Streptococcus* 119, 120, 121fc, 360
  diagnosis 120
  management 120
  prophylaxis 120fc
Growth
  factor, placental 98
  restriction intervention trial study 179

H

Harmonic scalpel 45
Haultan's repair 291
Hayman suture 249, 249f
Head 202
  circumference 174
Headache 333, 456
Heart
  disease 231
    coronary 231
    valvular 457
  failure 108, 137, 278, 280, 285
    acute left 195
    decompensated 112
    diagnosis of 111fc
    drug therapy, strategy for 284t
    etiology of 109
    magnitude of 109
    management of 110
    medications 113
    nonacute onset of 110
    population of 112
    pre-eclampsia with 282
    signs typical of 110t
    symptoms typical of 110t
    therapy 282
    types of 108, 108t
  rate 297
  sound, third 279
Helicobacter pylori infection 14
Hematocrit 71, 72, 218
Hematoma 480, 481f
  postcesarean 481
  puerperal 481
  subcapsular 481
Hematosalpinx 34
Hematuria 300, 488
Hemodynamic changes 459f, 460f
Hemofiltration 196
Hemoglobin 230, 459
  estimation 462
Hemogram 25
Hemolysis 100, 223, 467, 472
  elevated liver enzymes, and low platelet count syndrome 100, 116, 117, 223, 399, 402
  massive intravascular 399
Hemolytic reaction, delayed 442
Hemoperitoneum 34, 46
Hemoptysis 66
Hemorrhage 58, 472
  acute 165
  antepartum 155, 158, 164, 200, 216, 408, 411
  atonic postpartum 194, 196
  cerebral 472
  decidual 6, 143
  fetal-maternal 74
  intracerebral 294
  intracranial 73
  intraparenchymal 482f
  massive obstetric 216
  maternofetal 76
  obstetric 340
  postpartum 91, 155, 158, 168, 220, 243, 294, 368, 394, 399, 401, 472
  pulmonary 175
  risk of 61
  severe 155
  transplacental 200
  uncontrolled 62
  vaginal 208
Hemostasis
  commonly available tests of 402
  normal 398
Heparin 273, 403
  low-molecular-weight 273, 285, 404
Hepatic artery ligation 47
Hepatic failure, acute 447
Hepatitis
  A 121
    diagnosis 121
    management 121
    maternal and fetal effects 121
  B 121, 332, 335
    immunoglobulin 335
    surface antigen 6
    virus surface antigen 230
  C virus 6, 122, 230
    diagnosis 122
    management options 122
    maternal and fetal risks 122
  infection 121
  viral 115
  virus infections 121
Herbal supplements 431
Hernia surgery 327
Herpes simplex virus 174
Hormone metabolism disorders 142

Obstetric Emergencies

Hour-glass appearance 42f
Human chorionic gonadotropin 55, 56, 59, 62
　high levels of 323
　serum 4
Human endometrial stromal cells 7
Human immunodeficiency virus 6, 230, 278, 332, 335, 358, 468
Human papillomavirus 332
Human placental lactogen 323
Huntington's repair 291
Hydatidiform mole 55, 68, 399
　clinical presentation 58
　clinical signs 58
　complete 56t
　diagnosis 59
　management 61
　partial 56t
　pathogenesis 57
　pathology 58
　risk factors 55
Hydralazine 271
Hydroxyzine 275
Hypercapnia, severe 391
Hyperemesis gravidarum 14, 14t, 17
　clinical examination 15
　dual therapy 16
　history 15
　investigations 15
　management 15
　medications 16
　pathogenesis of 14
　risk factors 15
　severe 16
　single therapy 16
　transient hyperthyroidism of 15
Hyperglycemia 175
　uncontrolled 322
Hypertension 105, 218, 271, 425
　chronic 96
　drugs for treatment of 271t
　excessive 139
　gestational 95, 96
　mild-to-moderate 103
　persistent pulmonary 175
　postpartum 104
　pregnancy induced 332
　severe 104
　types of 96
Hypertensive crisis 103
Hypertensive disorders 95, 96, 96t, 223, 481
　classification of 95
　complications of 472
Hypertrophy, left ventricular 108

Hypocalcemia 175
Hypocapnia 72
Hypofibrinogenemia 196
Hypoglycemia 175
Hypotension 194, 195, 219, 442, 451, 455
　maternal 73
　sepsis induced 358
Hypothermia 175, 443, 455
Hypovolemia 399
　management of 370
Hypoxia 88
Hypoxic ischemic encephalopathy 489
　fractures 90
Hysterectomy 64, 155, 187
　definitive treatment 219
　subtotal 32 251t
Hysterotomy 64, 90, 393
　high vertical 487
　resuscitative 239, 295

I

Ibuprofen 275
Ibutilide 274
Iliac artery ligation, internal 250
Immune hemolytic disease 190
Immunity, humoral 98
Immunoglobulin
　E independent anaphylaxis 445
　G 445
　　role of 445
　intravenous 285
Implantable cardioverter-defibrillator 282
Implantation, secondary 37
In utero transfer 407, 408, 413
　feasibility of 412
　for spontaneous preterm labor 412fc
　roles and responsibilities 410fc
　staffing needs for 413
In vitro fertilization 21
Incarceration
　causes of 52
　clinical picture of 53
Incision
　classical 233
　small abdominal 328
　T-shaped 233
　types of 265
Indomethacin 147
Infections 119, 142, 368, 399, 468
　classification of 119

　congenital 123
　gene-environment interactions 143
　microbiology 142
　nonpregnancy-related 358
　nosocomial 358
　parasitic 119
　prevention of 113
　puerperal 469
　routes of 142
　systemic
　　manifestation of 359t
　　signs of 358
　viral 119
Inferior vena cava 239, 300
Infertility, secondary 394
Inflammation, acute 20
Inflammatory bowel disease 137
Injury
　abdominal 193
　electrical 76
　endothelial 398
　genital 332
　inhalation 75
　nongenital physical 332
　pattern of 71
　physical 334
　thermal 75
Inotropes 10
Inspired oxygen, fraction of 359
Insulin 273
　secretion of 323
　therapy 325
Intensive care unit 240, 299, 387, 417
Intermenstrual spotting 394
International Federation of Gynecology and Obstetrics 67
International normalized ratio 187, 244
International Society of Thrombosis and Haemostasis 402
Interval after index pregnancy 67
Intra-aortic balloon pump 196
Intrapartum
　management 178, 316
　monitoring 212f
　risk factors 88
　stillbirth 489
Intrauterine balloon tamponade 246
Intrauterine death 155, 201
Intrauterine device 309
Intrauterine fetal
　death 189, 432, 433
　demise 146, 399, 400, 401fc
　growth restriction 425, 432

Index

Intrauterine gestation 27f
  normal 19
Intrauterine growth
  intervention, disproportionate 179
  restriction 6, 58, 173, 173f, 176b, 200, 327, 332, 407
    asymmetrical 174, 174t
    complications 174
    diagnosis 177
    etiology of 173, 174t
    management 178
    neonatal complications of 175t
    pathogenesis 173
    prediction 174
    prevention 176
    symmetrical 174t
Intrauterine insemination 433
Intrauterine pregnancy
  absence of 473
  normal 48
Intravenous fluids, administration of 214
Inversion, degrees of 288f
Ipratropium 275, 390
  bromide 390
Iron
  deficiency 462
    anemia 58, 460, 462t, 464
    folic acid supplementation 3
    requirement, calculation of 464
    serum 462, 463
Ischemia, uteroplacental 142, 143
Isoniazid 275
Isoxsuprine 147
Itching 442

J

Jaundice 114, 117fc
  severe 456
Joel-Cohen incision 232
Johnson maneuver 290

K

Kadar principle 24
Karman cannula 63
Ketamine 219, 317
Ketoacidosis 323, 368
  euglycemic 323
Ketoconazole 275
Kidney 100
  disease, chronic 96
  injury, acute 447

Klebsiella pneumoniae 360
Kleihauer count 190
Kleihauer-Betke test 81
Krebs cycle 366

L

Labor
  abnormal progress of 436, 440
  abnormalities, types of 436
  after cesarean delivery, trial of 486, 487
  and delivery in emergency department 417
  augmentation of 208, 221, 265
  cessation of 219
  course of 380, 381
  dystocia 438t
  elective induction of 424
  first stage of 470
  induction of 260, 265, 317, 423, 424, 424fc, 424t, 425t, 432, 432t
  management during 202, 470
  methods of induction of 261, 424, 427
  monitoring of 262, 262b
  normal 141, 365
  obstructed 365, 487
  precipitate 439
  prolonged
    latent phase of 438b
    second stage of 88
  second stage of 243, 470
  spontaneous 260
  third stage of 169, 170, 204, 470
  trial of 259, 260
Lacerations, vaginal 91
Lactate dehydrogenase 467
Lactation failure 469
Lactic acid dehydrogenase 116
Lamotrigine 272, 313, 314
Laparoscopic approach over laparotomy, advantages of 29
Laparoscopic technique 31, 32, 33
Laparoscopy
  advantages of 328
  basic guidelines for 329
  diagnostic 26
  gasless 327
  hand-assisted 327
  in pregnancy 327
    complications 328
    contraindications 327

  indications 327, 328
  patient position 328
  premedication 328
  preoperative instructions 328
  types 327
  three-port 31
Laparotomy 44f
Last menstrual period 241
Late pregnancy 54
  loss 4
Left ventricular ejection fraction 108, 284, 285
Lethal fetal anomaly 146
Levalbuterol 390
Levetiracetam 272, 313, 314
Levonorgestrel-releasing intrauterine system 318
Levothyroxine 275
Lidocaine 274
Linezolid 273
Lipolysis 324
Liver 100, 481
  disease 115, 139
    chronic 35
    management of 116t
  enzymes, elevated 223, 472
  function test 15, 35, 61, 62, 244, 280, 335, 464
Lobectomy, partial 47
Loratadine 275
Lorazepam 317
Loveset maneuver 203, 204f
Lung injury, acute 441, 442
Lupus erythematosus 457

M

Macrolides 273
Macrosomia 87, 221, 394
Magnesium sulphate 146-148, 224, 342
  dosage regimen of 104
Mallory-Weiss syndrome 17
Malpresentation 366, 379, 383
Mass
  mixed echogenic 477f
  spectrometry 25
Mast cells 193
Mastitis 363
Maternal
  age, advanced 141, 394
  anaphylaxis 447fc, 448f
  and fetal risks 119, 122, 123

cardiac status 450fc
collapse 239, 239t, 293, 295
  causes 239
  management of 239
complications 150t, 368, 489
disease 176, 411
hemodynamic monitoring 218
morbidity 266, 369
mortality 48, 266, 369, 447
  causes of 95
sepsis, management of 484
trauma, causes of 71
Matrix metalloproteinases 7
Mauriceau maneuver 205f
Mauriceau-Smellie-Veit maneuver 203
Maylard incision 232
McRoberts maneuver 421
Mean amniotic fluid volume across normal pregnancy 182f
Mean arterial pressure 221, 358
Mechanical circulatory support and transplantation 282, 285
Meclizine 275
Meconium
  aspiration 175
  stained liquor 208
Medical and legal implications 372
Medical boards, role of 337
Medical professionals, role of 331
Medical Termination of Pregnancy amendment Bill 12
  Act 11, 12, 337
Medical treatment 344
  and care postsurgery 345
Medroxyprogesterone acetate injections 318
Membranes 151, 151fc
  artificial rupture of 304, 308, 428
  intact 141
  prelabor
    preterm rupture of 412, 413
    rupture of 155, 425, 432
  premature rupture of 141, 149, 150, 155, 200, 346, 347, 358
  preterm
    prelabor rupture of 425, 432
    premature rupture of 71, 151, 359
  rupture of 74, 201, 382
  spontaneous rupture of 304
  stripping 261, 424
Mental health, care of 191
Mesosalpinx 31
Metered-dose inhaler 386

Metformin 273
Methimazole 275
Methotrexate 34, 48, 68
  inhibits cellular proliferation 34
  therapy 35
Methyldopa 271
Methylenetetrahydrofolate 34
Methylergometrine 63, 187
Methylprednisolone 275
Metoclopramide 271
Metronidazole 273, 335
Microbiological tests 455
Mifepristone 11, 261, 431
Migraine 274
  drugs for treatment of 275t
Mineralocorticoid receptor antagonist 283, 284
Minimal access surgical procedure 327
Miscarriage 4, 5, 133, 327
  clinical examination 5
  complete 5
  delayed 4
  etiology 4
  incomplete 5
  inevitable 5
  laboratory investigations 6
  missed 5
  septic 5
  spontaneous 5
  threatened 5
  types of 4, 5t
Misgav Ladach technique 235
Misoprostol 11, 221, 234, 261
Molar pregnancy 55, 57, 59, 59f, 183f, 472
  clinical signs of 58, 59t
  complete 63, 64
  follow-up of 66fc
  management of 62fc, 63fc
  previous 55
Mole
  invasive 67
  partial 57f, 60
  types of 66
Morison's pouch 25
Morning sickness 14, 14t
Motor vehicle road accident 155
Müllerian duct anomalies 487
Multiple organ dysfunction syndrome 398
Muscles
  perineal 256f
  relaxants, nondepolarizing 225
Myocardial function 100

Myocardial infarction 186, 195, 294
Myocardial inflammation 279
Myocarditis, acute 282
Myomectomy 393
Myometrium, residual 487
Myosin light chain kinase 366

N

Naegele's formula 2
Naked eye appearance 58
Naratriptan 275
National Anemia Prophylaxis Programme 464
National Crime Records Bureau 332
National Institute for Health and Care Excellence 438
National Perinatal Epidemiology Unit Survey 408
Nausea 14, 271
  treatment of 271t
NCDRC's observations 346, 350, 352
Neck vein, engorged 279
Neglected shoulder presentation 369
Neonatal
  care 180
    after delivery 421
  infection, spectrum of 120
  intensive care unit 178, 263, 322, 408, 417
  morbidity, short-term 201
Neoplasia, gestational trophoblastic 61, 64, 67, 476
Neoplasm 462
Nephropathy 137
Nephrotic syndrome 137
Neural tube defects 313
Neuropathy, peripheral 17
New York Heart Association 279
Nifedipine 147
Nitrates 148
Nitrazine test 150
Nitric oxide 431
Nitrofurantoin 273
Nitroglycerin 147, 170
Nonmolar trophoblastic malignant neoplasms 55
Nonsteroidal anti-inflammatory drug 275, 329, 444
Nonstress test 179
N-terminal pro-brain type natriuretic peptide 108, 280
Nuchal cord 90, 304
Nystatin 275

Index

O

O'Sullivan method, modified 290, 290f
Obesity 236
    morbid 200
Obstetric
    complications 315
    consequences 332
    emergencies 23, 216, 339, 457, 472
        and trauma, managing 242
    management 112, 218, 222, 223
    thromboprophylaxis 138
        risk assessment and management 136
    ultrasound scanning 77
Obstructed labor 365, 487
    causes of 366
    etiology of 366t
    pathophysiology of 366
Oligohydramnios 200, 425
    management of severe 183
Omentum 48f
Ondansetron 271
Opioids analgesics 329
Optic atrophy 274
Organ dysfunction 359
Orthopnea 279
Ovarian hyperstimulation syndrome 297
Ovarian vein thrombosis 472, 483
Ovary, dermoid cyst of 376f
Oxidative stress 279
Oxygen 9
    mask 354
    partial pressure of 359
    saturation 63
    supplementation 388
Oxytocic agents, role of 63
Oxytocic drugs 113, 170, 290
Oxytocin 187, 221, 234, 261, 430
    augmentation 262
    dosage, protocol for 430t
    dose of 261
    infusion 64
    prophylactic 246
    receptor antagonists 147, 148
    risks of 430
    umbilical vein injection of 170

P

Packed red blood cell 196, 217, 441
Pain
    abdominal 46, 358, 488
    degree of lower abdominal 58
    localization of 298
    nature of 298
Pallor 2
Palmer's point 327
Palpation, abdominal 177
Palpitations 109
Pancreatitis 17
Paralytic ileus 368
Parenteral iron
    preparations 465t
    therapy 464
Parenteral nutrition, total 17
Partial molar pregnancy 63
    diagnosis of 60
Partial thromboplastin time 217
Parvovirus B$_{19}$ 174
Peak expiratory flow 386
Pelvic
    abscess 363
    bones 73
    examination 5, 39
        bimanual 21
    inflammatory disease 20, 298, 299
    pain, chronic 394
    surgeries 52
    tenderness 23
    vessels, engorgement of 73
Pelvis 73
Penicillin 273, 362
Pentoxifylline 285
Peptic ulcer disease 488
Peptide hormone 55
Pereira suture 249, 249f
Perimortem cesarean
    contraindications of 419
    delivery 239
    section 81, 419
Perinatal death 91, 201
    risk of 487, 487t
Perinatal morbidity 266
Perinatal mortality 266
    risk in 307
Perineal body 254
Perineal damage 91
Perineal tear 253
    degrees of 254
    first-degree 254f
    fourth-degree 255f
    second-degree 254f
    third-degree 255f
Perineal tissue, lack of elasticity of 254
Perineal triangle
    anterior 253f
    posterior 253f
Perineum 253
    lacerations of 253
    overstretching of 254
Peripartum cardiomyopathy 109, 113, 186, 195, 278, 280b, 280fc, 281b, 284t
    differential diagnosis of 281b
    medications for 283t
Peripartum collapse 293
    etiology 294
    incidence 293
    risk reduction 293
Peripheral blood
    film 462
    smear 464
Peripheral vein thrombosis 469
Peritoneum 234
    closure 234
    nonclosure 234
Peritonitis 394
Pethidine 317
Pfannenstiel incision 232, 488
Phenytoin 272, 314
Physical abuse 155
Pinard maneuver 203f
Pirbuterol 390
Placenta 244
    accreta 168, 169, 222, 288
        spectrum 472
    adherens 168, 169
    anterior 478
    control cord traction of 170
    cross-section of 171f
    fundal implantation of 288
    growth factor 101
    immature 55
    increta 169
    low-lying 160, 166
    management of retained 170fc
    manual removal of 171, 172f, 248, 487
    normal sized 38f
    percreta 169
    posterior 478, 478f
    prapped 168, 169
    previa 158, 200, 216, 236, 340, 381, 472, 478
        asymptomatic 164
        case study 341
        classification of 159, 160f
        clinical findings 161
        complications 164

diagnosis of 161, 478
etiology 159
incidence of 159
major 161
management 164
marginal 160, 160f, 216
minor 161
on color Doppler 162
partial 160, 160f, 216
prediction of 163
risk factors for 159b
signs of 479fc
symptomatic 164
total 159, 160f, 216
removal of piece of 341
removing 242
retained 168
Placental abruption 71, 74, 103, 155, 200, 201, 339
   clinical features 156
   complications 158
   history of 155
   management of 157, 157fc
   pathophysiology 155
   risk factors 155
   treatment 339
Placental extraction, Crede's method of 169, 170
Placental lacunae, abnormal 163f
Placentation, abnormal 263, 394
Plasma
   exchange transfusion 196
   volume 72
Platelet
   activating factor 445f
   concentrate 441
   count, low 488
   transfusions 196
Plethora 339
Plethysmography, impedance 130
Pneumomediastinum 327, 329
Pneumothorax 329
Polyarthropathy, inflammatory 137
Polycythemia 175, 456
Polyglactin 45
Polyhydramnios 155, 185f, 200, 221, 304
   acute severe 184
   delivery of 185
   symptom of 185f
Polymerase chain reaction 122, 468
   test 123
Polymerization, hypoxia-induced 454
Polymicrobial infection 360

Postabortion 12
Postmortem
   examination 190
   report 345
Postpartum hemorrhage 91, 155, 158, 168, 220, 243, 294, 368, 394, 399, 401, 472
   classification of 243b
   management of 245, 245fc, 246f
   pharmacological management of 247t
   prevent 234
   recognition of 220fc
Postsurgical excision 33
   laparotomy 33
Post-thrombotic syndrome 134
Potassium 323, 325
Pouch of Douglas 24, 40, 52, 53f, 473, 474
Prednisolone 275
Prednisone 275
Pre-eclampsia 2, 6, 17, 58, 95, 96, 98, 98f, 101, 110, 200, 223, 342, 399, 400, 408, 426, 451
   classical features in 99t
   management of severe 104
   mild 102t
   severe 58, 102t, 146, 456
   superimposed 96
   syndrome, development of 101t
   treatment 342
Pregnancy 96, 270, 297
   abdominal 36, 36f, 39, 475
   accurate dating of 177
   acute fatty liver of 114, 116, 117, 298
   advanced abdominal 38
   after rape, reporting with 335
   and bowel 300
   and childbirth 303
   and kidney 300
   anembryonic 60
   antecedent 67
   complications in 263
   cornual 45, 474
   cranial trauma during 75
   ectopic tubal 21f
   fatty liver of 17
   hepatic 46, 47, 47f
   heterotopic 27, 297, 327, 475
   interstitial 45, 46f, 474
   intrahepatic cholestasis of 115, 425
   location of 49
   management of subsequent 489

   multifetal 466
   multiple 155, 200, 304
   nonmolar 66
   omental 48
   ovarian 39, 40, 475
   pharmacokinetics of 269
   physiological alterations in 72t
   physiology of 276
   poses, types of 48
   postdated 87
   post-term 425
   presentation of 19
   primary abdominal 37
   prophylaxis 335
   rape-related 332
   related complications 1
   risk factors to 293
   scoring 2
   secondary abdominal 37
   singleton 303
   splenic 46, 47f
   subsequent 68, 286
   termination of 337
   therapeutic termination of 64
   trauma in 71, 301
   tubal 20, 49
   types of 46
Pregnant trauma victim 74, 76, 79
Prematurity 133
Prepregnancy 120
Pressure
   intra-abdominal 327
   intracranial 75
Preterm birth 6
   prevention of 148, 149fc
Preterm labor 74, 81, 327, 411, 412
   accurate tests for 411
   advanced 148
   diagnosis of 143
   early 145
   management of 144fc
   pathophysiology 141
   risk factors 141, 141b
   stage of 144
   stimulation of 201
Preterm premature rupture, management of 151, 151fc
Previous cesarean delivery 260
   number of 265
Previous cesarean section 263, 393, 432, 486
   effects of 263
   indication of 262
   number of 394
Procainamide 274

Index

Prochlorperazine 271, 275
Progesterone 323
   serum 25
   supplementation 149
Progestin-only, endometria of 7
Prolactin theory 279
Prolonged labor 221, 436
   causes of 436
Promethazine 271
Prophylaxis 466
   regimens 121t
Prostaglandin 187, 428
   E2 221, 261
      analog 428
      gel 178, 428
      alpha 221
   inhibitors 148
   umbilical vein injection of 170
   use of 487
Protection of Children from Sexual Offences 337
Proteins
   deficiency 462
   angiogenic 99
   antiangiogenic 99
Proteinuria 100
Prothrombin time 115
Proton pump inhibitors 275
Protraction disorders 436, 438
Pseudoephedrine 275
Pseudogestational sac 25, 473f
Pseudo-sinusoidal pattern 212, 212f
Psychological disorder 331, 333
Psychological distress, forms of 331
Puerperal sepsis 358
   clinical findings 360
   diagnosis 360
   effects 362
   management 361
   microbiology 360
   prevention 363
Puerperium 470
Pyelonephritis 399
Pyrexia, puerperal 359

Q

Quantifying amniotic fluid, methods of 181
Quinidine 274
Quinolones 273

R

Radiation, ionizing 77
Radiology, conventional 374
Raising plasma glucose levels 323
Rape
   pregnancy of 331, 338
   trauma syndrome 333
Rectus
   muscle 234
   sheath 234
      hematoma 74
Red blood cell 72, 457
   leukocyte reduced 441
Red cell indices 462t
Relaxin 431
Renal disease, chronic 462, 468
Renal disorder, serious 139
Renal failure 158
   acute 155, 218, 347
Renal function test 61, 62, 98, 244
   abnormal 35
Reproductive system 24
Resistant microorganism 363
   treatment of 362t
Respiratory
   distress 442
   medications 274, 275t
   support 195
   system 72, 420
   tract infection, upper 457
Resuscitation 361
   cardiopulmonary 79, 82, 227, 240, 295, 419
   hemostatic 187
   maternal 419fc
Retained placenta 168
   causes of 169t
   clinical features 169
   treatment 169
   types of 168, 168fc, 169
Retroplacental
   clot 480f
   collection 480
   sonolucent space, loss of 162, 163f
   space, normal 163f
Retroverted gravid uterus 51
   fate of 52
   manual correction of 54f
Retroverted uterus 51f, 52
   causes of 52
Rhesus isoimmunization 200
Ribonucleic acid 34
Ricinus communis 431
Rifampin 275
Ringer's lactate 221
Rubella virus 174
Rubin's criteria 43
Rudimentary horn, excision of 327

S

Saline
   infusion, intra-amniotic hypertonic 399
   solution, isotonic 325
Salpingectomy 30
   partial 30, 33, 33f
   total 32, 33f
Salpingostomy 30
   procedure, laparoscopic 32f
   technique of 30f
Salpingotomy 30
Saltatory pattern 210, 211f, 212, 212f
Scar
   dehiscence 393
      features of 264
      treatment of 395
   factors affecting integrity of 262
   lower segment 263t
   pregnancy 41
   rupture, features of 264
   tenderness, elicitation of 265
Seat belt, correct placement of 83f
Second trimester pulsatility index 175
Seizures 223
   absence 312
   common types of 312
   disorders
      classification of 311
      types of 312t
   effect of pregnancy on 314
   focal 312
   in labor, management of 316
   tonic-clonic 312
Sengstaken-Blakemore catheter 248
Sepsis 146, 158, 457
Septic abortion 8, 9, 399, 400
   investigations of 9
   management of 9
   types of 8
Septic pelvic vein thrombophlebitis 363
Septicemia 399
Serine protease 193
Serological tests 123, 190
Sexual assault 338
   victim of 335
Sexual dysfunction 332, 333
Sexual problems 333

Sexually transmitted
  disease 124, 334
  infections 12, 334
    risk of 332
Shock 368, 399
  absorber 73
  hemorrhagic 74, 218
  hypovolemic 158
  management of 9
  maternal 73
  neurogenic 289
  septic 358
Shoulder 202
  dystocia 86, 87b, 87t, 89, 90b, 91, 226, 347
    antepartum 87
    labor in 86
    management 88
    manipulations in 487
    maternal 91b
    preconceptual 87
    prevention of 91
    recurrence of 91
    resolve 88
    risk of 86, 87, 226
  posterior 89
Sickle cell
  anemia 454
    management of 468fc
  crisis 454
    complications of 454, 454t
    incidence 454
    investigation 455
    management 455
    pathophysiology 454
    precipitating factors 454
  disease 137, 231, 467
  hemoglobinopathies 462
  trait 467
Sinusoidal pattern 212, 212f
Skin 235
  disorders, inflammatory 466
  edges, approximation of 256f
  incision 232, 241
    types of 232f
Sleep
  active 212
  deep 212
  disorders 333
  pattern 212
Society for Maternal-Fetal Medicine Guidelines 187
Society of American Gastrointestinal Endoscopic Surgeons 300
Soft tissue 366

Sonography
  abdominal 77
  focused abdominal 77
  transabdominal 25, 217, 474
  transvaginal 25, 161
Speech abnormalities 456
Spherocytosis 462
Spironolactone 112
Sputum examination 464
Sterile speculum examination 150
Sterilization 266
  surgical 65
Steroids 10
  antenatal 145
  prophylactic 152
  rescue dose of 146
  role of 316
  therapy 470
Stomach 75
Stool examination 464
Streptococcus
  agalactiae 142
  pyogenes 359
Stress 141
  disorder, post-traumatic 191, 333
  incontinence 368
Stroke, repeated 456
Stroma, ovarian 41f
Subarachnoid block 222
Sudden cardiorespiratory collapse 452
Sulfonamides 273
Sulfonylurea 273
Sumatriptan 275
Swelling, soft globular 289
Symphyseal-fundal distance 177
Symphysiotomy 90
Synthetic protease inhibitor 404
Syphilis 334
Systemic inflammatory response syndrome 358
Systemic lupus erythematosus 96
Systemic vascular resistance 109, 297

T

Tachycardia 194, 209
  ventricular 295
Tamponade 42
  test 248
Targeted therapy 282, 285
Tear
  first-degree 254
  fourth-degree 254

repair
  first-degree 255
  second degree 255
  second-degree 254
  third-degree 254
Telangiectasis 134
Tenderness, abdominal 23
Terbinafine 275
Terbutaline 147, 275, 390
Tetanus
  diphtheria, and pertussis 3
  dose of 3
  toxoid 3
Tetracycline 273
Thalassemia 462, 462t, 467
Therapeutic dosage 3
Threatened preterm labor 410
  management of 120fc, 145fc
Thrifty gene hypothesis 175fc
Thrombin time 402
Thrombocytopenia 223
  maternal 100
Thromboelastography 244, 402
Thromboelastometry 244
Thromboembolic disorders 482
Thromboembolism
  acute pulmonary 484fc
  pulmonary 472
Thrombophilia 155
  diseases 190
Thromboprophylaxis, indications for 328
Thrombotic disorders 472
Thyroid
  diseases 190
  medications 274, 275t
  profile of mother 190
  stimulating hormone 6, 62
  storm 58, 64
Thyrotoxic crisis 17
Tinzaparin 133
  initial dose of 133b
Tiredness, chronic 333
Tissue
  hypoperfusion 359
  ovarian 41f
  subcutaneous 235
  trophoblastic 43f
Tocolysis 146, 148, 152
  prophylactic 328
Tocolytics 470
  agents 221, 317
  contraindications of 147t
  mechanism of action of 146, 146f
Topiramate 272, 314

Torsion ovary 297
Total iron binding capacity 463
Toxemia, pre-eclamptic 414
Toxic shock syndrome 359
Toxoplasma gondii 174
  isolation of 123
Toxoplasmosis 123
  diagnosis 123
  management 123
  maternal risk of 123
  transmission 123
Tranexamic acid 196, 234
Transcervical catheter 426
Transferrin receptor, serum 463
Transfusion reactions 441
  delayed 441t
  diagnosis 442
  etiology 441
  immune-mediated 441
  management 443
  pathophysiology 441
  symptoms and signs 442
  treatment 443
Transverse incision 232
  lower segment 232
Transverse lie 236, 381, 381f, 382, 383, 383fc
Trauma
  abdominal 79
  blunt abdominal 76, 81fc
  complicates 71
  during pregnancy 73
  etiology of 81
  minimize 49
  setting of 77
  severe 77
Treponema pallidum 174
Trophoblast
  endovascular 97
  proliferation, abnormal 55
  surgical excision of 41
  tissue 41
Trophoblastic disease, persistent gestational 66
Trophoblastic invasion 97f
  asynchronous 97
Trophotropism 159
Tubal ring 25, 473f
Tube muscularis layer 21
Tumor
  necrosis factor-alpha 323
  ovarian 327
  size, largest 67
  trophoblastic 68

Twin pregnancies 303
Tyrosine molecule 98

U

Ultrasonography
  role of 382
  transvaginal 395
Ultrasound, abdominal 46
Umbilical cord
  accidents 225
  prolapse 303, 304b, 305, 306, 306fc, 421
    consequences of 308, 308f
    diagnosis 305
    epidemiology 303
    incidence 303
    management of 306, 308, 309fc
    pathophysiology 305
    prevention 308
    risk factors 304
    types 303
United States Food and Drug Administration 77, 270
Ureaplasma urealyticum 142
Uric acid, serum 102
Urinary bladder rupture 74
Urinary tract infection 298, 332
Urine
  examination 464
  pregnancy test 64
Urogenital triangle 253
Urticaria 442
Uterine 51
  abnormalities 141
  anomalies 265
    metroplasty for 393
    septoplasty for 393
  artery
    Doppler 175
    embolization 44, 250
    ligation 219, 250
  atony 187, 220, 221
  bleeding
    abnormal 7
    profuse 58
  changes 23
  component 141
  compression
    bimanual 246
    sutures 248
  contractility 141
  contractions, maternal 208
  curettage 393

dehiscence 486
devascularisation, stepwise 248
displacement 218, 240
distention, excessive 142
dystonia 304
fundus 53f
gauze tamponade 246
hemorrhage 58
incision 232
  types of 233f, 265, 393t
inversion 223, 288, 289f
  anesthetic management of 223
  classification 288
  diagnosis 289
  etiology 288
  management 289
  prevention 291
  preventive measures for 291t
massage 246
overdistention 143
position 51
prolapse 291
relaxation, adequate 201
repair 219
retroversion 52
rupture 74, 91, 219, 263, 486, 487t, 488
  complete 219, 264t
  differential diagnosis 488
  during trial of labor, risk factors for 265
  incidence 486
  incomplete 264t
  management 488
  predicting 487
  prevention 489
  previous 486
  rate of 261t, 395, 395t
  risk of 265b, 486, 486t
  symptoms of 263
  terminology 486
scar dehiscence 219, 393
segment cesarean section 200
subinvolution 66
tenderness 218
vascular resistance 72
wall 187, 342
wound, healing of 266
Utero-vaginal packing 246
Uterus 27f, 40, 51, 72, 234
  anteverted 51f
  atonic 288
  clinical anatomy of 51

exteriorization of 234
hyperstimulated 213
incise 242
intact 369
inversion of 289*fc*
massage of 170
normal sized 38*f*
position of 51*f*
retroverted 51*f*
    gravid 51
rupture of 38, 351, 368, 370, 481
scarred 267
specimen of 43*f*

V

Vagina 289
    laceration of 91
    posterior 89
Vaginal birth after cesarean 259
    in twins, role of 267
    risks associated with 259
    section 258
        benefits of 259
        with preterm birth, role of 267
Vaginal birth, planned 201
Vaginal bleeding 218, 219, 368, 394, 488
    irregular 66
Vaginal breech delivery, indications for 202
Vaginal delivery
    operative 88
    spontaneous 286
Vaginal discharge 358

Vaginal evacuation, complications of 63
Vaginal examination 23, 169, 200, 289, 308, 367
Vaginal mucosa, closure of 255*f*, 256*f*
Vaginal swabs, high 359
Valproate 314
Valproic acid 272
Vancomycin 273
Varicose veins 134
Vasa previa 162*f*, 220, 472, 479
Vascular cell adhesion protein 457*f*
Vascular endothelial growth factor 101
Vasopressors 9, 187
    during labor and delivery 448
Vasospasm 99
Venereal disease 6
Venography 130, 131
Venous stasis 129, 455
Venous thromboembolism 134, 158, 231, 300, 404, 468
    risk assessment for 135
Ventilation, mechanical 391
Ventricular failure 109
Ventricular fibrillation 295
Ventricular function, normal 110
Vertical incision 232
    lower segment 232
Vesicles per vaginum, expulsion of 59*f*
Vesicoamniotic shunts, role of 184
Vessels, uteroplacental 327
Vincristine 68
Virchow's triad, constituents of 129

Visual disturbances 456
Vital signs 23, 143, 442
Vitamin
    B12 deficiency 462, 466
    K 404
        antagonist 133
        injection 421
        role of 316
Vomiting 14, 17, 271
    excessive 58
    treatment of 271*t*

W

Weight gain, excessive 87
Wernicke's encephalopathy 17
White blood cell 359, 363
Wood screw maneuver 89
World Health Organization 293, 365, 375
Wound infection 363

Z

Zavanelli maneuver 89
Zika
    syndrome, congenital 125
    virus 124
        diagnosis 125
        fetal risks 125
        management 125
        prevention 125
        transmission 125
Zolmitriptan 275

EU GSPR Authorised Reprsentative
Logos Europe, 9 rue Nicolas Poussin
1700, La Rochelle, France
Phone: +33 (0) 6 67 93 73 78
E-mail: contact@logoseurope.eu

www.ingramcontent.com/pod-product-compliance
Ingram Content Group UK Ltd.
Pitfield, Milton Keynes, MK11 3LW, UK
UKHW050430150426
5217IPUK00019B/1316